Personality Disorders

PRIMERS ON PSYCHIATRY

Stephen M. Strakowski, MD, Series Editor

Published and Forthcoming Titles:

Anxiety Disorders edited by Kerry Ressler, Daniel Pine, and Barbara Rothbaum

Autism Spectrum Disorders edited by Christopher McDougle

Schizoprehnia and Psychotic Spectrum Disorders edited by S. Charles Schulz, Michael F. Green, and Katharine J. Nelson

Mental Health Practice and the Law edited by Ronald Schouten

Borderline Personality Disorder edited by Barbara Stanley and Antonia New

Trauma and Stressor-Related Disorders edited by Frederick J. Stoddard, Jr., David M. Benedek, Mohammed R. Milad, and Robert J. Ursano

Depression edited by Madhukar H. Trivedi

Bipolar Disorder edited by Stephen M. Strakowski, Melissa P. Del Bello, Caleb M. Adler, and David E. Fleck

Public and Community Psychiatry edited by James G. Baker and Sarah E. Baker

Substance Use Disorders edited by F. Gerard Moeller and Mishka Terplan

Personality Disorders edited by Robert E. Feinstein

Personality Disorders

Edited by

ROBERT E. FEINSTEIN

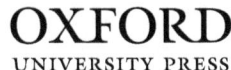

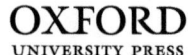

OXFORD
UNIVERSITY PRESS

Oxford University Press is a department of the University of Oxford. It furthers
the University's objective of excellence in research, scholarship, and education
by publishing worldwide. Oxford is a registered trade mark of Oxford University
Press in the UK and certain other countries.

Published in the United States of America by Oxford University Press
198 Madison Avenue, New York, NY 10016, United States of America.

Library of Congress Cataloging-in-Publication Data
Names: Feinstein, Robert E., editor.
Title: Personality disorders / [edited by] Robert E. Feinstein.
Other titles: Primer on.
Description: New York, NY : Oxford University Press, [2022] |
Series: Primer on series | Includes bibliographical references and index.
Identifiers: LCCN 2021031225 (print) | LCCN 2021031226 (ebook) |
ISBN 9780197574393 (pb) | ISBN 9780197574416 (epub) | ISBN 9780197574423
Subjects: MESH: Personality Disorders
Classification: LCC RC554 (print) | LCC RC554 (ebook) | NLM WM 190 |
DDC 616.85/81—dc23
LC record available at https://lccn.loc.gov/2021031225
LC ebook record available at https://lccn.loc.gov/2021031226

DOI: 10.1093/med/9780197574393.001.0001

Editorial Note

Dear Reader,

Robert E. Feinstein, MD Thank you for purchasing this primer on personality disorders. In this volume, Dr. Feinstein, as editor and expert in the field, recruited other international experts in personality constructs and disorders in order to provide a single source covering what are sometimes difficult and mystifying individuals to manage in our clinical practices. This book therefore introduces to early-stage and other practitioners the current evidence about how to conceptualize personality disorders, make diagnoses under current classification systems, and the multifactorial approach to management necessary for best outcomes. Although personality disorders are common and commonly comorbid in psychiatric and other mental health practices, they are often not well understood. This book, then, addresses this important knowledge gap. We believe you will find it to be exceptionally informative and helpful to you in your work.

This volume is part of the Oxford University Press "Primer On" series; I am honored to lead this series since 2016 and was particularly pleased to join an already successful venture. The "Primer On"' series has been designed specifically to support psychiatry residents, early-stage practicing psychiatrists, psychology graduate students, and other interested medical trainees and practitioners. Specifically, in this series we have asked international experts to create books that focus on a specific set of conditions to provide the basic science and clinical tools to diagnose, treat and manage these major psychiatric disorders. We have also expanded the scope of the series to provide this audience information and guidance to major aspects of mental health care practices. With these considerations in mind, each volume is written with an eye toward early-stage practitioners to present current evidence and recommendation in a format that is user-friendly and informative. These texts complement other resources, such as the Oxford American Psychiatry Library, by offering more comprehensive basic and clinical knowledge so that psychiatric and other trainees can better understand these disorders in ways that will prepare them for clinical practice and fellowships (and to take board exams). As they are released, each volume will be available in print, e-book, and Oxford Medicine Online (http://oxfordmedicine.com/). We have aimed to make these affordable books that bridge handbooks and more lengthy and expensive highly specialized textbooks. I hope you enjoy this text!

Best wishes
Steve Strakowski, MD
Vice Dean of Research
Associate Vice President, Regional Mental Health
Dell Medical School, University of Texas at Austin
Series Editor

Contents

Preface

Much has been written about personality disorders (PDs) and their treatments over the last 120 years. This began with descriptions of the PDs and psychoanalytic treatment early in the last century and progressed to the modern era of diverse conceptualization and treatments for patients with PDs (see Chapter 14 for a brief history). The PDs were diagnostically codified using the multiaxial system of the *Diagnostic and Statistical Manual of Mental Diseases* (DSM) *III* in 1980 and the DSM-IV in 1994. The multiaxial system, listing the PDs on Axis II, signaled the importance of treating the PDs in their own right as well as the importance of treating the PDs as comorbid disorders affecting the treatment and outcomes of other major mental conditions (Axis I disorders).

PDs have estimated worldwide prevalence rates of 12.6 percent, making them a cluster of very common disorders.[1] Psychosocial functioning of patients with PDs compared to patients with other mental disorders reveals that patients with PDs are more likely to be without partners, unemployed, disabled, and demonstrating significant impairments in social, occupational, leisure, and global functioning.[2] Patients with PDs have a more significant disability than the disability caused by any Axis I disorder, including major depressive disorder.[2] While PDs significantly affect the treatment and outcome of depression, bipolar disorder, eating disorders, addiction, and so on, treatments of these and other common mental disorders have *no ability* to modify personality functioning and have *no helpful impacts* on the treatment of PDs. However, since the 1990s there has been an explosion of many effective treatments for PDs.

The "Big Six," as I call them, are major evidence-based treatments for borderline personality disorders (BPDs). These treatments include transference-focused psychotherapy (TFP), mentalization-based treatment (MBT), cognitive behavioral therapy (CBT) for PDs, dialectical behavior therapy (DBT), schema therapy (ST), and good psychiatric management (GPM). There are now data from meta-analyses and some RCTs (see Chapter 5) that reveal these treatments are likely equally effective. This suggests that despite very different theoretical perspectives espousing treatment superiority, it may be that common factors across these approaches account for similar outcomes (see chapter 6). While the Big Six have much in common, it is also the case that each treatment has unique features that could be incorporated or borrowed from one evidence-based therapy (EBT) to another to improve therapeutic responsiveness to the needs of individual patients. The book explores this possibility.

While developed to treat BPD, these EBTs are also currently broadening their scope to see if these diverse psychotherapeutic modalities are also useful for the treatment of other PDs and other conditions. The data on the effectiveness of this approach, for all the

[1] Volkert J, Gablonski TC, Rabung S. Prevalence of personality disorders in the general adult population in Western countries: systematic review and meta-analysis. *Br J Psychiatry.* 2018: 213(6):709–715.
[2] Skodol AE. Impact of personality pathology on psychosocial functioning. *Curr Opin Psychol.* 2018: 1(21):33–38.

PDs, remain to be determined by further research. For clinicians, despite this current limitation, the authors of each chapter were encouraged travel in these uncertain waters recommending their treatment approach based on some evidence, the clinical literature, and/or their own expertise, when no clear definitive evidence for specific treatments for each of the PDs is available.

Many chapters in the book were written or co-authored by master clinicians and/or researchers and their students. This collaboration was intentionally encouraged, as I hoped it would make this book read more as a "how to understand" and "how to do psychotherapy" with patients suffering with PDs, rather than as a textbook on the PDs.

The book is divided into three sections.

Section 1 provides an overview of the diagnosis, assessment, clinical, and research approaches to working with PDs. It reviews prototypic personality syndromes, levels of personality organization, pathways from trauma to PDs, and a psychodynamic, integrated clinical and empirical approach to working with patients who have PDs.

Section II reviews multi-theoretical approaches to treatment of PDs. It covers six evidenced-based treatments designed to treat BPD, management of PDs in medical settings, psychopharmacology, and group therapy for the PDs. These diverse viewpoints help readers understand current theories about the origin and nature of the personality and how one can apply these principles to everyday care and treatment of patients.

Section III covers 10 major specific PDs, written from diverse theoretical perspectives. It is chock full of clinical illustrations and the wisdom from master clinicians when evidence-based treatment approaches are not yet known.

This book was written by 51 authors, representing diverse multi-theoretical viewpoints. I am especially appreciative of the good-natured and productive dialogue that emerged with all authors during the editorial process. I cannot thank the authors enough for their wonderful collaborative efforts and contributions.

It was very important to the editor and authors that this book contains theory and practices which could be widely applied to the treatment of our many patients who suffer with PDs. We hope that the book is comfortably accessible for use by mental health students, psychiatric residents, psychologists, social workers, faculty, and the widest scope of health professionals.

I am eager to know your reaction and comments about this work, as this kind of dialogue was the energy source for this book. Your reaction will ultimately determine the book's usefulness.

—Robert E. Feinstein, MD, Editor

Acknowledgments

I am very appreciative of my personal cyberspace editor Richard Carlin from New Jersey, whom I have never met in person because of Covid-19. His smarts, efficiencies, and detailed editing for style, formatting, and consistency was invaluable.

As in all my writing, I am exceeding grateful to my wife Marilyn for her encouragement, comments, and edits on my own chapters in this book.

I would also like to thank Oxford's Primer Series editor, Steven Strakowski, and all those working at Oxford University Press for offering me the opportunity and for ultimately making this publication possible.

ACKNOWLEDGMENTS

Contributors

Prof. Dr. Arnoud Arntz, PhD
Department of Clinical Psychology
University of Amsterdam
Amsterdam, The Netherlands

Elizabeth L. Auchincloss, MD
Professor and Vice-chair, Education
Department of Psychiatry
Weill-Cornell Medical College
New York, NY, USA

Aaron Stern MD, PhD
Professor of Psychodynamic Psychiatry
Department of Psychiatry
Weill-Cornell Medical College
New York, NY, USA

Brenda Berger, PhD
Clinical Assistant Professor of Medical
Psychology in Psychiatry
Columbia University Center for
Psychoanalytic Training and Research
Columbia University
New York, NY, USA

Curtis C. Bogetti, BS
Doctoral Student
Department of Psychology
The City College of New York, City University
of New York
New York, NY, USA

Robert F. Bornstein, PhD
Professor
Derner School of Psychology
Adelphi University
Garden City, NY, USA

Eve Caligor, MD
Clinical Professor of Psychiatry
Columbia University Vagelos College of
Physicians and Surgeons
New York, NY, USA

Gerardo Casteleiro, PhD
Adjunct Professor
Clinical Mental Health Counseling Program
Florida Atlantic University
Boca Raton, FL, USA

Samantha M. Catanzano, PharmD, BCCP
Clinical Assistant Professor
College of Pharmacy
The University of Texas
Austin, TX, USA

John F. Clarkin, PhD
Clinical Professor of Psychology in Psychiatry
New York Presbyterian Hospital-Weill
Medical College of Cornell University
White Plains, NY, USA

Sheila E. Crowell, PhD
Associate Professor
Department of Psychology, Department of
Psychiatry
Department of Obstetrics and Gynecology
University of Utah
Salt Lake City, UT, USA

Robert P. Drozek, LICSW
Therapist and Supervisor, Mentalization-
based Treatment Clinic, McLean Hospital
Teaching Associate, Department of Psychiatry,
Harvard Medical School
Belmont, MA, USA

Eva Fassbinder, MD
Department of Psychiatry and Psychotherapy
Christian-Albrechts-University Kiel
Niemannsweg, Kiel, Germany

Robert E. Feinstein, MD
Professor of Psychiatry
Department of Psychiatry
Donald and Barbara Zucker School of
Medicine at Northwell/Hofstra
Zucker Hillside Hospital
Long Island, NY, USA

Eric A. Fertuck, PhD
Associate Professor
Department of Psychology
The City College of New York, City University
of New York
New York, NY, USA

Gregory Fonzo, PhD
Assistant Professor
Department of Psychiatry and Behavioral
Sciences
Dell Medical School, University of Texas
Austin, TX, USA

**Isadora Fox, DNP, APRN, PMHNP-BC,
APRN-BC**
Doctor of Nursing Practice
Austin PsychCare
Austin, TX, USA

Glen O. Gabbard, MD
Clinical Professor
Department of Psychiatry
Baylor College of Medicine
Houston, TX, USA

Robert Alan Glick, MD
Professor of Clinical Psychiatry, Columbia
University
Former Director of the Columbia University
Center for Psychoanalytic Training and
Research
New York, NY, USA

Emma Golkin, MD
Fellow, Public Psychiatry
Department of Psychiatry
Columbia University/New York State
Psychiatric Institute
New York, NY, USA

Alyson A. Gorun, MD
Assistant Professor
Department of Clinical Psychiatry
Weill-Cornell Medical College
New York, NY, USA

Christopher Green, MD
Private Practice
New York, NY, USA

Jonathan T. Henry, MD, PhD
Medical Director, Addiction Treatment
Program
Department of Psychiatry
Jesse Brown Veterans Administration
Medical Center
Chicago, IL, USA

Richard G. Hersh, MD
Special Lecturer
Columbia University College of Physicians
and Surgeons
New York, NY, USA

Benjamin N. Johnson, MS
Doctoral Student
Department of Psychology
The Pennsylvania State University
University Park, PA, USA

Parisa R. Kaliush, MS
Department of Psychology
University of Utah
Salt Lake City, UT, USA

Royce Lee, MD
Associate Professor
Department of Psychiatry and Behavioral
Neuroscience
University of Chicago
Chicago, IL, USA

Kenneth N. Levy, PhD
Associate Professor
Department of Psychology
The Pennsylvania State University
University Park, PA, USA

Michelle Magid, MD, MBA
President, Austin Psychcare, PA
Associate Professor
University of Texas Dell Medical School
Austin, TX, USA
Adjunct Associate Professor
Texas A&M Health Science Center
Bryan, TX, USA

Benjamin McCommon, MD
Assistant Clinical Professor
Department of Psychiatry
Columbia University College of Physicians
and Surgeons
New York, NY, USA

Nancy McWilliams, PhD
Visiting Full Professor
Graduate School of Applied and Professional
Psychology
Rutgers University
Piscataway, NJ, USA

Nicolette Molina, BA
PhD Student
Department of Psychology
University of Utah
Salt Lake City, UT, USA

Adam P. Natoli, PhD
Assistant Professor
Department of Psychology and Philosophy
Sam Houston State University
Huntsville, TX, USA

Haruka Notsu, MS
Doctoral Student
Department of Psychology
Pennsylvania State University
University Park, PA, USA

Cynthia Playfair, MD
Private Practice, Affiliate Faculty, University
of Texas at Austin, Dell Medical School
Department of Psychiatry
Supervising and Training Psychoanalyst,
Center for Psychoanalytic Studies
Houston, TX, USA

Kenneth M. Pollock, PhD, CGP
Clinical Associate Professor (retired)
Department of Psychiatry
New York Medical College
Valhalla, NY, USA
Former Director of Group Psychotherapy
Training
Westchester Medical Center
Poughkeepsie, NY, USA

Alex Preston, MD
Resident
Department of Psychiatry
University of Arkansas for Medical Sciences
Little Rock, AR, USA

Emily Rosen, MD
Resident
Department of Psychiatry and Behavioral
Sciences
George Washington University
Washington, DC, USA

Valerie Rosen, MD
Associate Professor
Department of Psychiatry and Behavioral
Sciences
Dell Medical School, The University of Texas
at Austin
Seton Mind Institute
Austin, TX, USA

Edwin Santos
Research Intern
Department of Psychiatry and Behavioral
Neurosciences
Biological Sciences Division
The University of Chicago
Chicago, IL, USA

Shannon Sauer-Zavala, PhD
Assistant Professor
Department of Psychology
University of Kentucky
Lexington, KY, USA

Anja Schaich, Dr. rer. hum. biol. / MSc
Psychotherapist
Department of Psychiatry and Psychotherapy
University of Lübeck
Ratzeburger Allee, Lübeck, Germany
Department of Psychiatry and Psychotherapy,
Christian-Albrechts-University Kiel,
Niemannsweg, Kiel, Germany

Benjamin A. Scherban, MD
Resident Psychiatrist
New York Presbyterian Hospital
New York, NY, USA

Stephen A. Semcho, MS
Graduate Researcher
Department of Psychology
University of Kentucky
Lexington, KY, USA

Jonathan Shedler, PhD
Clinical Professor
Department of Psychiatry
University of California, San Francisco
San Francisco, CA, USA

Tawny L. Smith, PharmD, BCPP
Associate Professor
Department of Psychiatry and Behavioral
Sciences
Dell Medical School, The University of Texas
Austin, TX, USA

Jennifer Sotsky, MD
Consultation-Liaison Fellow
Columbia University Irving Medical Center
New York, NY, USA

Matthew W. Southward, PhD
Postdoctoral Scholar
Department of Psychology
University of Kentucky
Lexington, KY, USA

Julia F. Sowislo, PhD
Instructor of Psychology in Psychiatry
Department of Psychiatry
New York Presbyterian Hospital-Weill
Medical
College of Cornell University Westchester
Division
White Plains, NY, USA

Len Sperry, MD, PhD
Clinical Professor
Department of Psychiatry and Behavioral
Medicine
Medical College of Wisconsin
Milwaukee, WI, USA
Professor
Clinical Mental Health Counseling Program
Florida Atlantic University
Boca Raton, FL, USA

Robert D. Vlisides-Henry, MS
PhD Candidate
Department of Psychology
University of Utah
Salt Lake City, UT, USA

Frank Yeomans, MD, PhD
Clinical Associate Professor
Department of Psychiatry
Weill-Cornell Medical College
New York, NY, USA

I
OVERVIEW

1

The Personality Syndromes

Jonathan Shedler

Key Points

- Personality refers to an individual's characteristic patterns of thought, feeling, behavior, motivation, defense, interpersonal functioning, and ways of experiencing self and others.
- Clinical knowledge accrued over generations has given rise to a taxonomy of familiar personality syndromes.
- Personality syndromes exist on a continuum of functioning from healthy to severely disturbed. There is no discontinuity between normal and pathological personality.
- Understanding personality syndromes requires an understanding of underlying personality processes such as inner conflicts, defenses, and motives.
- A diagnostic prototype is provided for each personality syndrome, which describes the syndrome in its "ideal" or pure form.
- A practical diagnostic method based on pattern recognition is provided, whereby clinicians consider the overall resemblance between patients and diagnostic prototypes.
- The personality constructs provide the broad strokes of clinical case formulations. They can explain and contextualize presenting symptoms and disorders.
- Each personality syndrome is a distinct pathway to depression and requires a different treatment focus.

Introduction

Personality is not about what disorders you *have* but about who you *are*. It refers to a person's characteristic patterns of thought, feeling, behavior, motivation, defense, interpersonal functioning, and ways of experiencing self and others. All people have personalities and personality styles.

While there are as many personalities as people, clinical knowledge accrued over generations has given rise to a taxonomy of familiar personality styles or types. Most people, whether healthy or troubled, fit somewhere in the taxonomy. Empirical research over the past two decades has confirmed the major personality types and their core features.[1-5]

Most clinical theorists do not view the personality types as inherently disordered. They are generally discussed in the clinical literature as personality types, styles, or syndromes—not "disorders." Each exists on a continuum of functioning from healthy to severely disturbed. The term "disorder" is best regarded as a linguistic convenience for clinicians, denoting a degree of extremity or rigidity that causes significant dysfunction, limitation, or suffering. One can have, for example, a narcissistic personality *style* without having narcissistic personality *disorder*.

The same personality dynamics give rise to both strengths and weaknesses. A person with a healthy narcissistic personality style has the confidence to dream big dreams and pursue them; they can be visionaries, innovators, and founders. A person with a healthy obsessive-compulsive style excels in areas requiring precise, analytic thinking; they may be successful engineers, scientists, or academics. A person with a healthy paranoid style looks beneath the surface and sees what others miss; they may be investigative journalists or brilliant medical diagnosticians. Our best and worst qualities are often cut from the same psychological cloth.

Many psychodynamically influenced clinicians accept the broad outlines of an organizing framework proposed by Otto Kernberg,[6,7] which combines the concept of personality type with a "severity dimension" reflecting level of personality organization (healthy, neurotic, borderline, psychotic).[8-9] For example, we can speak of a patient with narcissistic personality organized at a neurotic level or at a borderline level. The approach presented here is consistent with this framework. (For discussion of levels of personality organization, see Chapter 2, Levels of Personality Organization: Theoretical Background and Clinical Applications.)

The recognition that personality styles exist on a continuum of functioning was undercut by the *Diagnostic and Statistical Manual of Mental Disorders*[10] (DSM) beginning with the publication of DSM-III.[11] To shoehorn personality styles discussed in the clinical literature into a categorical taxonomy of disorders, the framers of the DSM described them in pathological form, in some cases ratcheting up the severity to the point of caricature.[3,4] The DSM also disregarded the underlying personality processes at the core of the personality styles, such as internal conflict, defenses, and motives. It focused instead on outward behavior and readily observable symptoms. Thus, the DSM borrowed terminology and concepts from the clinical, chiefly psychoanalytic literature (obsessive-compulsive, narcissistic, paranoid, and so on) but disconnected them from the larger body of clinical knowledge.

Clinicians who are expert in treating personality have a working knowledge of personality syndromes that is richer, deeper, and more complex than the depictions in the DSM[8,9,12,13] and in some cases diverges from it.[3] This chapter provides an overview of the personality syndromes as understood by expert clinicians and verified by empirical research. The descriptions provided here go beyond overt behavior and symptoms and address the personality processes that underlie them. For many patients, they can provide roadmaps for effective treatment.

Diagnosis as Pattern Recognition

Each personality syndrome discussed in this chapter is represented by a paragraph-length description called a diagnostic prototype, which describes the personality syndrome in its "ideal" or pure form.[4,14-15] These diagnostic prototypes are evidence based. They were derived empirically, based on a national sample of N = 1,201 patients described by their clinicians using the Shedler-Westen Assessment Procedure (SWAP). They reflect empirically observable characteristics of actual patients, not just theoretical conjecture.

Naturally occurring diagnostic groupings were identified using statistical clustering methods, which largely confirmed the personality syndromes described in the clinical literature. The SWAP items (descriptive statements) that best describe each personality syndrome were likewise identified empirically, then arranged as paragraphs to create the diagnostic prototypes.[4] (The SWAP instrument is described in Chapter 4, Integrating Clinical and Empirical Approaches to Personality: The Shedler-Westen Assessment Procedure (SWAP). The instrument is available at https://swapassessment.org.)

The diagnostic prototypes have the advantage of being empirically based and also preserving the richness and complexity of accrued clinical knowledge. To make a personality diagnosis, a clinician rates the overall resemblance or match between a patient and a diagnostic prototype from 0 (no match) to 5 (very good match). Higher scores indicate more resemblance to the diagnostic prototype and more severity. The diagnostic prototypes are presented in Boxes 1.1 to 1.10 and the rating scale is included with each prototype.

If categorical diagnosis is desired for compatibility with the DSM-5 or International Classification of Diseases (ICD-10) diagnostic system, scores of 4 and 5 indicate a personality disorder diagnosis, and a score of 3 indicates traits or features of a disorder. Thus, if a patient receives a score of 5 for narcissistic personality and 3 for obsessive-compulsive personality, the categorical (DSM format) diagnosis is narcissistic personality disorder with obsessive-compulsive traits.

The premise of this approach is that a configuration or pattern of interrelated psychological characteristics defines a personality syndrome, not the presence or absence of separate characteristics. *Recognizing a personality syndrome is pattern recognition,* much as recognizing a face depends on pattern recognition, not tabulating separate features.[4,14,15]

Prototype matching provides reliable and valid diagnoses and works with the cognitive decision processes of clinicians, which rely on pattern recognition. It systematizes what expert clinicians already do in practice. In a consumer-preference study, psychologists and psychiatrists preferred this method of personality diagnosis to the DSM diagnostic system and to dimensional trait models of personality.[16]

Developing a Treatment Focus

In recent years, many clinicians have been trained to focus on presenting problems and DSM Axis I disorders (such as depression or generalized anxiety) and view them as encapsulated conditions separate from personality. Treatments that target specific DSM disorders implicitly assume all patients with a given DSM diagnosis have the "same" condition and will respond to the same interventions. Clinicians learn the hard way that things are rarely so simple.

Most often, the problems that bring people to mental health treatment are not encapsulated problems. They are woven into the fabric of their lives. They are embedded in, and inseparable from, the person's characteristic patterns of thinking, feeling, behaving, coping, defending, and relating to others: in other words, personality. This is true whether or not the person has a diagnosable "personality disorder." The patient needs the clinician to grasp something psychologically systemic about who they *are*, not just what disorders they *have,* to help them understand why they are repeatedly vulnerable to certain kinds of suffering and how to change it.

Meaningful and lasting change generally comes not from focusing on symptoms, but on the personality patterns that underlie them. Knowledge of personality styles provides a map of the personality terrain that expert clinicians navigate. Thus, each personality syndrome is not just description, but shorthand for the broad strokes of a clinical case formulation that can provide a treatment focus and address the underlying causes of many patients' suffering. The penultimate section of this chapter, Personality and Clinical Case Formulation, revisits this topic.

The Personality Syndromes

This section describes the major personality syndromes as understood by clinical theorists and confirmed by empirical research. The diagnostic prototypes and rating scales in Boxes 1.1 to 1.10 can be used for day-to-day clinical diagnosis.

Depressive Personality

Despite its omission from the DSM, depressive personality is the most common personality syndrome seen in clinical practice.[2] It is a personality syndrome in every sense of the term: an enduring pattern of psychological functioning evident by adolescence and encompassing the full spectrum of personality processes.

People with depressive personalities are chronically vulnerable to painful affect, especially feelings of inadequacy, sadness, guilt, and shame. They have difficulty recognizing their needs, and when they do recognize them, they have difficulty expressing them. They are often conflicted about allowing themselves pleasure. They may seem driven by an unconscious wish to punish themselves, either by getting into situations destined to cause pain or depriving themselves of opportunities for enjoyment. A psychologically insightful observer might describe the person as their own worst enemy.

Where there is an enemy, there is often anger and aggression. One underlying psychological theme in depressive personality is internal attacks against the self. The person is angry, defends against experiencing anger, and instead directs it at themselves in the form of self-criticism, self-deprivation, and self-punitiveness. The relevant SWAP item is, "Has trouble acknowledging or expressing anger toward others and instead becomes depressed, self-critical, self-punitive, etc." In short, the person treats themselves like someone they despise.

Clinicians can easily miss the patient's anger and aggression because people with depressive personalities tend to be overtly agreeable and put others' needs first, including the clinician's needs. If psychotherapy is to bring about meaningful psychological change, anger must be recognized, experienced, and explored in the therapy relationship.

A second psychological theme involves separation, rejection, and loss. The person may be preoccupied with, and painfully vulnerable to, disruptions in interpersonal relationships. They fear being abandoned and left unprotected and uncared for. As a result, they avoid interpersonal conflict and have difficulty asserting themselves. Undue people-pleasing and helpfulness protect against disapproval or rejection. In psychotherapy, they suppress legitimate criticisms and dissatisfactions for fear of hurting the clinician's feelings or damaging the therapy relationship. Instead of communicating their needs and wants, they accept what is offered and make do. This can lead to a relationship dynamic in which the clinician thinks things are going swimmingly and the patient does without, thereby recreating the patient's dysfunctional relationship pattern in the therapy relationship.

This pattern may have roots in relational disruption or insufficient emotional availability of a caretaker in early development, leaving the person feeling emotionally empty and incomplete, and believing their deprivation was caused by their own badness. Some patients have a pervasive sense that someone or something essential to their well-being has been lost and can never be recovered. These feelings can crystalize around, and be amplified by, subsequent experiences of loss. Rewards and pleasures that are realistically available may be experienced as a pale shadow of what was lost or could have been. Such patients may need the clinician's help to mourn what has been lost before they can invest emotionally in what life can offer now.

For some patients with depressive personalities, themes of unconscious anger and self-attack predominate. For others, themes of separation and loss predominate. These themes have been discussed in the clinical and research literature in terms of introjective (self-critical) and anaclitic (dependent) depression.[17,18] Both themes may be present in any blend.

Depressive personality is the most common personality style among people drawn to the mental health professions.[19] Clinical practitioners have endless opportunity to care for others instead of themselves, be unduly helpful, and fault themselves for falling short of unrealistic, self-imposed standards.

See Box 1.1, p. 8 for the depressive personality prototype.

Anxious-Avoidant Personality

The term "Avoidant Personality Disorder" is used by the DSM and is more familiar to clinicians, but the hyphenated term "anxious-avoidant" more accurately and telegraphically conveys the essence of this personality syndrome.

People with anxious-avoidant personalities are, first and foremost, anxious. Anxiety pervades their experience of themselves and their world. They ruminate and dwell on perceived dangers and past mistakes. Their predominant emotions are anxiety, shame, and embarrassment. They defend against sources of anxiety by avoidance. The problem is that the sources of anxiety are everywhere, including within. Ultimately, avoidant responses become bars in a psychological prison, constricting and limiting freedom of thought, feeling, choice, and action. As a result, people with anxious-avoidant personalities lead constricted lives and tend to adhere to familiar routines. Despite their avoidant

---

Box 1.1 Depressive Personality Prototype

Summary statement: Individuals with depressive personality are prone to feelings of depression and inadequacy, tend to be self-critical or self-punitive, and may be preoccupied with concerns about abandonment or loss.

Individuals who match this prototype tend to feel depressed or despondent and to feel inadequate, inferior, or a failure. They tend to find little pleasure or satisfaction in life's activities and to feel life has no meaning. They are insufficiently concerned with meeting their own needs, disavowing or squelching their hopes and desires to protect against disappointment. They appear conflicted about experiencing pleasure, inhibiting feelings of excitement, joy, or pride. They may likewise be conflicted or inhibited about achievement or success (e.g., failing to reach their potential or sabotaging themselves when success is at hand). Individuals who match this prototype are generally self-critical, holding themselves to unrealistic standards and feeling guilty and blaming themselves for bad things that happen. They appear to want to "punish" themselves by creating situations that lead to unhappiness or avoiding opportunities for pleasure and gratification. They have trouble acknowledging or expressing anger and instead become depressed, self-critical, or self-punitive. They often fear that they will be rejected or abandoned, are prone to painful feelings of emptiness, and may feel bereft or abjectly alone even in the presence of others. They may have a pervasive sense that someone or something necessary for happiness has been lost forever (e.g., a relationship, youth, beauty, success).

5 very good match (patient *exemplifies* this disorder; prototypical case)	**Diagnosis**
4 good match (patient *has* this disorder; diagnosis applies)	
3 moderate match (patient has *significant features* of this disorder)	**Features**
2 slight match (patient has minor features of this disorder)	
1 no match (description does not apply)	

---

defenses, anxiety still leaks out through a variety of channels, which can include somatic symptoms and concerns.

People with anxious-avoidant personalities are fearfully avoidant not only of the external, interpersonal world but also their own internal world. The former is manifested in social avoidance, self-consciousness, and social awkwardness. The latter is manifested in inhibition and constriction of emotional life and desire. They are motivated to avoid perceived harm, not to pursue their desires.

The challenge in psychotherapy is that patients with anxious-avoidant personality are avoidant in psychotherapy, too. They are likely to steer clear of difficult topics, change the subject when their thoughts lead in disturbing directions, and fend off the clinician's efforts to explore psychological experience beyond the most familiar, well-worn grooves. This creates a dilemma for clinicians: If they don't confront avoidant defenses, therapy will accomplish little; if they do, the patient may quit or shut down. Effective treatment involves a balancing act of support and confrontation. The clinician should help and

---

Box 1.2 Anxious-avoidant Personality Prototype

Summary statement: Individuals with anxious-avoidant personality are chronically prone to anxiety, are socially anxious and avoidant, and attempt to manage anxiety in ways that limit and constrict their lives.

Individuals who match this prototype are chronically anxious. They tend to ruminate, dwelling on problems or replaying conversations in their minds. They are more concerned with avoiding harm than pursuing desires, and their choices and actions are unduly influenced by efforts to avoid perceived dangers. They are prone to feelings of shame and embarrassment. Individuals who match this prototype tend to be shy and self-conscious in social situations and to feel like an outcast or outsider. They are often socially awkward and tend to avoid social situations because of fear of embarrassment or humiliation. They tend to be inhibited and constricted and to have difficulty acknowledging or expressing desires. They may adhere rigidly to daily routines, have trouble making decisions, or vacillate when faced with choices. Their anxiety may find expression through a variety of channels, including panic attacks, hypochondriacal concerns (e.g., excessive worry about normal aches and pains), or somatic symptoms in response to stress (e.g., headache, backache, abdominal pain, asthma).

5 very good match (patient *exemplifies* this disorder; prototypical case)	**Diagnosis**
4 good match (patient *has* this disorder; diagnosis applies)	
3 moderate match (patient has *significant features* of this disorder)	**Features**
2 slight match (patient has minor features of this disorder)	
1 no match (description does not apply)	

---

support the patient to put words to previously unarticulated feelings and fantasies. When they respond to situations (both inside and outside therapy) with fearful avoidance, they should be pressed for details about the presumed dangers ("And what would happen then?") so they can be examined in the light of day. When a secure working alliance is established, the clinician should encourage the patient to face feared situations and experiences in incremental steps. See Box 1.2 for the anxious-avoidant personality prototype.

Dependent-Victimized Personality

The term "Dependent Personality Disorder" is used by DSM, but the hyphenated term "dependent-victimized" communicates a core feature of the personality syndrome: the tendency to put oneself in harm's way. People with this personality syndrome are drawn to relationships in which they are mistreated, exploited, or abused.

People with dependent-victimized personalities are characterized by intense dependency, leading them to subordinate their needs to those of others in order to maintain desperately needed attachments. This leaves them vulnerable to mistreatment and exploitation. The person experiences the attachment relationship as essential to their existence and seems prepared to go to any length to preserve it, including agreeing to things they find objectionable and things that may be self-destructive. Externally, they are ingratiating, passive, and submissive. Internally, they experience themselves as unworthy, undeserving, and bereft without the connection to and approval of the other person. In severe cases, existence outside the relationship, however self-destructive, may seem unimaginable. Because of an inner experience of deep unworthiness, they may experience a person who demeans them as the only one who can understand them.

Subservience leads to anger and resentment, but overt anger must be suppressed because it threatens the attachment relationship they perceive as their lifeline. Disavowed anger and aggression leak out in the form of passive-aggressive behavior, which tends to elicit further mistreatment from others. These relationship patterns can play out in the therapy relationship via transference and countertransference. The patient may feel dependent on the clinician while passive-aggressively thwarting all efforts to help. Clinicians may initially respond to the patient's need with extra efforts to provide care, then find themselves becoming controlling or punitive after the patient has "helplessly" and repeatedly thwarted all their efforts. At this point, the therapy relationship comes to resemble the patient's other dysfunctional attachments. Understanding these patterns and how they come about can open the door to new ways of relating. See Box 1.3, p. 11 for the dependent-victimized personality prototype.

Obsessive-Compulsive Personality

Obsessive-Compulsive personality is among the most familiar and easily recognized of the personality syndromes. On the surface, people with obsessive-compulsive personality are conscientious, meticulous, regimented, and cerebral. They have little access to their emotional life and are more comfortable in the realm of thoughts and ideas than the realm of feelings. Ask a person with obsessive-compulsive personality what they feel, and they will likely tell you what they *think*, often at length, with careful weighing of pros and cons, arguments and counterarguments.

Their intellectualized discourse does not, however, lead to a decision or plan of action. Instead, they may digress into minutia or get caught up in intellectualized abstraction. Their thought processes do not lead to emotional clarity because their unconscious function is to defend against feelings, impulses, and desires. When confronted with the need to make a personal choice, they are likely to vacillate and equivocate. For every pro, there is a con of equal and opposite weight.

Because they come across as robotic and emotionally inaccessible, one theorist described people with obsessive-compulsive personality style as "living machines."[20] But defenses are proportionate to the impulses they defend against. Under the conscious surface, the person with obsessive-compulsive personality is waging epic emotional battles.

At the core of obsessive-compulsive personality is a conflict between obedience and defiance.[12] Obedience—obeying the rules, deference to authority—is experienced as submission and humiliation. This leads to rage and the urge to defy and humiliate the other. Defiance leads to guilt and fear of punishment, which leads back to obedience. Mundane, everyday issues lose proportion. The decision to come early or late to an appointment takes on the proportions of an epic battle between submission and defiance.

Box 1.3 Dependent-victimized Personality Prototype

Summary statement: Individuals with dependent-victimized personality are highly dependent and fearful of being alone, tend to show insufficient concern for their own well-being to the point of jeopardizing their welfare or safety, and have difficulty expressing anger directly.

Individuals who match this prototype tend to be needy and dependent, fear being alone, and fear rejection or abandonment. They tend to be ingratiating or submissive, often consenting to things they find objectionable in an effort to maintain support or approval. They tend to be passive and unassertive and to feel helpless and powerless. They tend to be indecisive, suggestible or easily influenced, and naïve or innocent, seeming to know less about the ways of the world than would be expected. They tend to become attached to people who are emotionally unavailable, and to create relationships in which they are in the role of caring for or rescuing the other person. Individuals who match this prototype tend to get drawn into or remain in relationships in which they are emotionally or physically abused, or needlessly put themselves in dangerous situations (e.g., walking alone or agreeing to meet strangers in unsafe places). They are insufficiently concerned with meeting their own needs and tend to feel unworthy or undeserving. Individuals who match this prototype have trouble acknowledging or expressing anger and instead become depressed, self-critical, or self-punitive. They tend to express anger in passive and indirect ways (e.g., making mistakes, procrastinating, forgetting) that may provoke or trigger anger or mistreatment from others.

5 very good match (patient *exemplifies* this disorder; prototypical case)	Diagnosis
4 good match (patient *has* this disorder; diagnosis applies)	
3 moderate match (patient has *significant features* of this disorder)	Features
2 slight match (patient has minor features of this disorder)	
1 no match (description does not apply)	

Acquiescing to another's preference or insisting on one's own can feel like being annihilated or annihilating. Minor decisions become emotionally fraught. With so much at stake, fear, shame, and rage constantly threaten to break through.

The overtly observable features of obsessive-compulsive personality derive from this conflict. Conscientiousness and orderliness derive from fear of authority and punishment. Defiance and rage "leak out" in the form of critical attitudes, controlling behavior, oppositionality, power struggles, stinginess, procrastination, and inevitable pockets of messiness and disorder. Intellectualization and emotional constriction serve to keep the conflict outside awareness.

People with obsessive-compulsive personality benefit from exploratory, interpretive psychotherapy. They benefit from insight into their defenses against emotional life and their high cost vis-à-vis their relationships and capacity for spontaneity and joy. The clinician should be alert to the patient's tendency to intellectualize and treat the clinician's comments as theories to ponder versus matters of immediate emotional import. For example, if the patient says the clinician's observation makes sense, the clinician might ask whether it just "makes sense" or whether they recognize it in themselves and feel it to be true. In this way, the clinician can draw attention to the patient's emotional life and the defenses that squelch it.

Obsessive-compulsive *personality* is different from obsessive-compulsive *disorder*, which is a distinct phenomenon requiring different treatment. See Box 1.4 for the obsessive-compulsive personality prototype.

Box 1.4 Obsessive-compulsive Personality Prototype

Summary statement: Individuals with obsessive-compulsive personality are intellectualized and overly "rational" in their approach to life, are emotionally constricted and rigid, and are critical of themselves and others and conflicted about anger, aggression, and authority.

Individuals who match this prototype tend to see themselves as logical and rational, uninfluenced by emotion. They tend to think in abstract and intellectualized terms, to become absorbed in details (often to the point of missing what is important), and prefer to operate as if emotions were irrelevant or inconsequential. They tend to be excessively devoted to work and productivity to the detriment of leisure and relationships. Individuals who match this prototype tend to be inhibited and constricted, and have difficulty acknowledging or expressing wishes, impulses, or anger. They are invested in seeing and portraying themselves as emotionally strong, untroubled, and in control, despite evidence of underlying insecurity, anxiety, or distress. They tend to deny or disavow their need for nurturance or comfort, often regarding such needs as weakness. They tend to adhere rigidly to daily routines, becoming anxious or uncomfortable when they are altered, and to be overly concerned with rules, procedures, order, organization, schedules, and so on. They may be preoccupied with concerns about dirt, cleanliness, or contamination. Rationality and regimentation generally mask underlying feelings of anxiety or anger. Individuals who match this prototype tend to be conflicted about anger, aggression, and authority. They tend to be self-critical, expecting themselves to be "perfect," and to be equally critical of others, whether overtly or covertly. They tend to be controlling, oppositional, and self-righteous or moralistic. They are prone to being stingy and withholding (e.g., of time, money, affection). They are often conflicted about authority, struggling with contradictory impulses to submit versus defy.

5 very good match (patient *exemplifies* this disorder; prototypical case)	Diagnosis
4 good match (patient *has* this disorder; diagnosis applies)	
3 moderate match (patient has *significant features* of this disorder)	Features
2 slight match (patient has minor features of this disorder)	
1 no match (description does not apply)	

Schizoid-Schizotypal Personality

The term "schizoid" is among the most confusing in the clinical literature, because different writers have used the same word to describe very different types of patients. Those impaired enough to be diagnosed with a DSM personality disorder have basic deficits in psychological capacities. They are characterized by impoverishments in interpersonal functioning, emotional life, and thought processes. The schizoid-schizotypal personality prototype presented here describes this deficit-based syndrome.

Psychoanalytic writers have also used the term "schizoid" to describe a very different and much healthier type of patient who does not suffer from such basic deficits, whose psychology is more conflict-based. These patients may have rich inner lives and deep capacity for empathy, even as they keep their distance from others. Their underlying psychological conflict is between longing for closeness and fear of engulfment, impingement, or overstimulation. (For discussion of this healthier, conflict-based version of "schizoid personality," see Chapter 17, Some Thoughts About Schizoid Dynamics.)

With respect to the more impaired (deficit-based) patients, research does not support the DSM distinction between schizoid and schizotypal personality disorders. The framers of DSM attempted to sharpen the boundaries between these diagnostic categories by emphasizing subsyndromal positive symptoms of schizophrenia in one (schizotypal) and subsyndromal negative symptoms in the other (schizoid). However, the distinction does not hold up empirically. Research with the SWAP instrument consistently identified a single diagnostic grouping with features of both schizoid and schizotypal personality disorders, hence the hyphenated term "schizoid-schizotypal."

Patients who match the schizoid-schizotypal prototype lack close relationships and appear indifferent to human company or contact. They lack social skills and tend to be socially awkward or inappropriate. They may seem odd or peculiar in appearance or manner; something about them seems "off." They tend to think in concrete terms and have little capacity to appreciate metaphor, analogy, or nuance. They have difficulty making sense of others' behavior and likewise have little insight into their own. Despite apparent detachment, they suffer inwardly, often greatly, and experience themselves as outcasts and outsiders. A subset of schizoid-schizotypal patients shows substantial aberrations in thinking, reasoning, and perception, and their speech and thought processes may be digressive and circumstantial.

The schizoid-schizotypal grouping, identified empirically by statistical clustering methods, may not describe a homogeneous group of patients best understood in terms of personality. The patients share surface similarities, notably absence of close relationships and deficits in interpersonal functioning. In some cases, this may reflect personality. But other patients in this diagnostic cluster may have subclinical schizophrenic spectrum disorders and others may be on the autistic spectrum. Clinicians tempted to diagnose schizoid-schizotypal personality should consider carefully whether the patient's difficulties might be better accounted for by factors other than personality per se.

Psychotherapy for deficit-based schizoid-schizotypal patients is largely supportive. Close interpersonal connections and emotional intimacy may not be attainable goals, but patients can work toward more harmonious and frictionless coexistence. Therapy should support ego functions (executive function) and assist patients with reasoning, interpreting events, interpreting others' behavior, planning, judgment, and decision processes. See Box 1.5, p. 14 for the schizoid-schizotypal personality prototype.

Box 1.5 Schizoid-schizotypal Personality Prototype

Summary statement: Individuals with schizoid-schizotypal personality are characterized by pervasive impoverishment of, and peculiarities in, interpersonal relationships, emotional experience, and thought processes.

Individuals who match this prototype lack close relationships and appear to have little need for human company or contact, often seeming detached or indifferent. They lack social skills and tend to be socially awkward or inappropriate. Their appearance or manner may be odd or peculiar (e.g., their grooming, posture, eye contact, or speech rhythms may seem strange or "off"), and their verbal statements may be incongruous with their accompanying emotion or non-verbal behavior. They have difficulty making sense of others' behavior and appear unable to describe important others in a way that conveys a sense of who they are as people. They likewise have little insight into their own motives and behavior, and have difficulty giving a coherent account of their lives. Individuals who match this prototype appear to have a limited or constricted range of emotions and tend to think in concrete terms, showing limited ability to appreciate metaphor, analogy, or nuance. Consequently, they tend to elicit boredom in others. Despite their apparent emotional detachment, they often suffer emotionally: They find little satisfaction or enjoyment in life's activities, tend to feel life has no meaning, and feel like outcasts or outsiders. A subset of individuals who match this prototype show substantial peculiarities in their thinking and perception. Their speech and thought processes may be circumstantial, rambling, or digressive, their reasoning processes or perceptual experiences may seem odd and idiosyncratic, and they may be suspicious of others, reading malevolent intent into others' words and actions.

5 very good match (patient *exemplifies* this disorder; prototypical case)	**Diagnosis**
4 good match (patient *has* this disorder; diagnosis applies)	
3 moderate match (patient has *significant features* of this disorder)	**Features**
2 slight match (patient has minor features of this disorder)	
1 no match (description does not apply)	

Antisocial-Psychopathic Personality

The DSM diagnosis of Antisocial Personality Disorder emphasizes criminality but largely ignores the personality processes and motives that define a personality syndrome. The empirically derived diagnostic prototype describes personality processes and more closely resembles the historical concept of psychopathy.[21-23] The hyphenated term "antisocial-psychopathic" serves as a bridge between the DSM construct and the clinical personality syndrome.

People engage in antisocial and criminal behavior for many reasons unrelated to personality pathology. Not all people who engage in criminal behavior (or meet DSM criteria for Antisocial Personality Disorder) have psychopathic personalities; not all people with psychopathic personalities engage in criminality. In some walks of life, psychopathic traits are rewarded. People with antisocial-psychopathic personality styles, given the right opportunities, may become business or political leaders, not criminals, and pursue their ruthless agenda with social approval and even admiration.

People with antisocial-psychopathic personality lack an internalized moral system. What is right is what they can get away with. They are out for personal gain, take advantage of other people, and manipulate and deceive without guilt or inhibition. They show reckless disregard for others' rights, property, or safety. They experience little remorse for the harm they cause. On the contrary, they take sadistic pleasure in dominating and exercising power over others.

People with antisocial-psychopathic personality experience little anxiety, and they show minimal autonomic reactivity in response to aversive events. Many have a high need for stimulation and seek thrills, novelty, and excitement. They push limits and act impulsively, because impulses are not checked by anxiety, empathy, or an internalized moral system. Non-impulsive variants of antisocial-psychopathic personality also exist but are less common. In these variants, sadistic aggression is planned, deliberate, and coldly emotionless, in a way that has been described as "reptilian."

People with antisocial-psychopathic personality are motivated by self-interest, sensation seeking, and desire for power and dominance. Others may puzzle over the person's motive for manipulation or cruelty where there seems little to be gained. The reason is: because they can. Dominance and exerting power over another are their own rewards.

People with antisocial-psychopathic personalities have little interest in self-exploration and rarely come to treatment of their own accord. They come when they perceive some immediate personal advantage to doing so (for example, inducing the clinician to intercede on their behalf, or to get out of legal or other trouble). They are expert at convincing others they have turned over a new leaf, only to revert to the same behavior once they have gotten out of trouble. They understand power, not empathy, and are likely to perceive the clinician's sympathetic attention and compassion as a weakness to exploit. Prognosis is poor. Therapeutic leverage, to the extent there is any, comes from a position of power and dominance few clinicians are comfortable assuming. See Box 1.6, p. 16 for the antisocial-psychopathic personality prototype.

Narcissistic Personality

The hallmark of narcissistic personality is the coexistence of feelings of grandiosity and feelings of inadequacy and emptiness. Grandiosity defends against and masks underlying feelings of inadequacy (but see the section on Malignant Narcissism for a possible exception).

When narcissistic defenses are working, patients with narcissistic personalities feel special and superior. They have an exaggerated sense of self-importance, feel privileged and entitled, expect preferential treatment, and seek to be the center of attention. Their inner life is dominated by fantasies of limitless success, power, glory, beauty, or talent. They tend to treat others as an audience (to witness their magnificence) or as extensions of themselves.

Idealization and devaluation are central defenses. When they idealize someone to whom they are connected, they feel special and important by association. When they devalue someone, they feel superior. They are relatively oblivious to others' actual

---

Box 1.6 Antisocial-psychopathic Personality Prototype

Summary statement: Individuals with antisocial-psychopathic personality exploit others, experience little remorse for harm or injury caused to others, and have poor impulse control.

Individuals who match this prototype take advantage of others, tend to lie or deceive, and to be manipulative. They show a reckless disregard for the rights, property, or safety of others. They lack empathy for other people's needs and feelings. Individuals who match this prototype experience little remorse for harm or injury they cause. They appear impervious to consequences and seem unable or unwilling to modify their behavior in response to threats or consequences. They generally lack psychological insight and blame their difficulties on other people or circumstances. They often appear to gain pleasure by being sadistic or aggressive toward others, and they may attempt to dominate significant others through intimidation or violence. Individuals who match this prototype tend to be impulsive, to seek thrills, novelty, and excitement, and to require high levels of stimulation. They tend to be unreliable and irresponsible and may fail to meet work obligations or honor financial commitments. They may engage in antisocial behavior, including unlawful activities, substance abuse, or interpersonal violence. They may repeatedly convince others of their commitment to change, leading others to think "this time is really different," only to revert to their previous maladaptive behavior.

5 very good match (patient *exemplifies* this disorder; prototypical case)	**Diagnosis**
4 good match (patient *has* this disorder; diagnosis applies)	
3 moderate match (patient has *significant features* of this disorder)	**Features**
2 slight match (patient has minor features of this disorder)	
1 no match (description does not apply)	

---

emotional experience unless it coincides with their own. Interpersonally, they have been described as having emotional transmitters but not receivers.

Grandiosity serves a defensive function, warding off and masking painful feelings of inadequacy, emptiness, smallness, anxiety, and rage. When narcissistic defenses fail, the person is at the mercy of these painful feelings and may lash out in rage or slump into depression and despair.

Deflated or depleted narcissists are less easily recognized than well-defended, grandiose narcissists (and not recognized at all by the DSM). However, they are common in clinical practice. Deflated narcissists are likely to be diagnosed with depressive disorders and may present as ashamed, defeated, and beaten down. When clinicians gain access to their internal world, they find the patient is preoccupied with fantasies of glory and aggrieved at a world that has failed to recognize their unique worth or provide the rewards to which they feel entitled. Behind a depressive presentation, one sometimes finds a deflated narcissist.

Effective treatment involves a careful balancing act, with a judicious blend of empathy and confrontation. Patients with narcissistic personalities benefit from empathic understanding of their underlying pain, insecurity, and vulnerability when these feelings are accessible. With the clinician's help, they can develop greater capacity to tolerate the feelings without resorting to grandiosity and devaluation. On the other hand, they benefit from tactful but systematic confrontation of narcissistic defenses, and exploration of the considerable cost of these defenses vis-à-vis relationships and their ability to find meaning and fulfillment in their lives.

Countertransference reactions include feeling disengaged, deskilled, or competitive with the patient (when devalued), or tempted to join them in a mutual admiration society (when idealized). The clinician's countertransference provides a window into the patient's relationship patterns and the responses they elicit from others. It is important to recognize and explore the relationship patterns as they arise in the therapy relationship, instead of simply repeating the patterns with a new person. People with narcissistic personalities may be most receptive to psychotherapy in mid-life or later, when fantasies of extraordinary success and glory have failed to materialize and they are forced to confront life's realistic limits. See Box 1.7, p. 18 for the narcissistic personality prototype.

Malignant Narcissism

Malignant narcissism is a variant of narcissistic personality that has gained public attention in recent years. It is, in fact, the intersection of narcissistic personality and antisocial-psychopathic personality, blending the characteristics of both. Malignant narcissism has also been described by clinical theorists as narcissism suffused with sadistic aggression.[6] It is not sufficient for the malignant narcissist to feel important and special; it is necessary for someone else to be demeaned or vanquished. The syndrome could plausibly be called "psychopathic narcissism" or "narcissistic psychopathy," but malignant narcissism is the historically and clinically familiar term.

When psychopathic deception, exploitation, sadistic aggression, and externalization combine with narcissistic grandiosity and self-importance, the result can be especially destructive. When there is no internalized moral system to counteract grandiose strivings, others' needs, rights, and well-being become irrelevant. Other people are used and discarded without guilt or remorse. Harmful consequences and disastrous outcomes are always someone else's fault.

Externalizing blame can have toxic effects on others and is often discussed by non-professionals as "gaslighting." The item in the SWAP assessment instrument that addresses externalization is: "Tends to blame own failures or shortcomings on other people or circumstances; attributes his or her difficulties to external factors rather than accepting responsibility for own conduct or choices." The psychological processes that give rise to gaslighting are straightforward. The underlying logic is something like, "The world exists for my aggrandizement and my personal benefit. I am not responsible for my actions or the harm they cause. *You* are responsible."

In extremis, people with severe malignant narcissism may appear to lose touch with reality. This comes about when external events starkly contradict their grandiose, defensively constructed self-image. It is as though the person, forced to choose between revising their self-image and revising reality, opts to revise reality. They may demand that others in their orbit also accept their revised version of reality.

Box 1.7 Narcissistic Personality Prototype

Summary statement: Individuals with narcissistic personality are grandiose and entitled, dismissive and critical of others, and often show underlying signs of vulnerability beneath a grandiose façade.

Individuals who match this prototype have an exaggerated sense of self-importance. They feel privileged and entitled, expect preferential treatment, and seek to be the center of attention. They have fantasies of unlimited success, power, beauty, or talent, and tend to treat others primarily as an audience to witness their importance or brilliance. They tend to believe they can only be appreciated by, or should only associate with, people who are high-status, superior, or "special." They have little empathy and seem unable to understand or respond to others' needs and feelings unless they coincide with their own. Individuals who match this prototype tend to be dismissive, haughty, and arrogant. They tend to be critical, envious, competitive with others, and prone to get into power struggles. They attempt to avoid feeling helpless or depressed by becoming angry instead, and tend to react to perceived slights or criticism with rage and humiliation. Their overt grandiosity may mask underlying vulnerability: Individuals who match this prototype are invested in seeing and portraying themselves as emotionally strong, untroubled, and emotionally in control, often despite clear evidence of underlying insecurity or distress. A substantial subset of narcissistic individuals tend to feel inadequate or inferior, to feel that life has no meaning, and to be self-critical and intolerant of their own human defects, holding themselves to unrealistic standards of perfection.

5 very good match (patient *exemplifies* this disorder; prototypical case)	Diagnosis
4 good match (patient *has* this disorder; diagnosis applies)	
3 moderate match (patient has *significant features* of this disorder)	Features
2 slight match (patient has minor features of this disorder)	
1 no match (description does not apply)	

In empirical research with the SWAP instrument, items addressing underlying inadequacy and inferiority did not emerge as descriptors of malignant narcissism.[24] It is unclear whether underlying feelings of inadequacy are not a component of malignant narcissism or were not evident to the clinicians who provided the data. It seems likely that when personality dynamics are predominantly narcissistic, underlying inadequacy is present, even if not readily observable; when personality dynamics are fundamentally antisocial-psychopathic, it may not be.

Depending on the blend of narcissism and psychopathy, people with malignant narcissism may or may not be amenable to psychotherapy. Where narcissism predominates and psychopathic traits are secondary, psychotherapy may be helpful, albeit difficult. When psychopathy predominates, prognosis is poor, for the same reasons it is poor for antisocial-psychopathic personality. There is little therapeutic leverage when patients lack an internalized value system or a basic capacity for mutuality.

Paranoid Personality

Patients with paranoid personalities are chronically suspicious, angry, and hostile. They read malevolent intent into others' words and actions and are quick to assume others mean them harm. They hold grudges, dwell on slights, and react to perceived threats with rage and aggression. They see their difficulties as externally caused and lack insight into their own role in shaping events.

At the core of paranoid personality is the defense of projection. People with paranoid personalities are filled with aggression and rage, which they project onto others and (mis)perceive as originating from them. People with paranoid personalities experience the world as cold, hostile, and dangerous because they see their own hostility wherever they look.

Paranoid personality style is found at healthy and neurotic levels of personality organization but is more often seen at borderline levels of organization, at least in clinical populations. Often underappreciated in the clinical literature (and neglected in the DSM) is the extent of cognitive and perceptual disturbances in patients with paranoid personalities. They tend to show disturbances in thinking, above and beyond paranoid ideas. Their perceptions and reasoning can be odd and idiosyncratic, and they may become irrational in the face of strong emotion. While the role of cognitive and perceptual disturbances has been historically underappreciated, it is perhaps not surprising given the pervasiveness of paranoid projection, which necessarily requires some confusion about what is internal versus external and what is reality versus fantasy.

Clinicians' strong emotional reactions to patients with paranoid personality give them a small taste of the fear and rage the patients experience chronically and seek to manage through externalization and projection. The clinician should assist the patient with reality testing when necessary, and help the patient recognize and find more adaptive ways to manage their anger and aggression. An overly friendly or sympathetic stance on the part of the clinician is likely to arouse the patient's suspicion and intensify paranoid thinking. A matter-of-fact stance, even to the point of brusqueness, is generally more effective. See Box 1.8, p. 20 for the paranoid personality prototype.

Hysteric-Histrionic Personality

The terms "hysteric" and "histrionic" evoke an era of patriarchy and gender inequality and are offensive to many, with reason. There is, however, a difference between the term and the phenomenon. Regardless of the label, a personality syndrome does exist. It is described repeatedly in the clinical literature and emerges in empirical research using statistical clustering methods. Objections to terminology should not blind us to the clinical phenomenon. Nomenclature is beyond the scope of this chapter, which addresses clinical issues.

Before DSM-III introduced the diagnosis of histrionic personality disorder, the term "hysteric" was used to describe higher-functioning people with this personality style and "histrionic" was used for more disturbed patients (such as those in the borderline range of functioning). The hyphenated term "hysteric-histrionic" encompasses higher- and lower-functioning variants of the personality syndrome and provides a bridge between the DSM construct and the extensive clinical literature.

Box 1.8 Paranoid Personality Prototype

Summary statement: Individuals with paranoid personality are chronically suspicious, angry and hostile, and may show disturbed thinking.

Individuals who match this prototype are chronically suspicious, expecting that others will harm, deceive, conspire against, or betray them. They tend to blame their problems on other people or circumstances, and to attribute their difficulties to external factors. Rather than recognizing their own role in interpersonal conflicts, they tend to feel misunderstood, mistreated, or victimized. Individuals who match this prototype tend to be angry or hostile and prone to rage episodes. They tend to see their own unacceptable impulses in other people instead of in themselves and are therefore prone to misattribute hostility to other people. They tend to be controlling, to be oppositional, contrary, or quick to disagree, and to hold grudges. They tend to elicit dislike or animosity and to lack close friendships and relationships. Individuals who match this prototype tend to show disturbances in their thinking above and beyond paranoid ideas. Their perceptions and reasoning can be odd and idiosyncratic, and they may become irrational when strong emotions are stirred up, to the point of seeming delusional.

5 very good match (patient *exemplifies* this disorder; prototypical case)	Diagnosis
4 good match (patient *has* this disorder; diagnosis applies)	
3 moderate match (patient has *significant features* of this disorder)	Features
2 slight match (patient has minor features of this disorder)	
1 no match (description does not apply)	

Hysteric-histrionic personality is a multifaceted syndrome encompassing the full spectrum of personality processes. On the surface, people with hysteric-histrionic personality styles exemplify gender stereotypes. They present as stereotypically feminine or masculine, like a leading lady or leading man in a stylized Hollywood movie. They are emotional and dramatic. They use their physical attractiveness and sexuality to gain attention. They are flirtatious, seductive, and sexually provocative. They may lead people on and make romantic conquests. They tend to become involved in romantic triangles involving rivals. They can charm and captivate members of the other sex (when both are heterosexual) but may annoy or threaten members of the same sex. Their emotions can seem simultaneously intense and shallow. They can develop intense infatuations which they describe as love, and lose interest when a new prospect arrives.

For people with hysteric-histrionic personality, facts and reason take a backseat to emotion. Their reactions tend to be based on feelings, not reason. If you ask a person with hysteric-histrionic personality what they think, they are likely to tell you how they feel. Their cognitive style tends to be glib, global, and impressionistic; they miss details and gloss over inconsistencies.[25] They come across as naïve and seem to know less about the ways of the world than might be expected. Their beliefs can seem cliché or stereotypical, as if taken from storybooks or movies. They tend to be suggestible. Their impressionistic cognitive style is unrelated to intelligence and serves a defensive function.

People with hysteric-histrionic personality do not look too closely at details or connect too many dots, for fear of seeing and knowing too much.

At the core of hysteric-histrionic personality are conflicts around gender and power. Unconsciously, they see their own gender as weak, defective, or inferior. They see the other gender as powerful, exciting, and frightening, and they are unconsciously envious. They use sexuality as a way to turn the tables and gain power over the other gender. Such use (or misuse) of sexuality helps to ward off feeling of weakness, powerlessness, and fear. They may flaunt their sexuality in exhibitionistic ways to counteract underlying shame, fear, and envy. Genuine sexual intimacy and satisfaction are difficult for the same reasons; it is hard to experience deep connection while feeling shamefully defective or frightened by one's partner. When underlying psychological conflicts cannot find expression in thoughts and words, they may find expression through somatic symptoms (conversion symptoms). Beneath the dramatic presentation and sexualization is a fear of being abandoned and left uncared for, and a yearning to be cared for and protected. Their tragedy is that they long for a caring relationship but find sexual relationships instead.

Patients with hysteric-histrionic personalities respond well to psychotherapy and benefit from both its exploratory, interpretive aspects and its relational aspects. The dependability of the therapist and safety of the therapeutic frame provide a context for self-exploration and insight into conflicts around gender, power, and sexuality. At the same time, the therapy relationship provides a new and different relationship template, one in which a therapist of the other gender is neither seductive nor seducible, and a therapist of the same gender is neither ineffectual nor competitive. Therapists should let the patient lead, allowing them to explore their needs, feelings, wishes, fears, and conflicts at their own pace. The patient does not need an authority figure explaining their experience to them; they benefit from exploring and explaining it to themselves. A didactic stance on the part of the therapist may reinforce feelings of defectiveness and powerlessness.

When both parties are heterosexual, high-functioning hysteric-histrionic patients may charm therapists of the other gender and annoy those of the same gender, at least initially. It is helpful to remember the patient unavoidably brings their relationship patterns into the therapy relationship, and this is what makes it possible to explore the thoughts, feelings, and experiences that underlie them. More disturbed patients (in the borderline range of functioning) with hysteric-histrionic personality may alarm and exasperate therapists with flagrant seductiveness or acting out in place of talking and reflecting. See Box 1.9, p. 22 for the hysteric-histrionic personality prototype.

Borderline-Dysregulated Personality

The term "borderline" dates back to a time when psychiatric classification distinguished primarily between neurotic and psychotic disturbance based on intact versus impaired reality testing. Over time, clinical writers began describing patients on the "border," who seemed neither neurotic nor psychotic. The diagnostic construct has evolved, but the term "borderline" remains. The hyphenated term "borderline-dysregulated" retains the familiar term and highlights the emotional dysregulation that is a hallmark of the personality syndrome.

People with borderline-dysregulated personality have been described as "stably unstable."[26] There is a pattern of instability in emotional life, self-concept, and relationships.

Box 1.9 Hysteric-histrionic Personality Prototype

Summary statement: Individuals with hysteric-histrionic personality are emotionally dramatic and cognitively impressionistic, sexually provocative, and interpersonally suggestible, idealizing of admired others, and paradoxically both intensely and superficially attached.

Individuals who match this prototype are emotionally dramatic and prone to express emotion in exaggerated and theatrical ways. Their reactions tend to be based on emotion rather than reflection, and their cognitive style tends to be glib, global, and impressionistic (e.g., missing details, glossing over inconsistencies, mispronouncing names). Their beliefs and expectations seem cliché or stereotypical, as if taken from storybooks or movies, and they seem naïve or innocent, seeming to know less about the ways of the world than would be expected. Individuals who match this prototype tend to be sexually seductive or provocative. They use their physical attractiveness to an excessive degree to gain attention and notice, and they behave in ways that seem to epitomize gender stereotypes. They may be flirtatious, preoccupied with sexual conquest, prone to lead people on, or promiscuous. They tend to become involved in romantic or sexual "triangles" and may be drawn to people who are already attached or sought by someone else. They appear to have difficulty directing both tender feelings and sexual feelings toward the same person, tending to view others as either virtuous or sexy, but not both. Individuals who match this prototype tend to be suggestible or easily influenced, and to idealize and identify with admired others to the point of taking on their attitudes or mannerisms. They fantasize about ideal, perfect love, yet tend to choose sexual or romantic partners who are emotionally unavailable or who seem inappropriate (e.g., in terms of age or social or economic status). They may become attached quickly and intensely. Beneath the surface, they often fear being alone, rejected, or abandoned.

5 very good match (patient *exemplifies* this disorder; prototypical case)	**Diagnosis**
4 good match (patient *has* this disorder; diagnosis applies)	
3 moderate match (patient has *significant features* of this disorder)	**Features**
2 slight match (patient has minor features of this disorder)	
1 no match (description does not apply)	

Core features include affect dysregulation, splitting, identity diffusion, projection, projective identification, and insecure attachment.

People with borderline-dysregulated personality have difficulty regulating affect. Their emotions can change rapidly and unpredictably and spiral out of control, leading to extremes of despair, anxiety, agitation, and rage. They experience episodes of deep depression in which they lose access to any glimmer of hope. They are often filled with rage, and they are prone to destroy relationships with hateful, rage-filled outbursts. Poor impulse control is an ongoing problem and leads to ill-considered actions and self-destructive behavior.

Splitting refers to compartmentalizing good and bad perceptions, feelings, and experiences, leading the person to experience self and others as all good or all bad. (The term "dichotomous thinking" in dialectical behavioral therapy also refers to this phenomenon.) Splitting results in extreme, wildly fluctuating views of self and others, depending on which "compartment" the person is experiencing. When distressed, people with borderline-dysregulated personality lose the capacity to see others as complex, three-dimensional human beings. Instead, they become one-dimensional heroes, saviors, victims, villains, and abusers.

The person may see certain people as all good ("good objects") and others as all bad ("bad objects"), or their experience of the same person may swing between contradictory extremes. This leads to unstable and chaotic relationships. For example, a person with borderline-dysregulated personality may see the clinician as a savior, until they disappoint. Then they may see the clinician as a "bad person" and attack them for their callousness or incompetence. Such shifts from idealization to devaluation are often precipitated by perceived criticism or rejection.

Splitting also refers to compartmentalized, contradictory experiences of self. The person may vacillate between experiencing themselves as a good person and as someone evil and rotten to the core. Self-concept depends on which of multiple, contradictory self-representations is being experienced. Shifts between different self-representations bring corresponding shifts in emotional state and keep the person on an emotional rollercoaster. Affect dysregulation and splitting therefore go hand in hand.

Because disparate self-representations are not integrated into a coherent whole, people with borderline-dysregulated personality have difficulty maintaining a consistent, stable sense of self ("identity diffusion"). Their attitudes, values, and self-concept are unstable and changeable. They may shift with relationships, circumstances, or emotional state. The person may present in strikingly different ways on different occasions, often to the consternation of clinicians. If they are feeling good, they may be blithely unconcerned that they were recently suicidal. If depressed, they may feel no connection to any part of themselves they have ever experienced as positive.

Primitive forms of projection are a hallmark of borderline-dysregulated personality. Split, disavowed representations of self and others and the feelings associated with them are projected wholesale onto other people with conviction and certainty. The projections often involve intensely negative emotions like anger, spite, hate, envy, and disgust. The person regards their projections as facts, not perceptions. It can be disorienting and maddening to others, including clinicians, to be seen and treated repeatedly as someone they are not.

Projective identification takes the defense of projection a step further. In addition to projecting disavowed parts of themselves, the person works to induce and evoke the feelings they have projected with such vehemence, so that the other person comes to feel and act in accord with the projection. Borderline-dysregulated patients are masterful in bringing this about, although they do not do it consciously. Clinicians describe experiences of not being able to think their own thoughts or feel their own feelings, as if their minds have been colonized by something alien.[27] Under the sway of projective identifications, clinicians may find themselves filled with hatred for their patient or impelled to cross professional boundaries to rescue them.

The transfer of thoughts and feelings from patient to clinician that occurs in projective identification is not mysterious or mystical. Observable behavior on the part of the patient pulls, pushes, coaxes, and coerces the clinician into their assigned role, although the clinician may be unaware of this as it is occurring. Generally, countertransference comes first, and understanding emerges after the fact.

Borderline-dysregulated patients with a history of abuse are prone to enacting scenarios involving shifting roles of abuser, victim, and rescuer.[27,28] Through processes of projection and projective identification, clinician and patient can inhabit any of the three roles. A common scenario begins with the patient in the role of victim and the clinician in the role of rescuer. As the patient's needs and demands escalate, the clinician overextends themselves to the point of feeling persecuted and victimized by the patient (for example, taking late night phone calls, allowing sessions to run overtime, not collecting fees). The clinician may become controlling and punitive as they try to reestablish boundaries, moving into the abuser role. Ideally, clinician and patient can examine the patient's shifting experience of self and other and how these role relationships are recreated in the therapy relationship, instead of just reenacting them with a new person.

Finally, people with borderline-dysregulated personality have insecure or disorganized attachment styles and are hypersensitive to rejection. They are needy and dependent, become attached quickly and intensely, yet anticipate rejection and abandonment. They are desperate to be cared for, but their concept of "caring" involves unrealistic levels of availability and attunement that no one can provide. When the other person inevitably falls short, they become enraged and lash out. This dynamic is captured by a pithy book title: *I Hate You—Don't Leave Me*.[29]

A number of therapy models have been developed for borderline-dysregulated personality and are described in other chapters. Work with borderline-dysregulated patients can be fast, furious, chaotic, and confusing. One supervisor likened it to "tumbling helplessly in a clothes dryer," never knowing what is coming or from where. In the early stages of treatment, the clinician's role may simply be to accept and tolerate the confusion, remain engaged with the patient, and maintain the treatment frame. A clear theoretical model provides direction and helps contain the clinician's anxieties.

All therapy models emphasize attention to boundary issues, attention to what is happening in the therapy relationship, and active management of behaviors potentially destructive to the therapy and the therapy relationship. Because borderline-dysregulated patients are prone to crises, therapy can easily be derailed if crisis management rather than work on underlying psychological issues becomes the focus. Therapy models for borderline-dysregulated personality include regular consultation and support for therapists, to help manage intense countertransference.

Borderline-dysregulated personality can be viewed as a personality syndrome in its own right (when no other personality syndrome is salient) or as a level of personality organization associated with any other personality syndrome. For example, a patient who matches the descriptions for narcissistic personality and borderline-dysregulated personality can be described as having narcissistic personality organized at a borderline level; a patient who matches the descriptions for paranoid personality and borderline-dysregulated personality can be described as having paranoid personality organized at a borderline level; and so on. This organizing framework brings considerable clarity to diagnostic formulations. See Box 1.10, p. 25 for the borderline-dysregulated personality prototype.

Box 1.10 Borderline-dysregulated Personality Prototype

Summary Statement: Individuals with borderline-dysregulated personality have impaired ability to regulate their emotions, have unstable perceptions of self and others that lead to intense and chaotic relationships, and are prone to act on impulses, including self-destructive impulses.

Individuals who match this prototype have emotions that can change rapidly and spiral out of control, leading to extremes of sadness, anxiety, and rage. They tend to "catastrophize," seeing problems as disastrous or unsolvable, and are often unable to soothe or comfort themselves without the help of another person. They tend to become irrational when strong emotions are stirred up, showing a significant decline from their usual level of functioning. Individuals who match this prototype lack a stable sense of self: Their attitudes, values, goals, and feelings about themselves may seem unstable or ever-changing, and they are prone to painful feelings of emptiness. They similarly have difficulty maintaining stable, balanced views of others: When upset, they have trouble perceiving positive and negative qualities in the same person at the same time, seeing others in extreme, black-or-white terms. Consequently, their relationships tend to be unstable, chaotic, and rapidly changing. They fear rejection and abandonment, fear being alone, and tend to become attached quickly and intensely. They are prone to feeling misunderstood, mistreated, or victimized. They often elicit intense emotions in other people and may draw them into roles or "scripts" that feel alien and unfamiliar (e.g., being uncharacteristically cruel, or making "heroic" efforts to rescue them). They may likewise stir up conflict or animosity between other people. Individuals who match this prototype tend to act impulsively. Their work life or living arrangements may be chaotic and unstable. They may act on self-destructive impulses, including self-mutilating behavior, suicidal threats or gestures, and genuine suicidality, especially when an attachment relationship is disrupted or threatened.

5 very good match (patient *exemplifies* this disorder; prototypical case)	Diagnosis
4 good match (patient *has* this disorder; diagnosis applies)	
3 moderate match (patient has *significant features* of this disorder)	Features
2 slight match (patient has minor features of this disorder)	
1 no match (description does not apply)	

Personality and Clinical Case Formulation

It should be clear that personality syndromes are not merely descriptive constructs, like DSM diagnoses; they are explanatory. The descriptions of the personality syndromes explicate underlying psychological processes that leave people vulnerable to a range of mental health problems. Mental health problems do not arise in a vacuum. More often than not, they arise in the matrix of personality dynamics.

The personality syndrome descriptions provide the broad strokes of clinical case formulations. They can provide a treatment focus and direct the clinician's attention to psychological processes underlying presenting symptoms and diagnoses. They are broad strokes because they are simplifications, especially when applied to people at higher (healthy and healthier neurotic) levels of functioning. People at higher levels of functioning have greater psychological flexibility and commonly show a blend of personality styles. Even so, it is possible to recognize areas where specific personality dynamics (depressive, obsessive-compulsive, narcissistic, and so on) prevail. "Purer" examples of personality styles are generally seen at lower levels of personality organization.

Clinical case formulations articulate cause and effect. For example, the person with depressive personality defends against anger, which finds indirect expression through self-criticism and self-punitiveness. The person with narcissistic personality inflates themselves to ward off underlying feelings of inadequacy and emptiness, but their defensively constructed self-image cuts off authentic connection with self and others. The person with borderline-dysregulated personality cannot reconcile contradictory perceptions and feeling states, and so vacillates between them. The person with paranoid personality sees their own projected hostility everywhere they look, and so experiences the world as cold and cruel.

Such statements describe cause-and-effect relationships that can form the nucleus of individualized, patient-specific case formulations that give treatment direction and focus. Without a coherent case formulation, treatment can devolve into a haphazard "spaghetti-on-the-wall" process, with the clinician trying one intervention after another, hoping something will "stick." It can also devolve into aimless, directionless "supportive therapy" in which the therapist has essentially given up on meaningful change. To recognize a personality syndrome is to begin to articulate a clinical case formulation.

Personality Pathways to Depression

The most common mental health diagnoses, at least in North America, are depressive disorders. Many depressed patients experience only minimal relief from symptom-focused treatments, or experience relief but then relapse. Depression is often considered a chronic condition. In many cases, it may appear chronic because the personality processes that give rise to it have never been addressed in psychotherapy.

Nearly all of the personality syndromes can be pathways to depression and require their own distinct treatment focus. I will briefly describe how several of the personality syndromes create vulnerability to depression and will touch even more briefly on some treatment implications. My purpose is to illustrate connections between personality processes and depression, not provide specific instructions for conducting treatment, which would require a book in its own right, or several.

Depressive Personality

Depressive personality refers to enduring personality dynamics, not mood state. People with depressive personalities may or may not experience clinical depression, and people with recurring or chronic depression may or may not have depressive personality styles.

Difficulty recognizing needs and desires can lead to clinical depression. It is difficult to meet your needs when you do not know what they are. Failure to meet basic emotional needs leads to depletion and depression. Work in psychotherapy should focus not just on expressing unrecognized and unarticulated needs, but on recognizing the psychological processes that interfere with recognizing them. The clinician should be alert to subtle ways the patient steers away from needs and desires, and help them articulate the fears that lead them to steer away.

Anger directed at the self can lead to depression. Being berated, punished, and scorned causes pain, and this is equally true when the person doing the punishing is oneself. To stop the self-torment, the person must recognize and consciously experience the anger they habitually disavow. This process cannot be merely academic or intellectual; the anger must be experienced in the "here and now" of the therapy relationship. The therapist should be alert to indirect indications of irritation or disappointment, or their absence where they might be expected, and actively invite them into the therapy relationship. "I'm sorry I was late" is not an invitation to explore disappointment or anger; "I notice you didn't say how it felt when I was not here" *is* an invitation.

Patients who have not internalized a reliably available caretaker remain dependent on others for emotional care and are vulnerable to depression when left to rely on their own internal resources. They benefit from experiencing and internalizing a relationship with an attuned and reliably available therapist. Brief therapies with arbitrary session limits can be destructive. Instead of helping them repair early experiences of relational disruption or loss, they can force the patient to relive them.

Avoidant Personality

Emotional well-being requires engagement in the world and at least a modicum of enjoyment and pleasure. People with anxious-avoidant personality styles cut themselves off from emotional sustenance through fearful avoidance. Their living space can become too restricted to meet basic needs, leading to depletion and depression. To make matters worse, the person finds little respite from their anxieties even when they avoid feared situations, because perceived dangers are internal as well as external. The effort to keep anxieties at bay is emotionally depleting and exhausting.

Therapy must help the patient confront what they avoid, internally and externally. They remain vulnerable to depression so long as their lives remain too constricted to meet their emotional needs, and so long as they devote their energies to avoiding harm at the expense of pursuing desires.

Obsessive-Compulsive Personality

People with obsessive-compulsive personalities are engaged in an ongoing internal conflict, which they defend against by constricting and inhibiting emotional awareness and expression. Unfortunately, it is impossible to selectively inhibit negative emotions. The defenses that inhibit shame, fear, and rage also inhibit spontaneity, joy, excitement, desire, and pleasure. Life becomes monotonized, routinized, and pleasureless.

Desires are forbidden, and when the person does pursue desire, it gives rise to so much guilt that they cannot enjoy it. Constant squelching of needs and desires, and excessive devotion to work and productivity at the expense of leisure and enjoyment, lead to depletion and depression. Underlying shame, humiliation, and rage constantly threaten to erupt, which can leave the person with a background feeling of impending doom.

Effective psychotherapy explores defenses against emotional life and allows the patient to discover through lived experience in the therapy relationship that emotion and desire can be met with acceptance and interest, not horror, and can be expressed without bringing about punishment, retaliation, or catastrophe.

Narcissistic Personality

People with narcissistic personality are inherently vulnerable to depression. One source of vulnerability is a chronic gap between grandiose expectations and what the world affords. Rewards that come the person's way fall short of those to which they feel entitled and are therefore devalued. Instead of feeling satisfaction and pleasure, the person ends up feeling disappointed and aggrieved. The gap between expectation and reality never closes, leading to dejection, hopelessness, and despair.

There is likewise a chronic gap between self-expectations and capabilities. The narcissistic person fantasizes about unlimited success, power, beauty, or talent. Instead of experiencing satisfaction and pride in legitimate accomplishments—which could provide a basis for realistic self-esteem—they perpetually feel they have fallen short.

Finally, their defensively constructed self-image represents a barrier to genuine intimacy and can cut them off from love and meaningful connection with others.

Effective psychotherapy can help these patients understand how they devalue life's pleasures, devalue their own legitimate abilities, and cut themselves off from intimate connections that make life meaningful and make its hardships bearable (including the connection potentially available with the therapist). If they develop enough trust in the therapy relationship, they may allow themselves to reveal the parts of themselves they experience as shameful and inadequate and keep hidden away. They may then slowly internalize the therapist's more accepting and benign view of their fundamental humanness. Ultimately, they must grieve the loss of the perfect person and perfect world of their fantasies, in order to live as they person they are in the world that is.

Paranoid Personality

People with paranoid personality are vulnerable to depression because they experience the world as cold, cruel, and hostile. They feel embattled and surrounded by enemies and dangers on all sides. They experience the world as hostile because they project their anger and aggression and see their own hostility wherever they look. The chronic experience of being embattled, persecuted, and excluded leads to depressive states. Additionally, the person is deprived of meaningful attachments and emotional support because they keep others at a distance, and their hostility and suspicion make others want to keep their distance.

Psychotherapy may help the person recognize that the aggression they experience as external emanates from within, understand its sources and its role as protection against deeper injuries, and understand their own role in creating hostile and adversarial interactions.

Borderline-Dysregulated Personality

People with borderline-dysregulated personality experience episodes of dark, deep depression. Their severe depressive states seem to encompass the entirety of their being. There can be a pervasive feeling that everything about them and everything about their world is dark and hopeless and always has been and always will be. The person may feel irreparably damaged, evil, or rotten to the core. Positive self-representations and experiences seem inaccessible.

These severe depressive states are rooted in splitting. At healthier levels of personality organization, good and bad self-representations and feeling states are integrated into a coherent whole and naturally modify and modulate one another. But when self-representations are split and compartmentalized, the current self-representation and feeling state is experienced as *all there is*. When painful feeling states are not modulated by other experiences, they are felt in their rawest form.

Other factors also contribute to severe depressive states. Identity diffusion, or difficulty maintaining a coherent and stable sense of self, leads to painful feelings of emptiness. Recurring relationship patterns in which the person relives experiences of helplessness and victimization lead to depression. Unstable relationships and rageful responses to others can leave them without emotional support when they need it most. Impulsive, ill-considered choices and actions can bring painful consequences.

Some therapy approaches emphasize management of dysregulated emotional states (for example, by learning and practicing self-regulation skills). Others address and work to change the underlying psychological processes that cause the dysregulated states. This requires creating a sturdy reflective space in which the patient's intense emotional reactions can be contained, examined, and understood.

Conclusion

The purpose of diagnosis is to provide more helpful treatment. When presenting complaints and diagnoses are rooted in personality dynamics, as they often are, meaningful change means addressing personality dynamics. Because personality dynamics tend to fall into recognizable patterns, personality diagnosis is largely a matter of pattern recognition. Clinicians who recognize these patterns have a tremendous advantage in navigating the clinical landscape. For example, they will recognize underlying psychological processes that create vulnerability to suffering, the defenses they are likely to encounter, and the roles they themselves are likely to be cast in (via transference and countertransference) as treatment unfolds. Treating patients without an understanding of personality syndromes is like navigating without a map.

The eleven personality syndromes described in this chapter reflect not only clinical knowledge accrued over generations of practice experience but also the findings of empirical research. The typology itself—the eleven diagnostic groupings or classifications—is derived via statistical clustering methods applied to large clinical samples. The core diagnostic features of the syndromes, summarized in the diagnostic prototypes, are also empirically derived. Clinicians who use this diagnostic system can be confident they are utilizing an evidence-based approach.

Perhaps most important, each personality syndrome provides the broad strokes of a clinical case formulation that therapist and patient, working together, can fill in,

---

Box 1.11 Resources for Clinicians and Researchers

- swapassessment.org.
  This is where to access the SWAP assessment instrument. Clinicians can complete an assessment online and receive a comprehensive assessment report with personality diagnoses, clinical case formulations, and treatment recommendations. There is an extensive bibliography with links to downloadable reprints.
- swapassessment.org/prototypes.
  This is a three-page quick reference guide (pdf file) containing all the diagnostic prototypes. It is available as a free reference resource to facilitate personality diagnosis in day-to-day clinical practice.

---

elaborate upon, and revise as new understandings emerge. This kind of case formulation gives treatment direction and focus that can lead to meaningful and lasting change for many patients.

For additional resources for clinicians and researchers review Box 1.11.

Conflict of Interest/Disclosure: The authors of this chapter have no financial conflicts and nothing to disclose.

References

1. Westen D, Shedler J. Revising and assessing axis II, Part I: developing a clinically and empirically valid assessment method. *Am J Psychiatry*. 1999 Feb;156(2):258–272.

2. Westen D, Shedler J. Revising and assessing axis II, Part II: toward an empirically based and clinically useful classification of personality disorders. *Am J Psychiatry*. 1999 Feb;156(2):273–285.

3. Shedler J, Westen D. Refining personality disorder diagnosis: integrating science and practice. *Am J Psychiatry*. 2004 Aug;161(8):1350–1365.

4. Westen D, Shedler J, Bradley B, DeFife JA. An empirically derived taxonomy for personality diagnosis: bridging science and practice in conceptualizing personality. *Am J Psychiatry*. 2012 Mar;169(3):273–284.

5. Shedler J. Integrating Clinical and Empirical Approaches to Personality: The Shedler-Westen Assessment Procedure (SWAP). (Chapter 4, this volume).

6. Kernberg, O. *Severe Personality Disorders: Psychotherapeutic Strategies*. New Haven, CT: Yale University Press; 1984.

7. Kernberg O. *Borderline Conditions and Pathological Narcissism*. Lanham, MD: Jason Aronson; 1975.

8. McWilliams N. *Psychoanalytic Diagnosis: Understanding Personality Structure in the Clinical Process*. 2nd ed. New York, NY: Guilford Press; 2011.

9. McWilliams N, Shedler J. Personality syndromes. In: Lingiardi V, McWilliams N, eds. *Psychodynamic Diagnostic Manual (PDM-2)*. 2nd ed. New York, NY: Guilford Press; 2017:15–67.

10. *Diagnostic and Statistical Manual of Mental Disorders*. 5th ed. Washington DC: American Psychiatric Association; 2013.

11. *Diagnostic and Statistical Manual of Mental Disorders*. 3rd ed. Washington DC: American Psychiatric Association; 1980.

12. MacKinnon R, Michels R. *The Psychiatric Interview in Clinical Practice*. Philadelphia, PA: WB Saunders; 1971.

13. Gabbard, GO. *Psychodynamic Psychiatry in Clinical Practice*. 5th ed. Washington, DC: American Psychiatric Publishing; 2014.

14. Westen D, Shedler J, Bradley R. A prototype approach to personality disorder diagnosis. *Am J Psychiatry*. 2006 May;163(5):846–856.

15. Westen D, Shedler J. A prototype matching approach to diagnosing personality disorders: toward DSM-V. *J Pers Disord*. 2000 Summer;14(2):109–126.

16. Spitzer RL, First MB, Shedler J, Westen D, Skodol AE. Clinical utility of five dimensional systems for personality diagnosis: a "consumer preference" study. *J Nerv Ment Dis*. 2008 May;196(5):356–374.

17. Blatt SJ, Zuroff DC. Interpersonal relatedness and self-definition: two prototypes for depression. *Clinical Psychology Review*. 1992:12(5):527–562.

18. Blatt SJ, Quinlan DM, Chevron, ES, McDonald C, Zuroff D. Dependency and self-criticism: psychological dimensions of depression. *J Consul Clin Psychol*. 1982;150:113–124.

19. Hyde J. *Fragile Narcissists or the Guilty Good? What Drives the Personality of the Psychotherapist?* Dissertation. Macquarie University; 2009.

20. Reich W. *Character Analysis*. New York, NY: Farrar, Straus & Giroux; 1972. Original work published 1933.

21. Cleckley H. *The Mask of Sanity*. St. Louis, MO: Mosby; 1941.

22. Hare RD. *Psychopathy: Theory and Research*. New York, NY: Wiley; 1970.

23. Meloy R, Shiva A. A psychoanalytic view of psychopathy. In: A Felthous, H Saß, eds. *The International Handbook of Psychopathic Disorders and the Law*. Hoboken, NJ: Wiley; 2007:335–346.

24. Russ E, Shedler J, Bradley R, Westen D. Refining the construct of narcissistic personality disorder: diagnostic criteria and subtypes. *Am J Psychiatry*. 2008;165:1473–1481.

25. Shapiro D. *Neurotic Styles*. New York, NY: Basic Books; 1965.

26. Schmideberg M. The borderline patient. In: Arieti S, ed. *American Handbook of Psychiatry*. Vol. 1. New York, NY: Basic Books; 1959:398–416.

27. Gabbard GO, Wilkinson SM. *Management of Countertransference with Borderline Patients*. Washington DC: American Psychiatric Press; 1994.

28. Davies JM, Frawley MG. Dissociative processes and transference-countertransference paradigms in the psychoanalytically oriented treatment of adult survivors of childhood sexual abuse. *Psychoanal Dialogues*. 1992;2(1):5–36.

29. Kreisman JK, Straus H. *I Hate You—Don't Leave Me: Understanding the Borderline Personality*. New York, NY: Avon; 1991.

2

Levels of Personality Organization

Theoretical Background and Clinical Applications

Eve Caligor, John F. Clarkin, and Julia F. Sowislo

Key Points

- Object relations theory provides a theoretically based, dimensional approach to understanding personality pathology that is useful to the clinician and is conceptually compatible with the DSM-5 Alternative Model of Personality Disorder (AMPD).
- The concept of *structure*, central to object relations theory, refers to an organization of psychological functions or processes that is relatively stable over time and organizes an individual's behavior and subjective experience.
- The structural diagnosis of the patient with personality pathology is made by the dimensional assessment of six domains of functioning (identity, object relations, defenses, aggression, moral functioning, and reality testing), which leads to determination of level of personality organization.
- Assessment of the levels of personality organization is crucial for treatment planning and implementation of treatment.
- Clinical vignettes of patients at different levels of personality organization are provided.
- There is empirical evidence of the object relations approach to assessment and treatment.

Introduction

The inclusion of personality disorder diagnoses in the *Diagnostic and Statistical Manual of Mental Disorders* (DSM-III)[1] resulted in a dramatic increase in the clinical and empirical study of personality disorders and led to significant advances in our understanding of personality functioning and personality pathology. At the same time, clinical and research experience with the personality disorders since DSM-III has highlighted central questions and controversies that remain.[2] Do the official personality-disorder categories hold up to empirical scrutiny? Why do so many patients meet criteria for multiple personality disorders, while other individuals with obvious interpersonal difficulties meet criteria for no personality disorder? Instead of multiple categories of personality disorder, is there one general factor of personality disturbance? Is personality dysfunction best conceived as a dimension, a category, or some hybrid of the two? What is the demarcation between normal personality functioning and personality disorder? And, most important and the focus of this chapter, what are the key behavioral patterns and their underlying mental states of patients with personality traits or disorders that require assessment, treatment, tracking, and change?

A central issue underlying these questions is: What are the essential features that define personality disorders as a group and that distinguish disordered from normal personality functioning? A growing consensus reflected in the *Diagnostic and Statistical Manual 5* (DSM-5) Alternate DSM-5 Model for Personality Disorders (AMPD)[3] suggests that: (1) pathology of self-functioning and functioning with others is the hallmark of personality disorders; and (2) general severity of pathology in these domains, in contrast to specific personality disorder diagnosis, is the most robust predictor of prognosis and clinical outcome.[4] This consensus highlights the need to identify core domains of functioning central to understanding self in relation to others.

Object relations theory provides a dimensional model of personality functioning and pathology that is both clinically near[5] and evidence based. Object relations theory identifies six domains of functioning essential to healthy and disordered personality functioning: (1) identity; (2) quality of object relations; (3) defensive operations; (4) quality and management of aggression; (5) moral functioning and internalized values; and (6) reality testing. Assessment of these domains provides a clinically relevant determination of self and interpersonal functioning and of severity of personality pathology; this assessment organizes treatment planning and clinical intervention for individuals with personality disorders.

It is the goal of this chapter to introduce the system of classification of personality disorders emerging from object relations theory, conceptualized in terms of levels of personality organization. We describe this model of classification and its underlying theoretical foundation based in the object relations theory understanding of personality functioning and pathology. We review empirical support for the model. We highlight the object relations model's relevance to assessment and treatment planning for patients with a range of personality dysfunction, providing in-depth clinical illustrations, and we compare the object relations model with the model introduced in the AMPD.

Personality and Personality Pathology Through the Lens of Object Relations Theory

Personality can be defined as the dynamic integration of repetitive patterns of behavior, emotion, and cognition characteristic of the individual. These patterns are born of a combination of constitutional endowments and developmental factors, reflecting in particular: the individual's temperament; constitutionally determined cognitive capacities; character and its subjective correlate, identity; and internalized value systems.[6] The object relations theory model of personality conceptualizes the entire range of personality functioning along a continuum, from normal personality through the most extreme personality disorders.

Personality Structure

The concept of "structure" is central to the object relations theory of personality. Structure refers to an organization of psychological functions or processes that is relatively stable and enduring over time. Psychological structures organize an individual's behavior and subjective experience. A distinction can be made between observable structures captured as traits, and deep structures, such as identity or defenses, that are not directly observable but can be observed through their impact on an individual's experience and behavior. Object relations theory emphasizes both traits and the mental structures that organize self-functioning and interpersonal functioning and account for both stability of personality functioning and the capacity for change.

Within the framework of object relations theory, internal object relations are considered the most basic psychological structures. An *internal object relation* is a mental representation of the self in relation to another person linked to a particular affect state. For example, a well-cared for self in relation to an attentive caretaker may be linked to feelings of gratification, or, conversely, a neglected self in relation to an unavailable caretaker could be linked to feelings of frustration. It is hypothesized that internal object relations are constructed from early interactions with caregivers, subsequently modified and organized on the basis of ongoing development and interpersonal experience. Internal object relations function as the organizers of subjective experience, and also as the building blocks of higher-order, or superordinate, structures: in particular, identity, the psychological structure that organizes the individual's sense of self and experience of significant others.

Nosology: Levels of Personality Organization

In contrast to familiar, categorical systems of classification of personality disorders that describe distinct disorders defined on the basis of a collection of observable traits and symptoms, the object relations model classifies personality pathology dimensionally, on the basis of severity of personality pathology and reflecting the nature and degree of integration of central psychological structures, or level of personality organization. Determination of level of severity can be combined with a prototypical classification of personality pathology based on a description of dominant traits or personality style.[5,6] The core psychological structures, or processes, that determine level of personality organization are described as: (1) identity; (2) defenses; (3) object relations; (4) moral functioning; (5) aggression; and (6) reality testing.

On the basis of assessment of these domains, personality functioning and pathology are characterized along a spectrum from healthiest through increasingly severe, as follows: (1) normal personality functioning; (2) subsyndromal personality disorder, described in terms of a neurotic level of personality organization; and (3) personality disorder, described in terms of a borderline level of personality organization (BPO).[6,7] The BPO classification is divided into mild (high BPO), severe (middle BPO), and extreme personality disorder (low BPO). In addition, some individuals with psychotic illness who present with the structural features of BPO in the setting of frank loss of reality testing may be described as having psychotic level of personality organization.[8] For a summary of the central features of the five levels of personality pathology, see Table 2.1, p. 36.

Table 2.1 Structural Approach to the Nosology of Personality Pathology

	Normal Personality Organization	Neurotic Personality Organization	High-Level Borderline Personality Organization	Middle Borderline Personality Organization	Low-Level Borderline Personality Organization
Identity	Consolidated, with stable and integrated sense of self and others	Consolidated, with stable and integrated sense of self and others	Mild–moderate identity pathology with some instability and distortion in sense of self and others	Severe identity pathology with polarized and affectively charged, distorted, and unstable experience of self and others	Severe identity pathology with polarized and highly affectively charged, distorted, and unstable experience of self and others
Object Relations	Deep, mutual relations; capacity for concern	Deep, mutual relations; capacity for concern; some conflict	Some capacity for dependent relations; highly conflictual or distant	Relations are based on need fulfillment with limited interest in the needs of the other independent of the needs of the self; limited to no capacity for dependent relations	Relations based on frank exploitation; others are used as a means to an end; no capacity for dependency
Predominant Defensive Style	Mature and repression-based	Repression-based	Repression- and splitting-based	Splitting-based	Splitting-based
Moral Functioning	Internalized, consistent, flexible	Internalized, consistent but rigid or demanding	Variable across individuals; may see marked rigidity combined with focal deficits	Moderate pathology with failure of internalized values; inconsistent or deficient moral functioning; may see circumscribed antisocial behavior	Extreme pathology with absent or corrupt moral system; prominent antisocial traits with frank antisocial behavior
Aggression	Modulated; appropriate	Modulated; inhibited	Verbal aggression; temper outbursts; self-directed aggression in the form of self-neglect	Poorly integrated and poorly modulated; potential for aggression against self and others; outbursts, threats, and self-injurious behavior	Severe aggression against self and others; assault, intimidation, and self-mutilation

Table 2.1 Continued

	Normal Personality Organization	Neurotic Personality Organization	High-Level Borderline Personality Organization	Middle Borderline Personality Organization	Low-Level Borderline Personality Organization
Reality Testing	Intact and stable	Intact and stable	Intact	Vulnerable to extreme stress with transient loss of reality testing; altered mental states without loss of reality testing such as dissociation, depersonalization	Vulnerable to extreme stress with transient loss of reality testing; altered mental states without loss of reality testing such as dissociation, depersonalization

It is important to appreciate the distinction between DSM-5 borderline personality disorder (BPD) and the borderline level of personality organization (BPO). BPD is a specific personality disorder, diagnosed on the basis of a constellation of descriptive features. BPO is a much broader category based on structural features: in particular, pathology of identity formation. The BPO diagnosis subsumes the DSM-5 BPD diagnosis as well as all of the severe personality disorders. For illustration of the relationship between the different levels of personality organization and the DSM-5 categorical diagnoses, see Figure 2.1.

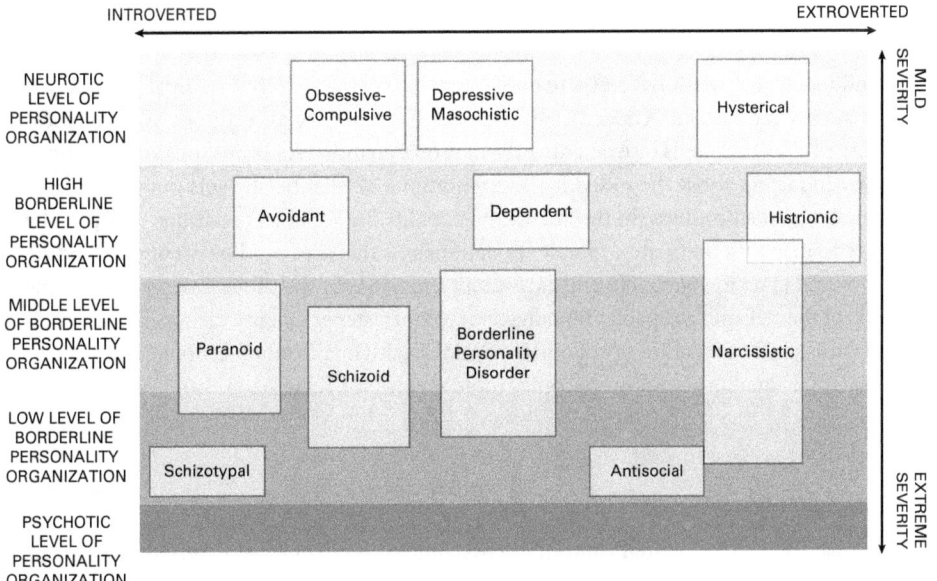

Figure 2.1. Relationship between Level of Personality Organization and DSM-5 Personality Disorder Diagnoses

Core Psychological Structures

Identity

"Identity" is defined as the higher-order, or supraordinate, psychological structure that organizes an individual's concept of self in relation to others. Identity is the cornerstone of the object relations model of personality disorders, with pathology of identity formation being the hallmark of all the personality disorders. In normal identity formation, individual object relations—representations of self and other linked to an affect state—coalesce to form an overarching, coherent, and integrated sense of self, associated with both positive and negative affective experiences of significant others that are not grossly distorted by defensive mechanisms. Normal identity formation, or *identity consolidation*, confers a core sense of self that is stable, coherent, realistic, and continuous across time; a corresponding stable and rich experience of significant others; and affective experience that is complex and well-modulated. A coherent and integrated conception of self and others contributes to relationships that involve empathy and mutual dependence, as well as the ability to mentalize: to realistically understand self and others in terms of intentions, motivations, and emotions.[9]

In contrast, individuals with personality disorders suffer from pathology of identity formation, reflecting failure of component object relations to form an overarching, integrated self-structure. Pathology of identity formation is reflected in the absence of a fully elaborated, stable, and coherent sense of self and others, which is instead unstable, distorted, extreme, discontinuous, and poorly contextualized. Affects are highly charged, poorly integrated, and poorly modulated. Failure of identity consolidation is also reflected in an incapacity to identify and sustain longer-term goals or to invest in relationships and personal interests. Capacity for empathy and ability to mentalize are impaired.

Object Relations

"Quality of object relations" refers to one's "working models of relationships," the internal beliefs, expectations, and capacities that organize interpersonal relations. We can assess quality of object relations by evaluating the nature of an individual's interpersonal relations and by inquiring about the individual's expectations of what he/she gets out of and gives to important relationships. In the normal personality, we see object relations in depth: the ability to maintain mutually dependent relationships that are based on an understanding of give and take; to appreciate and care about the needs of the other independent of the needs of the self; and a capacity for concern. In contrast, personality disorders are associated with significant pathology of object relations, with quality of object relations deteriorating as personality pathology becomes more severe (see Table 2.1, p. 36).

Defenses

"Defenses" are an individual's automatic psychological response to external stressors or psychological conflict. Defenses exist on a spectrum, from most to least adaptive.[10,11] At the most adaptive and flexible end of the spectrum, defenses are mature or healthy. These are followed by the repression-based defenses, which introduce rigidity into personality

---

Box 2.1 Classification of Defenses (ordered from most flexible and adaptive to most maladaptive)

Mature Defenses: Healthy adaptation and coping

- Suppression
- Anticipation
- Altruism
- Humor
- Sublimation

Repression-based Defenses: Conflictual aspects of internal experience are banished from consciousness

- Repression proper
- Reaction formation
- Neurotic projection
- Displacement
- Isolation of affect
- Intellectualization

Splitting-based Defenses: Aspects of conscious experience are dissociated to avoid conflict

- Splitting proper
- Primitive idealization
- Devaluation
- Projective identification
- Omnipotent control
- Primitive denial

Psychotic Defenses: Aspects of external reality are distorted

- Delusional projection
- Psychotic denial
- Psychotic distortion

---

functioning. Next are the highly maladaptive splitting-based, or image-distorting, defenses. Finally, at the most pathological end of the spectrum and most maladaptive, are the psychotic defenses. Box 2.1 lists the categories of defenses and their mode of action.

Moral Values

The normal personality is associated with a commitment to values and ideals. This person possesses a "moral compass" that is consistent, flexible, fully internalized (i.e., one plays by the rules even when no one is watching), and fully integrated into the individual's sense of self. In contrast, personality disorders are characterized by variable but clinically significant degrees of pathology in moral functioning, ranging from mild to extreme impairment (review Table 2.1, p. 36). At the most severe end of the spectrum, we see the absence of any internal moral compass and a lack of capacity for guilt or remorse, characteristic of patients functioning at a low BPO level, and in particular those with antisocial personality disorder or severe narcissistic pathology.

Aggression

Aggression in the normal personality is well-modulated and well-integrated, and is manifest in appropriate and measured expressions of anger as well as in self-assertion and competition. In the neurotic personality organization, aggression is also typically well-modulated and integrated, but the individual may demonstrate inhibitions in normal expressions of aggression. In contrast, in the personality disorders, difficulty managing aggression is central to psychological functioning. This is especially pronounced in the severe personality disorders where intense affects such as rage, hatred, and envy often predominate. Aggression may be directed toward others in the form of verbal outbursts or physical violence, sadism, or threat, and/or directed toward the self in the form of self-injurious behavior, suicide, risk-taking, self-neglect, or self-mutilation.

Reality Testing and Reflective Capacities

Sustained loss of perceptual reality testing is not a feature of personality disorders. However, transient loss of reality testing can be seen in some of the more severe personality disorders, especially in the setting of alcohol and substance misuse. Personality disorders may also be associated with disturbances in the sense of reality without frank loss of reality testing, such as dissociation, derealization, and depersonalization. In addition, in the setting of interpersonal conflict, individuals with severe personality disorders are vulnerable to highly concrete, although not frankly psychotic, mental states. Here the individual's experience in the moment leaves little room for entertaining alternative perspectives ("How I see it is how it is") or to reflect upon what might be happening. For example, Ms. B presented with unstable relationships with men. She noted that many of her breakups were precipitated by her conviction in the moment that her boyfriend was lying to her; in her mind, he was an untrustworthy, exploitative liar. These episodes, although very dramatic, were time limited, often followed by frantic attempts to reestablish the relationship. In personality disorders, as a rule, thinking tends to be more concrete in areas of conflict and interpersonal intensity. As pathology becomes more severe, so too does the vulnerability to concrete thinking, with a parallel decline in the capacity to reflect upon internal states in self and other (i.e., the capacity to mentalize).

Classification: Four Levels of Personality Pathology

Assessment of identity, defenses, object relations, moral functioning, and aggression leads to a determination of severity of personality pathology, described in terms of level of personality organization. We describe the core features of the four levels of personality organization used to characterize the range of personality disorders, and we provide extensive clinical examples.

Neurotic Personality Organization

Neurotic level of personality organization, the mildest, subsyndromal form of personality dysfunction, is characterized by: (1) consolidated identity; (2) the predominance of repression-based defenses and mature defensive operations (see Box 2.1, p. 39); as well as (3) relatively well-integrated, complex affect states.

Neurotic personality organization is distinguished from the normal personality on the basis of rigidity of personality functioning; whereas individuals with normal personality organization are able to flexibly and adaptively manage external stressors and internal conflicts, individuals with neurotic personality organization tend to rely on rigid and to some degree maladaptive responses that interfere with flexible adaptation. This rigidity reflects the impact of repression-based defenses on psychological functioning. As in the normal personality, individuals organized at a neurotic level benefit from a sense of self and also of significant others that is stable, well-differentiated, realistic, and coherent, along with a capacity for full, deep, and mutual relationships. Moral functioning is consistent and internalized in the neurotic personality, although it may be excessively rigid, leading to a propensity toward excessive self-criticism. In addition, there may be difficulty combining intimacy with sexuality. Aggression is for the most part well-integrated and adequately modulated, and reality testing is stable.

Borderline Personality Organization

BPO is characterized by: (1) pathology of identity formation; in conjunction with (2) predominance of splitting-based defenses; and (3) poorly integrated affect states with a preponderance of poorly modulated aggression, which may be either self-directed or directed toward others. BPO is associated with an experience of self and others that is more or less unstable, superficial, poorly differentiated, polarized ("black and white"), distorted, and discontinuous. Splitting-based defenses are responsible for maintaining this fragmented and poorly integrated experience of self and others. Individuals organized at a borderline level have pervasive difficulties that adversely compromise functioning in many if not all domains, and their maladaptive traits are more extreme and more rigid than those of individuals in the neurotic personality organization group.

Three Levels of BPO

The borderline level of personality organization covers a relatively broad spectrum of personality pathology (see Figure 2.1, p. 37); distinctions within the range of BPO are highly clinically significant. At the higher (healthier) end of the BPO spectrum (e.g., those with histrionic, dependent, avoidant, healthier narcissistic traits), individuals have some capacity for dependent, albeit troubled relationships; generally have only minor pathology of moral functioning, such as extreme rigidity coupled with focal deficits; and are not overtly aggressive in most settings. In contrast, individuals at the low end of the BPO spectrum (e.g., those having antisocial personality or malignant narcissism, the most severe presentations of narcissistic personality disorder, characterized by psychopathy, severe aggression, sadism, and paranoia[7]) have extreme pathology of object relations, based purely on ruthless exploitation and sadistic gratification; extreme pathology of moral functioning with prominent antisocial behavior; and extreme expressions of aggression that may be self- or other-directed. These expressions of aggression include, for example, making physical threats, committing assault, or self-mutilation. Individuals in the middle BPO spectrum (e.g., those with borderline, narcissistic, paranoid, and schizoid personality disorders) have severe pathology of object relations expressed in superficial, often chaotic relationships based on need fulfillment. They demonstrate variable impairment of moral functioning and significant pathology of aggression, although less severe than those characteristic of the low BPO spectrum.

Empirical Investigation of Object Relations Theory

Empirical research on object relations theory has shown that personality organization correlates in a theoretically meaningful way to both severity of personality pathology and treatment response. The studies reviewed in this section capture object relations theory–related constructs (such as identity and quality of object relations) by specific self-report measures (i.e., Inventory of Personality Organization for Adolescents [IPO-A[12]] or Inventory of Personality Organization [IPO[13]]) or clinical interviews (i.e., Structured Interview of Personality Organization [STIPO[14]] or Structured Interview of Personality Organization-Revised [STIPO-R[15]]).

Personality organization relates to severity of personality pathology as operationalized by the DSM-5. For instance, patients with DSM personality disorders were found to function on a lower level of personality organization in all domains compared to patients without personality disorders.[16] In a study of patients with chronic pain, there was a significant correlation between personality organization as measured by the STIPO and the number of DSM diagnoses.[17] A very close but not complete association was found between STIPO structural diagnoses and DSM personality pathology in a sample of patients with opiate addiction.[17]

Moreover, personality organization correlates with specific symptoms, such as higher negative affect, aggressive dyscontrol, dysphoria, lack of positive affect,[13] substance abuse,[18] and interpersonal[19] and sexual problems.[20,21] Individuals with lower personality organization also tend to have a higher number of negative life events,[22] suicide attempts, and psychiatric hospitalizations.[23] These latter results, seen in samples of adult participants, are mirrored by results showing that personality organization correlates with severity of pathology in adolescents as well. More precisely, low-level personality organization is associated with affective and conduct problems,[24] severe personality disorder symptoms, and low psychosocial functioning in adolescence.[25] Low personality organization in mothers is associated with higher levels of intrusive and aggressive maternal behaviors, adversely impacting parenting capacity.[26]

With regard to treatment response, pathology of personality organization has been shown to be a predictor of dropping out of treatment. Despite the significant association between personality organization difficulties and DSM diagnoses, treatment dropout among dual-diagnosis patients can be predicted more effectively based on level of personality organization than on personality disorder diagnoses.[27] Other results show that early dropping out from inpatient psychotherapy is predicted by the most severe and least severe levels of personality organization.[28]

Treatment studies have demonstrated that psychotherapy can lead to improvement in personality organization. Doering et al.[29] conducted a random clinical trial (RCT) comparing the efficacy of outpatient transference-focused psychotherapy in treatment by experienced community psychotherapists with a sample of BPD patients. After one year of psychotherapy, significant changes were found at the level of personality organization. Similarly, studies in patients with personality disorders and affective disorders showed improvements of personality organization after multimodal, psychodynamic, hospitalization-based treatment (with a maximum duration of 12 months[30] and a typical duration of one to three months[31]).

In sum, as predicted by the object relations model, empirical research demonstrates the relation of personality organization to both severity of pathology and treatment response, supporting the validity of the object relations model of personality disorders.

Clinical Illustrations of Levels of Personality Organization

In this section, we present illustrations of pathology of personality functioning organized at a normal, neurotic, high, middle, and low BPO. For comparison, we also present an illustration of the normal personality, as well as of the psychotic level of personality organization. These clinical vignettes should familiarize the reader with prototypical presentations of the different levels of personality organization.

Normal Personality Organization

A 28-year-old single, elementary school teacher, Ms. Y, is seen in consultation one month after the death of her mother, because she is experiencing acute distress. Ms. Y and her mother, a single parent, had sustained a close and loving relationship into Ms. Y's adulthood. When her mother was diagnosed with pancreatic cancer and passed away within months, Ms. Y had been devastated. Now, a month after the funeral, Ms. Y described painful feelings of loss and sadness that she could not get past, saying, "The world will never be the same." She spoke of finding herself unpredictably bursting into tears in the grocery store, in the street, with friends, and when alone. She told the interviewer that she comforted herself with memories of happy times spent with her mother over the years and of the deep love and friendship that they had maintained. Ms. Y acknowledged that she appreciated the efforts of her long-term boyfriend to provide support, but at the same time felt badly for him because "nothing can touch the ache inside of me."

Ms. Y acknowledged that this was the first time she had "hit a roadblock"; until this point, she had responded to adversity with flexible adaptation and coping, turning to her relationships, teaching, and many hobbies and interests to help her get through the rough patches. Throughout her mourning, she had continued to function in her job as a teacher, describing her work as both challenging and fulfilling, and she denied neurovegetative symptoms of depression.

Ms. Y was attractive and charming despite her grief. She described an intimate and sexually satisfying relationship with her boyfriend and expressed gratitude for the support she had received from her close group of friends who, she felt, "are always there for me." She saw herself as an overall optimistic and level-headed person. She had no difficulty asserting herself, enjoyed competitive sports, and noted that she rarely experienced anger. She described feelings of demoralization about her inability to get past her current sadness and worried that this was a sign of weakness. At the same time, she shared with the consultant that just the act of calling to make the appointment for an evaluation had begun to lift her spirits.

Identity: Fully Consolidated

Ms. Y's sense of herself and of significant others is realistic, stable, and nuanced. Even through her grief, she is able to clearly see her own strengths and limitations as well as those of her loved ones, and she demonstrates a capacity to realistically assess and to empathize with her boyfriend as he has unsuccessfully tried to cheer her up. She has been able to identify and pursue long-term goals for herself, both professional and personal, with plans to marry and start a family. She is deeply invested in her professional life, deriving great pleasure from her work with young children and from her hobbies of cooking and crafts.

Quality of Object Relations: Deep and Mutual with a Capacity for Concern

Ms. Y's object relations are marked by depth, concern, and a capacity to care about the needs of others, independent of the needs of herself. Interpersonally, she has maintained a mutually gratifying and emotionally caring relationship with her boyfriend, and she describes their sexual life as pleasurable, intimate, and fun. She has maintained close and caring, long-term friendships with both women and men from various phases of her life; when Ms. Y was in need, her friends rallied around her. She made it clear how much their support has meant to her in the face of her mother's illness and passing, as well as a shared understanding within the group that she would do the same for any of them.

Defensive Functioning: Higher Level; Mature and Repression-based

Ms. Y's stable and historically flexible emotional and interpersonal functioning reflect the impact of mature defenses with an admixture of repression-based defenses (see Box 2.1). The impact of repression-based defenses is most apparent in a tendency to be unaware of angry feelings in herself or in others. Her current state of grief did not strike the interviewer as an expression of defensive rigidity, but rather as part of a normal, albeit intense, mourning process.

Moral Values: Fully Internalized and Flexible

Ms. Y is honest, loyal, and conscientious. Her moral values are consistent, fully integrated into her sense of self, and not excessively rigid ("Sometimes I have to give myself a break and just kick back!"). She takes pleasure in "doing the right thing" and deeply values being part of a caring community.

Aggression: Well-integrated and Well-modulated, with Mild Inhibition

Ms. Y avails herself of healthy and adaptive expressions of aggression in her enjoyment of competitive sports. She has a self-assertive, "can-do" personal style. Angry feelings are often repressed, but this does not seem to have adversely impacted her functioning or well-being in any significant way.

Case Formulation

Ms. Y illustrates many of the features of the normal personality. Her sense of self and her sense of others are stable and realistic, complex, and multifaceted; throughout her life, she has been able to identify and pursue long-term goals; she is deeply invested in her relationships, career, and personal interests. She is able to sustain a mutually satisfying sexual and intimate relationship with her boyfriend. Although currently in mourning, she enjoys a full range of affects, with a predominance of positive affect states. Her moral functioning is fully internalized and flexible, although she is somewhat inhibited in the expression of aggression. Overall she is a resilient and optimistic person, likely to readily respond to supportive interventions to facilitate her mourning.

Neurotic Personality Organization

Mr. N is a 35-year-old married lawyer with two young children. He was seen in consultation with complaints of anxiety, "problems at work," and problems with self-esteem. Mr. N described his work as a junior partner at a competitive law firm as challenging, engaging, and intellectually fulfilling. Nevertheless, he often felt anxious and inadequate in the workplace, and had received feedback that a tendency to be "too detail oriented" was slowing his advancement in the firm.

In the interview, Mr. N was extremely reserved but conveyed a deeply felt attachment to his wife and young children, providing a lively, three-dimensional picture of his loved ones. He understood that his wife, and to some degree his children as well, experienced him as emotionally distant, and although deeply troubled by this, he found himself unable to change his behavior. Although free of sexual symptoms, he reported limited sexual interest. He had a small group of close friends dating back to high school and college, but by his own account was not especially social. After hearing Mr. N's story, the consultant found himself impressed by Mr. N's conscientiousness and by his motivation for treatment.

Identity: Fully Consolidated

Mr. N's sense of himself and of significant others is realistic, stable, and nuanced, accommodating both desirable (conscientious, loyal, reliable) and less desirable (emotionally constricted and distant) qualities. He demonstrated a capacity to realistically assess and to empathize with the experience of his loved ones. He has been able to identify and pursue long-term goals and is deeply invested in both his professional and personal life.

Quality of Object Relations: Mild Impairment

Mr. N's object relations are marked by depth, concern, and reciprocity, despite the reserve and emotional distancing that characterize his interpersonal relations. He has been able to maintain a stable marriage and long-term friendships characterized by depth and stability. He demonstrates a fully developed capacity to appreciate the needs of others independent of his own needs.

Defensive Functioning: Repression Based

Mr. N's stable but rigid emotional and interpersonal functioning reflect the impact of repression-based defenses. In particular, he relies heavily on isolation of affect. There is no evidence of contradictory experiences of self and other, frank denial of painful realities, or extreme affect states that would point to splitting-based defenses.

Aggression: Well-integrated, Largely Repressed, with Rigidity

Mr. N reports that, although he is able to be assertive, he rarely gets angry, and instead tends to become cold or to withdraw at times when he might be expected to experience anger.

Moral Values: No Impairment

Mr. N is honest, conscientious, and prides himself on being highly ethical in his professional and personal life. Moral values are internalized and consistent. He demonstrates some moral rigidity, expressed as excessive self-criticism when he does not live up to his own high internal standards.

Case Formulation

Mr. N illustrates many core features of neurotic personality organization with an obsessive-compulsive personality style. He benefits from a stable and realistic sense of self and others and is able to pursue and invest in long-term goals. Although emotionally constricted, he has a capacity for in-depth object relations and is able to empathize with the internal experience of his loved ones. Moral functioning is fully internalized although somewhat rigid, and he is inhibited in the expression of aggression and, to some degree, of sexuality as well. Although we would need to work with Mr. N over time to more fully understand his dynamics, it is likely that his low self-esteem and perfectionism reflect conflicts in relation to the expression of aggression ("If I am aggressive, I am bad, undeserving, inferior"), which is rigidly repressed. His emotional constriction can be understood in terms of more global anxieties about potentially "losing control of strong emotions."

High Borderline Personality Organization

Ms. H, a 45-year-old divorced nurse practitioner (NP) without children, was seen in consultation for her chronically depressed mood. She did not endorse tearfulness or neurovegetative symptoms of depression, but described a lifelong history of self-criticism, feelings of inferiority, and inadequacy: "I see myself as a waste of space. I don't live up to my potential, but maybe I have no potential."

At the same time, in her professional life, Ms. H was regarded as an effective, compassionate, and dedicated clinician. When confronted with the discrepancy between how she was viewed at work and how little she thought of herself, Ms. H was quietly dismissive, explaining that she was able to derive only limited pride or support of her self-esteem from her work, and was instead preoccupied ("tormented") by a failed aspiration, abandoned decades earlier, to become a physician.

Ms. H described a series of failed one- to three-year relationships with men whom she initially loved and felt passionate toward, but whom she ultimately found disappointing. The interviewer noted that Ms. H's descriptions of the men in her life were somewhat superficial, two-dimensional, self-referential, and vague ("a really good boyfriend, smart, good-looking" or "kind of a loser, in the end not much to offer"). In contrast, she maintained positive, mutually satisfying relationships with her work colleagues, both men and women, and had a small circle of long-standing female friends.

Despite her self-deprecation, Ms. H was appealing and engaging. The consultant found it easy to imagine that she was an asset to her clinical team, and also that she did not have difficulty attracting interest from men.

Identity: Moderate Identity Disturbance

Ms. H's sense of herself is consistently (negatively) distorted, and her view of the men in her life is somewhat superficial and unstable across time (initially idealized and then devalued). In contrast, in less conflictual areas of functioning, with her patients and friends, Ms. H can be empathic, capable of astutely inferring and responding to others' emotional needs. Although she has been able to pursue long-term goals in her profession, her capacity to derive a sense of satisfaction from her work is compromised; she is unable to fully invest in her identity as an NP or to feel proud of her accomplishments.

Quality of Object Relations: Moderate Impairment

Ms. H has moderate pathology of object relations, as demonstrated by a failure of intimacy and difficulty with dependence. Ms. H's friendships are stable if somewhat distant, and she demonstrates a capacity for concern outside of areas of conflict (intimacy and dependency). Her intimate relationships with men, in contrast, are marked by superficiality; she demonstrates little interest in or empathy for the experience of her partners as they move from an idealized to a devalued position in her eyes.

Defensive Functioning: Repression-based and Splitting-based Defenses

Ms. B's reliance on splitting-based defenses is most evident in her intimate relations, which are organized in relation to idealization and devaluation, supported by rationalization and denial. She demonstrates repression-based and higher-level defenses, including intellectualization, reaction formation, anticipation, and humor in her professional life, where she functions smoothly and consistently.

Aggression: Moderate Pathology

We see evidence of pathology in the management of aggression in Ms. H's vicious self-depreciation and her ultimately cool, at times callous treatment of her partners.

Moral Values: Mild Impairment

Ms. H is honest and conscientious in her work and friendships, and she holds herself to high standards of comport in these domains. In her relationships with men, she lets herself "off the hook," to some degree, for her callous rejections of former partners.

Case Formulation

Ms. H illustrates many core features of high BPO, reflecting both the relative strengths and vulnerabilities of individuals organized at this level. She presents with prominent narcissistic traits, although she does not meet criteria for DSM-5 narcissistic personality disorder. Although able to successfully pursue a career, her capacity to emotionally invest in and obtain satisfaction from her accomplishments is limited to some degree. In contrast to what we would expect to see in more severe pathology, Ms. H has a capacity for empathy and is able to maintain stable, if somewhat superficial, relationships with friends and colleagues. However, conflicts in intimacy and an inability to rely on others interfere with her functioning in her romantic life; she idealizes her partners to defend against underlying hostility and mistrust, ending the relationship when these defenses fail. Idealization and devaluation in relation to her sense of self lead to excessively high aspirations that cannot be met, coupled with devaluation of her accomplishments, ultimately leading to a poor self-image. There are no antisocial features, and pathology of aggression is largely limited to attacks on the self and devaluation of her partners.

Middle Borderline Personality Organization: Moderate Impairment

Ms. B, a 28-year-old, single, part-time receptionist presented with a chief complaint of "problems in my love life." Ms. B described how, upon meeting a man, she would feel that "This is the one who will solve all my problems," only to find herself within weeks enraged and frustrated. She explained that when her feelings toward a boyfriend changed, she found it difficult to control her anger with him; on one occasion, she had verbally assaulted and physically threatened a man whom she had been dating, to the point that he called the police (although she had no history of actual physical assaults). On other occasions, she had threatened to harm herself when men did not behave toward her as she felt they should.

Ms. B had few friends, "more acquaintances, actually," who came and went. She had been estranged from her parents since they discovered she had on one occasion taken "just 20 dollars" from her mother's purse ("I was desperate"). When the interviewer asked if Ms. B could empathize with her parents' feelings, Ms. B responded, "I know it looks bad, but you'd think they could give me a break!" She otherwise denied a history of stealing or of any other illegal activity, although she routinely spent time on the job doing online shopping and making social calls, and she frequently called in sick. She justified these behaviors on the basis of the boring and routine nature of her work. She had held a series of short-lived jobs, which she described as dreary, boring, and pointless, although she could not think of any other job that she would like to do.

Ms. B described feeling unhappy and resentful much of the time; she enjoyed shopping but otherwise had few interests. She felt her life was "going nowhere," and she was plagued by chronic feelings of emptiness. The consultant found himself feeling burdened by the profound and pervasive emptiness that characterized Ms. B's narrative and experience, along with the chaotic level of her functioning in multiple domains.

Identity: Extreme Identity Pathology

The superficiality and instability of Ms. B's sense of self and others is apparent in her grossly unstable experience of her partners and her corresponding sense of self (from loved, cared for, and fortunate to mistreated, neglected, and exploited). When asked for a self-description, she responded, "How can I describe myself when I have no idea who I am?" Other stigmata of identity pathology included feelings of emptiness, aimlessness, and an inability to pursue long-term goals or to invest in or derive satisfaction from pursuits or relationships.

Quality of Object Relations: Severe Pathology

Ms. B has few relationships, and those she does have are superficial, short-lived, and unstable, organized entirely around her own emotional needs, with no capacity for empathy.

Defensive Style: Splitting-based

Ms. B relies predominantly on splitting-based defenses, including idealization/devaluation, the corollary of her unstable and polarized experience of self and others.

Aggression: Severe Pathology

Ms. B presents with markers of poorly integrated and poorly regulated aggression, expressed as temper tantrums, verbal outbursts, and threats of assault and self-injury.

Moral Values: Moderate Pathology

Ms. B demonstrates significant deficits in moral functioning, illustrated by the antisocial behavior of taking money from her mother and exploiting her employers, for which she demonstrates no guilt or remorse. She has not been engaged in illegal activity nor has she been in trouble with the law.

Case Formulation

Ms. B illustrates many core features of the middle Borderline Personality Organization, which reflects a severe personality disorder. Dynamically, Ms. B struggles with poorly integrated and poorly modulated aggression, splitting-based defenses, and identity pathology manifested in an incapacity to invest in her career, relationships, or personal interests, as well as painful feelings of emptiness, aimlessness, and meaninglessness. She has no capacity for dependency or intimacy; superficial and fragile idealization of others quickly gives way to underlying rage and paranoia, expressed in hateful temper outbursts and efforts to control significant others in a hostile way.

While she demonstrates significant pathology of moral functioning, Ms. B's overall pathology is not as extreme as that seen in low BPO. Her antisocial traits are limited, and she is able to empathize with moral standards ("I know it looks bad, but . . . ") even while failing to change her behavior. Similarly, while aggressive outbursts and pathology of object relations are indicative of severe pathology, they do not reach the extreme level of physical assault, ruthless exploitation, or systematic intimidation characteristic of individuals functioning at a low BPO. Diagnostically, she has identity disturbance, affective instability, unstable relationships, anger outbursts, and chronic emptiness. Ms. B meets criteria for BPD with mild antisocial features.

Low Borderline Personality Organization

Mr. L, a 38-year-old married, unemployed, self-described "businessman," without children, was seen in consultation requesting stimulants "for my ADHD." Mr. L explained that he has challenges with time management, which had made it difficult for him to excel in his work. He had benefited from stimulants in the past.

As the interview proceeded, it emerged that since graduating from college, Mr. L had been let go from a series of jobs due to his hostile and combative behavior. He also has a history of misusing expense accounts in his jobs, as well as a criminal record for attempting to steal office equipment from a previous employer. Most recently, he was fired after physically threatening a coworker and then pushing him against a copy machine; an act he described as "fully justified under the circumstances." Mr. L explained that his coworkers were not showing him the kind of deference and respect he deserved based on his greater level of experience and intelligence.

Mr. L had lost sexual interest in his wife early in their marriage. He routinely visited prostitutes, engaging in sadomasochistic practices involving threatening and humiliating his partners, without penetration. He explained that he stayed in his marriage because his wife owned the apartment they lived in, and he enjoyed living off her income.

In the interview, although he was initially smooth-talking, his underlying hostility and contempt soon became overt, as did his derisive, challenging attitude toward the interviewer. Toward the end of the evaluation, the interviewer explained that he would need to see the results of formal testing before prescribing a stimulant, but in the interim they could discuss other treatment options for ADHD. At that point, Mr. L abruptly stood up and cursed at the interviewer for having deceived him and wasted his time. He announced, "There's no way you'll see a dime from me!" and stormed out of the office. The interviewer was left feeling shaken but also disdainful of Mr. L.

Identity: Severe Identity Pathology

Mr. L exhibited a superficial and grossly distorted, albeit stable grandiose sense of himself as being above the rules. His experience of others was also markedly superficial, vague, caricature-like, and grossly devalued. He was able to describe his wife in only the most superficial and derisive terms, saying she was "tedious" and "no longer attractive." He demonstrated an inability to pursue long-term goals or to invest in or derive satisfaction from any pursuits or relationships.

Quality of Object Relations: Extreme Pathology

Mr. L's only personal contacts are his wife and the prostitutes whom he solicits; these interactions are based on frank exploitation and sadistic gratification. He demonstrates a callous disregard for the needs of others, with no capacity for empathy.

Defensive Functioning: Splitting-based

Mr. L relies on splitting-based defenses–splitting proper, devaluation, and omnipotent control—with no capacity for idealization and gross denial of any realities that might confront his grandiosity.

Aggression: Extreme Pathology

Mr. L shows poorly modulated expression of poorly integrated aggression, expressed in chronic and hostile contempt for others, sadism, verbal outbursts, and physical assault.

Moral Values: Extreme Impairment

Mr. L evidences significant antisocial features. He has a criminal record for theft and has engaged in absenteeism, assault, exploitation, and cruelty, all with no remorse. He lies freely and demonstrates callous disregard for the needs or safety of others.

Case Formulation

Mr. L illustrates the core features of low BPO, the most extreme pathology within the spectrum of severe personality disorders. Poorly integrated ("primitive") and poorly modulated aggression in the setting of extreme pathology of object relations and deficits in moral functioning are the hallmark of low BPO. Mr. L's personality functioning and psychological life are organized largely in relation to expressions of aggression in the form of violent outbursts and rage, cruelty, sadism, hatred, and devaluation. He demonstrates no capacity for idealization—not even the fragile idealization seen with Ms. B, for example. His positive affects are essentially absent. Ruthless and pleasurable exploitation and intimidation of others and ego-syntonic sadism are his dominant sources of gratification; his sexual activity is of interest only if it provides sadistic pleasure. Typical ethical standards are not only disregarded, but even viewed with contempt. His engagement in antisocial behavior, including lawlessness, his consistently irresponsible and dishonest behavior, irritability, and global and callous lack of concern for others and lack of remorse, meets the diagnostic criteria for antisocial personality disorder.

Personality Disorders in DSM-5 and the Alternative Model of Personality Disorders

After much deliberation, the DSM-5 Personality Disorders Work Group decided to retain the categorical DSM-IV TR[32(pp.761-781)] definition and classification of personality disorders in Section II of the DSM-5, while introducing an alternative approach to personality disorders in Section III.[3(pp. 761-781)] The AMPD[3] represents a paradigm shift within the DSM approach to these disorders, introducing significant convergence with the object relations model. With the AMPD, for the first time, the DSM-5 does the following: (1) embraces a dimensional approach (in contrast to a categorical one) to personality disorders; (2) defines the essential nature of personality pathology in terms of personality *functioning*, in contrast to traits and symptoms; and (3) privileges the dimension of severity.

The AMPD introduces the following as general criteria for personality disorder: (1) significant impairments in self-functioning and interpersonal functioning (Criterion A); in conjunction with (2) the presence of one or more pathological personality traits (Criterion B). Self-functioning is conceptualized in terms of identity and self-direction; interpersonal functioning is conceptualized in terms of capacity for empathy and intimacy. Impairment in self and interpersonal functioning is classified dimensionally according to severity of impairment, from mild, or subsyndromal, through extreme, using the Level of Personality Functioning Scale (LPFS)[3(pp. 775-778)]; see Table 2.2, p. 52.

While the development of the object relations model[6,7] predated introduction of the AMPD by several decades, there is considerable overlap between the two models. The AMPD is in many ways compatible with the object relations model of personality pathology (see Table 2.2, p. 52). Both models embrace a dimensional approach, in contrast to a categorical one, to personality disorder diagnosis; identify self and interpersonal functioning as core features of healthy and pathological personality functioning; and privilege severity of impairment in the classification of personality pathology across the range of personality disorder presentation.

While the overlap between the object relations model and the AMPD model is significant, and it is possible to move between AMPD and object relations classifications with relative ease, there are also important distinctions between the two models, which are highly relevant to clinical work. Whereas both models focus on self and interpersonal functioning as essential features of personality pathology, the object relations model is unique in also identifying defensive operations, moral functioning, and management of aggression as central domains of personality functioning. In contrast, the AMPD characterizes moral functioning and aggression as traits, rather than as domains of functioning central to personality disorder, while omitting consideration of defenses entirely.

Table 2.2 Alternative Model of Personality Disorder and Level of Personality Functioning Scale Compared to ORT Levels of Personality Organization*

	AMPD LPFS Level 1	AMPD LPFS Level 2	AMPD LPFS Level 3	AMPD LPFS Level 4
Self-Functioning (Identity and self-direction)	Some difficulty with self-esteem; excessively focused on or conflicted about goals	Vulnerable self-esteem; goals are often a means of gaining others' approval	Weak sense of autonomy and agency; difficulty establishing or achieving personal goals	Weak or distorted self-image; unrealistic or incoherent personal goals
Interpersonal Functioning (Empathy and intimacy)	Inconsistent in perceiving impact on others; cooperation with others is conflicted	Excessively self-referential; generally unaware of effect of own behavior on others; cooperates with others for personal gain	Limited ability to understand others; significant impairment in capacity for positive and enduring connections with others	Pronounced inability to consider or understand others; relations with others limited by profound disinterest or expectation of harm
Comparable Level of Personality Organization*	Neurotic Personality Organization	High Borderline Personality Organization	Middle Borderline Personality Organization	Low Borderline Personality Organization

*Both ORT and AMPD describe self and interpersonal functioning as central domains of personality. ORT identifies defensive operations, moral functioning, and management of aggression as three additional domains of personality functioning. AMPD characterizes moral functioning and aggression as traits, without consideration of defenses.
Key

ORT = Object Relations Theory

AMPD = Alternative Model of Personality Disorder[3(pp. 761–781)]

LPFS = Level of Personality Functioning Scale[3(pp. 761–781)]

Levels of Personality Organization[5–8]

The neglect of defenses in the AMPD model reflects intention on the part of the DSM-5 work group to develop a model that is empirically based, purely descriptive, and purposefully a-theoretical. The object relations model, in contrast, is embedded in an overarching, psychodynamic theory of personality functioning emerging from decades of experience in intensive clinical work with patients with personality disorders;[5,6] this model attends not only to descriptive features, but also to the underlying structural and dynamic features that support and organize those descriptive features. Within the framework of object relations theory, defenses provide a conceptual model for dynamic factors that sustain personality pathology and interfere with identity consolidation. Furthermore, in this approach, the resolution of splitting to support identity integration organizes clinical objectives in the treatment of personality disorders.[5,33]

In its attention to moral functioning, the object relations model recognizes that varying degrees of deficits in moral functioning are involved not only in the antisocial personality disorder, but to a greater or lesser degree in all severe personality disorders; in particular, moral deficits are seen in patients presenting with borderline and narcissistic personality disorders and with malignant narcissism. As moral functioning deteriorates, one moves from high, to middle, to low BPO; severe pathology of moral functioning is a hallmark of low BPO, the most extreme disorders in the BPO spectrum. Similarly, pathological aggression, poorly integrated and poorly modulated, is viewed as central to personality functioning in the personality disorders, and increasingly so in the more severe range of the spectrum.

In sum, while compatible with the AMPD, the object relations model emphasizes the careful assessment of both moral functioning and aggression, alongside identity and object relations. This comprehensive assessment provides a highly specific and nuanced determination of the severity of pathology as it relates to prognosis, treatment planning, and treatment course, while enabling clinicians to anticipate problems (e.g., deception and withholding, destructive acting out) likely to emerge in the treatment of patients with severe to extreme personality pathology.[6]

Assessment of Levels of Personality Organization

Determination of the patient's level of personality organization is essential to guiding differential treatment planning.[5] As part of the detailed description of an object relations approach to personality pathology, Kernberg[7] developed the Structural Interview, a systematic but flexible clinical interview designed to evaluate not only the patient's symptoms and areas of difficulty, but also the level of personality organization. While obtaining necessary information about symptoms and current functioning, the Structural Interviewer focuses attention on areas of conflict that become activated in the exchange between therapist and patient. This process enables real-time observation and exploration of the patient's dominant defenses and associated object relations as part of the assessment process. (For an in-depth description of the Structural Interview, review Kernberg.[34])

Given the dependence of the Structural Interviewer on interviewing skills and clinical judgment, it can be difficult to reliably obtain consistency among different interviewers in terms of focus and diagnostic conclusions. This potential shortcoming led to the construction of the STIPO[14] and its shorter version, the STIPO-R.[15] These are semi-structured instruments that assess personality organization. These interviews provide standard questions, follow-up probes, and scoring guidelines to ensure reliability in structural assessment. For clinicians, the STIPO and STIPO-R offer a useful guide to the evaluation of personality organization; the interview can be incorporated into a standard clinical evaluation, where it is generally well received by patients. In a research setting, the STIPO and STIPO-R can be used to provide a reliable assessment of personality organization and change during treatment.

The STIPO-R systematically assesses five domains of functioning: (1) identity (including capacity to invest in work and studies, sense of self, sense of others); (2) object relations (interpersonal relations, intimate relations, internal working model of relationships); (3) defenses (splitting-based and higher level); (4) aggression (self-directed and other-directed); and (5) moral values. Each of these key domains involves both observable behavior and internal mental attitudes and complex perceptions and biases. The STIPO and STIPO-R can be downloaded at ISTFP.org

Levels of Personality Organization and
Treatment Planning

Diagnosis of level of personality organization has direct and reliable implications for treatment planning.[5,6] Individuals functioning at a neurotic level of personality organization have a very favorable prognosis and can benefit from relatively unstructured treatments. These patients typically do not have difficulty establishing and maintaining a therapeutic alliance, and transference distortions tend to be slow in developing, consistent, and subtle. In contrast, individuals organized at a borderline level, particularly those in the low borderline spectrum, require a highly structured treatment setting. These individuals have great difficulty establishing and maintaining a therapeutic alliance; transference distortions develop rapidly and are highly affectively charged and extreme, often leading to disruption of the treatment.

For patients functioning at a neurotic level, psychodynamic treatment is organized around the goal of reducing rigidity in personality functioning.[35] For patients at a borderline level of organization, the treatment goal is ameliorating identity diffusion and promoting normal identity consolidation.[5,33] More progress toward this goal is expected with high and middle BPO in comparison to low BPO. Progress toward these goals will be manifest in changes in the transference relationship between patient and therapist and in improved relationships with friends, intimates, and work associates. The technical approach is to explore the patient's internal object relations as they are activated in interpersonal relationships with significant others and with the clinician.[5]

Conclusion

In this chapter, we have presented the object relations model of personality disorders. Emerging from decades of clinical experience and convergent with the DSM-5 AMPD and with current empirical developments in the study of personality functioning and personality disorders, the object relations model of personality disorders provides clinicians with an important guide to understanding, evaluating, and classifying personality pathology.

The object relations model provides a three-faceted approach to personality pathology involving a theoretical orientation (object relations theory), a nosology (levels of personality organization), and methods of assessment. Consistent with the DSM-5 AMPD, the nosology of object relations theory emphasizes the primary role of pathology of self and interpersonal functioning in patient assessment and treatment planning, while at the same time retaining a role for identification of prototypical personality disorder presentations. Most important, as the detailed descriptions of individuals at different levels of personality organization in this chapter illustrate, the object relations approach is both nuanced and clinically near, guiding clinicians in determining patient prognosis and treatment planning and in anticipating clinical process.[36] See Box 2.2, p. 55 for relevant resources on personality structure and BPD.

Conflict of Interest/Disclosure: The authors of this chapter have no financial conflicts and nothing to disclose.

Box 2.2   Resources

- International Society of Transference-Focused Psychotherapy. www.ISTFP. org

  This website provides reader-friendly descriptions of personality pathology, including the severe form in BPD, that is helpful to the consumers of psychiatric treatment. This site also provides information helpful to the professional mental health worker, including a copy of the assessment instrument, the STIPO-R, referred to in this chapter.
- Borderline Disorder. www.BorderlineDisorders.com

  Provides information on the description and treatment of personality disorders.

References

1. *Diagnostic and Statistical Manual of Mental Disorders: DSM-III.* Washington, DC: American Psychiatric Publishing; 1980.

2. Wright AG, Zimmermann J. At the nexus of science and practice: answering basic clinical questions in personality disorder assessment and diagnosis with quantitative modeling techniques. In: Huprich SK, ed. *Personality Disorders: Toward Theoretical and Empirical Integration in Diagnosis and Assessment.* Washington, DC: American Psychological Association; 2015:109–144.

3. *Diagnostic and Statistical Manual of Mental Disorders: DSM-5.* Washington, DC: American Psychiatric Publishing; 2013.

4. Conway CC, Hammen C, Brennan PA. Optimizing prediction of psychosocial and clinical outcomes with a transdiagnostic model of personality disorder. *J Pers Disord.* 2016;30(4):545–566.

5. Caligor E, Kernberg OF, Clarkin JF, Yeomans FE. *Psychodynamic Therapy for Personality Pathology: Treating Self and Interpersonal Functioning.* Washington, DC: American Psychiatric Association Publishing; 2018.

6. Kernberg OF, Caligor E. A psychodynamic theory of personality disorders. In: Lenzenweger MF, Clarkin JF, eds. *Major Theories of Personality Disorder.* 2 ed. New York, NY: Guilford Press; 2005:114–156.

7. Kernberg OF. *Severe Personality Disorders: Psychotherapeutic Strategies.* New Haven, CT: Yale University Press; 1984.

8. Kernberg OF. Psychotic personality structure. *Psychodyn Psychiatry.* 2019;47(4):353–372.

9. Bateman A. *Mentalization-based Treatment for Borderline Personality Disorder: A Practical Guide.* Oxford, UK: Oxford University Press; 2006.

10. Vaillant GE. *The Wisdom of the Ego.* Cambridge, MA: Harvard University Press; 1995.

11. Vaillant GE. Ego mechanisms of defense and personality psychopathology. *J Abnorm Psychol.* 1994;103(1):44.

12. Biberdzic M, Ensink K, Normandin L, Clarkin JF. Psychometric properties of the inventory of personality organization for adolescents. *Adolesc Psychiatry.* 2017;7(2):127–151.

13. Lenzenweger MF, Clarkin JF, Kernberg OF, Foelsch PA. The Inventory of Personality Organization: psychometric properties, factorial composition, and criterion relations with affect, aggressive dyscontrol, psychosis proneness, and self-domains in a nonclinical sample. *Psychol Assess.* 2001;13(4):577.

14. Clarkin JF, Caligor E, Stern B, Kernberg OF. Structured Interview of Personality Organization (STIPO). Weill Medical College of Cornell University. Posted 2007. http://www.borderline-disorders.com/assets/Structured-Interview-of-Personality-Organization.pdf.

15. Clarkin JF, Caligor E, Stern BL, Kernberg OF. Structured Interview for Personality Organization-Revised (STIPO-R). Weill Medical College of Cornell University. Posted 2016. http://www.borderlinedisorders.com/assets/STIPO-R.pdf.

16. Doering S, Burgmer M, Heuft G, et al. Reliability and validity of the German version of the Structured Interview of Personality Organization (STIPO). *BMC Psychiatry.* 2013;13(1):210.

17. Fischer-Kern M, Kapusta ND, Doering S, Hörz S, Mikutta C, Aigner M. The relationship between personality organization and psychiatric classification in chronic pain patients. *Psychopathology.* 2011;44(1):21–26.

18. Fuchshuber J, Hiebler-Ragger M, Kresse A, Kapfhammer H-P, Unterrainer HF. Depressive symptoms and addictive behaviors in young adults after childhood trauma: the mediating role of personality organization and despair. *Front Psychiatry.* 2018;9:318.

19. De Meulemeester C, Lowyck B, Vermote R, Verhaest Y, Luyten P. Mentalizing and interpersonal problems in borderline personality disorder: the mediating role of identity diffusion. *Psychiatry Res.* 2017;258:141–144.

20. Prunas A, Bernorio R. Dimensions of personality organization and sexual life in a community sample of women. *J Sex Marital Ther.* 2016;42(2):158–164.

21. Prunas A, Di Pierro R, Bernorio R. The relationship between personality organization and sexual life in a community sample of men. *Psychoanal Psychother.* 2016;30(4):345–358.

22. Uji M, Nagata T, Kitamura T. The influence of borderline personality organization on trait depressive affects and the generation of negative life events. *Trauma Stress Disor Treat.* 2013;4:2.

23. Kampe L, Zimmermann J, Bender D, et al. Comparison of the structured DSM–5 clinical interview for the Level of Personality Functioning Scale with the Structured Interview of Personality Organization. *J Pers Assess.* 2018;100(6):642–649.

24. Fontana A, De Panfilis C, Casini E, Preti E, Richetin J, Ammaniti M. Rejection sensitivity and psychopathology symptoms in early adolescence: the moderating role of personality organization. *J Adolesc.* 2018;67:45–54.

25. Ammaniti M, Fontana A, Clarkin A, Clarkin JF, Nicolais G, Kernberg OF. Assessment of adolescent personality disorders through the interview of personality organization processes in adolescence (IPOP-A): clinical and theoretical implications. *Adolesc Psychiatry.* 2012;2(1):36–45.

26. Ensink K, Rousseau Me, Biberdzic M, Bégin M, Normandin L. Reflective functioning and personality organization: associations with negative maternal behaviors. *Infant Ment Health J.* 2017;38(3):351–362.

27. Preti E, Rottoli C, Dainese S, Di Pierro R, Rancati F, Madeddu F. Personality structure features associated with early dropout in patients with substance-related disorders and comorbid personality disorders. *Int J Ment Health Addiction.* 2015;13(4):536–547.

28. Ingenhoven TJ, Duivenvoorden HJ, Passchier J, van den Brink W. Treatment duration and premature termination of psychotherapy in personality disorders: predictive performance of psychodynamic personality functioning. *J Psychiatr Pract.* 2012;18(3):172–186.

29. Doering S, Horz S, Rentrop M, et al. Transference-focused psychotherapy v. treatment by community psychotherapists for borderline personality disorder: randomised controlled trial. *Br J Psychiatry.* 2010;196(5):389–395.

30. Vermote R, Lowyck B, Luyten P, et al. Patterns of inner change and their relation with patient characteristics and outcome in a psychoanalytic hospitalization-based treatment for personality disordered patients. *Clin Psychol Psychother.* 2011;18(4):303–313.

31. Kraus B, Dammann G, Rudaz M, Sammet I, Jeggle D, Grimmer B. Changes in the level of personality functioning in inpatient psychotherapy. *Psychother Res.* 2020: 31:117–131.

32. *Diagnostic and Statistical Manual of Mental Disorders:DSM-IV-TR.* Washington, DC: American Psychiatric Publishing; 2000.

33. Yeomans FE, Clarkin JF, Kernberg OF. *Transference-focused Psychotherapy for Borderline Personality Disorder: A Clinical Guide.* Washington, DC: American Psychiatric Publishing; 2015.

34. Kernberg OF. Structural interviewing. *Psychiatr Clin North Am.* 1981;4(1):169–195.

35. Caligor E, Kernberg OF, Clarkin JF. *Handbook of Dynamic Psychotherapy for Higher Level Personality Pathology.* Arlington, VA: American Psychiatric Publishing; 2007.

36. Bender DS, Morey LC, Skodol AE. Toward a model for assessing level of personality functioning in DSM–5, part I: a review of theory and methods. *J Pers Assess.* 2011;93(4):332–346.

3

Pathways Between Psychological Trauma and the Development of Personality Disorders

Valerie Rosen, Gregory Fonzo, Emily Rosen, and Alex Preston

Key Points

- Trauma in childhood and early adulthood is unfortunately quite prevalent.
- Trauma at an early age may leave long-lasting psychological and biological deficits.
- Trauma often paves the road for the development of personality disorders; multifactorial components exist for this pathway.
- Research with magnetic resonance imaging (MRI) demonstrates how trauma and biological vulnerabilities impart neuroanatomical changes that play a role in emerging character symptomatology.

Introduction

What are little boys made of
What are little boys made of
Snips & snails & puppy dogs tails
And such are little boys made of.

What are little girls made of
What are little girls made of
Sugar & spice & all things nice
And such are little girls made of.[1]

This old English nursey rhyme conjures up images of rosy cheeked, playful children. Regrettably, in today's world, the innocence of childhood is stolen from too many youth at the hands of abusers. The prevalence rate of child abuse and maltreatment today is alarming. The World Health Organization reports disturbing statistics: one in four adults were physically abused as children; one in five girls are sexually abused at least once in their life; and one out of two children suffered violence in the past year.[2] According to the Attorney General of Texas, at any one time in the state of Texas, there are 79,000 victims of youth domestic sex trafficking: Yes, you read it correctly, 79,000![3] New York and California report even larger numbers.

The nursery rhyme describes the "ingredients" that make up boys and girls. Clinical experience informs us that a multitude of factors are at play when a personality disorder is born. The recipe consists of genetics, epigenetic vulnerability, temperament, parent–child fit, and environmental stressors including childhood abuse. In addition to the typical consequences of trauma, early-life trauma carries with it the ability to damage or delay neurodevelopment in ways that can have long-lasting deleterious effects. As childhood and young adulthood are critical times in terms of personality development, it is no surprise that early trauma has effects on shaping personality traits and coping styles that often persist into adulthood.

The Association of Trauma with Personality Disorders

Many studies have shown a strong association with childhood abuse and personality disorders (PDs). A community-based longitudinal study spanning from 1975–1993 reported those with childhood abuse were greater than four times more likely than those not abused to develop a personality disorder even when controlling for age, parental psychiatric illness, and parental education. Specific type of abuse was also correlated with specific personality disorders: physical abuse correlated with higher symptoms of antisocial and depressive PDs; sexual abuse was more correlated with borderline PD; and neglect was associated with elevated symptoms of antisocial, avoidant, borderline, narcissistic, and passive-aggressive PDs. A reexamination of the same data demonstrated verbal abuse in childhood increased the risk of PD symptoms.[4,5] Results from the National Epidemiological Survey on Alcohol and Related Conditions demonstrated childhood abuse and neglect were most closely associated with Cluster A (paranoid, schizoid, and schizotypal) and B (antisocial, borderline, histrionic, and narcissistic) PDs after adjusting for mood, anxiety, substance use disorders, and differences in sociodemographics. Data from the same study from 2004–2005 described associations between antisocial PD and physical abuse and between borderline PD and emotional abuse.[6,7]

There are many inconsistencies in the literature regarding which types of trauma are most associated with particular PDs. Differences may be accounted for by the fact that details—such as the severity, onset, frequency, chronicity, and relation to abuser—are often not included in studies. In addition, many who have endured one type of trauma have endured multiple types, and may not report all of them, making it impossible to fully parse out and control for which type of trauma led to specific PDs. Further details about specific abuse and individual PDs will be discussed in depth later in this chapter.

The seminal Adverse Childhood Experiences Study (ACES) study put a spotlight on the frequency of adverse childhood experiences in the general population and highlighted that multiple types of adverse events exist. Approximately 70 percent of 17,337 adults presenting for an annual physical had experienced adverse childhood events. This study proved these events were associated with many physical and mental illnesses later in life and had additive effects on future adverse outcomes.[8]

Beyond emotional, sexual, and physical abuse, researchers have examined a variety of adverse events that impede healthy personality development. For example, the Barbados Nutrition longitudinal study looked at adults over a span of 47 years to determine the personality-development consequences of children with both malnutrition and childhood maltreatment. Malnutrition history was associated with paranoid, schizoid, avoidant, and dependent PDs; maltreatment history was associated with paranoid, schizoid, schizotypal, and avoidant PDs.[9]

In addition to studying lesser-recognized trauma types, studying populations outside of the United States is also critical. As one researcher noted, subjects from Western, educated, industrialized, rich, and democratic (WEIRD) societies are "some of the most psychologically unusual people on Earth."[9,10] In a 2008 survey of psychology journals, 96 percent of the subjects studied were from Western countries, which only accounted for 12 percent of the world's population.[11]

The effect of childhood trauma on personality development has been studied in more diverse populations with similar findings. An outpatient study in Ireland in 2014 reported of the 85/136 patients who met criteria for a personality disorder, 87 percent of them had experienced childhood trauma. The most prevalent were antisocial PD (100 percent had experienced trauma), passive-aggressive PD (97 percent), paranoid PD (97 percent), and borderline PD (84 percent). Only antisocial PD was significantly associated with childhood sexual abuse. They reported a dose-response relationship in terms of type, number, and severity of abuse with severity of symptomatology as an adult.[12] A study of outpatients from a counseling center in Shanghai, China, showed emotional abuse plus emotional neglect were predictive of Cluster A and B PDs, sexual abuse predicted Cluster B PDs, and emotional neglect alone was predictive of Cluster C (avoidant, dependent, and obsessive-compulsive) PDs.[13]

Trauma Influences the Development of Personality Disorders

While it is now clear that childhood trauma is linked to personality disorders, the mechanisms at play are less definitive. The literature is rich with hypotheses as to how trauma influences the development of PDs. Several studies have shown that deficits in mother–infant relatedness (caused by neglect or other abuse) resulted in deficiencies in skills such as social and emotional understanding and perspective-taking up to four years after infancy.[14] This dyadic responsivity is important for tuning in to internal states and the ability to differentiate oneself from others. Inherent in these tasks is the ability to understand what events might cause certain emotions and appropriate responses to others' shifts in mood. The maltreated child may not have any mirroring or modeling from an abusive caretaker or might receive conflicting signals from loving parents and abusive others. In a meta-analysis on abuse and social understanding, 16 of the 19 studies evaluated showed poorer performance on developmental age-specific emotional skills, such as the ability to recognize and understand the cause of emotions. Earlier childhood abuse resulted in the most severe deficits.[14] Difficulties with attachment can hinder the ability to form secure relationships, which often impacts identity integration, self-control, and social concordance.[15] Variables such as Intelligence Quotient (IQ) and age at the time of trauma can also mediate these difficulties. The multifactorial nature of personality development may help explain why some abused children have deficits and some do not.

Severity of childhood abuse and resultant low self-esteem increases the use of immature defense mechanisms leading to more psychopathology. Prolonged use of these defenses, such as acting out, splitting, or projection, is a likely risk factor for the development of a PD.[16] For example, the neurotic defense mechanism of repetition-compulsion may lead a survivor to engage with dangerous people as an attempt to repeat interactions with the wish of reparation or repair. This may lead to re-victimization and a repeating cycle of behavior that may manifest as fodder for developing a PD. Additional hypotheses concerning trauma and developing PDs will be discussed in the sections about specific PDs.

Psychological Effects of Trauma

How does trauma effect survivors psychologically?

Seventy percent of us will experience a traumatic event in our lifetime, while only approximately 20 percent of those who survive trauma will go on to develop post-traumatic stress disorder (PTSD).[17] Thankfully, resilience is the norm. The effects of trauma can be long-lasting even if one does not develop PTSD.

Cognitive Style and Trauma

Cognitive processing therapy (CPT), a first-line, evidence-based treatment for PTSD, can help elucidate the typical thinking of survivors of trauma and how that might impair personality growth. CPT combines expressing and feeling emotions about the trauma and cognitively challenging beliefs that emanate from ones' perception of why a trauma occurred. It is the meaning one ascribes to the trauma that is most important and often prevents recovery. Treatment involves teaching cognitive skills to challenge assumptions and applying skills to five areas that are impacted regardless of trauma type. These include: safety; trust; power and control; esteem; and intimacy.

We are born to be inquisitive. We all crave control. When faced with an outlier event, we have an innately strong desire to understand it. Like the *Sesame Street* jingle, "one of these things is not like the other," these events stand out and challenge our comfort level. How do we make sense of the world when the outlier is a traumatic event?

CPT posits people tend to do one of three things after a traumatic event:

1. Assimilation, which means changing details about how one perceives a trauma to make it fit within a prior belief system. This often leads to an erroneous line of thinking but allows one to keep one's prior belief system intact and often provides an illusion of control. The downside to assimilation is that it produces guilt, shame, and self-blame that can each be important causes of impaired personality development and PTSD.
2. Over-accommodation occurs when one completely changes their worldview to make sense of a trauma. For example, changing a pre-traumatic view that the world is safe to a view that the world is *never* safe. This line of reasoning leads to disruption in other vital aspects of personality development such as trust and relatedness to others.
3. Accommodation is the most adaptive option. Here one challenges the evidence behind their thoughts and recognizes they may have "connected the dots" about the trauma in ways that were not accurate in order to feel in control. To recognize one had no control, a hallmark of trauma, is more difficult but leads to resilience and more balanced, flexible thinking. Those that master this method may reduce post-traumatic symptoms or lose their diagnosis of PTSD and, importantly for the topic at hand, may reduce their risk of developing a personality disorder.

The salient point here is that unprocessed or untreated trauma shatters how people view themselves and humanity. Responses to trauma—such as nightmares, flashbacks, and intrusive thoughts—can impact one's ability to test reality and lead to symptoms that appear in the psychotic range. Hypervigilance and startle responses, in addition to a breach in trust, can lead to paranoia. Dissociative responses to trauma or detachment impede skills needed for relatedness and connectivity with others. Each of these aspects and other symptoms related to trauma will be covered in more detail in relation to specific PDs.

Neurobiological Effects of Trauma

What does trauma do from a neurobiological perspective?

There is accumulating evidence demonstrating that PDs are associated with abnormal structure and function of the brain. Evidence in specific disorders will be covered, but it is helpful to briefly review some key concepts that will aid the reader in better understanding these neuropsychiatric findings.

Methods Used to Study the Brain

What are the typical ways in which the human brain is studied? Researchers typically utilize noninvasive modalities of measuring the function and structure of the brain, which rely on measurements that are indirect indicators of the process of interest. Chief among these technologies is magnetic resonance imaging (MRI), which utilizes powerful magnetic fields to obtain computerized images of the brain. There are two broad subdivisions of imaging metrics: structural, and functional (see Boxes 3.1[18-20] and 3.2, and Table 3.1 for details, p. 64).

In recent years, psychiatric research has benefited greatly from the application of these noninvasive tools to study the structure and function of the brain. The study of PDs is no exception, with many studies now examining differences in brain structure, brain activation, and brain connectivity between individuals with and without a personality disorder.

Box 3.1 Structural Magnetic Resonance Imaging

Structural MRI relies on a high-resolution image to produce measurements regarding the gray matter and white matter of the brain.

- Gray matter encompasses the bodies of the brain's neurons (as well as dendrites, where the neuron's cell body connects with other neurons via neurotransmitter receptors).
- White matter is mainly the myelinated axons of neurons (composed mainly of fat, and thus appears more "white" on MRI images) as well as glial cells that support the functioning of neurons.
- Brain structure changes across the lifespan, initially increasing in gray matter and cortical thickness, followed by a leveling off, then an age-related decline.[18,19]
- Age-related changes are different between males and females.[20]

Box 3.2 Functional Magnetic Resonance Imaging

Functional MRI (fMRI) relies on a different type of MRI contrast to infer brain activity over time.

- In contrast to structural MRI, which is concerned primarily with differences in tissue types as revealed by variations in image intensity, fMRI is concerned with tracking changes in intensity over periods of time.
- This intensity change over time is known as the blood oxygenation level dependent (BOLD) response, which is sensitive to the degree to which blood in a particular area of the brain is oxygenated.
- Blood oxygen will initially dip in an active area (due to neurons drawing in more oxygen to support their firing activity), then drastically increase (as more fresh blood is delivered to that region to support ongoing neuronal firing), and eventually drop back down to a baseline level (after the neurons have stopped firing).
- This whole process begins about 1–2 seconds after the onset of the "activating" stimulus, reaches a peak at about 4–6 seconds, and then gradually declines back down to baseline at around 10–12 seconds.
- Tracking of the magnitude of this process allows researchers to infer what portions of the brain were "activated" by a given stimulus and the extent to which this brain structure was activated.

Table 3.1 MRI Definitions

Structural MRI

Gray-matter volume and density	The approximate volume of neuronal gray matter or density of gray matter in a particular fixed volume of space.
Cortical thickness and surface area	The approximate thickness or surface area of the gray-matter sheet that covers the outside of the brain.
Fractional anisotropy of white matter	The degree to which white matter in the brain inhibits the movement of water molecules in particular directions.

Functional MRI

BOLD (Blood oxygenation level dependent response)	The intensity change over time in an fMRI measured by the contrast sensitivity to blood oxygenation in a specific area.
Functional connectivity	The degree of spontaneous coherence between BOLD signal changes in two parts of the brain. The more correlated BOLD signal changes between two or more brain structures, the more "functionally connected" they are, and the greater the degree they are working together in a coordinated process.

Trauma and the Neurobiology of Specific Personality Disorders

With a basic understanding of trauma and relevant measurement tools, we can examine the relationship between early-life adversity (child abuse or neglect) and the development and manifestation of particular PDs. We will briefly review possible psychological etiologies of select PDs in regard to trauma's contributions to their development and review what is known about connections between trauma and neuroanatomical changes related to PDs via neuroimaging studies. We chose to highlight four PDs in terms of their relationship to trauma. We first describe borderline PD, because it is most recognized as having a trauma etiology. As a breach in trust is often a core component of trauma, we wanted to point out the less often recognized parallels with paranoid and schizotypal PDs, where mistrust is paramount. Antisocial PD patients are often stereotypically interpreted to be more malicious and manipulative. While true in many regards, calling attention to possible trauma etiologies in these patients may aid in building rapport and reducing negative countertransference.

Borderline Personality Disorder

Borderline personality disorder (BPD) is characterized by emotion dysregulation, fragile self-image, impulsivity, and troubled interpersonal relationships. Patients with BPD often have an intense fear of being abandoned and may exhibit suicidal or self-injurious behavior. The prevalence of BPD in the general population is 1.7 percent, and 15 and 28 percent among patients in psychiatric clinics or hospitals.[21]

Borderline Personality Disorder and Trauma

Prior to 2000, the association between childhood abuse and BPD was hotly debated; many argued it was not a contributing factor to the development of BPD. Retrospective studies were limited by not specifying the severity of trauma or if more than one trauma was present. A more recent study, confirming childhood trauma occurred by multiple adult sources, demonstrated that children who were sexually abused were four times more likely to exhibit borderline pathology than those who were not abused.[22]

We now know that adverse childhood experiences are strongly associated with and, according to some experts, are the most significant environmental risk factor for the development of BPD.[23] BPD is more consistently associated with child abuse and neglect than any other personality disorder. Child abuse occurs in 30 to 90 percent of BPD patients.[21] A recent review reported physical abuse, emotional abuse, sexual abuse, and neglect of children were independently associated with borderline features, with a higher symptom burden for more frequent and severe trauma.[24] However, although it is an important risk factor, childhood abuse is not necessary nor sufficient for a BPD diagnosis.

Etiologic Hypotheses

Marsha Linehan describes BPD as a disorder of emotion dysregulation that stems from both invalidating environments and biologic vulnerabilities.[25] Her biosocial theory emphasizes three emotional traits: heightened sensitivity; inability to regulate responses;

and a slow return to baseline. These threads are common in many of the hypothesized psychological etiologies for BPD and are more compelling in the advent of trauma.

Temperament

The hyperbolic temperament model focuses on the tendency to experience inner pain in response to perceived slights, coupled with impulsivity to seek attention, leading to a cycle of invalidation, chronic dysphoria, and dependency needs. It's easy to see how this temperament type would be amplified further if paired with trauma, where slights are not only real, but more severe. The interaction between temperament in general and trauma may influence the severity of BPD. A study of BPD patients and siblings found affective instability and impulsivity were better predictors of BPD severity than degree of trauma.[26] Similarly, children who have been abused exhibit personality traits distinguished by high neuroticism, low conscientiousness, and low agreeableness or openness to experiences that often manifest in analogous BPD traits in adulthood.[23] An innate difficult temperament may potentiate parental frustration and develop into ineffective parenting.

Invalidating Environments and Attachment

Unhealthy attachments to parental figures come in many forms, including parenting that is over- or under-involved, inconsistent, low in affection or empathy, aversive, or frankly abusive or neglectful. Without healthy parental mirroring and attunement, grasping the fundamental tools to relate to others may be impossible and may lead to a disorganized sense of self and the inability to self-soothe. Invalidating environments, where emotions are often ignored until they are expressed in an extreme manner, tend to reinforce the idea that emotions are unimportant. This can lead to deficits in understanding, labeling, and expressing emotions. Similarly, one's experience of trauma can be invalidated by family ("You should not have been drinking, so the rape is your fault"), friends ("You should be over that by now"), or the police ("Do you really want to ruin his life by accusing him of rape?"). If trauma is met with invalidation, it is common to exhibit symptoms consistent with BPD. A sense of detachment from others or dissociation may present as a lack of emotional expression, leading to disturbed interpersonal relationships. What may seem like emotional dysregulation may be a post-trauma vacillation between feeling numb and feeling intense trauma-related emotions. Self-loathing or blame may lead to suicidality or reckless behavior.

If emotional expression was never modeled, this may explain some BPD patients' inability to connect with or understand what others are feeling. For example, even in bipolar patients with neglect histories, facial recognition of anger has been shown to be impaired.[27] On the other hand, some BPD patients may have a keen ability to detect anger in others. This may represent an adaptive response to childhood trauma, particularly physical or sexual abuse, where the ability to sense anger in others was vital to learn for protection when anger signaled danger. In these survivors, a conflict may arise between a desire to connect, even if only through anger or abuse, and a fear of abandonment. Here, inciting anger in others can lead to turning inward and detachment in the BPD patient once the aggression is experienced: a recipe for relationship chaos.

Table 3.2 Overlapping Symptoms: Borderline Personality Disorder and Trauma Responses or PTSD[27]

Borderline Personality Characteristics	Responses to Trauma or PTSD
Patterns of unstable, intense interpersonal relationships	Instability of relationships due to erosion of trust in others secondary to trauma.
Unstable sense of self, self-hatred	Based on trauma-related shame, guilt, self-blame.
Impulsivity: indiscriminate sex, substance abuse, or other reckless behaviors that are potentially self-damaging	Actions that appear like promiscuity: "If I say yes to intimacy, no one can force it on me" leads to an illusion of control. Substance use to numb or avoid trauma reminders. Reckless behavior to regain adrenaline rush associated with some trauma experiences, "to feel something again" and not be numb.
Emotion dysregulation, inappropriate intense anger, reactive mood instability	Anger or irritability due to hyperarousal, alterations between numbness and feeling trauma-related emotions intensely.
Stress-induced, transient dissociative symptoms or psychotic symptoms	Trauma-related dissociation, flashbacks, or intrusive memories can be mistaken for auditory or visual hallucinations.
Suicidal ideation or gestures	Suicidal ideation as punishment for trauma-related guilt, shame, or self-blame.
Chronic feelings of emptiness	Detachment from others who can't understand the trauma they experienced.
Difficulty understanding the feelings and needs of others	Detachment often leads to trouble understanding others' stressors that pale in comparison to their trauma, can be seen as unempathetic and lead to conflicted relationships.
Black-and-white thinking	Overgeneralizing due to trauma, "All men are bad."

Overlap between Borderline Personality Disorder and Post-traumatic Stress Disorder

It's often difficult to assess whether the biological vulnerability inherent in BPD puts someone at risk for trauma, or if trauma is an etiologic factor for BPD. As just described, the symptoms of both disorders overlap and can be interpreted to be primary to either disorder. To confound matters further, both disorders are often comorbid (see Table 3.2[28] for diagnostic similarities and Box 3.3 (see p. 68) for a clinical example).

The development of BPD in the setting of trauma has multifactorial components. In addition to the psychological etiologies and invalidating environments, additional factors include developmental stage when a trauma occurs, changes in hypothalamic-pituitary-adrenal axis (HPA axis), epigenetics, inherent differences in neurocircuitry, and other genetic vulnerabilities and heritability.

Box 3.3 PTSD Masquerading as BPD

A medical student is seen for difficulty in school due to chaotic relationships and extreme mood shifts. She has had a few suicide attempts and has chronic intermittent suicidal ideation. She is impulsive in using substances regularly to excess. She worries friends will abandon her and feels "empty" inside. She was diagnosed with BPD and was not improving with dialectical behavioral therapy and psychodynamic work. After a year of treatment, she divulged a history of sexual abuse by her father. A shift to trauma-focused therapy revealed a core belief that she was damaged, and if anyone stayed with her long enough, they would recognize that and leave her. Her chaotic relationships were a result of her ambivalence of letting others truly know her, coupled with a fear of being abandoned. She was promiscuous because she felt if she always consented to sex, she would always be in control. Substances were used to numb and avoid thinking about her trauma. Her internal emptiness stemmed from feeling no one could understand what happened to her and was more accurately categorized as a detachment she felt from others. Once her core belief was challenged and she no longer felt guilty about her abuse, she was able to create lasting, stable relationships. She no longer needed to use substances to numb, she felt understood, and she excelled in school. In six months, she was engaged in a stable, supportive relationship.

Neurobiology of Borderline Personality Disorder

Structural MRI

Structural MRI has revealed some consistent patterns of anatomical alterations in BPD, most prominently, reduced structural volumes of the hippocampus[29-32] and the amygdala,[30,31] although no significant differences in amygdala volumes have also been reported.[28] Reductions in subcortical volumes are often attributed to stress-induced atrophy secondary to the release of stress hormones and are nonspecific markers also observed in disorders such as major depression and PTSD.[33] This is consistent with the high comorbidity of BPD with both major depression and PTSD, suggesting a shared underlying pattern of limbic neurobiological abnormalities that characterize the common affective disturbances.[34] Structural alterations have also been observed in cortical areas in BPD, such as increased gray-matter volume of the cingulate cortex and the precuneus[35] (a cortical area in the rear of the brain that is critically implicated in sense of self and autobiographical memory[36]), but decreased gray-matter volumes in the orbitofrontal cortices[37] (which are critically involved in decision-making[38]). These opposite patterns of structural abnormalities intriguingly reflect different aspects of the BPD symptomatology (i.e., disturbed sense of self and impulsivity/decision-making impairments).

This suggests a neuroanatomical basis for common clinical observations. Intriguingly, these patterns of structural alterations reflect those observed in survivors of early-life trauma,[39] which suggests potential neurobiological changes that might lead from early-life trauma to the development of BPD.

Functional MRI (fMRI)

Functional imaging studies of BPD have largely focused on task-based fMRI, wherein participants with and without BPD will complete a behavioral paradigm while undergoing scanning. Comparisons of brain activation during key contrasts of interest are utilized to identify areas of abnormal brain functioning in the patient group, which can give some indication of the potential disorder pathophysiology. Many of these task-based studies have focused on the processing of negative emotional stimuli, like facial expressions, due to the prominent affective disturbances that characterize the disorder. A brief summary on the processing of negative emotional stimuli reveals consistent evidence for hyperactivity of limbic structures implicated in the detection of emotional stimuli and generation of an emotional response.[34,40–42] In addition, a decreased engagement of frontal regions is also implicated in emotion regulation and top-down control of emotional responses.[34,42] This is a pattern of abnormalities that is shared with other disorders of negative affect often comorbid with BPD, such as major depression and PTSD.[34]

This exaggerated limbic engagement and deficient frontal response is often interpreted to be indicative of excessive emotional reactivity that is unable to be adaptively regulated. This is highly consistent with the BPD clinical presentation. Interestingly, some aspects of this pattern appear to be specifically related to adverse childhood experiences, such as a deficiency in habituating amygdala responses to negative stimuli over repeated presentations.[40] Thus, BPD represents both biologically and behaviorally one developmental endpoint of repeated and numerous early-life stressors, traumas, and adverse experiences. This undoubtedly detrimentally impacts the capacity of learning to adequately regulate one's emotional state in interpersonal relationships and other aspects of daily life.

Cluster A Personality Disorders and Trauma

Cluster A personalities include schizotypal, schizoid, and paranoid personality disorders. This cluster is characterized by eccentricity or oddness and mistrust, often leading to social isolation. We will focus on schizotypal PD and paranoid PD that cross over in terms of suspiciousness and general distrust of others, whereas with schizoid PD, patients prefer to be alone without necessarily having mistrust. Mistrust in these PDs is often the connecting strand to trauma in these patients, as a breach in trust is often a core component of trauma.

Schizotypal Personality Disorder

Schizotypal personality disorder (SPD) is characterized by an impaired sense of self, difficulty relating to others in terms of empathic deficits, avoidance of relationships usually out of suspiciousness and paranoia, and psychotic-like symptoms of odd or unusual beliefs and eccentric behavior including magical thinking and bizarre perceptions of reality.

Schizotypal Personality Disorder and Trauma

When focusing on type of trauma as a mediator of schizotypy, studies report conflicting results. A study of patients from general medical and obstetrical clinics showed emotional abuse alone predicted five out of eight criteria for SPD and was most significantly predicative of odd behavior or appearance. PTSD itself was predictive of four SPD symptoms: excessive social anxiety, lack of close friends, unusual perceptions, and eccentric appearance or behavior.[43] Looking at undergraduate students in China, neglect was positively correlated with schizotypy traits.[44] A literature review spanning 1806 to 2013 reported all forms of childhood abuse were associated with increased schizotypy, especially positive traits. Increased childhood trauma was experienced by a greater number of schizotypal individuals compared to controls, not accounted for by parental psychopathology or genetics alone.[45] To further disentangle contributing factors, Berenbaum measured the rate of first-degree relatives with psychotic disorders and signs of neurodevelopmental disorders to evaluate genetic risk factors. He investigated if PTSD, antisocial PD, and borderline PD were mediators between trauma and schizotypal symptoms. Trauma experiences were still associated with schizotypy when removing shared variances for all of the other factors. In terms of gender differences, childhood trauma and PTSD predicted schizotypal symptoms in women, whereas only childhood trauma, not PTSD, was predictive in men.[46]

Characteristics and Etiologic Psychological Hypotheses

The diagnostic criteria for SPD can be conceptualized as a multifactorial construct. For ease of pointing out components affected by trauma, it is helpful to use the three-factor construct consisting of (1) positive traits (odd perceptions, magical thinking, suspiciousness); (2) interpersonal or negative traits (lack of social connectedness and affect); and (3) disorganized traits (eccentric behavior).[47]

Positive Schizotypy Traits

In a study of patients with psychosis, their siblings, and controls, those with abuse compared to those without had a higher incidence of positive schizotypy traits. These traits were more closely associated with emotional, physical, or sexual abuse than neglect.[48] Paranoia and unusual beliefs have been associated with physical abuse and sexual abuse, whereas severe sexual abuse has been most associated with ideas of reference, magical thinking, and odd beliefs.[49,50] Trauma exposure has been linked with difficulty in discerning lies, sarcasm, and suspiciousness.[51]

Odd perceptions may be manifestations of intrusive thoughts that are not recognized as originating internally.[52,53] This external attribution bias, in terms of trauma, may be due to an aversion to intrusive thoughts and feeling more in control by attributing them to external loci rather than unwanted fragments of true, past reality. Patients who hallucinate show greater reality-monitoring errors for self-generated items if the task is emotionally charged.[54] This illustrates how intrusive, emotionally evocative triggers from trauma may lead to hallucinations. The developmental stage when trauma occurs may affect how memory is encoded; namely, a young child with no verbal memory may be left with fragmented memories which may, as an adult, lead to distortions and ultimately hallucinations. Alternatively, trauma may have deleterious effects on early neurodevelopment and predispose one to adult psychosis, especially if genetic vulnerability exists.

Schizotypal traits of paranormal beliefs may serve as a means to gain control over a traumatic situation. Believing external forces or entities are to blame may allow one to feel safe around an abusive parent from whom there is no escape.[55] Children use fantasy in play to express their thoughts and emotions. It's not a large jump to conclude that abused children may use fantasy as a means to create an environment where they attempt to make sense out of trauma by gaining control or numbing themselves to their true reality.

Uncommon or more bizarre traumatic experiences can also mimic positive schizotypy. Please see examples in Box 3.4, p. 71.

Box 3.4 Unusual Trauma Experiences

If the nature of one's trauma is unusual, ensuing behavioral responses may appear eccentric and implausible. For example, patients with PTSD stemming from being raised in a cult may express odd or eccentric beliefs that can be misattributed to schizotypy or SPD. Abused children whose caregivers brainwashed them may have difficulty letting go of untrue manipulative-based beliefs if they were strongly ingrained throughout childhood.

- "Because you are so bad, other people can sense that and won't like you."
- "The police know who you are, if you ever tell anyone about what happened, they will know and will be able to find you."
- "I put a microchip inside your head—so I will always know where you are."
- "The evil inside you is so strong, when anyone looks into your eyes, they will want to kill you."

Negative Schizotypy Traits

Physical abuse, emotional abuse, and severe emotional neglect have also been associated with social anxiety and constricted affect seen in patients with SPD.[43,50]

PTSD symptoms and responses to trauma may be misinterpreted as schizotypy or SPD. It is well known that trauma can lead to emotional numbing, which can mimic the constricted affect often associated with SPD. Responses to trauma—such as shame, blame, guilt, and a sense that one is forever damaged—may serve as barriers to developing meaningful relationships, which are often lacking in patients with SPD. Patients with trauma or SPD may fear being misunderstood, abandoned, or abused, which can lead to social defeat and exclusion, or feeling like an outsider. Traumas that involve intentional harm such as sexual, physical, or emotional abuse often lead to chronic self-denigration and social defeat, whereas traumas such as accidents or caregiver death may not.[56]

This sense of social defeat or feeling like an outsider increases paranoia, in that having less social connectedness alters one's ability to accurately appraise the risk of threat in social interactions.[57,58] Research on trauma and resiliency has revealed that perceived social support lowers the risk of developing PTSD. Both isolation due to trauma and schizotypy traits reduce the ability to create supports, deepening the risk for longer-term behavioral patterns, or developing PTSD and/or SPD.

Alternatively, one can argue that traits of negative schizotypy may be biologically or genetically mediated. Here a biological vulnerability may predispose one to trauma. In this case, someone who is innately odd or eccentric may easily show up on the radar of predators, enhancing their risk of victimization. Regardless of the cause, treatment of trauma is beneficial; see Box 3.5, p. 72 for a clinical illustration of this point.

Disorganized Schizotypy Traits

Physical or emotional abuse, neglect, and bullying have also been associated with eccentricity.[43,59,60]

> ### Box 3.5 The Chicken or the Egg: Primary Psychosis versus Trauma
>
> Despite which comes first—psychosis or PTSD/trauma—it is still paramount to treat trauma. Even in those with primary psychotic disorders, trauma-focused therapy can reduce symptoms significantly. After a course of cognitive processing therapy, a schizophrenic patient who was sexually and emotionally abused by her father still heard voices, but they were no longer critical of her as her father had been. Subsequently, the hallucinations bothered her less, which led to an improved quality of life and less overall impairment. She was medication and treatment compliant because she no longer believed the abuse was her fault. Because she valued herself more, she felt she deserved to be happy and therefore had a reason to engage in treatment.

Neurobiology of Schizotypal Personality Disorders

Like BPD, functional imaging studies of SPD have largely focused on task-based fMRI. For example, individuals with and without SPD underwent fMRI while completing a visual working-memory task. Those with SPD displayed less activation of various prefrontal and parietal regions that are typically recruited during task completion, suggesting a potential deficit in recruiting brain areas implicated in cognitive functions,[61] a feature that is often observed to be a sequelae of early-life trauma.[39] Healthy controls also performed better on the memory task, on average. An older study utilizing a different imaging modality, single photon emission computed tomography (SPECT), also observed abnormal prefrontal function (in this case measured by cerebral blood flow, another proxy measure for neuronal function) in SPD, but this time the authors observed increased blood flow in the right prefrontal cortex relative to healthy controls.[62] The disparate findings could be related to the type of cognitive task performed; in the latter study, individuals performed the Wisconsin Card Sorting Task, which is a common measure of executive function rather than memory processes per se. Taken together, the rather limited body of work suggests abnormal prefrontal function in SPD, which is also consistent with the effects of early-life trauma on the brain.[39]

Paranoid Personality Disorder

Paranoid personality disorder (PPD) consists of behaviors ruled by suspiciousness and lack of trust, including a preoccupation with mistrusting others, a tendency to hold on to perceived slights, and a pervasive fear of confiding in anyone due to perceived wanton maliciousness of others.

The prevalence of PPD is 1.21 percent to 4.4 percent of the US population and is more frequently diagnosed in males.[63,64] In a community-based adult study, African Americans (AA) had higher paranoid personality traits than Caucasians, which was related to socioeconomic status differences and trauma exposure.[65] In another study, AA college graduates had less mistrust than AA high school dropouts, pointing less to race and more to societal disadvantage leading to paranoia.[66] Living in a society where victimization and lack of control are prevalent can make developing mistrust and paranoia par for the course. Evolutionarily, survival of the fittest depends on a level of paranoia to ensure propagation of offspring.

Paranoid Personality Disorder and Trauma

Disagreements exist as to how to best categorize PPD, because it is generally accepted that paranoia exists along a spectrum, with less severity found in many non-clinical samples.

Trauma can represent the ultimate breach of trust. Suspiciousness is an adaptive response to some degree for protection, but it is no longer adaptive if taken to extremes. New relationships may be seen through the trauma lens where unjustified assumptions about others are made, prohibiting the formation of new connections. Due to the nature of PPD, with mistrust being paramount, these patients are less willing to seek out or accept opportunities to participate in research.[67,68] Therefore, less is known about the links between trauma and developing PPD. A few studies have identified childhood trauma as a risk factor for PPD along with other PDs.[63,69] In a group of adult survivors of serious childhood burn injuries, approximately 50 percent were found to have a PD, the most common was PPD at 19.4 percent. Prior trauma, parental loss in the fire, and dysfunctional parental–child interactions after the burn injury were not accounted for and may have contributed to the formation of PPD.[70]

Etiologic Psychological Hypotheses

Several theoretical viewpoints have been described concerning the etiology of PPD,[63] many of which are relevant in terms of trauma.

From a Freudian viewpoint, inward conflicts may be projected outwards as paranoia. Here inwardly, intolerable low self-esteem and shame may be at play. As discussed, trauma often leads to shame and self-blame in an effort to gain control. Esteem is one of the five core constructs affected by trauma. A study of teens and young adults who did not meet full criteria for schizophrenia but had significant paranoia demonstrated that shame moderated the association between stressful life events and paranoia.[71]

Bowlby's attachment theory depends on normal caregiver responses to develop a model of relatedness. Children abused at the hands of their parents develop an insecure attachment that may lead them to assume risk in future relations with a paranoid tint, hard-earned though past experience.[72,73]

A cognitive theory of PDs posits symptoms are perpetuated by strongly held cognitive beliefs. In regard to PPD, Aaron Beck proposed these patients continue to ruminate on beliefs where they feel they lack efficacy and that others have mal-intent toward them, leading to paranoia.[74] A bias may exist in PPD toward jumping to conclusions that has been predictive of paranoia in psychotic, non-psychotic clinical, and non-clinical samples.[68,75] In a study of undergraduates, those with PPD were intolerant of ambiguity and were more inclined to jump to conclusions quickly.[75] This ties in to post-trauma desires to make sense of outliers or ambiguity to gain control. Trauma leading to feeling one is vulnerable and others are dangerous often engenders paranoia. This is in line with the threat anticipation model of paranoia where persecutory ideation arises from a fear that one's safety is constantly at risk.[68] After trauma, avoidance or self-isolation creates an environment where there are no social contacts to vet these thoughts for validity, and they become absolute truths, or delusional in nature.

Neurobiological Correlates of Paranoia

A review of the literature revealed an absence of studies examining the neurobiology of PPD. This is likely due both to the relative rarity of the disorder, as well as the reasonable conclusion that individuals manifesting high levels of paranoid ideation are unlikely to devote themselves to participating in research and undergoing experiments.

Antisocial Personality Disorder

Antisocial personality disorder (ASPD) is characterized by an apparent disregard for others, manifesting as disobeying norms and laws, manipulation and deceit for personal gain or amusement, aggression toward others, impulsivity, irresponsibility, and typically a lack of remorse for all of these actions. Per DSM-5, the onset of these behaviors must be before the age of 15 and accompanied by conduct disorder. The annual prevalence rate for ASPD is reported to range from 0.02–3.3 percent.[64]

Antisocial Personality Disorder and Trauma

Multiple studies have demonstrated the connection between childhood abuse and antisocial behavior, with conflicting ideas about which type of abuse may be most significant in this population.

Physical and Sexual Abuse
Prospective data from 1000 young adults in New Zealand showed prevalence rates of ASPD among 18- to 25-year-olds were two to four times higher in those sexually abused and two to seven times higher in those regularly physically abused, compared to the non-abused.[76,77] In a study of adult criminal offenders, overall psychopathy was associated with more childhood maltreatment, with physical abuse most strongly related to antisocial features.[78] Similarly, in a group of federal offenders, physical abuse was a significant predictor of ASPD.[77]

Emotional Neglect
In a group of US juvenile offenders, emotional neglect was found to be more predictive of callousness traits than other types of abuse.[79]

Verbal Abuse and Caretaker Sexual Abuse
The Collaborative Longitudinal Personality Disorders Study examined patients aged 18–45 years, where meeting criteria for ASPD predicted higher verbal abuse and caretaker sexual abuse.[80]

Regardless of the type of abuse suffered, as an adaptation to trauma, future painful experiences may be desensitized. Less emotional or physiological responsiveness may lead to unresponsiveness to others' needs as a pathway to callousness and lack of empathy.[81] These are important connections, as ASPD can lead to violent behavior, and a greater understanding of potential causal factors may impart enhanced treatment and prevention options. A link between childhood abuse and violent perpetration was demonstrated by analyzing 22,575 delinquent youth referred to the Florida Department of Juvenile Justice. Each trauma or adverse childhood experience increased the risk of becoming a serious, violent offender by 35 percent after controlling for other risk factors for criminality.[82]

Antisocial Personality Disorder Characteristics and Psychopathy

An ASPD diagnosis does not necessarily lead to violence and criminality. Disagreement exists as to whether psychopathy is its own entity or part of a spectrum and considered a severe form of ASPD. Psychopathy is distinguished from ASPD by the additional traits of callousness, superficial charm, grandiosity, and a difference in emotion regulation. ASPD patients typically show dysregulation in response to abuse, whereas in psychopathy, emotional blunting and social dominance reign strong. Innate callousness and manipulative skills may serve as a defense against emotional regulation deficits secondary to childhood abuse in psychopathic patients.[78]

Types of Psychopathy
Akin to the nurture-versus-nature argument, several researchers have validated a dual theory of psychopathy. Lykken's hypothesis describes innate tendencies toward antisocial behavior as "psychopathy," and "sociopathy" as a trait for those in whom environmental factors shaped their turn toward criminality. He astutely hypothesized that the older generational cultural norm of children being reared by large extended families fared better in socializing youth than the overburdened one- or two-parent team taking on the daunting task. If the full-team approach failed, it was more likely that an inborn psychopath was at hand. If one or two parents cannot devote enough time and nurturing in terms of socialization, a sociopath may be created.[83]

Etiologic Hypotheses

Low Fear Pathway to Antisocial Personality Disorder
In terms of this innate component, one can hypothesize about children who are born fearless. Consequences and punishment are effective enforcers of societal rules unless one is born without fear.[83] The presence of an internalized conscience by age four was predicted by maternal gentle discipline in fearful but not in fearless children. For fearless children, a secure attachment from a mutually positive parent–child relationship predicted internal conscience formation.[84] This lends hope to the notion that children with innate fearless temperaments are not destined to develop ASPD or psychopathy. With secure attachments, fearlessness can translate into boldness rather than cruelty and/or criminality.[84,85]

Temperament

A fearless or aggressive temperament can be associated with ASPD because it can make the task of forming a positive parent–child bond difficult. Parents may simply give up or turn to abusive behaviors to control their child. Negative emotionality and lack of effortful control may serve as risk factors for antisocial behavior. There are two tendencies in this population: (1) forgoing socially appropriate responses in favor of instinctual responses due to lack of inhibition or impairments in effortful control; and (2) high levels of "hot" emotions such as anger, irritability, and hostility verses "cold" emotions such as anxiety or depression.[86] In juvenile offenders, after controlling for childhood abuse and psychopathy, temperament was a significant predictor of antisocial behavior. Hot or angry temperaments were more associated with violence than blunted or emotionless features.[87]

Attachment

Studies have shown conflicting results when looking at the relationship of parental style and attachment with antisocial behavior. Some conclude ASPD patients are not affected by parenting style, whereas others point to dysfunctional parenting as leading to callous traits and psychopathy. These differences might point to the prior mentioned innate versus environmentally driven subtypes of ASPD, and how temperament may impede healthy attachment. Trauma can lead to disorganized attachment that creates temporarily adaptive responses—such as aggression or detachment from emotions—to survive the traumatic relationship. Outside of trauma, these behaviors are no longer adaptive and may lead to ASPD. Attachment difficulty within the first 18 months of life has been shown to significantly predict ASPD 20 years later.[88] In terms of maternal or paternal influences, correlations between maternal rejection (but not maternal overprotection) and ASPD have been reported.[89] In a university population, physical abuse and neglect accounted for the greatest variance in ASPD symptoms, followed by father involvement in care and teasing, with subjects least affected by overprotective mothers. Alternatively, in a study of incarcerated adolescents, boys who reported less empathic mothers had higher callousness traits. Maternal warmth and affection appeared to be protective against aggression.[79] Empathy and morality are learned by modeling from attachment figures, internalizing their values and behavior and experiencing positive reciprocity.[90] When trauma prohibits secure attachment, the possibility of ASPD looms large.

Trauma Exposure Modulates Aggressive Behavior

As discussed, violence and aggression are often connected to ASPD. Trauma exposure may modulate what type of aggression ensues. Reactive aggression is in response to perceived threat, which ASPD patients tend to overestimate. This responsive aggression is committed as a protection, not as a random internally created objective.[91] The perception of intent, not actual intent, is the causal aspect behind whether a person chooses to act with reactive aggression.[92] A trauma history full of repeated breaches in trust naturally skews perception toward mal-intent. On the other hand, proactive aggression is unprovoked and more malicious, involving the desire to control others.[91,93] A group of

---

Box 3.6 Violent Trauma Leads to Violent Behavior

A child living in a rough neighborhood is attacked by a gang of children. Those who do not join the gang are continually victimized. Those who do join the gang are indoctrinated by becoming perpetrators of violence. If there are no positive parental role models, and adopting violence is the only means for safety or survival, violence becomes habitual and a learned way of responding to the world.

---

violent offenders with ASPD, with and without high levels of psychopathy, were studied to help distinguish what role childhood abuse played in violence in terms of reactive versus proactive aggression. The more violent offenders with ASPD and psychopathy reported more childhood physical abuse—but not sexual or emotional abuse—than those with ASPD without psychopathy and non-offenders. Higher psychopathy, but not childhood abuse, correlated with proactive aggression, whereas childhood physical abuse was associated with reactive aggression.[93] Interestingly, a study of African American boys in grade school in North Carolina showed proactively aggressive boys were deemed by their peers to be as dangerous and as irritating as reactively aggressive boys. However, only the proactive boys were seen as leaders who could have a sense of humor.[91] It may be this thread of positively perceived aggressive qualities that enables antisocial serial killers to use charm and charisma to lure their victims. See Box 3.6 for a clinical example.

Neurobiology of Antisocial Personality Disorder

In regard to brain structure, individuals with ASPD have been found to display reduced whole brain volumes and, more specifically, reduced volume of the temporal lobes; however, increased volumes were observed in the putamen (which are a portion of the basal ganglia). [94] Interestingly, some evidence suggests that the presence of psychopathy, in addition to the hallmark negative externalizing behavior, may reflect a unique biological subtype. One study observed that individuals with ASPD with psychopathy displayed reduced gray-matter volumes in the frontal and temporal poles relative to individuals with ASPD but without psychopathy, as well as healthy controls.[95] This is particularly interesting given the functional roles of the frontal and temporal poles in social cognition, empathic and moral reasoning, and prosocial emotions,[96,97] which are all processes deficient in psychopathic individuals. Volumes in the orbitofrontal cortex, a portion of the frontal lobes important for decision-making, have also been found to be reduced in individuals with psychopathic traits.[98] The impact of early-life stress on frontal lobe structure has been found to result in similar alterations (i.e., reductions in frontal lobe gray-matter volumes), which highlights a potential developmental pathway linking early-life trauma to the development of several PDs, including antisocial.[39]

ASPD has been shown to have a substantial heritability component, ranging from 38–69 percent.[77] This high degree of heritability suggests genetic and early shared environmental components may interact to produce this phenomenon. Relatedly, some individuals view antisocial PD as reflecting a neurodevelopmental abnormality. Evidence suggests this may be the case, as one study found that in a community sample those displaying a brain marker for fetal neural maldevelopment (cavum septum pellucidum) were more likely to display antisocial behaviors and psychopathic traits.[99] This does not, however, indicate that all cases of ASPD reflect neurodevelopmental abnormalities, but suggests that at least a subset do. Moreover, a specific genetic variant of the monoamine oxidase-A (an enzyme responsible for the breakdown of monoamine neurotransmitters) gene, in which low transcriptional activity is noted in vivo, was demonstrated to be associated with an abnormality in amygdala surface area for individuals with ASPD versus those without, suggesting this genetic feature may serve as a potential liability for the disorder via effects on amygdala structure,[100] perhaps in interaction with early-life stress.[101]

Implications for Treatment

Neuroimaging research is leading the way to a better understanding of changes that occur post-trauma to identify new targets for treatments. Current studies measuring brain changes after psychotherapy will enhance our understanding of how trauma-focused psychotherapy affects the brain and aids in enhancing treatment course and outcomes. Many effective psychotherapies exist today for PTSD. This chapter highlights the importance of developing better screening tools in childhood to assess for trauma so that early interventions may prevent character pathology. As with all psychotherapies, it may take months to years before a patient is fully comfortable sharing about trauma. A trauma-informed approach allows the clinician to be aware of clues that trauma exists and opens the door for the patient to feel more comfortable in disclosing what they are avoiding. If behaviors post-trauma are addressed early on, development may not be hindered and, for some, character pathology may be prevented.

Conclusion

Traumatic experiences can have profound effects on how a person thinks about themselves and the world. Adaptive responses to survive adverse experiences often shape new behaviors and consequently the way one interacts with others. When trauma occurs early in development, disruptions in parent–child interactions and human connection in general help pave the way for repetitive behaviors that may lead to PDs. Temperament, biology, genetic vulnerabilities, neuroanatomical differences, biological changes, and environmental stressors all contribute to the development of character pathology. Review Box 3.7, p. 79 for additional relevant resources.

Conflict of Interest/Disclosure: The authors of this chapter have no financial conflicts and nothing to disclose.

Box 3.7 Recommended Resources for Patients, Families, and Clinicians

For Patients and Families

- **Childhood trauma and how it impacts development:** Perry BD, Szalavitz M. *The Boy who was Raised as a Dog.* 3rd ed. New York, NY: Basic Books; 2017.
- **Trauma for lay readers and clinicians:** Van der Kolk B. *The Body Keeps the Score.* Reprint ed. NY: Penguin Books; 2015.
- **Borderline Personality Disorder:** Mason PT, Kreger R. *Stop Walking on Eggshells: Taking Your Life Back When Someone You Care About Has Borderline Personality Disorder.* 3rd ed. Oakland, CA: New Harbinger Books; 2020.
- **Antisocial Personality Disorder and Psychopathy:** Hare RD. *Without Conscience: The Disturbing World of the Psychopaths among Us.* New York, NY: Guilford Press; 1999.
- **Resiliency and Trauma:** A self-biography of a psychologist who treats PTSD and survived the holocaust: Eger EE. *The Choice: Embrace the Possible.* Reprint ed. New York: Scribner; 2018.

For Therapists

- Monson CM, Chard KM, Resick, PA. *Cognitive Processing Therapy for PTSD: A Comprehensive Manual.* New York: Guilford Press; 2016.

For Details about PTSD Treatment Options:

- US Department of Veterans Affairs PTSD: National Center for PTSD. https://www.ptsd.va.gov/appvid/video/index.asp.
  White Board Cartoon Videos that explain the three most evidenced-based psychotherapies: Cognitive Processing Therapy (CPT), Prolonged Exposure (PE), and Eye Movement Desensitization and Reprocessing (EMDR)—in addition to medications for PTSD.
- "This American Life."
  NPR podcast that summarizes and plays snippets of a patient going through a course of CPT: https://www.thisamericanlife.org/682/ten-sessions.

References

1. Opie I, Opie P, eds. *The Oxford Dictionary of Nursery Rhymes*, new ed. Oxford: Oxford University Press; 1997.

2. Violence against children. World Health Organization website. https://www.who.int/health-topics/violence-against-children.

3. Human Trafficking. Ken Paxton, Attorney General of Texas website. https://www.texasattorneygeneral.gov/initiatives/human-trafficking.

4. Johnson JG, Cohen P, Brown J, Smailes EM, Bernstein DP. Childhood maltreatment increases risk for personality disorders during early adulthood. *Arch Gen Psychiatry*. Jul 1999; 56(7): 600–606. doi:10.1001/archpsyc.56.7.600

5. Johnson JG, Cohen P, Smailes EM, Skodol AE, Brown J, Oldham JM. Childhood verbal abuse and risk for personality disorders during adolescence and early adulthood. *Compr Psychiatry*. Jan-Feb 2001; 42(1):16–23. doi:10.1053/comp.2001.19755

6. Afifi TO, Mather A, Boman J, et al. Childhood adversity and personality disorders: results from a nationally representative population-based study. *J Psychiatr Res*. Jun 2011; 45(6): 814–822. doi:10.1016/j.jpsychires.2010.11.008

7. Waxman R, Fenton MC, Skodol AE, Grant BF, Hasin D. Childhood maltreatment and personality disorders in the USA: specificity of effects and the impact of gender. *Personal Ment Health*. Feb 2014; 8(1): 30–41. doi:10.1002/pmh.1239

8. Anda RF, Felitti VJ, Bremner JD, et al. The enduring effects of abuse and related adverse experiences in childhood: A convergence of evidence from neurobiology and epidemiology. *Eur Arch Psychiatry Clin Neurosci*. Apr 2006; 256(3): 174–186. doi:10.1007/s00406-005-0624-4

9. Hock RS, Bryce CP, Fischer L, et al. Childhood malnutrition and maltreatment are linked with personality disorder symptoms in adulthood: Results from a Barbados lifespan cohort. *Psychiatry Res*. Nov 2018; 269: 301–308. doi:10.1016/j.psychres.2018.05.085

10. Henrich J, Heine SJ, Norenzayan A. Most people are not WEIRD. *Nature*. Jul 1 2010; 466(7302): 29. doi:10.1038/466029a

11. Arnett JJ. The neglected 95 percent: Why American psychology needs to become less American. *Am Psychol*. Oct 2008; 63(7): 602–614. doi:10.1037/0003-066x.63.7.602

12. Wota AP, Byrne C, Murray I, et al. An examination of childhood trauma in individuals attending an adult mental health service. *Ir J Psychol Med*. Dec 2014; 31(4): 259–270. doi:10.1017/ipm.2014.49

13. Zhang T, Chow A, Wang L, Dai Y, Xiao Z. Role of childhood traumatic experience in personality disorders in China. *Compr Psychiatry*. Aug 2012; 53(6): 829–836. doi:10.1016/j.comppsych.2011.10.004

14. Luke N, Banerjee R. Differentiated associations between childhood maltreatment experiences and social understanding: A meta-analysis and systematic review. *Dev Rev*. 2013; 33(1): 1–28. doi:10.1016/j.dr.2012.10.001

15. Cohen LJ, Ardalan F, Tanis T, et al. Attachment anxiety and avoidance as mediators of the association between childhood maltreatment and adult personality dysfunction. *Attach Hum Dev*. Feb 2017; 19(1): 58–75. doi:10.1080/14616734.2016.1253639

16. Finzi-Dottan R, Karu T. From emotional abuse in childhood to psychopathology in adulthood: a path mediated by immature defense mechanisms and self-esteem. *J Nerv Ment Dis*. Aug 2006; 194(8): 616–621. doi:10.1097/01.nmd.0000230654.49933.23

17. Traumatic Stress Disorder Fact Sheet. Sidran Institute Traumatic Stress Education and Advocacy website. https://www.sidran.org/wp-content/uploads/2018/11/Post-Traumatic-Stress-Disorder-Fact-Sheet-.pdf.

18. Gogtay N, Giedd JN, Lusk L, et al. Dynamic mapping of human cortical development during childhood through early adulthood. *Proc Natl Acad Sci U S A*. May 25 2004; 101(21): 8174–8179. doi:10.1073/pnas.0402680101

19. Lenroot RK, Gogtay N, Greenstein DK, et al. Sexual dimorphism of brain developmental trajectories during childhood and adolescence. *Neuroimage*. Jul 15 2007; 36(4): 1065–1073. doi:10.1016/j.neuroimage.2007.03.053

20. Shaw P, Kabani NJ, Lerch JP, et al. Neurodevelopmental trajectories of the human cerebral cortex. *J Neurosci.* Apr 2 2008; 28(14): 3586–3594. doi:10.1523/jneurosci.5309-07.2008

21. Cattane N, Rossi R, Lanfredi M, Cattaneo A. Borderline personality disorder and childhood trauma: Exploring the affected biological systems and mechanisms. *BMC Psychiatry.* Jun 15 2017; 17(1): 221. doi:10.1186/s12888-017-1383-82

22. Zelkowitz P, Paris J, Guzder J, Feldman R. Diatheses and stressors in borderline pathology of childhood: the role of neuropsychological risk and trauma. *J Am Acad Child Adolesc Psychiatry.* Jan 2001; 40(1): 100–105. doi:10.1097/00004583-200101000-00022

23. Gunderson JG, Herpertz SC, Skodol AE, Torgersen S, Zanarini MC. Borderline personality disorder. *Nat Rev Dis Primers.* May 24 2018; 4: 18029. doi:10.1038/nrdp.2018.29

24. Ibrahim J, Cosgrave N, Woolgar M. Childhood maltreatment and its link to borderline personality disorder features in children: A systematic review approach. *Clin Child Psychol Psychiatry.* Jan 2018; 23(1): 57–76. doi:10.1177/1359104517712778

25. Lynch TR, Chapman AL, Rosenthal MZ, Kuo JR, Linehan MM. Mechanisms of change in dialectical behavior therapy: theoretical and empirical observations. *J Clin Psychol.* 2006; 62(4): 459–480. doi:10.1002/jclp.20243

26. Laporte L, Paris J, Guttman H, Russell J. Psychopathology, childhood trauma, and personality traits in patients with borderline personality disorder and their sisters. *J Pers Disord.* Aug 2011; 25(4): 448–462. doi:10.1521/pedi.2011.25.4.448

27. Russo M, Mahon K, Shanahan M, et al. The association between childhood trauma and facial emotion recognition in adults with bipolar disorder. *Psychiatry Res.* Oct 30 2015; 229(3): 771–776. doi:10.1016/j.psychres.2015.08.004

28. Rosen V, Ayers G. An update on the complexity and importance of accurately diagnosing post-traumatic stress disorder and comorbid traumatic brain injury. *Neurosci Insights.* 2020; 15: 2633105520907895. doi:10.1177/2633105520907895

29. Brambilla P, Soloff PH, Sala M, Nicoletti MA, Keshavan MS, Soares JC. Anatomical MRI study of borderline personality disorder patients. *Psychiatry Res Neuroimaging.* 2004/07/30/ 2004; 131(2): 125–133. doi:https://doi.org/10.1016/j.pscychresns.2004.04.003

30. Driessen M, Herrmann J, Stahl K, et al. Magnetic resonance imaging volumes of the hippocampus and the amygdala in women with borderline personality disorder and early traumatization. *Arch Gen Psychiatry.* 2000; 57(12): 1115–1122. doi:10.1001/archpsyc.57.12.1115

31. Weniger G, Lange C, Sachsse U, Irle E. Reduced amygdala and hippocampus size in trauma-exposed women with borderline personality disorder and without posttraumatic stress disorder. *J Psychiatry Neurosci.* 2009/09; 34(5): 383–388.

32. Irle E, Lange C, Sachsse U. Reduced size and abnormal asymmetry of parietal cortex in women with borderline personality disorder. *Biol Psychiatry.* 01/15/2005; 57(2): 173–182. doi:https://doi.org/10.1016/j.biopsych.2004.10.004

33. Logue MW, van Rooij SJH, Dennis EL, et al. Smaller hippocampal volume in posttraumatic stress disorder: a multisite ENIGMA-PGC study: subcortical volumetry results from posttraumatic stress disorder consortia. Biol Psychiatry. Feb 1 2018; 83(3): 244–253. doi:10.1016/j.biopsych.2017.09.006

34. Schulze L, Schulze A, Renneberg B, Schmahl C, Niedtfeld I. Neural correlates of affective disturbances: a comparative meta-analysis of negative affect processing in borderline personality disorder, major depressive disorder, and posttraumatic stress disorder. *Biol Psychiatry.* 2019/03/01; 4(3): 220–232. doi:https://doi.org/10.1016/j.bpsc.2018.11.004

35. Jin X, Zhong M, Yao S, et al. A voxel-based morphometric MRI study in young adults with borderline personality disorder. *PLOS ONE.* 2016; 11(1): e0147938. doi:10.1371/journal.pone.0147938

36. Hebscher M, Ibrahim C, Gilboa A. Precuneus stimulation alters the neural dynamics of autobiographical memory retrieval. *NeuroImage* 2020/01/20; 2020: 116575. doi:https://doi.org/10.1016/j.neuroimage.2020.116575

37. Nenadic I, Voss A, Besteher B, Langbein K, Gaser C. Brain structure and symptom dimensions in borderline personality disorder. *Eur Psychiatry.* Feb 7 2020; 63(1): e9. doi:10.1192/j.eurpsy.2019.16

38. Walton M, Rudebeck PH, Behrens T, Rushworth MF. Cingulate and orbitofrontal contributions to valuing knowns and unknowns in a changeable world. In: Delgado MR, Phelps EA, Robbins TW, eds. *Decision Making, Affect, and Learning: Attention and Performance XXIII.* New York: Oxford University Press; 2011:235.

39. Pechtel P, Pizzagalli DA. Effects of early life stress on cognitive and affective function: an integrated review of human literature. *Psychopharmacology (Berl).* Mar 2011; 214(1): 55–70. doi:10.1007/s00213-010-2009-2

40. Bilek E, Itz ML, Stößel G, et al. Deficient amygdala habituation to threatening stimuli in borderline personality disorder relates to adverse childhood experiences. *Biol Psychiatry.* 2019/12/15; 86(12): 930–938. doi:10.1016/j.biopsych.2019.06.008

41. Herpertz SC, Dietrich TM, Wenning B, et al. Evidence of abnormal amygdala functioning in borderline personality disorder: a functional MRI study. *Biol Psychiatry.* 2001/08/15; 50(4): 292–298. doi:https://doi.org/10.1016/S0006-3223(01)01075-7

42. Minzenberg MJ, Fan J, New AS, Tang CY, Siever LJ. Fronto-limbic dysfunction in response to facial emotion in borderline personality disorder: An event-related fMRI study. *Psychiatry Res Neuroimaging.* 2007/08/15; 155(3): 231–243. doi:10.1016/j.pscychresns.2007.03.006

43. Powers AD, Thomas KM, Ressler KJ, Bradley B. The differential effects of child abuse and posttraumatic stress disorder on schizotypal personality disorder. *Compr Psychiatry.* Jul-Aug 2011; 52(4): 438–445. doi:10.1016/j.comppsych.2010.08.001

44. Liu J, Gong J, Nie G, et al. The mediating effects of childhood neglect on the association between schizotypal and autistic personality traits and depression in a non-clinical sample. *BMC Psychiatry.* Oct 25 2017; 17(1): 352. doi:10.1186/s12888-017-1510-0

45. Velikonja T, Fisher HL, Mason O, Johnson S. Childhood trauma and schizotypy: a systematic literature review. *Psychol Med.* Apr 2015; 45(5): 947–963. doi:10.1017/s0033291714002086

46. Berenbaum H, Thompson RJ, Milanek ME, Boden MT, Bredemeier K. Psychological trauma and schizotypal personality disorder. *J Abnorm Psychol.* Aug 2008; 117(3): 502–519. doi:10.1037/0021-843x.117.3.502

47. Reynolds CA, Raine A, Mellingen K, Venables PH, Mednick SA. Three-factor model of schizotypal personality: invariance across culture, gender, religious affiliation, family adversity, and psychopathology. *Schizophr Bull.* 2000; 26(3): 603–618. doi:10.1093/oxfordjournals.schbul.a033481

48. Heins M, Simons C, Lataster T, et al. Childhood trauma and psychosis: a case-control and case-sibling comparison across different levels of genetic liability, psychopathology, and type of trauma. *Am J Psychiatry.* Dec 2011; 168(12): 1286–1294. doi:10.1176/appi.ajp.2011.10101531

49. Steel C, Marzillier S, Fearon P, Ruddle A. Childhood abuse and schizotypal personality. *Soc Psychiatry Psychiatr Epidemiol.* Nov 2009; 44(11): 917–923. doi:10.1007/s00127-009-0038-0

50. Velikonja T, Velthorst E, McClure MM, et al. Severe childhood trauma and clinical and neurocognitive features in schizotypal personality disorder. *Acta Psychiatr Scand.* Jul 2019; 140(1): 50–64. doi:10.1111/acps.13032

51. Quidé Y, Cohen-Woods S, O'Reilly N, Carr VJ, Elzinga BM, Green MJ. Schizotypal personality traits and social cognition are associated with childhood trauma exposure. *Br J Clin Psychol.* Nov 2018; 57(4): 397–419. doi:10.1111/bjc.12187

52. Morrison AP, Frame L, Larkin W. Relationships between trauma and psychosis: a review and integration. *Br J Clin Psychol.* Nov 2003; 42(Pt 4): 331–353. doi:10.1348/014466503322528892

53. Steel C, Fowler D, Holmes EA. Trauma-related intrusions and psychosis: an information processing account. *Behav Cogn Psychother.* 2005; 33(2): 139–152. doi:10.1017/S1352465804001924

54. Larøi F, Van der Linden M, Marczewski P. The effects of emotional salience, cognitive effort and meta-cognitive beliefs on a reality monitoring task in hallucination-prone subjects. *Br J Clin Psychol.* Sep 2004; 43(Pt 3): 221–233. doi:10.1348/0144665031752970

55. Lawrence T, Edwards C, Barraclough N, Church S, Hetherington F. Modelling childhood causes of paranormal belief and experience: childhood trauma and childhood fantasy. *Pers Individ Differ.* 1995; 19(2): 209–215. doi:10.1016/0191-8869(95)00034-4

56. Selten JP, van der Ven E, Rutten BP, Cantor-Graae E. The social defeat hypothesis of schizophrenia: an update. *Schizophr Bull.* Nov 2013; 39(6): 1180–1186. doi:10.1093/schbul/sbt134

57. Valmaggia LR, Day F, Garety P, et al. Social defeat predicts paranoid appraisals in people at high risk for psychosis. *Schizophr Res.* Oct 2015; 168(1-2): 16–22. doi:10.1016/j.schres.2015.07.050

58. Seo J, Choi JY. Social defeat as a mediator of the relationship between childhood trauma and paranoid ideation. *Psychiatry Res.* Feb 2018; 260: 48–52. doi:10.1016/j.psychres.2017.11.028

59. Irwin HJ. The relationship between dissociative tendencies and schizotypy: an artifact of childhood trauma? *J Clin Psychol.* Mar 2001; 57(3): 331–342. doi:10.1002/jclp.1015

60. Raine A, Mellingen K, Liu J, Venables P, Mednick SA. Effects of environmental enrichment at ages 3-5 years on schizotypal personality and antisocial behavior at ages 17 and 23 years. *Am J Psychiatry.* Sep 2003; 160(9): 1627–1635. doi:10.1176/appi.ajp.160.9.1627

61. Koenigsberg HW, Buchsbaum MS, Buchsbaum BR, et al. Functional MRI of visuospatial working memory in schizotypal personality disorder: a region-of-interest analysis. *Psychol Med.* 2005; 35(7): 1019–1030. doi:10.1017/S0033291705004393

62. Buchsbaum MS, Trestman RL, Hazlett E, et al. Regional cerebral blood flow during the Wisconsin Card Sort Test in schizotypal personality disorder. *Schizophr Res.* Oct 17 1997; 27(1): 21–28. doi:10.1016/s0920-9964(97)00081-9

63. Lee R. Mistrustful and misunderstood: a review of paranoid personality disorder. *Curr Behav Neurosci Rep.* Jun 2017; 4(2): 151–165. doi:10.1007/s40473-017-0116-7

64. *Diagnostic and Statistical Manual of Mental Disorders: DSM-5*, 5th ed. Washington, DC: American Psychiatric Association; 2013.

65. Iacovino JM, Jackson JJ, Oltmanns TF. The relative impact of socioeconomic status and childhood trauma on Black-White differences in paranoid personality disorder symptoms. *J Abnorm Psychol.* Feb 2014; 123(1): 225–230. doi:10.1037/a0035258

66. Whaley AL. Cross-cultural perspective on paranoia: a focus on the black American experience. Psychiatr Q. Winter 1998; 69(4): 325–343. doi:10.1023/a:1022134231763

67. Turkat ID, Banks DS. Paranoid personality and its disorder. *J Psychopathol Behav Assess.* 1987; 9(3): 295–304. doi:10.1007/BF00964558

68. Freeman D. Suspicious minds: the psychology of persecutory delusions. *Clin Psychol Rev.* May 2007; 27(4): 425–457. doi:10.1016/j.cpr.2006.10.004

69. Johnson JG, Smailes EM, Cohen P, Brown J, Bernstein DP. Associations between four types of childhood neglect and personality disorder symptoms during adolescence and early adulthood: findings of a community-based longitudinal study. *J Pers Disord.* Summer 2000; 14(2): 171–187. doi:10.1521/pedi.2000.14.2.171

70. Thomas CR, Russell W, Robert RS, Holzer CE, Blakeney P, Meyer WJ. Personality disorders in young adult survivors of pediatric burn injury. *J Pers Disord.* Apr 2012; 26(2): 255–266. doi:10.1521/pedi.2012.26.2.255

71. Johnson J, Jones C, Lin A, Wood S, Heinze K, Jackson C. Shame amplifies the association between stressful life events and paranoia amongst young adults using mental health services: Implications for understanding risk and psychological resilience. *Psychiatry Res.* Dec 15 2014; 220(1-2): 217–225. doi:10.1016/j.psychres.2014.07.022

72. Natsuaki MN, Cicchetti D, Rogosch FA. Examining the developmental history of child maltreatment, peer relations, and externalizing problems among adolescents with symptoms of paranoid personality disorder. *Dev Psychopathol.* Fall 2009; 21(4): 1181–1193. doi:10.1017/s0954579409990101

73. Bowlby J. *Attachment and Loss: Vol 2. Loss.* New York: Basic Books, 1980.

74. Beck AT, Butler AC, Brown GK, Dahlsgaard KK, Newman CF, Beck JS. Dysfunctional beliefs discriminate personality disorders. *Behav Res Ther.* Oct 2001; 39(10): 1213–1225. doi:10.1016/s0005-7967(00)00099-1

75. Thompson-Pope SK, Turkat ID. Reactions to ambiguous stimuli among paranoid personalities. *J Psychopathol Behav Assess.* 1988; 10(1): 21–32. doi:10.1007/BF00962982

76. Fergusson DM, Boden JM, Horwood LJ. Exposure to childhood sexual and physical abuse and adjustment in early adulthood. *Child Abuse Negl.* Jun 2008; 32(6): 607–619. doi:10.1016/j.chiabu.2006.12.018

77. DeLisi M, Drury AJ, Elbert MJ. The etiology of antisocial personality disorder: The differential roles of adverse childhood experiences and childhood psychopathology. *Compr Psychiatry.* Jul 2019; 92: 1–6. doi:10.1016/j.comppsych.2019.04.001

78. Dargis M, Newman J, Koenigs M. Clarifying the link between childhood abuse history and psychopathic traits in adult criminal offenders. *Personal Disord.* Jul 2016; 7(3): 221–228. doi:10.1037/per0000147

79. Kimonis ER, Cross B, Howard A, Donoghue K. Maternal care, maltreatment and callous-unemotional traits among urban male juvenile offenders. *J Youth Adolesc.* Feb 2013; 42(2): 165–177. doi:10.1007/s10964-012-9820-5

80. Battle CL, Shea MT, Johnson DM, et al. Childhood maltreatment associated with adult personality disorders: findings from the Collaborative Longitudinal Personality Disorders Study. *J Pers Disord.* Apr 2004; 18(2): 193–211. doi:10.1521/pedi.18.2.193.32777

81. Weiler BL, Widom CS. Psychopathy and violent behaviour in abused and neglected young adults. *Crim Behav Ment Health.* 1996; 6(3): 253–271. doi:10.1002/cbm.99

82. Fox BH, Perez N, Cass E, Baglivio MT, Epps N. Trauma changes everything: examining the relationship between adverse childhood experiences and serious, violent and chronic juvenile offenders. *Child Abuse Negl.* Aug 2015; 46: 163–173. doi:10.1016/j.chiabu.2015.01.011

83. Lykken DT. Psychopathy, sociopathy, and crime. *Society (New Brunswick)*. 1996; 34(1): 29–38. doi:10.1007/BF02696999

84. Kochanska G. Multiple pathways to conscience for children with different temperaments: from toddlerhood to age 5. *Dev Psychol*. Mar 1997; 33(2): 228–240. doi:10.1037//0012-1649.33.2.228

85. Patrick CJ, Fowles DC, Krueger RF. Triarchic conceptualization of psychopathy: developmental origins of disinhibition, boldness, and meanness. *Dev Psychopathol*. Summer 2009; 21(3): 913–938. doi:10.1017/s0954579409000492

86. DeLisi M, Vaughn MG. Foundation for a temperament-based theory of antisocial behavior and criminal justice system involvement. *J Crim Justice*. 2014; 42(1): 10–25. doi:10.1016/j.jcrimjus.2013.11.001

87. DeLisi M, Fox BH, Fully M, Vaughn MG. The effects of temperament, psychopathy, and childhood trauma among delinquent youth: A test of DeLisi and Vaughn's temperament-based theory of crime. *Int J Law Psychiatry*. Mar-Apr 2018; 57: 53–60. doi:10.1016/j.ijlp.2018.01.006

88. Shi Z, Bureau JF, Easterbrooks MA, Zhao X, Lyons-Ruth K. Childhood maltreatment and prospectively observed quality of early care as predictors of antisocial personality disorder features. *Infant Ment Health J*. Jan 2012; 33(1): 55–96. doi:10.1002/imhj.20295

89. Russ E, Heim A, Westen D. Parental bonding and personality pathology assessed by clinician report. *J Pers Disord*. Dec 2003; 17(6): 522–536. doi:10.1521/pedi.17.6.522.25351

90. Levy T, Orlans M. Kids who kill: attachment disorder, antisocial personality and violence. *The Forensic Examiner*. 1999; 8(3-4): 19–24.

91. Dodge KA, Coie JD. Social-information-processing factors in reactive and proactive aggression in children's peer groups. *J Pers Soc Psychol*. Dec 1987; 53(6): 1146–1158. doi:10.1037//0022-3514.53.6.1146

92. Dodge KA, Murphy RR, Buchsbaum K. The assessment of intention-cue detection skills in children: implications for developmental psychopathology. *Child Dev*. Feb 1984; 55(1): 163–173.

93. Kolla NJ, Malcolm C, Attard S, Arenovich T, Blackwood N, Hodgins S. Childhood maltreatment and aggressive behaviour in violent offenders with psychopathy. *Can J Psychiatry*. Aug 2013; 58(8): 487–494. doi:10.1177/070674371305800808

94. Barkataki I, Kumari V, Das M, Taylor P, Sharma T. Volumetric structural brain abnormalities in men with schizophrenia or antisocial personality disorder. *Behav Brain Res*. 2006/05/15/ 2006; 169(2): 239–247. doi:https://doi.org/10.1016/j.bbr.2006.01.009

95. Gregory S, ffytche D, Simmons A, et al. The antisocial brain: psychopathy matters: a structural MRI investigation of antisocial male violent offenders. *Arch Gen Psychiatry*. 2012; 69(9): 962–972. doi:10.1001/archgenpsychiatry.2012.222

96. Olson IR, Plotzker A, Ezzyat Y. The enigmatic temporal pole: a review of findings on social and emotional processing. *Brain*. Jul 2007; 130(Pt 7): 1718–1731. doi:10.1093/brain/awm052

97. Bludau S, Eickhoff SB, Mohlberg H, et al. Cytoarchitecture, probability maps and functions of the human frontal pole. *Neuroimage*. Jun 2014; 93 Pt 2: 260–275. doi:10.1016/j.neuroimage.2013.05.052

98. Boccardi M, Frisoni GB, Hare RD, et al. Cortex and amygdala morphology in psychopathy. *Psychiatry Res*. Aug 30 2011; 193(2): 85–92. doi:10.1016/j.pscychresns.2010.12.013

99. Raine A, Lee L, Yang Y, Colletti P. Neurodevelopmental marker for limbic maldevelopment in antisocial personality disorder and psychopathy. *Br J Psychiatry*. 2018; 197(3): 186–192. doi:10.1192/bjp.bp.110.078485

100. Kolla NJ, Patel R, Meyer JH, Chakravarty MM. Association of monoamine oxidase-A genetic variants and amygdala morphology in violent offenders with antisocial personality disorder and high psychopathic traits. *Sci Rep*. 2017/08/29; 7(1): 9607. doi:10.1038/s41598-017-08351-w

101. Tottenham N, Hare TA, Quinn BT, et al. Prolonged institutional rearing is associated with atypically large amygdala volume and difficulties in emotion regulation. *Dev Sci*. Jan 1 2010; 13(1): 46–61. doi:10.1111/j.1467-7687.2009.00852.x

4

Integrating Clinical and Empirical Approaches to Personality

The Shedler-Westen Assessment Procedure (SWAP)

Jonathan Shedler

Author's Note: This chapter is adapted from: Shedler J. Integrating clinical and empirical perspectives on personality: The Shedler-Westen Assessment Procedure (SWAP). In: Huprich SK, ed. *Personality Disorders: Toward Theoretical and Empirical Integration in Diagnosis and Assessment*. Washington, DC: American Psychological Association; 2015. The case of Melania is adapted from Lingiardi V, Shedler, J, Gazillo, F. Assessing personality change in psychotherapy with the SWAP-200: a case study. *J Pers Assess*. 2006; 86: 23–32.

> It is well known that [Paul Meehl] not only thinks it important for a psychologist to work as a responsible professional with real-life clinical problems but, further, considers the purely 'theoretical' personality research of academic psychologists to be unusually naïve and unrealistic when the researcher is not a seasoned, practicing clinician.
> —Paul Meehl, *Why I Never Attend Case Conferences*

Key Points

- There has been a disconnect between clinical and research approaches to personality. Empirical research has not built on clinical knowledge and understanding.
- The Shedler-Westen Assessment Procedure (SWAP) is an assessment method that integrates the strengths of clinical and empirical approaches.
- SWAP provides a standard vocabulary for clinical case description, preserving the richness and complexity of clinical case formulation while allowing clinicians to describe personality functioning in a systematic and quantifiable way.
- SWAP relies on what clinicians do best: describe individual patients they know well. It relies on statistical methods to do what they do best: combine information optimally to maximize reliability and validity.
- SWAP research in large patient samples has identified a taxonomy of personality diagnoses that is empirically based and captures the richness and complexity

of clinical understanding. The empirically based diagnostic taxonomy validates descriptions of personality syndromes found in the clinical literature.

- The SWAP instrument provides diagnostic scores for DSM-5 personality disorder diagnoses, diagnostic scores for the empirically based diagnostic taxonomy, and narrative case descriptions that can guide clinical treatment.
- The use of SWAP for both diagnosis and clinical case formulation is illustrated via a case of a patient in treatment for personality pathology.
- The clinical richness and relevance of the empirically derived personality taxonomy is illustrated via the borderline personality diagnosis.
- Evidence for reliability and validity is reviewed.

Introduction

There is often a disconnect between clinical knowledge and empirical research. This disconnect is pronounced when it comes to conceptualizing personality. For expert clinicians, personality assessment generally means *clinical case formulation*: understanding the patterns of thought, feeling, motivation, defenses, interpersonal functioning, experiencing self and others, and so on, that make a person unique and (if they are a patient) underlie their suffering.

Expert clinicians attend not only to what patients say but *how* they say it, drawing inferences from patients' accounts of their lives and relationships, from their interactions with the clinician in the consulting room, and from their own emotional responses to the patient.[1,2,3]

For example, skilled clinicians do not assess lack of empathy, a central feature of narcissistic personality, by administering questionnaires or asking direct questions about empathy. A moment's reflection reveals the dilemma: it would be a rare narcissistic patient who could report their own lack of empathy. More likely, the patient would describe themselves as a wonderful friend, perhaps the best ever. An initial sign of lack of empathy on the part of the patient may be a subtle feeling *in the clinician* of being interchangeable or replaceable, of feeling devalued, or being used as little more than a sounding board.[1,3,4]

The clinician's emotional responses become a data source for generating clinical hypotheses. The clinician might go on to consider whether they frequently feel this way with this patient and whether such feelings are usual in their clinical role. They might then become aware that the patient describes others more in terms of the functions they serve than who they are as people. The clinician might go on to consider how these observations dovetail with the patient's history and the problems that brought them to treatment. This kind of thinking lies at the heart of clinical case formulation.

In contrast, research-based approaches to personality eschew clinical judgment and inference. In psychiatry, successive editions of the *Diagnostic and Statistical Manual of Mental Disorders* (DSM) have minimized the role of inference, treating personality diagnosis as an essentially technical task of tabulating readily observable diagnostic criteria.[5]

In academic psychology, personality research has focused on dimensional trait models, notably the Five Factor Model and its variants.[6] The model derives from factor analysis of questionnaires and was developed without input from clinical practitioners. While it has been useful for many purposes and generative for research, clinicians expert in treating personality pathology see it as removed from their clinical understanding and concerns.[7-10]

The Science–Practice Schism

There is no reason we must choose between clinical depth and scientific rigor. Good clinical case formulation and good science have much in common. Clinical case formulation involves an ongoing, cyclical process of data collection, hypothesis generation, hypothesis testing, and hypothesis revision. Empirical research involves clinically informed (one hopes) judgment and inference at every step, from what to study, to how to conceptualize and operationalize it, to how to interpret findings and revise hypotheses as new data emerge.

Ideally, both activities involve a reciprocal interplay between the observations and judgments necessary to generate sound hypotheses and the investigation necessary to test them—what philosopher of science Hans Reichenbach[11] termed the *context of discovery* and the *context of justification*. Without a credible context of justification, clinical personality theory can look to empirical researchers like unfalsifiable conjecture. Without a credible context of discovery, empirical personality research can be clinically naïve and unhelpful to practitioners.[12,13]

Diagnosis and Case Formulation, Clinical and Statistical

The approach to personality described here, based on the *Shedler-Westen Assessment Procedure* (SWAP), bridges clinical and empirical approaches to personality and integrates the strengths of each. The approach relies on clinicians to do what clinicians do best: observe and describe individual patients they know well. It relies on statistical methods to do what they do best: combine information optimally to maximize reliability, validity, and predictive accuracy.[14-16] The goal is to provide a means of conceptualizing and assessing personality that is both clinically relevant and scientifically sound.

The remainder of this chapter will (a) discuss the challenges of incorporating clinical observation and inference in research; (b) describe the development of the SWAP as a method for systematizing clinical case description; (c) illustrate its use for both diagnosis and clinical case formulation; and (d) describe a diagnostic system for personality that is both empirically and clinically valid.

The Challenge of Clinical Data

It is a truism that "clinical judgment is unreliable," but truisms are not truths. The problem with clinical observation and inference is *not* that they are unreliable, as researchers often repeat.[16] The problem, rather, is that they come in a form difficult to work with. Rulers measure in inches and scales measure in pounds, but what metric do clinical assessors share? Consider three clinicians describing the same case. One might speak of beliefs and schemas, another of learning and conditioning, and the third, perhaps, of transference and resistance. It is not readily apparent whether the clinicians can or cannot make the same observations and inferences.

There are three possibilities: (1) The clinicians may be observing the same thing but using different language and metaphor systems to describe it; (2) they may be attending to different aspects of the clinical material, as in the parable of the elephant and the blind men; or (3) they may not, in fact be able to make the same observations. *To find out whether the clinicians can make the same observations and inferences, we must ensure they speak the same language and attend to the full range of relevant clinical phenomena.*

A Standard Vocabulary for Case Description

The Shedler-Westen Assessment Procedure (SWAP) is a tool for personality diagnosis and case formulation that provides clinicians of all theoretical orientations with a common vocabulary for case description.[5,17–21] The vocabulary consists of 200 personality-descriptive statements, each of which may describe a given patient very well, somewhat, or not at all. A clinician describes a patient by ranking the statements into eight categories, from most descriptive of the patient (scored 7) to not descriptive or irrelevant (scored 0). Thus, SWAP yields a score from 0 to 7 for 200 personality-descriptive variables.

The "standard vocabulary" of the SWAP allows clinicians to provide comprehensive, in-depth psychological descriptions of patients in a form that is systematic and quantifiable. SWAP statements stay close to the clinical data (e.g., "Tends to get into power struggles," or "Is capable of sustaining meaningful relationships characterized by genuine intimacy and caring"), and statements that require inference or deduction are written in clear, jargon-free language (e.g., "Tends to express anger in passive and indirect ways [e.g., may make mistakes, procrastinate, forget, become sulky, etc.]" or "Tends to see own unacceptable feelings or impulses in other people instead of in him/herself").

The major editions of the SWAP instrument are the SWAP-200 and the revised SWAP-II (their precursor was the SWAP-167).[22] In this chapter, I use the acronym *SWAP* to refer to concepts and findings that apply to both major editions of the instrument and specify SWAP-200 or SWAP-II where the information applies to a specific edition. Clinicians can complete a SWAP-200 assessment online and receive a comprehensive assessment report at www.SWAPassessment.org. (Versions of the SWAP have also been developed for adolescent personality assessment[23,24] but are beyond the scope of this chapter.)

SWAP Item Set

The initial SWAP item pool was drawn from a range of sources including: clinical literature on personality pathology written over the past 50 years[4,25–28]; DSM Axis II diagnostic criteria included in DSM-III through DSM-5; selected DSM Axis I criteria that could reflect enduring dispositions (for example, depression and anxiety); research on coping, defense, and affect regulation[13,29–31]; research on interpersonal functioning in patients with personality disorders[32,33]; research on personality traits in non-clinical populations[34–36]; research on personality pathology conducted since the development of DSM Axis II[37]; pilot studies in which observers watched videotaped interviews of patients with personality disorders and described them using draft versions of the SWAP item set; and the clinical experience of the SWAP authors.

Most important, the current SWAP item set is the product of a 16-year iterative item revision process that incorporated the feedback of thousands of clinician-consultants of all theoretical orientations who used earlier versions of the instrument to describe their patients. We asked each clinician-consultant one crucial question: "Were you able to describe the things you consider psychologically important about your patient?" If the answer was "no," we asked the clinician to describe what they could not express with the SWAP items. We added, rewrote, and revised items based on this feedback, then asked new clinician-consultants to describe new patients. We repeated this process over many iterations until most clinicians could answer "yes" most of the time.[21]

The methods used to develop and refine the SWAP item set ensured inclusion of clinically crucial concepts that are not addressed by other personality item sets. For example, virtually all clinical theorists regard the defense of projection as a central, defining feature of paranoid personality, but neither DSM nor dimensional trait models address it. SWAP captures and quantifies projection with the item, "Tends to see own unacceptable feelings or impulses in other people instead of in himself/herself."

Similarly, clinical theorists have identified the phenomena of *splitting* and *projective identification* as central, pathognomonic features of borderline personality,[2,4,25,38,39] but they are strikingly absent from both the DSM and from dimensional trait models of personality. SWAP-II addresses splitting with items like, "When upset, has trouble perceiving both positive and negative qualities in the same person at the same time (e.g., may see others in black or white terms, shift suddenly from seeing someone as caring to seeing him/her as malevolent and intentionally hurtful, etc.)," and "Expresses contradictory feelings or beliefs without being disturbed by the inconsistency; has little need to reconcile or resolve contradictory ideas." It addresses projective identification with items like, "Manages to elicit in others feelings similar to those s/he is experiencing (e.g., when angry, acts in such a way as to provoke anger in others; when anxious, acts in such a way as to induce anxiety in others)," and "Tends to draw others into scenarios, or 'pull' them into roles, that feel alien or unfamiliar (e.g., being uncharacteristically insensitive or cruel, feeling like the only person in the world who can help, etc.)."

I provide these examples to illustrate that it is possible to conduct systematic empirical research without sacrificing clinical richness and complexity, and possible to operationalize clinical (in this instance, psychodynamic) constructs that many empirical investigators dismiss as not researchable. I am not (yet) making claims about the validity of the underlying clinical theories. I am making the point that such clinical concepts, which reflect the accrued experience of generations of clinically skilled observers, *deserve to be taken seriously as research hypotheses to test.* Neither DSM-based structured interviews nor Five Factor Model instruments can provide data to confirm or disconfirm the clinical hypotheses because they make no effort to address them.

The methods used to develop and refine the SWAP item set were successful in creating a relatively comprehensive vocabulary for clinical case description. In a sample of 1,201 psychologists and psychiatrists who used SWAP-II to describe a current patient, 84 percent agreed or strongly agreed "The SWAP-II allowed me to express the things I consider important about my patient's personality" (fewer than 5 percent disagreed).

Scoring SWAP

The SWAP is based on the Q-Sort method which requires assessors to assign each score (0 to 7) a specified number of times (i.e., it uses a "fixed" score distribution). The fixed score distribution is asymmetric, with many items receiving low scores and progressively fewer items receiving higher scores. The shape of the fixed distribution mirrors the naturally occurring distribution in the population. Use of a fixed distribution has psychometric advantages, including reducing measurement error or noise inherent in standard rating scales (for discussion of this and other psychometric issues see [40-42]).

When SWAP is used in the context of psychotherapy, an experienced clinician can score the instrument after a minimum of six clinical contact hours with a patient. If a patient or subject is seen for assessment only—for example, in research, forensic, or personnel assessment contexts—SWAP can be scored on the basis of the Clinical Diagnostic Interview (CDI; available at www.SWAPassessment.org), which systematizes and compresses into an approximately 2½-hour time frame the kind of interviewing expert clinicians engage in to assess personality.[16,43-45] SWAP can also be scored reliably from other comparably psychologically rich interview sources.[46]

Capturing Complexity and Nuance

Just as academic researchers tend to be skeptical about clinical inference, clinicians sometimes express skepticism that *any* structured instrument can do justice to the richness, complexity, and uniqueness of a person's psychology. However, SWAP statements can be combined in virtually infinite patterns to capture complex, nuanced psychological phenomena, and convey meanings that transcend the content of individual items. The configuration of items is more than the sum of its parts.

Consider the meaning of the SWAP item, "Tends to be sexually seductive or provocative." Considered in isolation, the implications for personality diagnosis are unclear. However, if a patient receives a high score on this item along with high scores on the items, "Has an exaggerated sense of self-importance (e.g., feels special, superior, grand, or envied)" and "Seems to treat others primarily as an audience to witness own importance, brilliance, beauty, etc.," a portrait begins to emerge of a narcissistically organized person who seeks sexual attention to bolster their sense of importance and desirability.

If the same patient also receives high scores on the items, "Tends to feel s/he is not his/her true self with others; may feel false or fraudulent" and "Tends to feel s/he is inadequate, inferior, or a failure," a more complex portrait begins to emerge. The items, in combination, indicate that grandiosity co-exists with feelings of inadequacy, and suggests the clinical hypothesis that grandiosity masks or compensates for painful feelings of inadequacy. This duality is central to narcissistic personality dynamics.[47]

If the item "Tends to be sexually seductive or provocative" is instead combined with the items, "Tends to fear s/he will be rejected or abandoned," "Appears to fear being alone; may go to great lengths to avoid being alone," and "Tends to be ingratiating or submissive (e.g., consents to things s/he does not want to do, in the hope of getting support or approval)," a portrait begins to emerge a person with a dependent personality style who may rely on sexuality as a means of maintaining attachments in the face of feared rejection.

If the sexual seductiveness item is instead combined with the items, "Tends to act impulsively (e.g., acts without forethought or concern for consequences)," "Takes advantage of others; has little investment in moral values (e.g., puts own needs first, uses or exploits people with little regard for their feelings or welfare, etc.)," and "Experiences little or no remorse for harm or injury caused to others," a portrait begins to emerge of a person with a psychopathic personality style who seeks immediate gratification and has no qualms about exploiting others sexually.

These examples illustrate how SWAP items can be combined to communicate complex clinical concepts, and how a single SWAP item can convey a range of different meanings depending on the items that surround and contextualize it. I will further illustrate this with a case example (see section, Bridging Diagnosis and Clinical Case Formulation).

Diagnosis, Syndromal and Dimensional

SWAP-200 generates 37 diagnostic scale scores organized into three score profiles. (Computational algorithms for SWAP-II differ from those of SWAP-200.[21,48]) The score profiles provide (1) dimensional scores for DSM-5 personality disorder diagnoses; (2) dimensional scores for an alternative set of empirically identified personality syndromes (see the section, An Improved System for Personality Diagnosis, below); and (3) dimensional trait scores derived via factor analysis of the SWAP item set.[49] SWAP also provides a Psychological Health Index which measures adaptive psychological resources and capacities, or ego strengths. The SWAP *National Security Edition* includes the Dispositional Indicators of Risk Exposure (DIRE) scale, developed in collaboration with agencies of the United States federal government to assess potential for destructive or high-risk behavior in personnel being evaluated for sensitive positions such as those requiring access to classified information.[50]

SWAP diagnostic scores are expressed as T-scores (Mean = 50, SD = 10) and graphed to create score profiles (see Figure 4.1, p. 94). Each Personality Disorder scale score measures the similarity or "match" between a patient and a *diagnostic prototype* representing each DSM personality disorder in its pure or "ideal" form (for example, a prototypical patient with paranoid personality disorder). Thus, personality disorders are assessed on a continuum: low scores indicate that the patient does not resemble or match the diagnostic prototype, and high scores indicate a strong match.

Where categorical diagnosis is desired (e.g., to facilitate clinical communication, or for "backward compatibility" with the categorical approach of DSM), a score of T ≥ 60 provides a threshold for assigning a categorical diagnosis and a score of T ≥ 55 warrants a diagnosis of "traits" or "features" of a personality disorder. Thus, the patient represented by the solid line in Figure 4.1, p. 94 would receive a DSM diagnosis of "borderline personality disorder with antisocial and histrionic traits."

This approach to dimensional diagnosis preserves a *syndromal* understanding of personality. That is, it views personality as a configuration of functionally interrelated psychological processes (encompassing, for example, interrelated patterns of thinking, feeling, motivation, interpersonal functioning, coping, and defending), not as independent dimensions. *Functionally related* means the personality processes are interdependent, causally linked, and form a psychologically coherent and recognizable configuration or pattern.[51-53]

Dimensional diagnosis follows from the recognition that all personality syndromes fall on a continuum from relatively healthy through severely disturbed. For example,

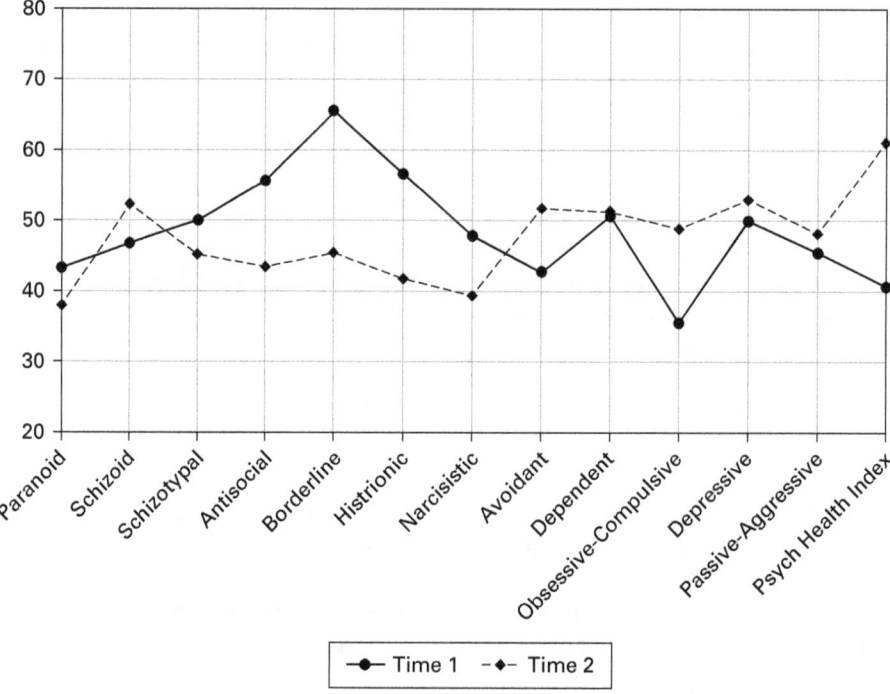

Figure 4.1. SWAP-200 Personality Disorder Score Profile (DSM-5 diagnoses)

a relatively healthy person with an obsessional personality style might be precise, orderly, logical, more comfortable with ideas than feelings, a bit more concerned than most with authority and control, and somewhat rigid in certain areas of thought and behavior. Toward the more severe end of the obsessional continuum, we find individuals who are rigidly dogmatic, have little access to affect, are preoccupied with control, and misapply logic in ways that lead them to miss the forest for the trees. The latter might properly be described as having a "disorder," but the threshold for diagnosing a disorder is a somewhat arbitrary point on a continuum. This is similar to many medical diagnoses, where variables like blood pressure are measured on a continuum, but certain ranges are described categorically as "borderline" or "high."

Although I am emphasizing here the utility of a syndromal approach to personality, SWAP also provides dimensional trait scores, derived via factor analysis of the SWAP item set. Factor analysis of the SWAP item sets yields clinically and empirically coherent personality factors, 12 in the case of SWAP-200[18] and 14 in the case of SWAP-II.[48] These dimensional trait or factor scores provide additional information to supplement syndromal diagnoses and offer another lens through which to view a person.

Syndromal and trait models of personality serve different purposes. Among other things, the former is *person-centered* (focusing on kinds of people) and the latter is *variable-centered* (focusing on kinds of variables). Elsewhere, I have suggested that a diagnostic system is like a good map, in that it must accurately depict the territory.[9] However, sometimes one requires a roadmap, sometimes a topographical map depicting elevations, and sometimes a political map. A roadmap, regardless of its validity, is of little use to a mountaineer. A topographical map is of little use to a motorist. One consequence of the science–practice schism in the field of personality is that there has been virtually no constructive discussion about what kind of map is useful to whom. Academic researchers have lobbied for maps that serve their purposes, citing reliability and validity but failing to recognize that the wrong kind of reliable and valid map may be useless to a clinician who needs a map for a different purpose.

The Case of Melania: Bridging Diagnosis and Clinical Case Formulation

Descriptive diagnosis and clinical case formulation are often viewed as separate activities. SWAP bridges these activities, allowing clinicians and investigators to both make psychiatric diagnoses and derive detailed clinical case formulations from the same data set. I will illustrate with a clinical case example.

Background

Melania is a 30-year-old woman with chief complaints of substance abuse and inability to extricate herself from an abusive relationship. She was diagnosed with substance abuse based on the SCID structured interview, and diagnosed with Borderline Personality Disorder with histrionic traits on the SCID-II. She received a Global Assessment of Functioning score of 45 at intake, indicating significant impairment in functioning.

Melania's early family environment was one of neglect and family strife. A recurring scenario is illustrative: Melania's mother would scream at her husband and say she was leaving him, then lock herself in her room, leaving Melania frightened and in tears. Both parents would then ignore Melania and often forget to feed her. By adolescence, Melania was skipping school and spending her days sleeping or wandering the streets. At age 18 she left home and began "life on the streets," entering a series of chaotic sexual relationships, abusing street drugs, and engaging in petty theft. In her mid-twenties, she moved in with her boyfriend, a small-time drug dealer. She periodically prostituted herself to obtain money or drugs for him.

Melania began psychodynamic therapy at a frequency of three sessions per week. The first 10 sessions were recorded and transcribed. Two clinicians, blind to other data, reviewed the transcripts and scored the SWAP-200 based on the session transcripts. The SWAP-200 item scores were averaged across the two clinical judges to enhance reliability. After two years of psychotherapy, 10 consecutive psychotherapy sessions were again recorded and transcribed, and the SWAP evaluation was repeated.

Descriptive Diagnosis

The solid line in Figure 4.1, p. 94 (Time 1) shows Melania's SWAP-200 scores profile for DSM-5 personality disorder diagnoses. Higher scale scores indicate more severe personality pathology. The Psychological Health Index is graphed as well, which reflects clinicians' consensual understanding of healthy personality functioning.[19] Higher scores on the Psychological Health Index indicate greater psychological strengths and resources.

Melania's score profile shows a marked elevation for borderline personality (T = 65, or one and a half standard deviations above the mean of the clinical reference sample), with secondary elevations for histrionic personality PD (T = 57) and antisocial personality (T = 56). Applying the recommended cut-scores of T ≥ 60 for making a categorical personality disorder diagnosis and T ≥ 55 for diagnosing traits or features, Melania's DSM-5 diagnosis at the start of treatment (Time 1) is "borderline personality disorder with histrionic and antisocial traits." Also noteworthy is the low T-Score of 41 on the Psychological Health Index, nearly a standard deviation below the mean in a reference sample of patients with personality disorder diagnoses. The low score indicates significant dysfunction.

Narrative Case Description

To move from diagnosis to individualized case description, we shift our focus from diagnostic scale scores to individual SWAP items. We can create a narrative description simply by listing the 30 SWAP items with the highest scores (i.e., those scored 5, 6, or 7) and arranging them in paragraph form.

The narrative description for Melania, below, illustrates this approach. The description is constructed exclusively from the 30 SWAP items with scores of 5 or above. To aid the flow of the text, I have grouped conceptually related items, made minor grammatical edits, and added some topic sentences and connecting text (italicized).

Melania experiences severe depression and dysphoria. She tends to feel unhappy, depressed, or despondent, appears to find little or no pleasure or satisfaction in life's activities, feels life is without meaning, and tends to feel like an outcast or outsider. She tends to feel guilty, and to feel inadequate, inferior, or a failure. Her behavior is often self-defeating and self-destructive. She appears inhibited about pursuing goals or successes, is insufficiently concerned with meeting her own needs, and seems not to feel entitled to get or ask for things she deserves. She appears to want to "punish" herself by creating situations that lead to unhappiness or actively avoiding opportunities for pleasure and gratification. *Specific self-destructive tendencies include* getting drawn into and remaining in relationships in which she is emotionally or physically abused, abusing illicit drugs, and acting impulsively and without regard for consequences. She shows little concern for consequences generally.

Melania has personality features associated specifically with borderline personality. Her relationships are unstable, chaotic, and rapidly changing. She has little empathy and seems unable to understand or respond to others' needs and feelings unless they coincide with her own. Moreover, she tends to confuse her own thoughts, feelings, and personality traits with those of others. She often acts in such a way as to elicit her own feelings in other people (for example, provoking anger when she herself is angry, or inducing anxiety in others when she herself is anxious), and she tends to draw people into scenarios or "pull" them into roles that they experience as alien and unfamiliar (e.g., being uncharacteristically cruel, or feeling like the only person in the world who can help).

When upset, Melania has difficulty perceiving positive and negative qualities in the same person at the same time (e.g., she sees others in black or white terms and may shift suddenly from seeing someone as caring to and seeing them as malevolent). She expresses contradictory feelings without being disturbed by the inconsistency and seems to have little need to reconcile or resolve contradictory ideas. She lacks a stable image of who she is or would like to be (e.g., her attitudes, values, goals, and feelings about self are unstable and changing), and she tends to feel empty inside. *Her affect regulation is poor:* She tends to become irrational when strong emotions are stirred up and shows a noticeable decline from her customary level of functioning. She seems unable to soothe or comfort herself when distressed and requires the involvement of another person to help her regulate affect. Both her living arrangements and her work life tend to be chaotic and unstable.

Finally, *Melania's attitudes toward men and sexuality are problematic and conflictual.* She tends to be hostile toward members of the opposite sex (whether consciously or unconsciously), and she associates sexual activity with danger (e.g., injury or punishment). She appears afraid of commitment to a long-term love relationship, instead choosing partners who seem inappropriate in terms of age, status (e.g., social, economic, intellectual), or other factors.

This narrative case description provides an in-depth portrait of a troubled patient with borderline personality pathology, highlighting personality features such as splitting, projective identification, identity diffusion, and affect dysregulation. The description illustrates the difference between descriptive psychiatry (aimed at establishing a diagnosis) and clinical case formulation (aimed at understanding the psychological makeup of a specific individual). However, all the findings presented here are derived from the same quantitative SWAP data.

Melania's case has a happy ending. The dashed line in Figure 4.1, p. 94 shows Melania's personality disorder scores after two years of psychodynamic psychotherapy (Time 2). Her scores on the Borderline, Histrionic, and Antisocial dimensions have dropped below T = 50, and she no longer warrants a DSM-5 personality disorder diagnosis. Her score on the Psychological Health Index has increased by two standard deviations, from 41 to 61, indicating the development of substantial psychological resources and capacities.[54]

Reliability and Validity

Inter-rater reliability of SWAP diagnostic scale scores is above .80 in all studies to date and often above .90.[40,45,46] Median test-retest reliability of SWAP-II personality disorder scales over four to six months is .90, with a range of .86 to .96 for individual scales. Median test-retest reliability for SWAP-II factor (dimensional trait) scales is .85, with a range of .77 to .96.[41] Median alpha reliability (Cronbach's *alpha*) for diagnostic scales for SWAP-II empirically derived personality syndromes is .79, with a range of .72 to .94 (see the section, An Improved System for Personality Diagnosis). These reliability coefficients are at least as strong as those of structured interviews and questionnaires that seek to minimize or eliminate clinical inference. The take-home message is that clinical judgment is highly reliable—when "harnessed" and quantified with appropriate methods.

With respect to validity, SWAP diagnostic scales show predicted relations with an extensive range of external criterion variables in both adult and adolescent samples, including genetic history variables such as psychosis and substance abuse in first- and second-degree biological relatives; developmental history variables such as childhood physical abuse, sexual abuse, animal torture, fire setting, truancy, and other school-related problems; life events such as psychiatric hospitalizations, suicide attempts, arrests, violent criminal behavior, and perpetrating domestic abuse; ratings of occupational functioning, social functioning, and global adaptive functioning; response to mental health treatment; and numerous other measures.[16,18–20,24,41,43,45,46]

There is a well-established literature on the inadequacies of clinical judgment, and it is fair to ask why SWAP yields strong reliability and validity findings that are inconsistent with this literature. The answers are straightforward. First, studies of "clinical judgment" have too often asked clinicians to make predictions about things that fall well outside their legitimate expertise[16] (unfortunately, some clinicians have been all too willing to offer such prognostications). In contrast, SWAP does not ask clinicians to *predict* anything, only to describe patients they know, based on psychological information readily available to them. Second, studies of clinical judgment rarely use appropriate psychometric methods to quantify clinical judgment in a reliable way. Third, studies of clinical judgment typically conflate clinicians' ability to provide accurate information about their patients (which they do well) with their ability to combine and weight variables to make predictions (a task *necessarily* performed better by statistical methods).

In fact, a substantial literature documents the reliability and validity of clinical observation and inference *when it is quantified and utilized appropriately*.[15] It is unfortunate, and telling, that research on the limitations of clinical judgment is widely cited by researchers, while compelling research on its strengths often goes overlooked.

The SWAP differs from other assessment approaches in that it harnesses clinical judgment using psychometric methods designed for this purpose, then applies statistical and actuarial methods to the resulting quantitative data. In short, it relies on clinicians to do what they do best, namely describing individual patients they know well. It relies on statistical algorithms to do what they do best, namely combining data optimally to derive reliable and valid scales and maximize prediction. In the framework of Paul Meehl's classic text on *Clinical Versus Statistical Prediction*, SWAP would be considered an example of *statistical* prediction.[14]

An Improved Taxonomy for Personality Diagnosis

The system for personality diagnosis provided by DSM finds little favor with either clinicians or researchers.[8,17,19] The DSM-5 Personality and Personality Disorders Work Group attempted to replace it entirely, but ideological conflicts prevented the Work Group from producing a viable alternative. As a result, DSM-5 diagnostic categories and criteria remained unchanged from DSM-IV and the opportunity for an improved and officially sanctioned system for personality diagnosis was lost.

An optimal diagnostic system should (1) "carve nature at the joints" as closely as nature reveals them and available research methods permit; (2) provide descriptions of personality syndromes that are *clinically* useful and relevant—ideally, they should facilitate a level of understanding that can guide treatment; and (3) provide a sound, workable method for making diagnoses in day-to-day clinical practice. In this section, I describe the findings of a 25-year research effort aimed at developing a diagnostic system meeting these requirements.[21]

An alternative to developing a diagnostic system by committee (with the unavoidable influences of group dynamics, politics, ideology, and other biases) is to derive a diagnostic taxonomy empirically, by conducting comprehensive assessments of personality in large, clinically representative patient samples, then employing statistical methods to identify and describe naturally occurring diagnostic groupings, assuming such groupings exist.

My co-investigators and I first described a diagnostic system based on such an approach in 1999, identifying naturally occurring diagnostic groupings in a national sample of personality-disordered patients assessed with the SWAP-200.[20] In this section, I summarize the findings of newer research using the SWAP-II in a larger, more representative sample of N = 1,201 adult patients.[21] We used the method of Q-factor analysis to identify naturally occurring diagnostic groupings in the patient sample. Q-factor analysis is computationally identical to factor analysis, with the difference that factor analysis identifies groupings of similar *variables*, whereas Q-factor analysis identifies groupings of similar *cases* or *people*. The resulting diagnostic groupings are data-driven and not the product of theoretical conjecture or decision by committee.

Data were provided by 1,201 licensed psychologists or psychiatrists, each of whom used the SWAP-II to describe a single, randomly selected current patient. The clinicians were instructed to describe "an adult patient you are currently treating or evaluating who has enduring patterns of thoughts, feelings, motivation, or behavior—that is, personality patterns—that cause distress or dysfunction." To ensure a clinically representative sample, the instructions emphasized that patients need *not* have a DSM personality disorder diagnosis. The methods are described in our original research report.[21]

An Empirically Derived Personality Taxonomy

The analysis identified 10 distinct, empirically and clinically coherent personality syndromes (Q-factors) organized hierarchically under superordinate groupings or broad personality spectra. Figure 4.2 illustrates the hierarchical structure of the empirically derived diagnostic system. At the level of broad superordinate groupings, the analysis identified an *internalizing* spectrum of personality syndromes, an *externalizing* spectrum, a *borderline-dysregulated* spectrum, and a spectrum we labeled *neurotic styles*.

Individuals with syndromes in the *internalizing* spectrum experience chronic painful emotions, especially depression and anxiety; tend to be emotionally constricted and socially avoidant; and tend to blame themselves for their difficulties. The spectrum subsumes the diagnoses of Depressive Personality, Anxious-Avoidant Personality, Dependent-Victimized Personality, and Schizoid-Schizotypal Personality.

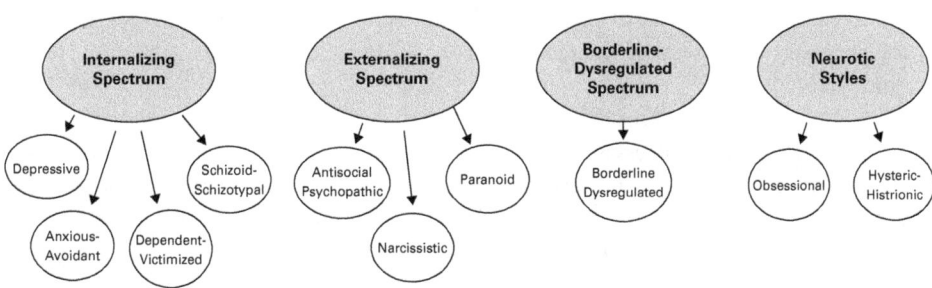

Figure 4.2. Hierarchical Structure of Personality Diagnoses

Individuals with syndromes in the *externalizing* spectrum cause others pain. They are angry or hostile, self-centered and lacking in empathy, and blame others for their difficulties. The spectrum subsumes the diagnoses of Antisocial-Psychopathic Personality, Narcissistic Personality, and Paranoid Personality.

Individuals in the *borderline-dysregulated* spectrum are qualitatively distinct from stable internalizers or stable externalizers. Their perceptions of self and others are unstable and changeable, and they have difficulty regulating emotion. As a result, they tend to oscillate between emotions characteristic of both internalizing and externalizing spectrum pathology (for example, depression, anxiety, rage). They may best be described as "stably unstable."[55] The salience of affect dysregulation in the clinical picture led us to hyphenate the name of the syndrome and add *dysregulated* to the more familiar term *borderline*.

The *neurotic styles* spectrum subsumes the diagnoses of Obsessional Personality and Hysteric-Histrionic Personality. The name of the spectrum reflects the recognition that individuals with these personality syndromes are, on average, higher functioning than those in the other diagnostic groupings and often do not show a level of dysfunction that warrants the term *disorder*. The two personality syndromes resemble "neurotic styles" described in the clinical literature[2,28,56] more than they resemble DSM descriptions of obsessive-compulsive and histrionic personality "disorders." The framers of DSM-III amplified the level of pathology of these two personality syndromes to fit them into a medical-model taxonomy of "disorders." Unfortunately, the resulting diagnostic DSM criterion sets described caricatures, not the characteristics of patients most often seen in real-world practice.

Empirically Derived Descriptions of Personality Syndromes

In addition to identifying naturally occurring personality syndromes, our research method allowed us to generate an empirically derived description of each personality syndrome. A description of the core, defining features of each diagnostic grouping or syndrome is obtained simply by listing the SWAP items with the highest factor scores for the syndrome. I will use borderline-dysregulated personality for illustration.

Box 4.1 (see p. 101) lists the 24 SWAP items with the highest factor scores for borderline-dysregulated personality (the items most central to the syndrome). To facilitate understanding of this complex syndrome, I have grouped the items under several broad themes. A number of findings are noteworthy. First, the empirical emergence of this diagnostic grouping validates the concept of borderline personality as a diagnostic entity. It confirms the existence of a distinct group of patients with common psychological characteristics. Second, the SWAP items describe a psychologically richer and more complex syndrome than described by DSM. Third, the description addresses internal psychological processes and aspects of inner experience crucial to understanding and treating this syndrome.

The findings validate clinical theories that view splitting, projective identification, and related psychological processes as central to borderline personality. Overall, the empirically derived personality syndrome more closely resembles the concept of borderline personality *organization* described in the clinical literature than the DSM description of borderline personality *disorder*. [2,4,25,38]

Box 4.1 Empirically Derived Description of Borderline-Dysregulated Personality

Affect Dysregulation
Emotions tend to change rapidly and unpredictably.

Emotions tend to spiral out of control, leading to extremes of anxiety, sadness, rage, etc.

Tends to become irrational when strong emotions are stirred up; may show a significant decline from customary level of functioning.

Is prone to intense anger, out of proportion to the situation at hand (e.g., has episodes of rage).

Is unable to soothe or comfort him/herself without the help of another person (i.e., has difficulty regulating own emotions).

Tends to "catastrophize"; is prone to see problems as disastrous, unsolvable, etc.

Tends to feel unhappy, depressed, or despondent.

Splitting
When upset, has trouble perceiving both positive and negative qualities in the same person at the same time; sees others in black or white terms (e.g., may swing from seeing someone as caring to seeing him/her as malevolent and intentionally hurtful).

Tends to stir up conflict or animosity between other people (e.g., may portray a situation differently to different people, leading them to form contradictory views or work at cross purposes).

Projective Identification
Manages to elicit in others feelings similar to those s/he is experiencing (e.g., when angry, acts in such a way as to provoke anger in others; when anxious, acts in such a way as to induce anxiety in others).

Tends to draw others into scenarios, or "pull" them into roles, that feel alien or unfamiliar (e.g., being uncharacteristically insensitive or cruel, feeling like the only person in the world who can help, etc.).

Identity Diffusion
Lacks a stable sense of who s/he is (e.g., attitudes, values, goals, and feelings about self seem unstable or ever-changing).

Is prone to painful feelings of emptiness (e.g., may feel lost, bereft, abjectly alone even in the presence of others, etc.).

Insecure Attachment
Tends to be needy or dependent.

Appears to fear being alone; may go to great lengths to avoid being alone.

Tends to fear s/he will be rejected or abandoned.

Tends to become attached quickly or intensely; develops feelings, expectations, etc. that are not warranted by the history or context of the relationship.
Tends to feel misunderstood, mistreated, or victimized.

Self-Harm (Desperate efforts to self-regulate)
Tends to engage in self-mutilating behavior (e.g., self-cutting, self-burning, etc.).
Tends to make repeated suicidal threats or gestures, either as a "cry for help" or as an effort to manipulate others.
Struggles with genuine wishes to kill him/herself.

Behavioral Sequelae
Relationships tend to be unstable, chaotic, and rapidly changing.
Work life and/or living arrangements tend to be chaotic or unstable (e.g., job or housing situation seems always temporary, transitional, or ill-defined).
Tends to be impulsive.

The items or personality features comprising the description of Borderline-Dysregulated Personality (and all other empirically identified syndromes) cannot be explained away as artifacts of clinicians' theoretical preconceptions. They emerged repeatedly when we stratified the sample by the theoretical orientation of the reporting clinicians, with the same items ranked highly by psychodynamic, cognitive-behavioral, humanistic, and biologically oriented clinicians.

Psychometric Assessment with the SWAP

We developed SWAP-II diagnostic scales to assess the empirically derived diagnostic syndromes by summing the most descriptive SWAP-II items for each syndrome (thus, the diagnostic scale for borderline-dysregulated personality comprises the 24 items listed in Box 4.1, p. 101). The number of scale items ranges from a low of 14 (for paranoid personality) to a high of 24 (for borderline-dysregulated personality), with the number of items reflecting the complexity of the syndrome. Alpha reliabilities for the diagnostic scales range from .72 to .94 with a median reliability of .79. To facilitate test interpretation, all diagnostic scores are scaled as normalized T-scores (Mean = 50, SD = 10).

An empirically derived Psychological Health Index was created by the same method, yielding an additional scale assessing global personality health/dysfunction. All personality syndromes fall on a continuum of functioning, and the score on the Psychological Health Index provides a context for interpreting other SWAP scale scores. An elevated score for a personality syndrome, coupled with a high Psychological Health Index score, indicates that the person is functioning at the healthier end of the health–pathology continuum for that syndrome, and a low score on the Psychological Health Index indicates the opposite. For example, a patient with an elevated score for paranoid personality and a high Psychological Health Index score has meaningful psychological resources or ego strengths and may be able to make constructive use of psychotherapy. A patient with the same paranoid personality score and a low Psychological Health Index score may prove untreatable. Both patients are likely to incorporate the therapist into a paranoid world-view and suspect the therapist of nefarious motives. However, the first patient will likely retain a capacity to reflect on their experience of the therapist and call their perceptions into question, whereas the second patient may not.

Diagnosis in Day-to-Day Practice

When maximum psychometric precision is required or where there are challenging diagnostic dilemmas, assessors can describe patients using the SWAP and obtain quantitative diagnostic scale scores for all the empirically derived personality syndromes (as well as for DSM-5 personality disorder diagnoses, and for SWAP factors or personality trait dimensions). For day-to-day diagnosis, my co-investigators and I have proposed a diagnostic system based on "prototype matching."[57]

In prototype matching diagnosis, the descriptions of the empirically derived personality syndromes are presented in paragraph rather than list form, to create a narrative description of each syndrome. The narrative descriptions constitute *diagnostic prototypes* that describe each personality syndrome in its "ideal" or pure form. The diagnostic prototypes are made up of the SWAP-II items that are empirically most defining of each syndrome (the same items used to construct the psychometric scales), organized and edited to create narratively coherent paragraphs. Each prototype description is preceded by a single-sentence summary statement intended to orient the diagnostician and convey telegraphically the core features of the syndrome.

The diagnostician's task is to consider the prototype description as a whole—as a configuration or pattern—and rate the *overall* similarity or match between a specific patient and the diagnostic prototype. The resulting diagnosis is dimensional (a 1–5 rating), but the scale can be dichotomized when a categorical (present/absent) diagnosis is desired, with ratings ≥ 4 indicating "caseness."

Box 4.2 (see p. 104) illustrates the prototype matching approach to personality diagnosis using depressive personality as an example. Despite its omission from DSM, depressive personality emerged consistently in our research as the most prevalent personality syndrome seen in clinical practice.[20] Diagnostic prototypes for all of the empirically derived personality syndromes are presented in Chapter 1 as well as in our original research report.[21] A quick reference guide containing all the prototypes is available for download from www.SWAPassessment.org/prototypes.

Prototype matching works *with*, rather than against, naturally occurring cognitive decision processes of diagnosticians and has considerable advantages over the criterion-counting approach of DSM. Among other advantages, it results in improved diagnostic reliability and validity and reduces comorbidity among personality disorder diagnoses. In head-to-head comparisons, clinicians rated SWAP prototype matching as more clinically useful and relevant than both the DSM diagnostic system and dimensional trait models of personality.[8,10] The conceptual rationale for the prototype matching method, and the research evidence supporting it, are described in detail elsewhere.[17,58–60]

Box 4.2 Depressive Personality Prototype

Summary statement: Individuals with Depressive Personality are prone to feelings of depression and inadequacy, tend to be self-critical or self-punitive, and may be preoccupied with concerns about abandonment or loss.

Individuals who match this prototype tend to feel depressed or despondent and to feel inadequate, inferior, or a failure. They tend to find little pleasure or satisfaction in life's activities and to feel life has no meaning. They are insufficiently concerned with meeting their own needs, disavowing or squelching their hopes and desires to protect against disappointment. They appear conflicted about experiencing pleasure, inhibiting feelings of excitement, joy, or pride. They may likewise be conflicted or inhibited about achievement or success (e.g., failing to reach their potential or sabotaging themselves when success is at hand). Individuals who match this prototype are generally self-critical, holding themselves to unrealistic standards and feeling guilty and blaming themselves for bad things that happen. They appear to want to "punish" themselves by creating situations that lead to unhappiness or avoiding opportunities for pleasure and gratification. They have trouble acknowledging or expressing anger and instead become depressed, self-critical, or self-punitive. Individuals who match this prototype often fear that they will be rejected or abandoned, are prone to painful feelings of emptiness, and may feel bereft or abjectly alone even in the presence of others. They may have a pervasive sense that someone or something necessary for happiness has been lost forever (e.g., a relationship, youth, beauty, success).

Please form an overall impression of the type of person described, then rate the extent to which your patient matches or resembles this prototype.

5 very good match (patient *exemplifies* this disorder; prototypical case)	**Diagnosis**
4 good match (patient *has* this disorder; diagnosis applies)	
3 moderate match (patient has *significant features* of this disorder)	**Features**
2 slight match (patient has minor features of this disorder)	
1 no match (description does not apply)	

Conclusion: Integrating Clinical and Empirical Perspectives

A clinically useful diagnostic system should encompass the spectrum of personality syndromes seen in clinical practice and have meaningful treatment implications. An empirically sound diagnostic system should facilitate reliable and valid diagnoses: independent clinicians should be able to arrive at the same diagnosis, diagnoses should be distinct, and each diagnosis should be associated with conceptually meaningful correlates, antecedents, and sequelae.

An obstacle to achieving this ideal has been the persistent schism in the mental health professions between science and practice. Too often, empirical research has been conducted in isolation from the crucial data of clinical observation. Too often, clinical

---

Box 4.3 Resources

- Clinicians can complete a SWAP assessments on line and receive computer-generated interpretive reports at https://swapassessment.org/.
- A bibliography of SWAP research with downloadable PDFs is available at https://swapassessment.org/bibliography/.
- A three-page Quick Reference Guide containing all the diagnostic prototypes can be downloaded from https://swapassessment.org/prototypes/.

---

theory has developed without regard for empirical credibility. Empirical researchers and clinical practitioners tend to talk past rather than with one another.

SWAP research represents an effort to bridge the science–practice schism by quantifying clinical observation and expertise, making clinical constructs accessible to empirical study. It relies on clinicians to make observations and inferences about individual patients they know, and on quantitative methods to reveal relationships and combine data in optimal ways.

The SWAP provides a "language" for clinical case description that is both psychometrically sound and clinically rich enough to describe the complexities of real patients. There remains a sizeable schism between science and practice. The SWAP instrument provides a language all parties can speak.

See Box 4.3 for additional resources.

Conflict of Interest/Disclosure: The author of this chapter have no financial conflicts and nothing to disclose.

References

1. Betan E, Heim AK, Zittel Conklin C, Westen D. Countertransference phenomena and personality pathology in clinical practice: an empirical investigation. *AJP*. 2005;162(5):890–898.

2. McWilliams N. *Psychoanalytic Diagnosis: Understanding Personality Structure in the Clinical Process*. 2nd ed. New York: Guilford Press; 2011.

3. Peebles MJ. *Beginnings: The Art and Science of Planning Psychotherapy*. 2nd ed. New York: Routledge; 2012.

4. Kernberg O. *Borderline Conditions and Pathological Narcissism*. New York: Jason Aronson; 1975.

5. Shedler J, Westen D. The Shedler-Westen Assessment Procedure (SWAP): making personality diagnosis clinically meaningful. *J Pers Assess*. 2007;89:41–55.

6. Widiger TA, Simonsen ES. Alternative dimensional models of personality disorders: finding common ground. *J Pers Disord*. 2005;19:110–130.

7. Kernberg O. A psychoanalytic theory of personality disorders. In: Clarkin JF, Lenzenweger MF, eds. *Major Theories of Personality Disorder*. New York: Guilford; 1996:114–146.

8. Rottman BM, Ahn WK, Sanislow CA, Kim NS. Can clinicians recognize DSM-IV personality disorders from five-factor model descriptions of patient cases? *Am J Psychiatry*. 2009;166:427–433.

9. Shedler J, Beck AT, Fonagy P, Gabbard GO, Gunderson J, Kernberg O, Michels R, Westen, D. Editorial: personality disorders in DSM-5. *Am J Psychiatry.* 2010;167:1026–1028.

10. Spitzer RL, First MB, Shedler J, Westen D, Skodal A. Clinical utility of five dimensional systems for personality diagnosis: A "consumer preference" study. *J Nerv Ment Dis.* 2008;196:3567–374.

11. Reichenbach H. *Experience and Prediction.* Chicago: University of Chicago Press; 1938.

12. Cousineau TM, Shedler J. Predicting physical health: implicit mental health measures versus self-report scales. *J Nerv Ment Dis.* 2006;194(6):427–432.

13. Shedler J, Mayman M, Manis M. The illusion of mental health. *Am Psychol.* 1993;48:1117–1131.

14. Meehl PE. *Clinical Versus Statistical Prediction: A Theoretical Analysis and a Review of the Evidence.* Minneapolis: University of Minnesota Press; 1954.

15. Sawyer J. Measurement and prediction, clinical and statistical. *Psychol Bull.* 1966;66:178–200.

16. Westen D, Weinberger J. When clinical description becomes statistical prediction. *Am Psychol.* 2004;59:595–613.

17. Shedler J, Westen D. Refining DSM-IV Personality Disorder Diagnosis: Integrating science and practice. *Am J Psychiatry.* 2004;161:1350–1365.

18. Shedler J, Westen D Dimensions of personality pathology: an alternative to the five factor model. *Am J Psychiatry.* 2004;161:1743–1754.

19. Westen D, Shedler J. Revising and assessing Axis II: I. Developing a clinically and empirically valid assessment method. *Am J Psychiatry.* 1999;156(2):258–272.

20. Westen D, Shedler J. Revising and assessing Axis II: II. Toward an empirically based and clinically useful classification of personality disorders. *Am J Psychiatry.* 1999;156(2):258–272.

21. Westen D, Shedler J, Bradley B, DeFife J. An empirically derived taxonomy for personality diagnosis: bridging science and practice in conceptualizing personality. *Am J Psychiatry.* 2012;169:273–284.

22. Shedler J, Westen D. Refining the measurement of Axis II: a Q-sort procedure for assessing personality pathology. *Assessment.* 1998;5(4):333–353.

23. Westen D, Dutra L, Shedler J. Assessing adolescent personality pathology: quantifying clinical judgment. *Br J Psychiatry.* 2005;186:227–238.

24. Westen D, Shedler, J, Durrett, C, Glass, S, Martens, A. Personality diagnosis in adolescence: DSM-IV axis II diagnoses and an empirically derived alternative. *Am J Psychiatry.* 2003;160:952–966.

25. Kernberg O. *Severe Personality Disorders.* New Haven, CT: Yale University Press; 1984.

26. Kohut H. *The Analysis of the Self.* New York: International Universities Press, 1971.

27. Linehan MM. *Cognitive-behavioral Treatment of Borderline Personality Disorder.* New York: Guilford; 1993.

28. Shapiro D. *Neurotic Styles.* New York: Basic; 1995.

29. Perry JC, Cooper SH. Empirical studies of psychological defense mechanisms. In: Cavenar J, Michels R, eds. *Psychiatry.* Philadelphia: JB Lippincott; 1987:444–452.

30. Vaillant G, ed. *Ego Mechanisms of Defense: A Guide for Clinicians and Researchers.* Washington, DC: American Psychiatric Press; 1992.

31. Westen D, Muderrisoglu S, Fowler C, Shedler J, Koren D. Affect regulation and affective experience: individual differences, group differences, and measurement using a Q-sort procedure. *J Consult Clin Psychol.* 1997;65:429–439.

32. Westen D. Social cognition and object relations. *Psychol Bull*. 1991;109:429–455.

33. Westen D, Lohr N, Silk K, Gold L, Kerber K. Object relations and social cognition in border-lines, major depressives, and normals: a TAT analysis. *Psychol Assess*. 1990;2:355–364.

34. Block J. *Lives Through Time*. Berkeley, CA: Bancroft; 1971.

35. John O. The 'big five' factor taxonomy: dimensions of personality in the natural language and in questionnaires. In: Pervin L, ed. *Handbook of Personality: Theory and Research*. New York: Guilford Press; 1990:66–100.

36. McCrae R, Costa P. *Personality in Adulthood*. New York: Guilford Press; 1990.

37. Livesley WJ, ed. *The DSM-IV Personality Disorders*. New York: Guilford Press; 1995.

38. Clarkin JF, Yeomans FE, Kernberg OF. *Psychotherapy for Borderline Personality: Focusing on Object Relations*. Washington, DC: American Psychiatric Publishing; 2006.

39. Gabbard GO. *Psychodynamic Psychiatry in Clinical Practice*. 4th ed. Washington, DC: American Psychiatric Publishing; 2005.

40. Westen D, Shedler J. Personality diagnosis with the Shedler-Westen Assessment Procedure (SWAP): Integrating clinical and statistical measurement and prediction. *J Abnor Psychol*. 2007;116:810–822.

41. Blagov PS, Bi W, Shedler J, Westen D. The Shedler-Westen Assessment Procedure (SWAP): evaluating psychometric questions about its reliability, validity, and impact of its fixed score distribution. *Assessment*. 2012;19(3):370–382.

42. Block J. *The Q-Sort Method in Personality Assessment and Psychiatric Research*. Springfield: Charles C Thomas; 1961.

43. Westen D. Muderrisoglu S. Reliability and validity of personality disorder assessment using a systematic clinical interview: evaluating an alternative to structured interviews. *J Pers Disord*. 2003;17:350–368.

44. Westen D. *Clinical Diagnostic Interview*. Atlanta, GA: Emory University, Departments of Psychology and Psychiatry and Behavioral Sciences; 2004.

45. Westen D, Muderrisoglu S. Clinical assessment of pathological personality traits. *Am J Psychiatry*. 2006;163:1285–1297.

46. Marin-Avellan L, McGauley G, Campbell C, Fonagy P. Using the SWAP-200 in a personality-disordered forensic population: is it valid, reliable and useful? *J Crim Behav Ment Health*. 2005;15:28–45.

47. Russ E, Bradley R, Shedler J, Westen D. Refining the construct of narcissistic personality disorder: Diagnostic criteria and subtypes. *Am J Psychiatry*, 2008;165:1473–1481.

48. Westen D, Waller N, Shedler J, Blagov P, Bradley R. Dimensions of personality and personality pathology: factor structure of the Shedler-Westen Assessment Procedure-II (SWAP-II). *J Pers Disord*. 2012;28(2):281–318.

49. Shedler J. *Guide to SWAP-200 Interpretation*. Denver: SWAP assessment LLC; 2009.

50. Shecter O, Lang E. *Identifying Personality Disorders that Are Security Risks: Field Test Results*. Defense Personnel Security Research Center, Technical Report 11-05; 2011.

51. Ahn W-K. Effect of causal structure on category construction. *Mem Cogn*. 1999;27(6):1008–1023.

52. Cantor N, Genero N. Psychiatric diagnosis and natural categorization: A close analogy. In: Millon T, Klerman L, eds. *Contemporary Directions in Psychopathology: Toward the DSM-IV*. New York, NY: Guilford; 1986: 233–256.

53. Kim NS, Ahn W. Clinical psychologists' theory-based representations of mental disorders predict their diagnostic reasoning and memory. *J Exp Psychol.* 2002;131(4):451–476.

54. Lingiardi V, Shedler, J, Gazillo, F. Assessing personality change in psychotherapy with the SWAP-200: a case study. *J Pers Assess.* 2006;86: 23–32.

55. Schmideberg M. The borderline patient. In: Arieti S, ed. *American Handbook of Psychiatry.* New York: Basic Books; 1959:398–416.

56. MacKinnon R., Michels R., Buckley P. *The Psychiatric Interview in Clinical Practice.* 2nd ed. Washington, DC: American Psychiatric Publishing; 2009.

57. Westen D, Shedler J. A prototype matching approach to personality disorders: toward DSM-V. *Journal of Personality Disorders.* 2000;14:109–126.

58. Westen D, DeFife JA, Bradley B., Hilsenroth MJ. Prototype personality diagnosis in clinical practice: a viable alternative for DSM-5 and ICD-11. *Prof Psychol Res Pr.* 2010;41(6):482–487.

59. Ortigo KM, Bradley B., Westen D. An empirically based prototype diagnostic system for DSM-V and ICD-11. In: Millon T, Krueger R, Simonsen E, eds. *Contemporary Directions in Psychopathology: Scientific Foundations of the DSM-V and ICD-11.* New York, Guilford; 2010:374–390.

60. Westen D, Shedler J, Bradley R. A prototype approach to personality diagnosis. *Am J Psychiatry.* 2006;163:846–856.

II

MULTI-THEORETICAL
TREATMENTS OF PERSONALITY
DISORDERS

5

Crossing the Alphabet Divide

Navigating the Evidence for DBT, GPM, MBT, ST, and TFP for BPD

Kenneth N. Levy, Benjamin N. Johnson, and Haruka Notsu

Key Points

- Borderline personality disorder (BPD) is prevalent, complex, and historically difficult to treat.
- A number of treatments—primarily from cognitive-behavioral and psychodynamic traditions—have been developed and show efficacy in treating BPD.
- The "Big Five" empirically supported treatments for BPD are: dialectical behavior therapy (DBT); mentalization-based therapy (MBT); transference-focused psychotherapy (TFP); schema therapy (ST); and good psychiatric management (GPM).
- DBT is a behavioral, skills-focused treatment that targets self-harm and other behavioral manifestations of emotion dysregulation.
- MBT aims to improve clients' capacity to mentalize: to think about mental states in oneself and others.
- TFP addresses unintegrated internal representations of self and others to make more coherent clients' identity and foster enhanced self-regulation.
- ST aims to alter maladaptive schemas that generate and maintain dysfunctional views of oneself and others.
- GPM targets interpersonal sensitivity in BPD and is designed as a generalist treatment available to all manner of practitioners, rather than the specialist treatments DBT, MBT, TFP, and ST.
- The evidence for treating BPD as captured in randomized controlled trials (RCTs) and meta-analyses is strong and growing.
- RCTs have been conducted finding support for DBT, MBT, TFP, ST, and GPM.
- At least 14 RCTs have been conducted on DBT, finding significant reduction in behavioral symptoms of BPD, such as self-harm and suicide in particular.
- Two large-scale and four smaller RCTs have been conducted on MBT, finding significant improvement in social and interpersonal functioning in BPD, as well as other related symptoms.
- Three RCTs have been conducted on TFP, finding improvement in a range of primary and secondary features of BPD, particularly reflective functioning and attachment security.

- Three RCTs conducted on ST have found improvement in diagnostic criteria for BPD and improvement in quality of life.
- One original RCT of GPM, with two-year follow-up, suggests improvements in self-harm, hospitalizations, BPD symptoms, and secondary features, though examinations of the current standalone treatment have yet to be conducted.
- A number of meta-analyses of BPD treatments of various formats (e.g., individual, group) suggest treatments are moderately effective, no treatment modality claims superiority, and that psychotherapy—rather than medication management—is the optimal treatment approach for BPD.
- Treatments for BPD are generally long-term, intensive, and often include multiple formats (e.g., individual plus group).
- Therapists treating BPD generally require peer support/supervision and specialized training.
- BPD treatment is generally active, integrative, collaborative, flexible, and focused on emotion regulation and views of self and/or other.
- Given that a range of efficacious treatments exist, but without a clear "gold standard," we propose a number of integrative principles that cut across interventions.
- More research is needed to empirically evaluate how best to sequence or combine treatments and their elements.

Introduction

Borderline personality disorder (BPD) is a complex psychological disorder and one of the most vexing problems to treat in psychology and psychiatry. Historically, BPD has been thought to be difficult to treat because patients frequently do not adhere to treatment recommendations, use services chaotically, and repeatedly drop out of treatment. Many of the core difficulties associated with BPD—such as the chaotic relationships, vacillations between idealizations and derogations, tendency toward angry outbursts, and of course the suicidality and non-suicidal self-injury with its unpredictability—present special challenges to the therapist working with such patients. Individuals with BPD often present with extreme dependence, hostility, or confusing vacillations, and experience frequent, sometimes even "unrelenting" crises.[1] Clinicians are often intimidated by the prospect of treating BPD patients and are pessimistic about the outcome of treatment. Additionally, in settings with multiple care providers, patients with BPD may tend to split providers into idealized and devalued groups, which, if not well-managed, can impact the treatment team's ability to collaborate effectively.[2,3] Consequently, therapists treating patients with BPD have displayed high levels of burnout and have been known to be prone to enactments and even engagement in iatrogenic behaviors.[4,5]

However, over the last decade there has been a burgeoning empirical literature on the treatment of BPD suggesting that it can indeed be treated. Beginning with Linehan's seminal randomized controlled trial (RCT) of dialectical behavior therapy (DBT),[1] there are now a range of treatments—deriving from both the cognitive-behavioral and psychodynamic traditions—that have shown efficacy in RCTs and are available to clinicians. Among the available treatments for BPD are DBT, as well as mentalization-based treatment (MBT)[6]; transference-focused psychotherapy (TFP)[7]; schema therapy (ST),[8] and good psychiatric management (GPM).[9] These treatments have been referred to as the "Big Five."[10] In addition to the Big Five, there are several other treatments available to clinicians, including dynamic deconstructive psychotherapy (DDP)[11]; Systems Training for Emotional Predictability and Problem Solving (STEPPS)[12]; emotion regulation group therapy (ERGT)[13]; motive-oriented therapeutic relationship (MOTR)[14]; structured clinical management (CM),[15] and stepped care management (SC).[16] Adding to the expansive list of available treatments of BPD, there has also been one RCT of manual assisted cognitive treatment (MACT),[17] a highly structured adaptation of cognitive behavioral therapy (CBT), which has shown benefit for self-harm but has not been evaluated for other BPD symptoms.[18] Other approaches include psychoeducation.[19]

The results of the efficacy studies suggest several important evidence-based principles. First, BPD is a treatable disorder, although with specifically defined treatments. Second, therapists have a range of treatment options available to them. These options cut across psychodynamic and cognitive-behavioral theoretical orientations. Additionally, there is now enough data from numerous RCTs, including a few direct comparisons, and from several meta-analyses to suggest that no one approach is superior to another.[20-22] These findings suggest two corollary ideas. First, despite often espousing very different perspectives, there may be common factors that cut across the various approaches[23] (see Chapter 6, The Big Six: Evidenced-based Therapies for the Treatment of Personality Disorders, for additional discussion). Second, there may be many "roads to Rome," that is, multiple distinct treatments for BPD may be equally effective in producing desired outcomes.[23,24] However, in part due to the findings suggesting equivalence of outcomes, clinicians are left with a high degree of uncertainty about treatment selection, determining which patients will benefit from which specific or range of treatments, and how best to sequence or combine treatments and their elements.

The primary goal of this chapter is to summarize evidence for the various treatments for BPD, provide an overarching perspective by integrating findings from RCTs and meta-analyses to derive principles for treatment, and discuss strategies for integrating various approaches. Because of the many acronyms employed for the various treatments for BPD (e.g., DBT, MBT, TFP), we refer to the problem of treatment selection, derivation of principles, and psychotherapy integration as navigating or crossing the "alphabet divide." In this spirit, we encourage clinical researchers to begin examining treatments more broadly, including how elements of various approaches may be combined or sequenced to better help patients. We hope that the approach taken in this chapter and in Chapter 6 is helpful to patients and their families in seeking services, and that it may impact policymakers and insurance companies to consider a more complete evidence base.

The importance of thinking and treating across the alphabet divide is underscored not only by the findings of equivalent effects among different treatments, but also because even though many patients improve in these treatments, many others do not. Additionally, many patients who *do* show symptomatic improvement and even diagnostic remission still experience significant social and functional impairment over the long term. Both those who fail to improve and those who show partial or limited improvement may benefit and be better served from the inclusion of elements from other treatment approaches across the alphabet divide.[25] Finally, given the heterogeneity of BPD, it is unlikely that any one treatment will be useful for all patients, and thus having different treatment options is essential to clinicians in providing personalized care.

Evolution and Characterization of Treatments for BPD

DBT, MBT, TFP, ST, and GPM are referred to as the Big Five because they are theory-based, comprehensive approaches that have been broadly tested and well-disseminated. DBT, MBT, TFP, and ST are considered specialized treatments because they are adapted or modified from broader psychotherapy traditions such as CBT or psychodynamic psychotherapy (PDT), based on the specific psychopathology believed to underlie BPD. In doing so, Marsha Linehan[1,26] and Otto Kernberg,[3,27] from their respective traditions, were prescient of Kazdin's[28,29] later recommendations that treatment approaches should be based on the underlying developmental psychopathology of the problem being addressed. Thus, rather than a "one size fits all" philosophy, these clinical scholars followed a "different strokes for different folks" approach.[30] Jeff Young and Peter Fonagy employed the same philosophy in developing ST and MBT, respectively. Although Fonagy shares in many of the same psychodynamic theoretical bases as Kernberg (e.g., the importance of object relations, Kleinian theory, and ego psychology), he deviated from Kernberg in several important ways, some of which were consistent with the emphasis of Kohut[31] and Adler and Buie,[32,33] and others in ways that are based on his own articulation within psychoanalysis.[34] Young, a student of Aaron Beck, adapted cognitive therapy for patients suffering from BPD in developing ST. Coming from the Beckian tradition, his model is more cognitive in its focus compared to Linehan, which stressed more behavioral aspects. Each of these approaches is also considered specialized because, in addition to being developed specifically for BPD (or personality disorders more broadly), these treatments are intensive and, in addition to having a substantial commitment to treating this population of patients, are conducted by specially trained clinicians who need to devote many hours over several years toward developing adherence and competence in complex models. Often these treatments occur within specialized clinics or programs and are carried out by certified therapists.

In contrast, Gunderson's GPM is considered a generalist approach because it is rolled out more broadly to hospital and clinic staff and represents a distillation and application of the American Psychiatric Association's Practice Guidelines for the treatment of BPD.[35] It is an approach that is meant to be disseminated broadly to staff to guide interactions with patients suffering from BPD, and it is meant for those patients who may not require or do not have specialized treatments such as DBT, MBT, TFP, and ST available to them. Gunderson and colleagues[36] note that there are not enough treaters trained in the time-consuming specialized treatments for BPD and, similar to Paris,[16,37] suggest that not every BPD patient is in need of or can utilize a specialized treatment.

We will provide more specific, although brief, reviews of each of the Big Five treatments, including both the conceptual foundations of each treatment and the existing state of the literature on treatment efficacy. A complete consideration of the adjunctive treatments and generalists approaches beyond GPM is beyond the scope of this chapter.

Dialectical Behavioral Therapy (DBT)

DBT was initially developed in the 1980s by Marsha Linehan as a treatment program for women with parasuicidal and suicidal behaviors.[26] It was while applying for funding that program officers at NIMH suggested to Linehan that she had actually developed a treatment for BPD (Irene Elkin, Ph.D., conversation, June 20, 2007). These program officers suggested that she develop expertise in BPD. After a sabbatical semester at Cornell working with Otto Kernberg and John Clarkin, Linehan completed her treatment manual[1] and tested her treatment in a sample of women with BPD.[38] Although DBT is admittedly integrative[39] and shares aspects with even divergent approaches such as TFP,[40] it evolved out of a behavioral tradition (hence the initial focus on behaviors like parasuicidal and suicidal attempts) with integration of modified CBT skills modules and Buddhist philosophies. Linehan recognized that traditional CBT skills were not as relevant to the difficulties seen in BPD that led to self-injury and suicidality, and identified behavioral techniques and skills training to alleviate behavioral manifestations of emotion dysregulation in BPD as well as improve interpersonal functioning.[1,26] The focus of DBT lies in replacing maladaptive behaviors such as self-harm with adaptive skills, emphasizing a balance between change-focused techniques (e.g., cognitive modification) and acceptance-focused practices (e.g., mindfulness training).[41,42] See Chapter 11 for a broad discussion of DBT.

Mentalization-based Treatment (MBT)

Bateman and Fonagy[43] developed MBT based on the developmental theory of mentalizing, which integrates philosophy (theory of mind), ego psychology, Kleinian theory, and attachment theory.[34,44-47] Fonagy and Bateman's[48] MBT posits that the mechanism of change in all effective treatments for BPD involves the capacity for mentalizing—the capacity to think about mental states in oneself and in others in terms of wishes, desires, and intentions. Mentalizing involves both (1) implicit or unconscious mental processes that are activated along with the attachment system in affectively charged interpersonal situations, and (2) coherent integrated representations of mental states of self and others. The core goal of MBT is to improve clients' capacity to mentalize by helping them to "regain mentalizing when it is lost, maintain it when it is present, and to increase clients' ability to maintain a mentalizing stance in situations where it might otherwise be lost."[22] Given that clients with BPD are particularly likely to lose mentalizing in interpersonal situations, the relationship between client and therapist is a key area of focus.

MBT involves a collaborative and structured approach to working to gently expand mentalizing and helping clients to identify mental states that were previously outside of their awareness. This approach involves the therapist exhibiting empathy and providing validation of the client's experience, clarifying and exploring the client's narrative, and identifying the affective focus of the session. The therapist then helps broaden the client's perspective on the events presented in their narrative by presenting alternative perspectives. The work to expand the client's mentalizing primarily focuses on the here and now of the session and gradually comes to involve relationships with core attachment figures and other key people in the client's life, how these relationships become activated with the therapist, and how they influence mentalizing. The therapist works to encourage mentalizing the therapeutic relationship, and takes into account both transference and countertransference reactions that are specifically defined in terms of technical application. As mentalizing improves, the client becomes increasingly able to generate alternative representations of important relationships.

The beginning of treatment in MBT involves the establishment of goals with the client. Initial goals are to include commitment to and engagement in treatment, as well as an agreement to reduce harmful and self-destructive behaviors. Attachment strategies activated in relationships are mapped out with the client and a joint formulation agreed. A long-term goal is the improvement of personal and social relationships, as well as engagement in constructive activity. MBT was initially developed and tested as an 18-month treatment program including both group and individual sessions; however, in clinical settings, it has been offered for shorter periods of time and in formats that include only individual or group therapy. Currently, there is no research evidence regarding the optimal format or length of MBT treatment. See Chapter 9 for a broad discussion of MBT.

Transference-focused Psychotherapy (TFP)

TFP is a modified psychodynamic psychotherapy designed for use with patients suffering from severe personality disorders, most prototypically borderline and narcissistic personality disorders.[49,50] Otto Kernberg, based on his experiences with the Menninger Psychotherapy Research Project, began modifying standard psychodynamic psychotherapy. Initially, he referred to this therapy as "exploratory psychotherapy," in an effort to distinguish it from more supportive psychotherapies.[50] These modifications were based on Kernberg's articulation of the developmental psychopathology underlying severe personality disorders and the clinical realities of treating those with these disorders. Over the subsequent decades, Kernberg and colleagues, particularly Frank Yeomans and John Clarkin at the Personality Disorders Institute of Cornell University, further articulated and developed the treatment in a series of treatment manuals.[7,51]

The overarching goals of TFP are to improve self-control, reduce impulsivity, increase emotion-regulation abilities, increase intimacy in relationships and relationship satisfaction, and improve capacity to realize life goals (that are consistent with the patient's abilities and desires). More specific goals include improvements in the symptoms central to BPD, especially suicidal and parasuicidal behaviors, angry outbursts, and impulsive behavioral difficulties. Improvements in these areas are hypothesized to lead to reduction of emergency service use, hospitalizations, and difficulties in relationship. These changes are posited to follow from the integration of disparate, contradictory, and incoherent internal mental representations of self and others.

Fundamental to the TFP model is that BPD derives from a failure to develop internal representations of self and others that are complex and realistic and characteristic of healthy psychological maturation. These fragmented representations of self and others impede the person's capacity to reflect on interactions with others as well as their own beliefs and to behave in a thoughtful and consistent goal-directed manner. Additionally, this lack of integration leads to fluctuations between extreme positive or negative emotions that impairs an individual's perception of day-to-day interactions. The inconsistent sense of self and others is called "identity diffusion" in the TFP model, and is analogous to identity disturbance defined in DSM-5[52] as well as psychological processes regarding identity formation described by Blatt and Blass,[53] Erikson,[54] Marcia,[55] and McAdams.[56]

In the TFP model, identity diffusion is considered the source for emotion dysregulation seen in BPD. Thus, the treatment focuses on the integration of one's sense of self and others and the emotions linking them. This integration is hypothesized to lead to representational and affective experiences becoming more nuanced, enriched, and modulated. The increased differentiation and integration of these internal representations result in the patient developing the capacity to think more flexibly and positively about the therapist, significant others, and themselves. The integration of these internal representations is achieved by exploring and understanding the patient's contradictory experiences of self and others, but particularly of the therapist.

TFP begins with a thorough assessment called a structural interview.[57] Based on the information gathered during this process as well as from collateral sources (e.g., referrals, significant others, previous treaters), the therapist forms their initial diagnostic impressions of the patient's difficulties that will be shared with them. Therapists do not want to impose their impressions on the patient or for the patient to acquiesce to their point of view. Likewise, the therapist does not want to abandon their own point of view. Instead, the initial work often involves the patient and therapist collaboratively developing a shared view or understanding of the nature of the patient's difficulties. With a shared understanding of the patient's difficulties, the therapist and patient discuss the structure of the treatment; essentially, how the treatment is thought to work and what each party's roles and responsibilities are in it. Expected obstacles and threats to the treatment are raised and discussed, as are how emergencies and crises will be handled by the patient and therapist.

Once the evaluation and frame of the therapy are established, the treatment can start. In the beginning, the patient may test the treatment frame to see if the therapist is trustworthy. In session, the therapist attends to or focuses on the dominant affect to guide their attention. The therapist then listens for relational themes in the patient's narrative, which are called object relation dyads. These themes are conceptualized as relational dyads because there is a representation of the self and the other in the patterns expressed (as well as the self in relation to the other and the affect that connects these representational dyads). These representations of self and others tend to vacillate in patients with BPD. Initially the patient might see themselves as the victim of a cold, uncaring other, but then in the narrative they might portray themselves as uninterested and unaffected by the other, who may be seen as needy or desperate. The therapist articulates these dyads, notes their vacillation, and works with the patient to understand their function or underlying motives. In the process of doing so, the therapist clarifies the patient's experience, gently brings disparate aspects of the patient's experience into their awareness, and tactfully interprets the patient's dominant affect-laden themes as they are expressed in the here-and-now of the relationship between the two (conceptualized as transference). This interpretative process is hypothesized to integrate incoherent and polarized representations of the self and others, resulting in better affect regulation and behavioral control. See Chapter 8 for a broad discussion of TFP.

Schema Therapy (ST)

A fourth treatment modality with support for BPD is Young's schema-focused therapy, or schema therapy, developed in the early 1990s. ST draws from the domains of CBT, gestalt therapy, and psychodynamic theory in an attempt to alter maladaptive schemas formed early in development that generate and maintain dysfunctional views of oneself and others.[50,58,59] ST catalogues a number of primary "modes" or ways in which individuals with BPD may see themselves vis-à-vis others in a given moment or mental state (e.g., "abandoned and abused"), which tend to shift from moment to moment and contribute to the emotional and behavioral dysregulation characteristic of the disorder. ST uses a number of mode-specific interventions to increase the individual's awareness of being in a given mode, bring the therapist into the interpersonal space as a genuine, reliable, and supportive other, and reduce "flipping" between modes.[58] See Chapter 12 for a broad discussion of ST.

Good Psychiatric Management (GPM)

Gunderson with Links[9] developed what was originally called general psychiatric management, and is now named good psychiatric management. GPM was originally developed as an active and credible control condition for an RCT examining the efficacy of DBT[60] and was based on recommendations from the *Guidelines for the Treatment of BPD* published by the American Psychiatric Association in 2001.[35] Based on the APA treatment guidelines, GPM consisted of three modes of intervention, including (1) case management, (2) individual psychotherapy, and (3) symptom-targeted medication management. In the initial trial, therapist-provided psychotherapy was informed by John Gunderson's psychodynamic approach treating BPD.[61] GPM has evolved since the original trial, and what follows is a description of the treatment as it was evaluated in 2001.

In the GPM model, clients are viewed and treated as competent adults, and therapists are encouraged to be flexible in terms of the treatment focus. Much attention is accorded to the client's role functioning.[62] GPM conceptualizes disturbed attachment relationships in terms of interpersonal sensitivity[63] and intolerance of aloneness[64] as the core problem underlying BPD. Emotion-processing problems figure centrally in disturbed attachment relationships, and consequently GPM has an emotion focus.[65] There are a variety of treatment strategies in the model, including: responding to crises; safety monitoring; establishing and monitoring a therapeutic framework and alliance; educating the client and his/her family about the disorder; facilitating adherence to the treatment regimen; coordinating multimodal therapies; and monitoring clinical status and treatment plans. Ancillary treatments are tailored to the client's needs. In the GPM model, therapists are not available outside of working hours, and clients are instead encouraged to exercise control over their behavior and seek out emergency services as needed. GPM incorporates aspects of a variety of therapy orientations, including interpretations of anger and acting out (PDT/TFP), psychoeducation, fostering social skills (CBT/DBT), and focusing on theory of mind and reflective functioning (MBT). What primarily sets GPM apart from these other treatments is that it does not claim to be a standalone specialized treatment for BPD but, with roots in Winnicott's[66] ideas of "good enough mothering," is instead designed as a "generalist" treatment, which can be implemented by all manner of practitioners, with more severe cases of BPD potentially being referred to "specialist" treatments such as TFP and DBT. See Chapter 13 for a broad discussion of GPM.

Evidence Base for Treatments

In this section, we consider the evidence base for the various treatments by reviewing the evidence from RCTs and meta-analyses.

Randomized Controlled Trials for Treatment of BPD

Evidence for Dialectical Behavior Therapy for Treatment of BPD

To date, DBT is the most frequently studied treatment for BPD, with at least 14 RCTs having been conducted on the full DBT program in BPD-diagnosed samples. In general, when compared to treatment-as-usual (TAU), DBT has been shown to significantly reduce behavioral symptoms often present in BPD, including non-suicidal self-injury[67–72] and both suicide attempts and hospitalizations.[68,69] However, several studies have found no difference between DBT and TAU in behavioral symptom decrease,[60,73–75] suggesting that the efficacy of DBT for this symptom cluster has yet to be determined. Furthermore, comparison trials of DBT against other active treatments for BPD, such as TFP or GPM, have found generally comparable outcomes for these treatments.[60,76] There is some evidence to suggest that DBT may reduce dropout rates among patients with BPD, with at least three studies specifically finding lower rates of dropout compared to TAU or community treatment by experts.[68,72,77] DBT has shown moderate effect size in comparison with TAU,[78] but when compared to alternative treatments,[60,76,79,80] there is no difference in outcome or effect size.[20,78]

Unfortunately, given the focus on change in behavioral symptoms as outcome in DBT treatment studies, less is known regarding DBT's effectiveness in other BPD-relevant symptom domains, such as identity disturbance, emptiness, and relationship chaos. Some RCT evidence suggests that DBT may provide little benefit in terms of the identity-relevant construct of reflective functioning (i.e., one's capacity to reflect on the mental states of self and other) compared to TFP, a treatment that directly targets identity disturbance, another core feature of BPD.[76] A variety of quasi-experimental and uncontrolled studies have shown varying levels of support for DBT, but these tend to focus solely on TAU as comparison (if one is present), and the implications of these findings are therefore limited.

Evidence for Mentalization-based Treatment for Treatment of BPD

Bateman and Fonagy have conducted two large-scale RCTs of MBT supporting its use for BPD. In the first,[6] the effectiveness of 18 months of an MBT day-hospital program was compared with routine general psychiatric care for BPD patients. Patients randomly assigned to MBT showed statistically significant improvement in depressive symptoms and better social and interpersonal functioning, as well as significant decreases in suicidal and parasuicidal behavior and number of inpatient days. Follow-up assessment also showed that gains were maintained and increased remittance in the MBT condition compared to TAU.[81] The findings of this RCT were especially strong; however, the MBT treatment in this RCT occurred in a 30-hour-a-week comprehensive MBT day-hospital treatment, and the TAU group, although having had ecological validity, consisted of twice monthly medication management. Thus, the comparison between the two conditions differ quite a bit in terms of dose (30 hours a week compared to 2 hours a month).

The second RCT[82] compared 18 months of outpatient MBT with structured clinical management (SCM), which focused on problem-solving skills and providing support. The number of suicidal and parasuicidal events and hospitalizations decreased at a significantly greater rate by post-treatment follow-up among the MBT participants compared with those in the SCM condition. MBT participants also had greater declines in secondary symptom severity over 18 months of treatment, including depression, interpersonal function, social adjustment, and global assessment of functioning ratings.

Furthermore, use of medication dropped significantly more in the MBT group than in the SCM group. While these findings provide support for MBT as an efficacious treatment for BPD, further follow-up analyses are needed to ascertain maintenance of treatment effects.

Evidence for Transference-focused Psychotherapy for Treatment of BPD

There is now accumulating evidence for the effectiveness and efficacy of TFP. At least three RCTs have examined the efficacy of TFP for BPD. The initial RCT by the Kernberg group[76,83] comparing TFP with two other active conditions (DBT and supportive psychotherapy [SPT][84]) found that TFP and DBT decreased suicidality over and above SPT; and TFP and SPT showed improvements in anger and impulsivity, whereas DBT did not. The TFP condition also showed unique improvements in a variety of aspects of aggression. The study further found roughly equivalent changes among the conditions in secondary features of depression, anxiety, and global level of functioning. In a second paper, this group[83] reported unique changes for TFP in comparison with DBT and SPT in reflective functioning (mentalizing) and attachment security. In sum, TFP appears at least as efficacious as DBT, but TFP may also provide unique and theoretically consistent improvements in areas such as attachment, identity, mentalizing, and aggression.

In a subsequent study by an independent group, Doering and colleagues[85] found that one year of TFP outperformed treatment provided by experienced community psychotherapists treating BPD, in terms of hospitalizations, suicide rates, BPD symptoms, psychosocial functioning, personality organization, secondary symptoms (e.g., anxiety and depression), and dropout rate. Although self-harm fell from 29.33 acts the year prior to 16.94 acts during the treatment year, this difference was not significant because of a large standard deviation, nor was it different from the reduction seen in the treatment by experienced community psychotherapists. TFP was also examined as a control condition in a study of ST.[86] Both treatments were quite effective at reducing the range of BPD symptoms and improving quality of life, yet the authors found that several BPD symptoms (e.g., impulsivity, fears of abandonment, relationship chaos) by year three of treatment improved more in ST over TFP. However, some concerns regarding the adequacy of the TFP implementation in this study[87,88] indicate that results may be unfairly partial toward ST, casting some doubt on the generalizability of the study in terms of TFP's efficacy for BPD.

Evidence for Schema Therapy for Treatment of BPD

Giesen-Bloo and colleagues[86] provide initial support for ST, as described in the discussion on TFP, although these results must be considered preliminary given the concerns we have outlined already. However, more recent data provide continued evidence for ST provided in a group format as an efficacious treatment for BPD. Farrell, Shaw, and Webber[89] report data from a small sample of women with BPD (N = 32), comparing eight months of group-based ST with TAU. At the end of treatment, 94 percent of the women in the ST group no longer met diagnostic criteria for BPD, a significantly greater reduction than in the 16 percent who no longer met criteria in the TAU group. Furthermore, ST led to significantly greater improvements on levels of general functioning and psychopathology in comparison to TAU. This study, therefore, provides further evidence for the efficacy of ST for BPD, although further research with larger samples and increased methodological rigor is needed to confirm this treatment's utility.

Evidence for Good Psychiatric Management for Treatment of BPD

Empirical support for GPM comes primarily from the original RCT using GPM as a credible control condition against DBT. Despite initial study hypotheses, GPM was found to be as effective as DBT across all outcome measures, including self-harm, hospitalizations, BPD symptoms, a range of secondary clinical correlates such as depression, and functioning variables.[60] A two-year follow-up study[90] found that these improvements either continued or were sustained over follow-up. Once again, neither treatment was found to be superior to the other. These results suggest that GPM may be a viable alternative to specialized treatments for BPD, especially in contexts in which such treatments are not available. However, GPM has evolved since the original trial and has not been examined in its current iteration, that is, as a generalist approach without a once-weekly dynamically oriented psychotherapy component.

Meta-analyses for Treatment of BPD

Meta-analysis is a procedure for statistically combining the results of many different research studies by aggregating data though the conversion of divergent outcomes into a common metric, called an effect size. The effect sizes represent the strength of an effect (on the dependent variable) and standardizes findings across studies such that they can be directly compared. Meta-analyses focus on the *direction* and *magnitude* of the effects across studies; by combining results from multiple studies, meta-analysis allows for the statistical examination of potential moderators. Several stage- or level-based evidence rating systems place systematic reviews and meta-analytic studies at the top of the evidence hierarchy,[91–93] because they can protect against the biases or chance findings that may occur in any one study. Additionally, such studies can protect against allegiance effects,[94,95] which might persist across several studies carried out by one group of investigators, and allow for the exploration of moderators. Both systematic reviews and meta-analytic ones, like all research, can be subject to critique, but over the last decade there have been several guidelines developed to facilitate the conduct and reporting of such studies (A Measurement Tool to Assess Systematic Reviews, AMSTAR[96]; Meta-Analysis Reporting Standards, MARS[97]; and Preferred Reporting Items for Systematic Reviews and Meta-Analyses, PRISMA[98,99]).

To date there have been five published meta-analyses examining the treatment outcome for individual psychotherapies for BPD;[20,78,100–102] two published meta-analyses examining dropout;[103,116] one published meta-analysis examining outcome for group treatment of BPD;[104] several meta-analyses of medication use; as well as several other meta-analyses of DBT in various contexts (e.g., inpatient).[100,101,105–108,114–115,117–118]

The first meta-analysis[100] included seven studies of 262 patients. Six of the studies were of DBT and one was for MBT. The authors found that there were no differences between active treatments and TAU for many outcomes such as remission of diagnosis, anxiety, and depression; there was some evidence for reduction of suicidality and para-suicidality. The authors concluded that some problems experienced by BPD patients may be amendable to "talk" and behaviorally oriented therapies; however, they warned that the wide confidence intervals around the effect sizes render the findings unreliable. Hence, the authors suggested that all talk/behavioral treatments at that time should be considered experimental. These conclusions ran counter to the acceptance of DBT as a treatment of choice and its wide dissemination across the United States and Europe between 1991 and the early 2000s.

The next published meta-analysis, by Kröger and colleagues,[78] reported findings examining 16 RCTs for DBT. They found an overall effect size of 0.39 for suicidal and parasuicidal behavior, which corresponds to a moderate effect.[109] However, their meta-regression model showed a negligible between-group effect size of 0.01 for trials in which DBT was compared with an active control or specific treatment for BPD.[60,76,79,110] This finding points to the presence of a possible moderator of effect size—the stringency of the control group against which the experimental treatment is measured—and suggests that clinicians may have options available to them in treating BPD besides DBT. Nevertheless, this meta-analysis focused only on DBT and included only RCTs, limiting the authors' conclusions and prohibiting them from examining treatment type and study design factors as moderators of effect size.

Stoffers and colleagues[101] for the Cochrane Collaboration published an updated quantitative review examining RCTs of psychotherapy for BPD. The authors noted that DBT was the most studied treatment, followed in no specific order by MBT, TFP, and ST. The authors conducted a number of subgroup analyses, separating effect size estimates by treatment and by outcome; however, this strategy resulted in only four treatment-outcome combinations that could be pooled across studies (DBT for anger, parasuicidality, mental health, and dropout). The rest of the treatment-outcome subgroups contained only single estimates. The authors concluded that DBT was helpful for these outcomes relative to TAU but, because of low power in these subgroup analyses (and thus low reliability of findings), could draw few other strong conclusions. Despite the conclusions, some people have interpreted the statement that DBT was the most studied treatment to mean that DBT had the most empirical support. However, that would be an erroneous conclusion. In fact, the opposite conclusion is perhaps more accurate. Given that there are more studies of DBT, we can feel more confident in its effect size and its equivalence to other active treatments, but there is no evidence for its superiority.

In a study of 20 RCTs with 1,375 participants, Oud et al.[102] found medium effects on overall BPD severity (ES = 0.59) and small-to-medium effects for DBT on self-injury (ES = 0.40). Other effects were inconclusive. The comprehensive published meta-analysis was conducted by Cristea et al.[20] It included 33 trials and over 2,000 patients. Similar to previous meta-analyses, the best-represented approach was DBT (12 trials). PDT had eight trials, and CBT had five trials. Effect sizes ranged from small to moderate = 0.32–0.44 across outcomes and across types of therapies. There were no differences between DBT and PDT treatments. In fact, the effect sizes were slightly (but non-significantly) higher for PDT ($g = 0.41$; 95 percent CI, 0.12 to 0.69 [seven trials]) than for DBT ($g = 0.34$; 95 percent CI, 0.15 to 0.53 [nine trials]). Both DBT and PDT were more effective than control interventions, while CBT ($g = 0.24$; 95 percent CI, −0.01 to 0.49 [five trials]) and other interventions ($g = 0.38$; 95 percent CI, −0.15 to 0.92 [six trials]) were not. There were no differences in dropout between DBT and PDT. The authors conclude that psychotherapy, particularly DBT and PDT, are effective for BPD symptoms; nonetheless, effects are small, inflated by risk of bias and publication bias, and unstable at follow-up.

Barnicot et al.[103] used meta-analysis to examine dropout from treatments for BPD. The authors concluded that although there was substantial dropout, it was not much higher than what is typical for other disorders, and that BPD, when treated with specialized psychotherapies, should no longer be thought of as a high-dropout disorder. Despite this conclusion, the completion rates varied quite a bit, and this variation was unexplained. Additionally, the findings of Barnicot et al.[103] run counter to a recent meta-analysis examining premature discontinuation in adult psychotherapy by Swift and

Greenberg.[111] They found that a personality disorder diagnosis was predictive of premature dropout. One way to understand this discrepancy between Baricot et al.[103] and Swift and Greenberg[111] is that specialized treatments for BPD may result in significantly less dropout than non-modified and specialized approaches, which was more common in Swift and Greenberg's[111] samples. This interpretation is consistent with the dropout rates in the RCTs for BPD, which tend to be about 20–25 percent as compared with early reports which were in the 50–65 percent range.[112]

More recently, McLaughlin et al.[104] examined group psychotherapy for BPD. The authors found 24 RCTs with 1,595 patients that compared group psychotherapy for BPD with TAU. The group treatment conditions included STEPPS, MBT, DBT, and ST. The authors concluded that group treatments were associated with greater symptom reduction when compared with TAU. However, there was a moderating effect for the context of the group. Two of the highest effect sizes were obtained from groups that were part of a comprehensive day program,[6,82] and thus groups used adjunctive to TAU, or as standalone, do not appear to have the same effect. See Chapter 14 on group therapy for patients with PDs

Regarding medications, the evidence for their efficacy from RCTs and meta-analyses suggests that the widespread use of medications in the treatment of BPD is not supported by the evidence.[101,105–108] Binks, et al.[100] examined ten studies of 554 patients, finding few and small differences between medications and placebo. They concluded that pharmacological treatment of people with BPD was not based on good evidence. Nosè et al.[106] reviewed 20 RCTs of 818 patients and found no differences between any medication examined and placebo for 22 drug–placebo comparisons. This included comparisons for instability and anger with antipsychotics and antidepressants, interpersonal relationship functioning treated with antidepressants, suicidality treated with antidepressants, mood stabilizers, or antipsychotics. A 2010 review of 21 pharmacological treatment studies of BPD and STPD suggested that antipsychotics were moderately effective for cognitive or perceptual symptoms, as well as for reducing anger.[105] Antidepressants had a small effect on anxiety symptoms, but were not effective for depression among these patients or for treating core PD symptomatology. In the most recent meta-analysis examining new studies since 2015, Storebø et al.[107] caution that antidepressants such as fluoxetine did not show efficacy for reducing suicidality and self-harm in BPD patients. This finding is consistent with Vita et al.,[108] who found no evidence that antidepressants reduce BPD dimensions. Thus, although some studies have found modest and small positive effects of medications, the findings are far from consistent and are associated with significant risks. As such, medications are often seen as adjunctive and to be used with caution. See Chapter 15 on Psychopharmacology of Personality Disorders for additional information.

Review Table 5.1 (see p. 124) for a summaries of meta-analyses and RCTs demonstrating effectiveness of various psychotherapies for BPD.

Crossing the Alphabet Divide: Deriving Evidence-based Principles

Given that there are several treatments available that have shown evidence of efficacy, often in multiple studies, what is a clinician to do? How is one to make sense of this alphabet soup of treatment and findings? There are several treatment implications of our review. First, there are multiple treatments available to patients with BPD and the

Table 5.1 Levels of Evidence for the Effectiveness of Various Psychotherapies for Borderline Personality disorder

Treatment	Primary Citation	Overall Level of Evidence	Summary of Levels of Evidence
Dialectical behavior therapy (DBT)	Linehan (1993)[1]	Level A	• Level I: Seven meta-analyses[20,78,102,107,114–118] and two systematic reviews find support for DBT on diagnostic remission, BPD symptoms, behaviors such as self-harm and suicide, and secondary features such as depression and anxiety. • Level II: 14 RCTs[38,60,68,72,73,75–77,79,119–123] find support for DBT for a range of symptoms, including behavioral symptoms such as self-harm and suicide in particular.
Mentalization-based treatment (MBT)	Bateman & Fonagy (1999)[6]	Level A	• Level I: Three meta-analyses[20,102,107] and three systematic reviews[117,124,125] find support for MBT on improving clinical outcomes of BPD, including symptom severity, comorbid disorders, and quality of life. • Level II: Six RCTs[81,82,126–129] find support for MBT in improving suicidal and parasuicidal behaviors, medication use, social and interpersonal functioning.
Transference-focused psychotherapy (TFP)	Yeomans, Clarkin, & Kernberg (2006)[7]	Level A	• Level I: Three meta-analyses[20,102,107] find support for TFP to be effective in treating BPD symptoms including suicidality and parasuicidality. • Level II: Three RCTs[76,85,86] find support for TFP in a range of primary and secondary BPD features, particularly reflective functioning and attachment security.
Schema therapy (ST)	Young (1994)[8]	Level A	• Level I: Two systematic reviews [130,131] of ST find support for improvement in BPD symptoms, including reduction of early maladaptive schema. • Level II: Three RCTs[86,89,132] find support for ST in diagnostic criteria for BPD and quality of life.
Good psychiatric management (GPM)	Gunderson & Links (2008)[9]	Level B	• Level II: One RCT[60] for a version of GPM finds improvement in self-harm, hospitalizations, BPD symptoms, and secondary features.

Note:
Criteria Levels of Evidence:
Level of Evidence A: Good quality patient-oriented evidence.
Level of Evidence B: Limited quality patient-oriented evidence
Level of Evidence C: Based on consensus, usual practice, opinion, disease-oriented evidence, or Case series for studies of diagnosis treatment prevention or screening
Level I: Systematic review or meta-analysis of randomized controlled trials
Level II: Randomized controlled trial
Level III: Controlled trial without randomization
Level IV: Case controlled or cohort studies

clinicians who treatment them. Although these treatments derive out of different theoretical orientations and do have some historical and conceptual differences, they all tend to be integrative, either explicitly or implicitly. Despite the use of different terms and jargon, there are more similarities across these treatments than is often recognized. This may be in large part because they are derived from similar clinical experiences in adapting to the challenge of treating clients with BPD, as treatments have been developed and refined in the context of knowledge derived from the broader literature on psychotherapy for BPD.

We will distill principles that clinicians can use to guide their work with individuals with BPD. First with regard to the research literature:

1) There are five empirically supported treatments available to the practicing clinician for treating borderline personality disorder. The Big Five are DBT, MBT, TFP, ST, and GPM.

2) Outcome data, direct comparisons, and meta-analyses all suggest few reliable differences between these treatments and that *no one treatment is more effective than the other.*

3) In addition, there are several adjunctive treatments (DBT skills group, STEPPS, MOTR) that may be useful when combined with specialized treatments.

4) Despite this evidence, at this point there are few prescriptive indicators suggested in literature.

There are several similarities between treatments that are useful for therapists to reflect upon. These include:

1) Treatment is not expected to be brief, casual, or designed to be intermittent. All of these treatments are designed and conceptualized to be long-term, with clinical trials lasting one to three years and naturalistic treatment often lasting longer. Each of these treatments is designed to be weekly and for multiple hours per week. For example, TFP is twice weekly; DBT includes one hour of therapy per week plus a 3-hour group and available phone consultation.

2) These treatments include the provision of supervision and consultation for therapists (or intervision—that is, supervision by peers—for more experienced therapists), with the explicit goal of providing the therapist with support and protecting against therapist burnout, enactments in the treatment, passivity, iatrogenic behaviors, and colluding with clients' pathology.

3) Therapists treating patients with BPD should strongly consider training in one or more of the evidence-based treatments: DBT, MBT, TFP, ST, and GPM. All have books and training material available and have organized workshops, trainings, supervisions, and even online training modules available.

4) Given that BPD is heterogeneous, that only 50–60 percent of patients improve within one year, and that even those patients who do improve only do so partially, it is useful for a therapist to know more than one treatment approach, especially approaches that may cut across theoretical orientations.

5) Many of the evidence-based treatments for BPD utilize concomitant treatments (e.g., 12-step programs, skills groups) and group therapy in addition to individual therapy: DBT includes skills groups; MBT has traditionally included

group therapy. Although TFP does not have a formal group component yet, adjunctive group treatments, including skills-based ones, are considered useful as long as there is communication between treaters and shared understanding of treatment goals. In fact, depending on the patient's issue, a TFP therapist may not only encourage but require involvement in group psychotherapy.

6) To avoid splitting across providers, each treatment emphasizes integration of different services received by clients and communication among providers. Related to this, there is some evidence that different treatment services provided within institutions are more effective than treatments across institutions.[113]

7) In these treatments, therapists tend to take an active role in treatment and are not passive listeners.

8) The therapist takes a thorough history from the patient, including past treatments. It is important to speak with informants, including referral sources, significant others, past treaters, and possibly others. Patients should provide permission to speak with such individuals. This may take some time to work through patients' ambivalence to involve others.

9) Once all information is obtained, and the therapist feels confident about their understanding of the patient's difficulties, this understanding should be explicitly shared with the patient. This typically includes the diagnosis, which of course needs to be done sensitively and without unnecessary stigmatizing of the patient. The patient's feedback should be considered, and a shared understanding of the difficulties should be sought and established. It is important to share the diagnosis with the patient for ethical reasons, but also because the patient may inadvertently find out or suspect the diagnosis. The therapist's withholding of the diagnosis can be interpreted as the diagnosis being dangerous and stigmatizing.

10) There is significant value in establishing a strong and explicit structure and frame for the treatment and clear roles and responsibilities of patient and therapist. Patient and therapist should strive to mutually agree on a hierarchy of priorities in treatment. The frame is set collaboratively. The therapist should try not to impose rules on the patient and should be vigilant to prevent patient acquiescence. Likewise, the therapist should not acquiesce to the patient if doing so feels uncomfortable or runs counter to the therapist's professional opinion.

11) The therapist adopts a nonjudgmental and flexible stance and empathizes with the client without reinforcing distortions in their perception of self or others.

12) Additionally, there is a common focus on emotion regulation, on views of self and others, and on addressing unintegrated or polarized mental states. The specific form this takes may differ by treatment; for instance, DBT focuses on dialectical thinking, TFP focuses on observing extreme vacillations in object-relations dyads (affectively charged mental representations of self and others in a relationship) and in integrating these extremes into a coherent whole, while ST focuses on abrupt shifts between schema modes (thoughts, behaviors, and emotions that reflect the emotional/behavioral state of the person at any given moment). MBT emphasizes awareness of shifts in mentalizing from effective mentalizing processes to non-mentalizing modes.

13) There is a common focus on helping clients to link and integrate their emotions, thoughts, and behaviors, generally including a focus on self-observation as well as considering alternative perspectives.

Conclusion

A number of psychotherapeutic treatments exist for BPD. These treatments hail from disparate theoretical foundations and come in a variety of formats, including individual and group therapies and as augmentation to other treatments. The evidence base for psychotherapy for BPD is strong, yet growing, showing moderate efficacy but with no one treatment consistently surpassing others. Consequently, clinicians and researchers should understand the similarities and differences among these approaches and begin to more effectively and coherently integrate across them. More work is needed to empirically evaluate the effectiveness of integrative approaches to treating BPD and how best to sequence or combine treatments and their elements. See Box 5.1 for relevant information for patients, families, and clinicians.

Conflict of Interest/Disclosure: The authors of this chapter have no financial conflicts and nothing to disclose.

Box 5.1. Resources for Patient Families and Clinicians

National Organizations for BPD

- BPD Resource Center. www.bpdresourcecenter.org.
- Treatment and Research Advancements for Borderline Personality Disorder (TARA4BPD). www.tara4bpd.org
- National Education Alliance for BPD (NEA-BPD). www.borderlinepersonalitydisorder.org

Self-Help Books for BPD

- Chapman AL, Gratz KL. *The Borderline Personality Disorder Survival Guide.* Oakland, CA: New Harbinger Publications; 2007.
- Friedel RO. *Borderline Personality Disorder Demystified: An Essential Guide for Understanding and Living with BPD.* rev. ed. New York: Da Capo Lifelong Books; 2018.
- Green T. *Self-Help for Managing the Symptoms of Borderline Personality Disorder.* Self-published; 2008.
- Kreisman JJ, Straus H. *I Hate You, Don't Leave Me: Understanding Borderline Personality Disorder.* Updated, rev. ed. New York: TarcherPerigree; 2014.
- Lee, T. (2016). Stormy Lives: A Journey Through Personality Disorder (Muswell Hill Press).
- Mason PTT, Kreger R. *Stop Walking on Eggshells: Taking Your Life Back When Someone You Care About Has Borderline Personality Disorder.* 3rd ed. Oakland, CA: New Harbinger Publications; 2020.
- Reiland R. *Get Me Out of Here: My Recovery from Borderline Personality Disorder.* Center City, MN: Hazelden Publishing; 2004.

Books for Families of Individuals with BPD

- Gunderson JG, Hoffman PD. *Understanding and Treating Borderline Personality Disorder: A Guide for Professionals and Families.* Washington, DC: American Psychiatric Association Publishing; 2006.
- Kreger R. *The Essential Family Guide to Borderline Personality Disorder.* Center City, MN: Hazelden Publishing; 2008.
- Lee, T. (2016). Stormy Lives: A Journey Through Personality Disorder (Muswell Hill Press).
- Manning SY. *Loving Someone with Borderline Personality Disorder.* New York: Guilford Press; 2011.
- Porr V. *Overcoming Borderline Personality Disorder: A Family Guide for Healing and Change.* New York: Oxford University Press; 2010.
- Tusiani P, Tusiani V, Tusiani-Eng P. *Remnants of a Life on Paper: A Mother and Daughter's Struggle with Borderline Personality Disorder.* Baroque Press, 2014.

Other Online Resources

- BDP Central. Accessed Feb. 10, 2021. www.bpdcentral.com
- BPDWORLD. Providing information advice and support to those affected by personality disorders. Accessed Feb. 10, 2021. www.bpdworld.org
- National Institute of mental health. Borderline personality disorder. Accessed Feb. 10, 2021. www.nimh.nih.gov/health/topics/borderline-personality-disorder/index.shtml
- BPD Family. Facing emotionally intense relationships. Accessed Feb. 10, 2021. www.bpdfamily.com

References

1. Linehan MM. *Cognitive-behavioral Treatment of Borderline Personality Disorder.* Guilford Press; 1993.

2. Gabbard GO. Splitting in hospital treatment. *Am J Psychiatry.* 1989 Apr;146(4):444–451. doi:10.1176/ajp.146.4.444

3. Kernberg O. Borderline personality organization. *J Am Psychoanal Assoc.* 1967;15(3):641–685. doi:10.1177/000306516701500309

4. Lewis G, Appleby L. Personality disorder: the patients psychiatrists dislike. *Br J Psychiatry J Ment Sci.* 1988;153:44–49. doi:10.1192/bjp.153.1.44

5. Paris J. The nature of borderline personality disorder: multiple dimensions, multiple symptoms, but one category. *J Personal Disord.* 2007;21(5):457–473. doi:10.1521/pedi.2007.21.5.457

6. Bateman A, Fonagy P. Effectiveness of partial hospitalization in the treatment of borderline personality disorder: a randomized controlled trial. *Am J Psychiatry.* 1999;156(10):1563–1569. doi:10.1176/ajp.156.10.1563

7. Yeomans FE, Clarkin JF, Kernberg OF. *Transference-Focused Psychotherapy for Borderline Personality Disorder: A Clinical Guide.* Washington, DC: American Psychiatric Publishing; 2015.

8. Young JE. *Cognitive Therapy for Personality Disorders: A Schema-Focused Approach*, rev. ed. Sarasota, FL: Professional Resource Press/Professional Resource Exchange; 1994.

9. Gunderson JG., Links PS. *Borderline Personality Disorder: A Clinical Guide.* 2nd ed. Washington, DC: American Psychiatric Publishing; 2008:xvi, 350.

10. Levy KN, Draijer N, Kivity Y, Yeomans FE, Rosenstein LK. Transference-focused psychotherapy (TFP). *Curr Treat Options Psychiatry.* 2019;6(4):312–324. doi:10.1007/s40501-019-00193-9

11. Gregory RJ, Chlebowski S, Kang D, et al. A controlled trial of psychodynamic psychotherapy for co-occurring borderline personality disorder and alcohol use disorder. *Psychotherapy.* 2008;45(1):28–41. doi:10.1037/0033-3204.45.1.28

12. Blum N, Pfohl B, John DS, Monahan P, Black DW. STEPPS: a cognitive-behavioral systems-based group treatment for outpatients with borderline personality disorder—a preliminary report. *Compr Psychiatry.* 2002;43(4):301–310. doi:10.1053/comp.2002.33497

13. Gratz KL, Gunderson JG. Preliminary data on an acceptance-based emotion regulation group intervention for deliberate self-harm among women with borderline personality disorder. *Behav Ther.* 2006;37(1):25–35. doi:10.1016/j.beth.2005.03.002

14. Kramer U, Rosciano A, Pavlovic M, et al. Motive-oriented therapeutic relationship in brief psychodynamic intervention for patients with depression and personality disorders. *J Clin Psychol.* 2011;67(10):1017–1027. doi:10.1002/jclp.20806

15. Bateman AW, Krawitz R. *Borderline Personality Disorder: An Evidence-based Guide for Generalist Mental Health Professionals.* New York, NY: Oxford University Press; 2013.

16. Paris J. Stepped care: an alternative to routine extended treatment for patients with borderline personality disorder. *Psychiatr Serv Wash DC.* 2013;64(10):1035–1037. doi:10.1176/appi.ps.201200451

17. Tyrer P, Tom B, Byford S, et al. Differential effects of manual assisted cognitive behavior therapy in the treatment of recurrent deliberate self-harm and personality disturbance: the POPMACT study. *J Personal Disord.* 2004;18(1):102–116. doi:10.1521/pedi.18.1.102.32770

18. Weinberg I, Gunderson JG, Hennen J, Cutter Jr CJ. Manual assisted cognitive treatment for deliberate self-harm in borderline personality disorder patients. *J Personal Disord.* 2006;20(5):482.

19. Zanarini MC, Frankenburg FR. A preliminary, randomized trial of psychoeducation for women with borderline personality disorder. *J Personal Disord.* 2008;22(3):284–290. doi:10.1521/pedi.2008.22.3.284

20. Cristea IA, Gentili C, Cotet CD, Palomba D, Barbui C, Cuijpers P. Efficacy of psychotherapies for borderline personality disorder: a systematic review and meta-analysis. *JAMA Psychiatry.* 2017;74(4):319. doi:10.1001/jamapsychiatry.2016.4287

21. Ellison WD. Psychotherapy for borderline personality disorder: does the type of treatment make a difference? *Curr Treat Options Psychiatry.* 2020;7(3):416–428. doi:10.1007/s40501-020-00224-w

22. Levy KN, McMain S, Bateman A, Clouthier T. Treatment of borderline personality disorder. *Psychiatr Clin North Am.* 2018;41(4):711–728. doi:10.1016/j.psc.2018.07.011

23. Levy KN, Scala JW. Integrated treatment for personality disorders: a commentary. *J Psychother Integr.* 2015;25(1):49–57. doi:10.1037/a0038771

24. Gabbard GO. Do all roads lead to Rome? New findings on borderline personality disorder. *Am J Psychiatry.* 2007;164(6):853–855. doi:10.1176/ajp.2007.164.6.853

25. Levy KN. Psychotherapies and lasting change. *Am J Psychiatry.* 2008;165(5):556–559. doi:10.1176/appi.ajp.2008.08020299

26. Linehan MM. Dialectical behavior therapy for borderline personality disorder: theory and method. *Bull Menninger Clin.* 1987;51(3):261–276.

27. Kernberg OF. Technical considerations in the treatment of borderline personality organization. *J Am Psychoanal Assoc.* 1976;24(4):795–829. doi:10.1177/000306517602400403

28. Kazdin AE. Bridging child, adolescent, and adult psychotherapy: directions for research. *Psychother Res.* 1995;5(3):258–277. doi:10.1080/10503309512331331376

29. Kazdin AE. Developing a research agenda for child and adolescent psychotherapy. *Arch Gen Psychiatry.* 2000;57(9):829–835. doi:10.1001/archpsyc.57.9.829

30. Blatt S, Felsen I. Different kinds of folks may need different kinds of strokes: the effect of patients' characteristics on therapeutic process and outcome. *Psychother Res.* 1993;3(4):245–259. doi:10.1080/10503309312331333829

31. Kohut H. *The Analysis of the Self: A Systematic Approach to the Psychoanalytic Treatment of Narcissistic Personality Disorders.* Chicago, IL: University of Chicago Press; 1971:xvi, 368.

32. Adler G, Buie DH. Aloneness and borderline psychopathology: the possible relevance of child development issues. *Int J Psychoanal.* 1979;60(1):83–96.

33. Buie DH, Adler G. Definitive treatment of the borderline personality. *Int J Psychoanal Psychother.* 1982;9:51–87.

34. Fonagy P. Thinking about thinking: some clinical and theoretical considerations in the treatment of a borderline patient. *Int J Psychoanal.* 1991;72 (Pt 4):639–656.

35. Oldham J, Phillips K, Gabbard G. Practice guideline for the treatment of patients with borderline personality disorder. *Am J Psychiatry.* 2001;158(10 Suppl):1–52.

36. Unruh BT, Gunderson JG. "Good enough" psychiatric residency training in borderline personality disorder: challenges, choice points, and a model generalist curriculum. *Harv Rev Psychiatry.* 2016;24(5):367–377. doi:10.1097/HRP.0000000000000119

37. Paris J. *Stepped Care for Borderline Personality Disorder: Making Treatment Brief, Effective, and Accessible.* New York, NY: Academic Press; 2017.

38. Linehan MM, Armstrong HE, Suarez A, Allmon D, Heard HL. Cognitive-behavioral treatment of chronically parasuicidal borderline patients. *Arch Gen Psychiatry.* 1991;48(12):1060–1064.

39. Heard HL, Linehan MM. Dialectical behavior therapy: an integrative approach to the treatment of borderline personality disorder. *J Psychother Integr.* 1994;4(1):55–82. doi:10.1037/h0101147

40. Swenson CR. Kernberg and Linehan: Two approaches to the borderline patient. *J Personal Disord.* 1989;3(1):26–35. doi:10.1521/pedi.1989.3.1.26

41. Koerner K, Linehan MM. Research on dialectical behavior therapy for patients with borderline personality disorder. *Psychiatr Clin North Am.* 2000;23(1):151–167. doi:10.1016/s0193-953x(05)70149-0

42. Robins CJ. Zen principles and mindfulness practice in dialectical behavior therapy. *Cogn Behav Pract.* 2002;9(1):50–57. doi:10.1016/S1077-7229(02)80040-2

43. Bateman A, Fonagy P. Mentalizing and borderline personality disorder. In: Allen, JG, Fonagy, P, eds. *The Handbook of Mentalization-Based Treatment.* Hoboken, NJ: Wiley; 2006:185–200. doi:10.1002/9780470712986.ch9

44. Fonagy P, Steele M, Steele H, Moran GS, Higgitt AC. The capacity for understanding mental states: the reflective self in parent and child and its significance for security of attachment. *Infant Ment Health J.* 1991;12(3):201–218. doi:10.1002/1097-0355(199123)12:3<201::AID-IMHJ2280120307>3.0.CO;2-7

45. Fonagy P, Target M. Playing with reality: I. Theory of mind and the normal development of psychic reality. *Int J Psychoanal.* 1996;77(Pt 2):217–233.

46. Target M, Fonagy P. Playing with reality: II. The development of psychic reality from a theoretical perspective. *Int J Psychoanal.* 1996;77(Pt 3):459–479.

47. Fonagy P, Gergely G, Jurist EL, Target M. *Affect Regulation, Mentalization, and the Development of the Self.* New York, NY: Other Press; 2002:xiii, 577.

48. Fonagy P, Bateman AW. Mechanisms of change in mentalization-based treatment of BPD. *J Clin Psychol.* 2006;62(4):411–430. doi:10.1002/jclp.20241

49. Levy KN, Kivity Y. Transference-focused psychotherapy. In: Zeigler-Hill V, Shackelford TK, eds. *Encyclopedia of Personality and Individual Differences.* Cham, Switzerland: Springer International; 2020:1–5. doi:10.1007/978-3-319-28099-8_2297-1

50. Johnson BN, Clouthier TL, Rosenstein LK, Levy KN. Psychotherapy for personality disorders. In: Zeigler-Hill V, Shackelford TK, eds. *Encyclopedia of Personality and Individual Differences.* Cham, Switzerland: Springer International Publishing; 2020:4216–4234. doi:10.1007/978-3-319-24612-3_925

51. Caligor E, Kernberg OF, Clarkin JF, Yeomans FE. *Psychodynamic Therapy for Personality Pathology: Treating Self and Interpersonal Functioning.* Washington, DC: American Psychiatric Association Publishing; 2018.

52. *Diagnostic and Statistical Manual of Mental Disorders (DSM-5®).* Washington, DC: American Psychiatric Association; 2013.

53. Blatt SJ, Blass RB. Attachment and separateness: a dialectic model of the products and processes of development throughout the life cycle. *Psychoanal Study Child.* 1990;45:107–127.

54. Erikson EH. *Childhood and Society.* New York, NY: Norton; 1950:397.

55. Marcia JE. Development and validation of ego-identity status. *J Pers Soc Psychol.* 1966;3(5):551–558. doi:10.1037/h0023281

56. McAdams DP. *The Person: An Introduction to Personality Psychology.* Fort Worth, TX: Harcourt Brace Jovanovich; 1990:ix, 677.

57. Kernberg OF. Structural interviewing. *Psychiatr Clin North Am.* 1981;4(1):169–195. doi:10.1016/S0193-953X(18)30944-4

58. Young JE. Schema-focused cognitive therapy and the case of Ms. S. *J Psychother Integr.* 2005;15(1):115–126. doi:10.1037/1053-0479.15.1.115

59. Young J, Flanagan C. Schema-focused therapy for narcissistic patients. In: Ronningstam, EF, ed. *Disorders of Narcissism: Diagnostic, Clinical, and Empirical Implications.* Washington, DC: American Psychiatric Association; 1998:239–262.

60. McMain SF, Links PS, Gnam WH, et al. A randomized trial of dialectical behavior therapy versus general psychiatric management for borderline personality disorder. *Am J Psychiatry.* 2009;166(12):1365–1374. doi:10.1176/appi.ajp.2009.09010039

61. Gunderson JG. *Borderline Personality Disorder: A Clinical Guide.* Washington, DC: American Psychiatric Association Publishing; 2001:xxii, 329.

62. Links PS. *Clinical Assessment and Management of Severe Personality Disorders.* Washington, DC: American Psychiatric Association Publishing; 1996.

63. Gunderson JG, Lyons-Ruth K. BPD's interpersonal hypersensitivity phenotype: a gene-environment-developmental model. *J Personal Disord.* 2008;22(1):22–41. doi:10.1521/pedi.2008.22.1.22

64. Gunderson JG. The borderline patient's intolerance of aloneness: insecure attachments and therapist availability. *Am J Psychiatry.* 1996;153(6):752–758. doi:10.1176/ajp.153.6.752

65. Gunderson JG. *Handbook of Good Psychiatric Management for Borderline Personality Disorder*. Washington, DC: American Psychiatric Association Publishing; 2014:xii, 168.

66. Winnicott DW. Transitional objects and transitional phenomena; a study of the first not-me possession. *Int J Psychoanal*. 1953;34(2):89–97.

67. Bohus M, Haaf B, Simms T, et al. Effectiveness of inpatient dialectical behavioral therapy for borderline personality disorder: a controlled trial. *Behav Res Ther*. 2004;42(5):487–499. doi:10.1016/S0005-7967(03)00174-8

68. Linehan MM, Comtois KA, Murray AM, et al. Two-year randomized controlled trial and follow-up of dialectical behavior therapy vs therapy by experts for suicidal behaviors and borderline personality disorder. *Arch Gen Psychiatry*. 2006;63(7):757–766. doi:10.1001/archpsyc.63.7.757

69. Pasieczny N, Connor J. The effectiveness of dialectical behaviour therapy in routine public mental health settings: an Australian controlled trial. *Behav Res Ther*. 2011;49(1):4–10. doi:10.1016/j.brat.2010.09.006

70. Pistorello J, Fruzzetti AE, Maclane C, Gallop R, Iverson KM. Dialectical behavior therapy (DBT) applied to college students: a randomized clinical trial. *J Consult Clin Psychol*. 2012;80(6):982–994. doi:10.1037/a0029096

71. Priebe S, Bhatti N, Barnicot K, et al. Effectiveness and cost-effectiveness of dialectical behaviour therapy for self-harming patients with personality disorder: a pragmatic randomised controlled trial. *Psychother Psychosom*. 2012;81(6):356–365. doi:10.1159/000338897

72. Verheul R, Van Den Bosch LMC, Koeter MWJ, De Ridder MAJ, Stijnen T, Van Den Brink W. Dialectical behaviour therapy for women with borderline personality disorder: 12-month, randomised clinical trial in The Netherlands. *Br J Psychiatry J Ment Sci*. 2003;182:135–140. doi:10.1192/bjp.182.2.135

73. Carter GL, Willcox CH, Lewin TJ, Conrad AM, Bendit N. Hunter DBT project: randomized controlled trial of dialectical behaviour therapy in women with borderline personality disorder. *Aust N Z J Psychiatry*. 2010;44(2):162–173. doi:10.3109/00048670903393621

74. Feigenbaum JD, Fonagy P, Pilling S, Jones A, Wildgoose A, Bebbington PE. A real-world study of the effectiveness of DBT in the UK National Health Service. *Br J Clin Psychol*. 2012;51(2):121–141. doi:10.1111/j.2044-8260.2011.02017.x

75. Koons CR, Robins CJ, Lindsey Tweed J, et al. Efficacy of dialectical behavior therapy in women veterans with borderline personality disorder. *Behav Ther*. 2001;32(2):371–390. doi:10.1016/S0005-7894(01)80009-5

76. Clarkin JF, Levy KN, Lenzenweger MF, Kernberg OF. Evaluating three treatments for borderline personality disorder: a multiwave study. *Am J Psychiatry*. 2007;164(6):922–928. doi:10.1176/ajp.2007.164.6.922

77. Soler J, Pascual JC, Tiana T, et al. Dialectical behaviour therapy skills training compared to standard group therapy in borderline personality disorder: a 3-month randomised controlled clinical trial. *Behav Res Ther*. 2009;47(5):353–358. doi:10.1016/j.brat.2009.01.013

78. Kliem S, Kröger C, Kosfelder J. Dialectical behavior therapy for borderline personality disorder: a meta-analysis using mixed-effects modeling. *J Consult Clin Psychol*. 2010;78(6):936–951. doi:10.1037/a0021015

79. Linehan MM, Dimeff LA, Reynolds SK, et al. Dialectical behavior therapy versus comprehensive validation therapy plus 12-step for the treatment of opioid dependent women meeting criteria for borderline personality disorder. *Drug Alcohol Depend*. 2002;67(1):13–26. doi:10.1016/s0376-8716(02)00011-x

80. Sachdeva S, Goldman G, Mustata G, Deranja E, Gregory RJ. Naturalistic outcomes of evidence-based therapies for borderline personality disorder at a university clinic: a quasi-randomized trial. *J Am Psychoanal Assoc*. 2013;61(3):578–584. doi:10.1177/0003065113490637

81. Bateman A, Fonagy P. 8-year follow-up of patients treated for borderline personality disorder: mentalization-based treatment versus treatment as usual. *Am J Psychiatry*. 2008;165(5):631–638. doi:10.1176/appi.ajp.2007.07040636

82. Bateman A, Fonagy P. Randomized controlled trial of outpatient mentalization-based treatment versus structured clinical management for borderline personality disorder. *Am J Psychiatry*. 2009;166(12):1355–1364. doi:10.1176/appi.ajp.2009.09040539

83. Levy KN, Meehan KB, Kelly KM, et al. Change in attachment patterns and reflective function in a randomized control trial of transference-focused psychotherapy for borderline personality disorder. *J Consult Clin Psychol*. 2006;74(6):1027–1040. doi:10.1037/0022-006X.74.6.1027

84. Appelbaum AH. Supportive psychotherapy. In: Skodol AE, Oldham JM, eds. *The American Psychiatric Publishing Textbook of Personality Disorders*. Washington, DC: American Psychiatric Publishing, Inc.; 2005:335–346.

85. Doering S, Hörz S, Rentrop M, et al. Transference-focused psychotherapy v. treatment by community psychotherapists for borderline personality disorder: randomised controlled trial. *Br J Psychiatry J Ment Sci*. 2010;196(5):389–395. doi:10.1192/bjp.bp.109.070177

86. Giesen-Bloo J, van Dyck R, Spinhoven P, et al. Outpatient psychotherapy for borderline personality disorder: randomized trial of schema-focused therapy vs transference-focused psychotherapy. *Arch Gen Psychiatry*. 2006;63(6):649–658. doi:10.1001/archpsyc.63.6.649

87. Levy K. Psychodynamic and psychoanalytic psychotherapy. *Clin Psychol Assess Treat Res*. Published online 2009:181–214.

88. Yeomans F. Questions concerning the randomized trial of schema-focused therapy vs transference-focused psychotherapy. *Arch Gen Psychiatry*. 2007;64(5):609–610; author reply 610–611. doi:10.1001/archpsyc.64.5.609-c

89. Farrell JM, Shaw IA, Webber MA. A schema-focused approach to group psychotherapy for outpatients with borderline personality disorder: a randomized controlled trial. *J Behav Ther Exp Psychiatry*. 2009;40(2):317–328. doi:10.1016/j.jbtep.2009.01.002

90. McMain SF, Guimond T, Streiner DL, Cardish RJ, Links PS. Dialectical behavior therapy compared with general psychiatric management for borderline personality disorder: clinical outcomes and functioning over a 2-year follow-pp. *Am J Psychiatry*. 2012;169(6):650–661. doi:10.1176/appi.ajp.2012.11091416

91. Centre for Evidence-Based Medicine (CEBM), University of Oxford. Levels of evidence: an introduction. https://www.cebm.ox.ac.uk/resources/levels-of-evidence/levels-of-evidence-introductory-document.

92. Spring B. Evidence-based practice in clinical psychology: what it is, why it matters; what you need to know. *J Clin Psychol*. 2007;63(7):611–631. doi:10.1002/jclp.20373

93. Cochrane and Systematic Reviews. http://cochrane-and-systematic-reviews.

94. Robinson LA, Berman JS, Neimeyer RA. Psychotherapy for the treatment of depression: a comprehensive review of controlled outcome research. *Psychol Bull*. 1990;108(1):30–49. doi:10.1037/0033-2909.108.1.30

95. Luborsky L, Diguer L, Seligman DA, et al. The researcher's own therapy allegiances: a "wild card" in comparisons of treatment efficacy. *Clin Psychol Sci Pract*. 1999;6(1):95–106. doi:10.1093/clipsy.6.1.95

96. Shea BJ, Hamel C, Wells GA, et al. AMSTAR is a reliable and valid measurement tool to assess the methodological quality of systematic reviews. *J Clin Epidemiol.* 2009;62(10):1013–1020. doi:10.1016/j.jclinepi.2008.10.009

97. Appelbaum M, Cooper H, Kline RB, Mayo-Wilson E, Nezu AM, Rao SM. Journal article reporting standards for quantitative research in psychology: the APA Publications and Communications Board task force report. *Am Psychol.* 2018;73(1):3–25. doi:10.1037/amp0000191

98. Moher D, Liberati A, Tetzlaff J, Altman DG, PRISMA Group. Preferred reporting items for systematic reviews and meta-analyses: the PRISMA statement. *PLoS Med.* 2009;6(7):e1000097. doi:10.1371/journal.pmed.1000097

99. Moher D, Shamseer L, Clarke M, et al. Preferred reporting items for systematic review and meta-analysis protocols (PRISMA-P) 2015 statement. *Syst Rev.* 2015;4:1. doi:10.1186/2046-4053-4-1

100. Binks CA, Fenton M, McCarthy L, Lee T, Adams CE, Duggan C. Psychological therapies for people with borderline personality disorder. *Cochrane Database Syst Rev.* 2006;(1):CD005652. doi:10.1002/14651858.CD005652

101. Stoffers JM, Völlm BA, Rücker G, Timmer A, Huband N, Lieb K. Psychological therapies for people with borderline personality disorder. *Cochrane Database Syst Rev.* 2012;(8):CD005652. doi:10.1002/14651858.CD005652.pub2

102. Oud M, Arntz A, Hermens ML, Verhoef R, Kendall T. Specialized psychotherapies for adults with borderline personality disorder: a systematic review and meta-analysis. *Aust N Z J Psychiatry.* 2018;52(10):949–961. doi:10.1177/0004867418791257

103. Barnicot K, Katsakou C, Marougka S, Priebe S. Treatment completion in psychotherapy for borderline personality disorder: a systematic review and meta-analysis. *Acta Psychiatr Scand.* 2011;123(5):327–338. doi:10.1111/j.1600-0447.2010.01652.x

104. McLaughlin SPB, Barkowski S, Burlingame GM, Strauss B, Rosendahl J. Group psychotherapy for borderline personality disorder: a meta-analysis of randomized-controlled trials. *Psychotherapy.* 2019;56(2):260–273. doi:10.1037/pst0000211

105. Ingenhoven T, Lafay P, Rinne T, Passchier J, Duivenvoorden H. Effectiveness of pharmacotherapy for severe personality disorders: meta-analyses of randomized controlled trials. *J Clin Psychiatry.* 2010;71(1):14–25. doi:10.4088/jcp.08r04526gre

106. Nosè M, Cipriani A, Biancosino B, Grassi L, Barbui C. Efficacy of pharmacotherapy against core traits of borderline personality disorder: meta-analysis of randomized controlled trials. *Int Clin Psychopharmacol.* 2006;21(6):345–353. doi:10.1097/01.yic.0000224784.90911.66

107. Storebø OJ, Stoffers-Winterling JM, Völlm BA, et al. Psychological therapies for people with borderline personality disorder. *Cochrane Database Syst Rev.* 2020;5:CD012955. doi:10.1002/14651858.CD012955.pub2

108. Vita A, De Peri L, Sacchetti E. Antipsychotics, antidepressants, anticonvulsants, and placebo on the symptom dimensions of borderline personality disorder: a meta-analysis of randomized controlled and open-label trials. *J Clin Psychopharmacol.* 2011;31(5):613–624. doi:10.1097/JCP.0b013e31822c1636

109. Cohen J. *Statistical Power Analysis for the Behavioral Sciences.* New York, NY: Academic Press; 2013.

110. Turner RM. Naturalistic evaluation of dialectical behavior therapy-oriented treatment for borderline personality disorder. *Cogn Behav Pract.* 2000;7(4):413–419. doi:10.1016/S1077-7229(00)80052-8

111. Swift JK, Greenberg RP. Premature discontinuation in adult psychotherapy: a meta-analysis. *J Consult Clin Psychol*. 2012;80(4):547–559. doi:10.1037/a0028226

112. Waldinger RJ, Gunderson JG. Completed psychotherapies with borderline patients. *Am J Psychother*. 1984;38(2):190–202. doi:10.1176/appi.psychotherapy.1984.38.2.190

113. Harley RM, Baity MR, Blais MA, Jacobo MC. Use of dialectical behavior therapy skills training for borderline personality disorder in a naturalistic setting. *Psychother Res*. 2007;17(3):362–370. doi:10.1080/10503300600830710

114. Bloom JM, Woodward EN, Susmaras T, Pantalone DW. Use of dialectical behavior therapy in inpatient treatment of borderline personality disorder: a systematic review. *Psychiatr Serv Wash DC*. 2012;63(9):881–888. doi:10.1176/appi.ps.201100311

115. DeCou CR, Comtois KA, Landes SJ. Dialectical behavior therapy is effective for the treatment of suicidal behavior: a meta-analysis. *Behav Ther*. 2019;50(1):60–72. doi:10.1016/j.beth.2018.03.009

116. Dixon LJ, Linardon J. A systematic review and meta-analysis of dropout rates from dialectical behaviour therapy in randomized controlled trials. *Cogn Behav Ther*. 2020;49(3):181–196. doi:10.1080/16506073.2019.1620324

117. Juanmartí FB, Lizeretti NP. The efficacy of psychotherapy for borderline personality disorder: a review. *Papeles Psicólogo*. 2017;38(2):148–156.

118. Panos PT, Jackson JW, Hasan O, Panos A. Meta-analysis and systematic review assessing the efficacy of dialectical behavior therapy (DBT). *Res Soc Work Pract*. 2014;24(2):213–223. doi:10.1177/1049731513503047

119. Harned MS, Chapman AL, Dexter-Mazza ET, Murray A, Comtois KA, Linehan MM. Treating co-occurring Axis I disorders in recurrently suicidal women with borderline personality disorder: a 2-year randomized trial of dialectical behavior therapy versus community treatment by experts. *J Consult Clin Psychol*. 2008;76(6):1068–1075. doi:10.1037/a0014044

120. Harned MS, Korslund KE, Linehan MM. A pilot randomized controlled trial of Dialectical Behavior Therapy with and without the Dialectical Behavior Therapy Prolonged Exposure protocol for suicidal and self-injuring women with borderline personality disorder and PTSD. *Behav Res Ther*. 2014;55:7–17. doi:10.1016/j.brat.2014.01.008

121. Linehan MM, Schmidt H, Dimeff LA, Craft JC, Kanter J, Comtois KA. Dialectical behavior therapy for patients with borderline personality disorder and drug-dependence. *Am J Addict*. 1999;8(4):279–292. doi:10.1080/105504999305686

122. Linehan MM, Korslund KE, Harned MS, et al. Dialectical behavior therapy for high suicide risk in individuals with borderline personality disorder: a randomized clinical trial and component analysis. *JAMA Psychiatry*. 2015;72(5):475–482. doi:10.1001/jamapsychiatry.2014.3039

123. McCauley E, Berk MS, Asarnow JR, et al. Efficacy of dialectical behavior therapy for adolescents at high risk for suicide: a randomized clinical trial. *JAMA Psychiatry*. 2018;75(8):777–785. doi:10.1001/jamapsychiatry.2018.1109

124. Vogt KS, Norman P. Is mentalization-based therapy effective in treating the symptoms of borderline personality disorder? a systematic review. *Psychol Psychother*. 2019;92(4):441–464. doi:10.1111/papt.12194

125. Malda-Castillo J, Browne C, Perez-Algorta G. Mentalization-based treatment and its evidence-base status: a systematic literature review. *Psychol Psychother Theory Res Pract*. 2019;92(4):465–498. doi:https://doi.org/10.1111/papt.12195

126. Carlyle D, Green R, Inder M, et al. A randomized-controlled trial of mentalization-based treatment compared with structured case management for borderline personality disorder in a mainstream public health service. *Front Psychiatry*. 2020;11:561916. doi:10.3389/fpsyt.2020.561916

127. Laurenssen EMP, Luyten P, Kikkert MJ, et al. Day hospital mentalization-based treatment v. specialist treatment as usual in patients with borderline personality disorder: randomized controlled trial. *Psychol Med*. 2018;48(15):2522–2529. doi:10.1017/S0033291718000132

128. Philips B, Wennberg P, Konradsson P, Franck J. Mentalization-based treatment for concurrent borderline personality disorder and substance use disorder: a randomized controlled feasibility study. *Eur Addict Res*. 2018;24(1):1–8. doi:10.1159/000485564

129. Rossouw TI, Fonagy P. Mentalization-based treatment for self-harm in adolescents: a randomized controlled trial. *J Am Acad Child Adolesc Psychiatry*. 2012;51(12):1304–1313.e3. doi:10.1016/j.jaac.2012.09.018

130. Sempértegui GA, Karreman A, Arntz A, Bekker MHJ. Schema therapy for borderline personality disorder: a comprehensive review of its empirical foundations, effectiveness and implementation possibilities. *Clin Psychol Rev*. 2013;33(3):426–447. doi:10.1016/j.cpr.2012.11.006

131. Jacob GA, Arntz A. Schema therapy for personality disorders—a review. *Int J Cogn Ther*. 2013;6(2):171–185.

132. Nadort M, Arntz A, Smit JH, et al. Implementation of outpatient schema therapy for borderline personality disorder with versus without crisis support by the therapist outside office hours: A randomized trial. *Behav Res Ther*. 2009;47(11):961–973. doi:10.1016/j.brat.2009.07.013

6

The Big 6

Evidence-based Therapies for the Treatment of Personality Disorders

Robert E. Feinstein

Key Points

- All evidence-based therapies (EBPs) suggest there are genetic and adverse or traumatic early-life experiences and/or environments that are responsible for the development of a personality disorder.
- The seven themes commonly described by six EBPs to treat personality disorders (PDs) are: (1) structuring the treatment; (2) developing therapist self-awareness; (3) managing countertransference or countertherapeutic reactions; (4) developing therapist responsiveness or adaptations; (5) recognizing missteps, mistakes, and therapeutic ruptures; (6) repairing the therapeutic alliance; and (7) supervision.
- The "Big Six" EBPs were originally developed for the treatment of borderline personality disorder (BPD) and have been subsequently applied to the treatment of other PDs. The "Big Six" include: transference-focused psychotherapy (TFP); mentalization-based treatment (MBT); cognitive therapy (CT); dialectical behavior therapy (DBT); schema therapy (ST); and good psychiatric management (GPM).
- TFP is based on ego psychology, object relations, and attachment theories. It focuses on changing self and other object representations to help patients develop a consolidated identity. The therapeutic alliance is seen as a crucial holding environment designed to help patients manage their emotional storms and create an environment for change. Countertransference is an essential focus as part of the treatment. The treatment uses a structured assessment and sets a treatment frame followed by an exploratory treatment phase. Patients develop the capacity to manage their emotions and behaviors, develop healthy dependency on others, develop the ability to sustain interpersonal relationships, and realize life goals. See Tables 6.1, p. 152 and 6.7, p. 169.
- MBT integrates ideas from psychoanalytic and attachment theory and the neurosciences. Defects in mentalization of self and others are responsible for the manifestations of the PDs. The therapeutic alliance and a stance of "not knowing" is essential. MBT focuses on developing the capacity to accurately mentalize self and others. The initial assessment phase engages the patient by evaluating their attachment style, mentalizing ability, and interpersonal functioning while providing psychoeducation about the PD and establishing a therapeutic contract.

The treatment phase enhances the patient's capacity to sustain accurate mentalizing of the self and others during periods of distress and translates this ability to form secure attachments, emotional stability, and improved interpersonal relationships. See Tables 6.2, p. 155 and 6.8, p. 169.

- CT focuses on the evaluation and treatment of core beliefs or schemas associated with each PD which influence current automatic thoughts, emotions, behaviors, and interpersonal relationships. The therapeutic alliance is based on collaborative empiricism. CT focuses on modifying the therapist's countertherapeutic reactions which can adversely impact treatment. CT has a structured assessment phase and a treatment phase designed to change core beliefs and maladaptive coping, leading patients to develop emotional control, self-sufficiency, and adaptive interpersonal relationships. They use psychoeducation and teach specific cognitive and behavioral skills. See Tables 6.3, p. 158 and 6.9, p. 170.

- DBT is a third-wave CBT treatment, primarily focused on behavioral change. It is based on dialectical philosophy, behavioral science, and mindfulness practices adopted from Buddhist traditions. DBT focuses on acceptance and change. DBT describes the therapeutic alliance as a nonjudgmental coaching relationship. DBT therapeutic relationship is used as a contingency, focused on remediation of patient treatment-interfering behaviors and helps the patient develop skills for facilitating behavioral change. It also acknowledges the need to remediate therapist-interfering behaviors. DBT teaches mindfulness, distress tolerance, emotional regulation, and interpersonal effectiveness as aids to develop a life worth living. See Tables 6.4, p. 161 and 6.10, p. 170.

- ST is an eclectic therapy based on cognitive, behavioral, psychodynamic, and experiential therapies. ST focuses on early maladaptive schemas, dysfunctional coping styles, and maladaptive modes of behavior. The therapeutic alliance is characterized as limited reparenting. ST utilizes the countertransference to help explain the patient's problematic interpersonal relationships. ST has a structured assessment and education phase based on a co-constructed case formulation. The treatment phase is designed to help patients give up maladaptive modes for a healthy adult mode. See Tables 6.5, p. 164 and 6.11, p. 171.

- GPM is a supportive psychodynamic psychotherapy using case-management strategies for the treatment of BPD. It is based on psychodynamic, cognitive, and behavioral theories. The alliance is supportive. Countertransference is sometime utilized as a way to help patients explore dysfunctional interpersonal relations. GPM has a structured treatment frame which begins with psychoeducation, and reducing suicidal behaviors. BPD is framed as "a problem with interpersonal hypersensitivity." Treatment is flexible following general psychiatric treatment principles and relying heavily on case-management strategies. See Tables 6.6, p. 167 and 6.12, p. 171.

- The different unique interventions of each of the six EBPs are listed together to make it easier for clinicians and researchers with a single orientation to explore the options for using intervention borrowed from other EBPs. See Tables 6.7–6.12, pp. 169–171.

Introduction

The literature on evidence-based treatment of personality disorders (PDs), which has exploded in the last 50 years, began in an effort to treat patients with borderline personality disorders (BPDs). The first major disseminated work was Otto Kernberg's widely publicized 1975 book on *Borderline Conditions and Pathological Narcissism*.[1] This laid the early foundations for the development of transference-focused psychotherapy (TFP).[2] In 1976, Aaron Beck, considered the father of cognitive behavioral therapy (CBT), began his work on cognitive therapy (CT) for the treatment of the PDs,[3] followed in 1995 by the work of his daughter, Judith Beck.[4] Mentalization-based therapy (MBT), developed by Peter Fonagy and Anthony Bateman, began in 1999 as a successful treatment of patients with BPD in a partial hospital-based program.[5] In 1991, Marsha Linehan (who had worked with Dr. Kernberg) introduced and began documenting the evidence for dialectical behavior therapy (DBT) as a treatment for BPD.[6] In 2003, Jeffery Young et al. began widespread dissemination of an eclectic treatment for BPD, called schema therapy (ST).[7] Good psychiatric management (GPM) was initially described by John Gunderson in 2001. Its widespread dissemination as a generalist treatment approach for BPD began in 2014.[10] I have named these treatments collectively as the "Big Six," as these are the treatments that are the most widely researched and disseminated.

The Big Six treatments for BPD have substantially grown, expanding their scope to treatment of other PDs and psychiatric conditions. A group of meta-analyses and clinical trials suggest that these treatments are all relatively effective in treating BPD, with little difference in efficacy across treatment modalities.[11] The evidence basis for the treatments for BPD can be reviewed in Chapter 5, as well as within each chapter covering these six modalities. There is no definitive evidence suggesting a preferential treatment for one kind of therapy over another in the treatment of BPD.[11] Current evidence-based approaches to the treatment for BPD are being applied clinically to treatment of the other PDs while we await further research evidence demonstrating the effectiveness of this approach, and the relative benefits and disadvantages of one treatment over another for each of the PDs.

Common Themes in the Evidence-based Treatments of PDs

There are common themes across all of the Big Six EBPs for PD. Patients with PDs commonly have deficits in higher-order brain processes: they experience difficulty regulating their ability to observe, reflect, describe, and comprehend their own emotional state and those of others. They also have deficits in predicting and understanding their own/others' behavior, cannot easily distinguish between their internal experiences and external reality, and struggle to reconcile conflicting thoughts and mental states.[12] In a narrower sense, treatments for the PDs describe dysregulation or over/under-regulation of emotions. Also, patients with PDs have deficits in the capacity to know themselves and others. They evidence maladaptive behaviors that interfere with interpersonal relationships, disrupting their ability to love, work, and play. In other words, PDs prevent a healthy life well lived.

All six EBPs for PDs share a general treatment approach, emphasizing acceptance of emotional experience. This approach helps patients become aware of moment-to-moment emotional, cognitive, behavioral, and interpersonal processes that cause emotional dysregulation, emotional reactivity, or hypersensitivity. During treatment, patients learn to act less impulsively and are encouraged to develop and sustain meaningful interpersonal relationships.

Common themes that are part of the EBPs for PDs include the need to: (1) recognize that patients with personality disorders have constitutional/genetic and environmental factors contributing to their origins; (2) establish the treatment frame and structure the treatment; (3) manage countertransference or countertherapeutic reactions; (4) develop therapist responsiveness to patients with PDs and/ or make treatment adaptations; (5) acknowledge missteps, mistakes, and therapeutic ruptures; (6) repair the working alliance; and (7) encourage therapist self-reflection, supervision, and/or team consultation.

Genetics of PDs

Genetic epidemiologic studies indicate that all ten of the PDs listed in the *Diagnostic and Statistical Manual of Mental Disorders–Fifth Edition* (DSM-5)[13] are modestly to moderately heritable, with broad trait vulnerability that is primarily based on one or more traits: (1) negative emotionality; (2) high impulsivity/low agreeableness; and (3) introversion.[14] While a detailed review of all PD genetics is beyond the scope of this chapter, a sampling of specific constitutional factors affecting a few PDs may suffice. Patients with a BPD show substantial heritability scores of 0.65 to 0.76, and decrease in volume in the anterior cingulate gyrus, hippocampus, amygdala, and surrounding areas of the temporal lobe, compared with healthy individuals.[15] Obsessive-compulsive personality disorders (OCPD) have a heritability rate of 0.78. Genetic effects account for 27 percent of the variance of OCPD symptoms.[16] Antisocial PD (ASPD) studies of family, twin, and adoption suggest that antisocial spectrum disorders and psychopathy have approximately a 51 percent heritability (95 percent CI = 40–67 percent).[17] Other studies suggest that ASPDs show reduced prefrontal volumes, serotonergic dysregulation in the septohippocampal system, developmental or acquired abnormalities in the prefrontal brain systems, and reduced autonomic activity. These deficits in ASPD may be responsible for low arousal, poor fear conditioning, and decision-making deficits.[18] In general, a wide array of genetic and neurobiological studies of all the PDs have some heritable traits, overlapping or specific neurobiology, or can be conceived of as neuro-developmental disorders.[19] For more information about the specific genetics of each PD, review the relevant sections in Chapter 3 and Chapters 16 to 25.

Environmental Factors in the Development of PDs

All EBP treatments describe the origins of the PDs based (in part) on adverse early-life experiences, trauma, and/or in invalidating environments (i.e., dysfunctional parenting, abuse, neglect, etc.). A community-based longitudinal study reported that those with childhood abuse were four times more likely than those not abused to develop a personality disorder, even when controlling for age, parental psychiatric illness, and parental education.[20-21] Specific types of abuse have also been correlated with specific PDs: physical abuse shows some correlation with traits of the antisocial, paranoid, and depressive PDs; sexual abuse was more correlated with borderline PD; and neglect was associated with elevated symptoms of antisocial, avoidant, borderline, narcissistic, and passive-aggressive PDs.[20-21] For more information about the relationship between trauma and PDs, review Chapter 3.

Treatment Frame and Structuring Personality Disorder Treatments

A treatment frame sets rules for the psychotherapeutic contract and fosters clear communication between patient and therapist, establishes treatment priorities, limits the patient's acting out, discourages boundary violations, promotes treatment for relevant comorbidities, and permits the needed structure to manage therapeutic disagreements and suicidal and homicidal risk. The treatment structures the practical arrangements for fees, scheduling, session time allotted, frequency, ground rules for medication use, and involvement of others.

Otto Kernberg's experiences, based on treating patients with BPD, led him to develop the first structured psychodynamic treatment approach, based on object relations, ego psychology, and transference analysis.[22] He was the first to describe the treatment frame as an essential requirement for managing the chaotic lives and treatment of patients with BPD. The treatment frame is necessary to protect the patient and others, as well as preserve a safe and consistent space where the work of psychotherapy can proceed. Box 6.1 contains elements of Kernberg's treatment frame,[22] as well as elements from TFP,[2] which are often incorporated in treatment frames for all patients with PDs.

All the other EBPs for PDs use similar approaches to tailoring their treatment to their theoretical models. Linehan discussed the importance of setting a therapeutic structure and contract, originally framed as setting the structure for the management of

---

Box 6.1 Setting the Treatment Frame

- Use a safe and consistent space where the work of psychotherapy can proceed.
- Describe the patient's and therapist's specific roles.
- Determine and set the goal(s) and problems to be addressed.
- Begin defining the patient's life choices (e.g., work, school, marriage, spirituality, etc.).
- Set the boundaries of the treatment relationship (e.g., confining all psychotherapeutic work within the session, managing phone calls and medications, discuss confidentiality, contact with others, etc.).
- Prioritize treatment focus on suicidal or homicidal threats over other maladaptive behaviors.
- Address acting out such as substance use, eating disorders, gambling, etc.
- Address other threats to the therapy such as not paying fees, missing sessions, or travel.
- Address patient's lying, withholding, or omitting information.
- Address patient's avoidance of meaningful subjects and emotional topics.
- Make sure there is no secondary gain from the psychotherapy.
- Allow the therapy to anchor the patient's life.

parasuicidal behavior.[6] She felt that there needed to be a contract with BPD patients that set the parameters for managing therapy-interfering behavior (TIB). An explicit definition of TIB is "any intentional or unintentional, strategic or automatic, calculated or absent-minded behavior" that interferes with therapy.[23] In the broadest sense, TIB refers to normal, understandable, or ordinary life events (not intentional behaviors) that still interfere with treatment (e.g., taking care of a child, needing to go to school, having to work extra shifts, an eating disorder, etc.) Other TIBs are intentional, often unconscious patient behaviors designed to interfere with therapy (i.e., coming late, missing sessions, not practicing skills, not paying fees, substance use).

All six EBPs identify and manage TIBs within a structured treatment frame. The importance of managing all resistances to therapy are openly discussed with the patient. Subsequently, TIBs and other resistance to treatment are strictly limited by the therapist to enable and facilitate a non-crisis, safe space for the ongoing work of psychotherapy. Ultimately, therapists strive to sets limits on all patient acting out, so treatment can proceed without interruption. All the EBPs for PD prioritize the management and treatment of suicidal/homicidal ideation or behaviors as their first and most important TIB target. Many EBPs for PDs have added variations in the kinds of TIBs, all of which are also limited. Other TIBs include self-injurious behaviors (SIBs); life (threatening) interfering behaviors (LIBs; e.g., overdose, crimes), quality-of-life-interfering behaviors (QIBs; e.g., homelessness), and treatment-destroying behaviors (TDBs; e.g., threatening a therapist or making sexual advances).

Self-awareness

EBPs for PDs highlight the importance of the therapist's emotional self-awareness and attunement to patient emotions as a prerequisite for delivering effective psychotherapy. Open and curious therapists, who question the patient and their own reactions, are well poised to avoid or limit countertherapeutic traps leading to countertherapeutic interventions. Self-aware therapists have better patient therapy outcomes.[24,25] Self-awareness can be broadly defined as the extent to which people are consciously aware of their internal states and their interactions or relationships with others.[26] Self-awareness also encompasses the abilities to focus on and reflect on one's own psychological processes and inner experiences, as well as the ability to understand one's relationships to others. While self-awareness has not directly been studied because the concept is so broad, covering so much territory, aspects of self-awareness have been researched. Genuineness, mindfulness, affect consciousness (AC), and mentalization have all been studied, and, when used by therapists, show trends toward improving therapist effectiveness and patient outcomes.

Genuineness

Genuineness, also called congruence, is an aspect of self-awareness defined as being authentically, freely, and deeply oneself; open to pleasurable and painful experiences, without defensiveness; accepting of contradictory feelings; and ultimately being one's self in all responses and verbalizations.[27] Genuineness also implies thoughtful reflection, measured judgments, and the capacity to skillfully convey the authentic self to a patient through words and actions. The relationship between therapist genuineness (implying part of self-awareness) and psychotherapy outcome has been researched, with mixed results, although it leans toward the positive. In one study, genuineness accounts for approximately 5.3 percent of the variance in treatment outcome.[27] Two meta-analyses[27,28] indicate a moderate relationship between therapist genuineness and the therapeutic alliance, with effect sizes between 0.45 and 0.71.

Mindfulness

Mindfulness, the most extensively researched intervention, is defined as the deliberate direction of attention to the senses, in the present moment, with an attitude of acceptance.[29] It may be further characterized as a kind of self-awareness or nonjudgmental attention to emotion, which consciously attempts to reduce or eliminate cognitive elaboration in order to reduce preconceptions of the self. Mindfulness is an essential practice for management of emotional dysregulation as part of DBT and, to a lesser extent, CT. Mindfulness is also recommended for therapists treating patients with PDs, to assist them in managing their own countertherapeutic practices or therapist-interfering behaviors. The majority of evidence for its use with PDs focuses on BPD treatment. There are positive associations between mindful practices used by patients with BPD and reduced psychiatric and clinical symptoms; patients show less emotional reactivity and impulsivity.[30] Fewer studies examine the generally positive results of using mindfulness for other PDs. Emerging case studies have applied mindfulness techniques to treatment with antisocial, avoidant, paranoid, and obsessive-compulsive personality disorders.[30]

Research examining mindfulness benefits for psychotherapists has also demonstrated benefits such as reducing stress and greater self-compassion.[31,32] In addition, it has been shown that mindfulness fosters the development of psychotherapy skills, such as increased comfort with silence and the ability to show empathy.[31,33]

Affect Consciousness (AC)

AC is defined as degrees of awareness, tolerance, nonverbal expression, and conceptual expression of nine specific affects.[34] These basic human affects provide emotional self-state information and show interactions and relationship with the external world. Like mindfulness, when applied to the treatment of PDs, AC is related to affect regulation. In addition, AC considers how emotions, cognition, motivation, and behavior are brought into consciousness. As a concept, AC is integrated within GPM and parts of TFP and MBT, which all focus on how affective storms can lead to interpersonal difficulties. To date, there is little empiric research on this subject, but applications of this concept may prove useful.

Mentalization

Mentalization, also called reflective functioning, encompasses aspects of mindfulness and AC. Mentalization is defined as the capacity to understand human behavior in terms of underlying mental states; that is, thoughts, feelings, wishes, needs, intentions of self and others.[35] It is typically measured by the reflective functioning scale.[36] Mentalization is the broadest of these three concepts because it incorporates aspects of genuineness, mindfulness, and AC.[37]

There is a significant relationship between mentalization and mindfulness. Some degree of mindfulness is needed for mentalization, because awareness of self (a mindfulness capacity) is required for mentalization. However, mentalization involves more than attention to self-states, because it also requires a focus on affect states, cognition, behavior, intentions of others, and interpersonal relatedness, which are not part of mindfulness. On the other hand, mindfulness includes attention to a broader range of phenomena than just mental states of self, because it also focuses on any here-and-now sensory impressions of the world.[38]

TFP, MBT, GMP, and perhaps ST consider mentalization a foundational process of change in psychotherapy, especially for patients with BPD and likely with the other PDs as well.[39] Reflective functioning (RF), often used as a measure of the capacity to mentalize, has important impacts on psychotherapy process and outcome. There is some evidence that RF has implications for how patients initially experience psychotherapy. Katznelson's findings suggest that patients with less capacity for RF may have an increase in psychotherapy dropout rates.[36] There is other evidence suggesting that 70.5 percent of the variance in therapist effectiveness is also accounted for by the therapist's capacity for RF.[38,40] Therapists with higher RF capacities had significantly better patient outcomes. Therapist RF is also thought to facilitate growth in the patient's reflective functioning. It is thus considered by some to be foundational as a common factor to all forms of psychotherapy.[41-43] These findings collectively suggest that deficits in RF are associated with core aspects of personality pathology, and the therapist's capacity for RF is an important factor, improving therapist effectiveness and psychotherapy outcomes.[38,40]

Managing Countertransference or Countertherapeutic Reactions

From a transtheoretical perspective, all therapists treating patients with PDs need to be aware of and address their reactions to patients to avoid any negative treatment impacts. This is also necessary to maintain the therapeutic alliance, avoid early patient dropout, maintain all other aspects of the treatment itself, and ultimately to optimize psychotherapy outcomes. All six EBPs for PDs recognize the importance of therapist's managing their countertherapeutic or countertransference reactions. However, they vary, according to their theoretical perspective, on the relative contributions of the therapist and patient in creating countertherapeutic reactions and on what management strategies should be used to resolve them.

This can be conceptualized as a continuum with the therapists being predominately responsible for their countertherapeutic contribution on one end (e.g., therapy goes awry due to the therapist's difficulties) to a middle ground where countertherapeutic reactions are co-created by the patient and therapist (all EBPs accept this to some degree) to the opposite end of the continuum, with the patient predominantly responsible for eliciting the therapist's countertherapeutic or countertransference reaction.

Kernberg conceptualizes countertransference as either "classical countertransference" or "totalistic countertransference."[44] Classic countertransference, also called therapist-originated transference to the patient (on the therapist's side of the countertransference continuum), can be defined as the therapist's unhelpful unconscious reactions to the patient that become an impediment to treatment. Totalistic countertransference (emanating from the patient's side of the continuum) includes emotional reactions experienced by the therapist that are unconsciously transmitted by the patient to the therapist via projection, projective identification, and enactments.[25,45] Psychodynamic therapists utilize aspects of their totalistic countertransference reactions as important communications revealing the patient's self and other representations that become the templates for their current interpersonal relationships.

Cognitive and behavioral therapists see their reactions to patients as mostly being generated by patients who display TIBs. They manage patient TIBs by setting firm limits on the patient's destructive behaviors. Cognitive and behavioral therapists acknowledge countertherapeutic reactions to patients that they call therapist TIBs. A therapist TIB is any therapist behavior that adversely affects the process or outcomes of psychotherapy or that has a negative impact on the therapeutic relationship. This includes therapist's mistakes or regrets for doing too much or not doing enough. A therapist's TIB is managed by setting realistic goals and limits for what a therapist can or cannot accomplish with a patient.[23]

Develop Therapist Responsiveness or Adaptations to the Patient

Responsiveness is the ability to adapt and tailor interventions to patient needs, characteristics, and behaviors. Evidence that therapeutic adaptations improve psychotherapy outcomes is extensive and can be reviewed elsewhere.[46] Gordon Paul's question summarizes the issue: "What treatment, by whom, is most effective for an individual with a specific problem, and under which set of circumstances?"[47]

Anyone working with patients who have PDs is certainly aware that no two patients with the same diagnosis or problems are alike. Common adaptations used by all the EBPs for the PDs include treating the patient as a capable, active, and competent person. All the EBPs share a strong emphasis on (1) the need for close collaboration, (2) setting the optimal boundaries between the patient and therapist, and (3) the importance of empathic validation, setting expectations for behavioral change, and the need for therapist flexibility.

Other needed adaptations include taking into account patient preference, the kind of therapeutic relationship needed, the therapist's style of communication, and the patient's attachment, coping style, and motivation or resistance to change. In addition, it is increasingly necessary to adapt treatments according to the patient's religion or spiritual beliefs, culture, gender identity, and sexual orientation.[46,48]

The need for therapeutic diversity, or a broader definition of what therapeutic responsiveness or adaptation means, is commonly acknowledged.[46,48] Each form of therapy discusses relative indications and contraindications for their treatments and acknowledges that different patients with different PDs may need different EBP approaches.[46,48] There is also some acknowledgment that each EBP may need to adapt its own treatment to cover a wider scope of patients, diagnoses, and problems. This trend to tailor our treatments of PDs is further manifested (although generally not expressed) by the fact that newer EBPs for PDs are becoming increasingly eclectic; one EBP may borrow from another therapy's interventions. In many ways, ST and GPM are exemplars of this approach because they both use multiple interventions, based on various combinations, coming from psychodynamic, TFP, CT, DBT, experiential therapies, and case-management strategies.

While the need for greater therapeutic responsiveness is acknowledged, at this stage the focus remains largely limited to adapting treatments for different diagnoses or problems. There is scant literature considering adjustments needed by each of the EBPs for PDs based on other, previously mentioned patients' needs, and the growing need for cultural and diversity adaptations. This dilemma for all the EBPs is best expressed by John Norcross's general comment about all forms of psychotherapy:

> The desire to be responsive with patients, frequently gives rise to a clinical dilemma. Therapist flexibility to patient preferences, values, and cultures, promises that psychotherapy "fits" with the patient, but not necessarily that the resulting treatment has any research support. Therapist fidelity to research, promises that psychotherapy works, but not necessarily with a particular client in a particular context. Errors in either direction can portend clinical failure.[48]

This dilemma leaves the EBPs for PDs in uncertain territory; utilizing different interventions from the various EBPs will often initially lack demonstrated efficacy. However, this is not a usual space for psychotherapists, as our efforts to use new clinical approaches or interventions are often the starting point for where new research needs to begin.

Recognize and Repair Missteps, Mistakes, and Therapeutic Ruptures

Patients with personality disorders have been identified as a likely group to have more alliance ruptures than other patients.[49-51] This probably represents how patients with PDs have difficulties in their real-world interpersonal relationships that are reflected in the alliances with their therapists. Therapeutic ruptures may also occur due to previously discussed countertherapeutic reactions in the therapist.

Bordin defined three elements of the working alliance between therapist and patient as goals, tasks, and bonds.[52] Missteps, mistakes, and therapeutic ruptures can occur when: (1) the goals of the treatment are not specified or agreed upon; (2) the tasks to accomplish the goals are vague, incorrectly chosen, or when there are disagreements; and (3) when the bonds between patient and therapist are weak or ineffective.

Ruptures have sometimes been organized into two main types: withdrawal and confrontation.[53] Withdrawal ruptures typically occur when a patient moves away or avoids the work of the therapy or interaction with the therapist. Withdrawal may also be revealed when patients offer minimal responses, are overly appeasing, use avoidant storytelling, or hide dissatisfactions. Confrontation ruptures occur when the patient moves against the therapist by expressing hostility, anger, defeat, or dissatisfaction with the therapist, or makes efforts to control the therapist. Some ruptures can include elements of both types.

There is general agreement across diverse theories of psychotherapy that intense reactions to patients require therapist competence to resolve these difficulties for effective psychotherapy outcomes to be maintained.[49] These difficulties have been widely recognized in the treatment of patients with PDs across the many schools of therapy.[54] Alliance problems in patients with PDs typically reflect their problematic interpersonal relationships in the real world.[53]

Ambivalence, Resistance, Reactance, and Ruptures
When Treating Patients with PDs

Problems in the working alliance vary along an intensity continuum, from minor tensions, miscommunications, and miss-attunement; to transient or temporary disruptions, impasses or stalemates; to major miscommunications, threats to the treatment; and to therapeutic ruptures, which are typically impulsive, premature, or unplanned termination of treatment. The literature also describes this continuum as ambivalence, resistance, reactance, and ruptures.

Ambivalence

Ambivalence about beginning treatment is ubiquitous in patients with PDs.[55,56] Many patients find it difficult to accept (1) an accurate description of their diagnosis or problems, (2) a suggestion that their problems are chronic in nature, and (3) a recommendation for a relatively long and expensive treatment. Ambivalence is typically managed by all EBPs for PDs through clear statements and psychoeducation about diagnosis, problem identification, benefits and disadvantages of various treatments, case formulations, and by attending to strong bond/alliance development with the patient.[55-57]

Resistance

Resistance emerges in treatment when the patient begins to unconsciously or consciously opposes the therapist.[55-57] Direct requests by a therapist or subtle suggestions that a patient modify or change their thoughts, emotions, and especially behavior is what generates resistance. Resistance may manifest as non-adherence, the patient maintaining or worsening their symptoms, consistently correcting the therapist, expressions of differences of opinions, the emergence of internal or interpersonal conflicts, and/or delays in practicing skills or doing homework

Resistance may be generated by cognitive or behavioral treatment for PDs that directly asks patients to manage or stop their suicidal tendencies, or asks for compliance with requests to practice skills or do homework.[55] Resistance may also be generated by psychodynamic treatments with subtle suggestions for change, made by the use of interpretations, requests for reflection, mentalization, or insight.[54] All EBPs for PDs anticipate that eliciting resistance is an essentially unavoidable part of treating all patients with PDs. Virtually all EBPs for PDs rely on empathy, validation, and the development of a strong working alliance as primary interventions for reducing resistance.[57,58] Patients with PDs need to be heard and understood, first, before suggesting any changes.

Reactance

Reactance is a more severe form of resistance, in which a patient intentionally opposes all of what the therapist recommends, says, or does.[57] The high-reactant PD patients are the most likely to develop therapeutic ruptures and abruptly terminate treatment. This is well known by practitioners, who all tend to prioritize and attempt to resolve all negative therapeutic reactions to treatment as soon as they emerge.

Two meta-analyses have demonstrated that high-reactant patients benefit from relatively low-directive treatments, whereas low-reactant patients benefit from relatively more-directive treatments.[57,58] As applied to PDs, this mean patients with Cluster A PDs and those with narcissistic PD and antisocial PD may benefit from more low-directive treatments (TFP, MBT, GMP), while patients with histrionic personality disorder and Cluster C diagnoses may benefit from more directive treatment, such as CT and DBT.

Rupture and Repairing the Therapeutic Alliance

While there is no shared model across EBPs for the PDs as to how to address ruptures and repair them, the literature reveals some common themes and clinical recommendations (see Box 6.2).

Across diverse theories of psychotherapy, there is general agreement that intense reactions of patients require therapist competence to resolve these difficulties for effective psychotherapy outcomes to be maintained.[59] Two meta-analyses reveal that rupture resolution processes are positively associated with the good psychotherapy outcome.[53,60]

Box 6.2 Repairing Ruptures and the Therapeutic Alliance

- Prophylactically, take a detailed history from the patient and others of disruptions in prior therapy relationships, significant early-life relationships, and current interpersonal relationships.
- Recognize and anticipate that patients with PDs will commonly have ambivalence, resistance, reactance, and even ruptures in the opening and later phases of treatment.
- Therapists new to treating patients with PDs can expect that alliance disturbances may evoke feelings of confusion, ambivalence toward the patient, feeling of incompetence, and/or guilt.
- Focus on developing a strong working alliance with special attention to bonds by using empathy and validation, to help the patient feel accepted and to minimize patient defensiveness.
- When ambivalence emerges, consider rolling with the ambivalence and focusing on change talk.
- Acknowledge the patient's courage and the strength it takes to have discussions about the treatment relationship.
- When resistances emerge, role play both sides: the wish not to change and the need to change. Foster an open discussion of where and how the alliance went awry.
- When resistance occurs, remind and repeat the purpose of treatment, treatment goals, and the rationale for a particular approach.
- Modify treatment tasks or goals to reduce resistances.
- Set limits on treatment-interfering behaviors.
- Negotiate differences by searching for new ways to acknowledge each other's intersubjectivity.
- Find new ways to be with others when you disagree.
- Therapists should accept responsibility, explain, or apologize for countertherapeutic reactions that are disturbing the alliance.
- Eventually try to link disturbances in the alliance to patient's prior disruptions in their interpersonal relationships.

Supervision

Most, if not all, beginning therapists who are treating patients with the PDs need supervision to foster self-reflection, to avoid countertherapeutic reactions, and to prevent boundary or ethical violations. Because of the wear and tear of treating patients with PDs, supervision is also considered essential as a safeguard for preserving the therapeutic relationship. It is important for committed, experienced therapists who work with PD patients to become supervisors and pass on their specialized expertise. Supervisors can offer and encourage supervisees to enroll in intensive, didactic seminars and review PD treatment protocols. It is also extremely important that inexperienced clinicians obtain regular (often weekly) practical learning by case supervision, role plays, audio-video supervision, live, or the apprenticeship model of supervision.[61] The best supervisors are often those who also assess their trainees' adherence to a treatment modality and evaluate competence.[62,63] Ongoing supervision of experienced practitioners can help them maintain their skills (which may deteriorate over time), practice new skills, and add new knowledge about an existing EBP through continuing education.

Following these general supervision guidelines, all six EBPs for the treatment of BPD advise that their brand of psychotherapy cannot be effectively delivered unless therapists are supported by education, share the specific treatment philosophy, get adequate training, and enroll in individual or group supervision, or team consultation.

Training in the EBP for PDs

Each EBP for PDs has its own training and supervision approach, generally offered by experts often related to the founder of the treatment approach. Experts teach theory, model clinical practice, require trainees to have hands-on experience with patients, and generally recommend continuing education. Some trainings also offer adherence and competence assessments. It is important to note that training and certification in all of these treatment approaches are offered not only to train clinicians to treat patients, but also to disseminate their approaches, preserve their brand, and for monetary gain. None of these EBP's trainings have been extensively researched for their efficacy at producing qualified therapists. Consonant with the state of our profession, it remains somewhat controversial if supervision "necessarily" leads to better patient outcomes.[64] With those caveats in mind, and the author's declaration that he has no disclosures or conflict of interest in these domains, resources for training are described in each section associated with each modality.

Overview of Six Evidence-based Treatments for the PDs

This section offers an overview of six EBPs that were originally designed to treat patients with BPD. These EBPs have subsequently been expanded and utilized in the treatment of other PDs, symptom clusters, and other psychiatric disorders. These include TFP, MBT, CT, DBT, ST, and GPM. Each EBP is briefly described and is followed by a table which summarizes key aspects of each treatment modality.

Transference-focused Psychotherapy (TFP)

TFP was developed as an evidenced-based treatment for BPD[2,22,65] and has also evolved as a treatment for narcissistic PD.[66] TFP is also being clinically applied to the treatment of other PDs.[66] TFP has been developed based on the integration of the ego psychological perspective, object relations, and attachment theory. Multiple complex positive and negative self and object representations, and the affect connecting them, form the basic building blocks of internal experiences and interpersonal relationships. TFP helps patients with PDs integrate their split-off self and object representations, leading to a consolidated stable identity. This treatment is designed to foster growth from a borderline personality organization to a neurotic or healthy personality organization (see Chapter 2 on the levels of personality organization). TFP creates change by focusing on transference analysis while using totalistic countertransference as a vital source of unconscious information about the patient's internal world and their ways of relating to others.

The first phase of TFP involves assessment, communication of the diagnosis, and establishment of the treatment frame and therapeutic contract. Review setting the treatment frame in Box 6.1, p. 141.

The second exploratory phase uses transference interpretations, encouraging multiple internal images of self (self-representations) to become integrated, organized, and consistent.[2] This organized integration leads to one's ability to regulate emotions, especially aggression, and a self capable of accurately reading reality (e.g., consistently capable of distinguishing between self and others, and one's internal and external worlds). In addition, this integration leads to stable self-esteem, behavioral self-control, and a healthier adult with realistic ideals, stable ethical standards, and a moral compass. With treatment, internal images of others (object representations) become similarly consistent and integrated, as the patient's primary attachments become secure and interpersonal relations generally become cooperative, intimate, and growth enhancing. Integrated images leading to a consolidated identity, a capacity for self-control, and greater ability to manage emotions (especially aggression), reduces impulsivity, permits a healthy dependency on others, and enhances the capacity for satisfying interpersonal and sexual relations and ability to realize life goals.

TFP and the Therapeutic Alliance

In TFP, the relationship between patient and therapist is the primary vehicle to mobilize change. The primary mechanism of change is not positive human regard, warmth, or a giving relationship, although all these relationship factors may be present. Instead, with therapeutic skills, the therapist provides the alliance as a holding environment to accept and contain the patient's emotional intensity and dysregulated emotional storms without getting frightened, defensive, withdrawing, or punishing the patient.[2] The therapeutic stance of TFP is described as "technical neutrality."[1,2,22] The therapist allies with the patient's ability to observe all internal forces involved in conflict (e.g., drives, impulses, prohibitions, relationship to reality, and moral and ethical standards and ideals), as well as all processes that facilitate negotiating internal and external reality. In TFP, early attachment relationships are inevitably recreated, repeated, and emerge within the therapeutic relationship, through transference and countertransference. These object relations of self and other represent the experiences of early-life relationships (and the kinds of early-life attachments) and form the basis for current attachment relationships. The containment function of the alliance, and focus on transference and countertransference patterns, allows transference analysis and interpretations to recognize, name, and understand the split-off object relations as they are playing out in therapy, with accompanying intense affect states. Through this awareness and interpretation, a patient with a PD begins to consider that a new healthy relationship, practiced with the therapist, can be mutually helpful. This kind of modeling empowers the patient to pursue gratifying, intimate, growth-enhancing relationships outside of therapy, ultimately essential to a more functional and happier life.

TFP and Countertransference

TFP therapists recognize that patient communication comes through three channels: verbal, behavioral, and the countertransference.[2] In TFP, totalistic countertransference is embraced from the viewpoint that what the therapist feels emanates from the patient. TFP borrows this concept of totalistic countertransference from Racker, who described that therapists could use their unconscious countertransference reactions to better understand the patient's unconscious.[67,68] Racker viewed the relational experiences of childhood as reflected in concordant and complementary countertransference.[68] In a "concordant" countertransference, via introjection and projections from the patient, the therapist identifies with the patient's central emotions (self-object). The therapist empathically feels whatever the patient feels. In "complementary" countertransference, the patient engenders, via projection, projective identification and enactments the opposite of what the therapist feels (object representation). For example, the patient acts masochistically (self-representation), while the analyst feels sadistic (the patient's object representation). TFP requires constant monitoring of totalistic countertransference as an aid to diagnosis of specific PDs.[69,70] Totalistic countertransference is also an early predictor of the nature of the therapeutic alliance, and an essential source to discover and better understand the patient's self/other representations and their interpersonal relations.[2,65]

TFP also recommends that therapists consider and/or receive their own therapy to manage their own "classic countertransference" (e.g., aspects of their own experiences, or transferences to the patient, which interfere with the patient's treatment). Many in the TFP camp would also acknowledge that, in addition to the transference relationship, it is also important to have elements of a real relationship with the patient[2] (e.g., finding something genuinely likeable in the patient). This is helpful, because the therapeutic attachment must be strong enough to weather the inevitable emotional storms. The real relationship component allows the therapist and patient to share common courtesies, sensibilities, genuine interest and hope for each other (their humanity), and to acknowledge and accept a common universal need to be able to realistically depend on others.

A summary of TFP concepts, core strategies, therapeutic relationship, countertransference, and treatment goals is described in Table 6.1, p. 152. Interventions used by the TFP therapist will be described in a later section. Review Chapter 8 for additional information and clinical illustration of TFP practices.

Table 6.1. Transference-focused Psychotherapy

Key Concepts	Definitions, Description, Use
Object-Relations Theory of Personality Disorders	Constitutional factors and early-life adverse experiences lead to the PDs. Unstable, distorted, and split images of self/others leads to emotional instability, aggression, deficits in identity formation create dysfunctional interpersonal relationships.
Self-Representation: Your view of yourself as a child and currently	Used to understand internal representation of self. These images vary across different points in time and in relation to different people. These become the template for interpersonal relationships.
Other-Representation: Describe your view of significant others	Used to understand internal representation of others and the feelings the patient has toward them. Internal images of others and the attached feelings vary at different time points and with varying self-images.
Affect: Describe the feeling between self and other	Images of self and others are connected by an affect or feeling (e.g., self-images as unwanted/bad child – fear – uncaring, self-involved parent; or a happy-self – joy– proud, admiring therapist).
Core Strategies	*Definitions, Description, Use*
Conceptualize, identify and modify object relations	Define the dominant object relations; name the self-representations and the feeling(s) linked to others; observe/interpret role reversals of the object relations dyads, and one dyad's defense against another.
Therapeutic Relationship	*Definitions, Description, Use*
Therapeutic Stance	Technical neutrality.
Working Alliance	Collaborative therapeutic relationship between patient and therapist which enables safe space for psychological work.
Classic countertransference	The therapist's transference to the patient based on the therapist's past history which is an impediment to treatment. Can be managed by self-reflection, supervision, or a personal treatment.
Totalistic Countertransference	All emotional reactions felt by the therapist, which communicates data about the patient's inner experience of either self/others, which can aid in the diagnosis and may characterizes the initial transferences.
Concordant Countertransference	Therapist identifies/feels similar to the patient. Therapist learns about how the patient feels about the self.
Complementary Countertransference	Therapist identifies with the significant other or feels the opposite of what the patient describes (e.g., the patient experiences self as a victim, the therapist experiences self as an abuser).
Interventions	See Table 6.7, p. 169
Treatment	*Definitions, Description, Use*
Individual Treatment	Twice per week for 1 to 2 years.
Treatment Goals	Integrate images of self/other leading to a consolidated identity; leads to a capacity for self-control, ability to manage emotions (especially aggression), reduces impulsivity, permits a healthy dependency on others and the capacity for intimate partnerships/sexually satisfying relations, a moral compass, and ability to realize life goals.

TFP Training

Training in TFP is offered by experts, and includes review of object-relations theory, core principles, use of TFP techniques, and supervision.[71] Theory, case material, and master therapist videos are used to present and illustrate common situations. After the initial basics, a course in TFP typically continues to discussions and supervision of participant cases. TFP training is available for a fee. It runs for 34 sessions per year and is available for one or two years. Participants receive a certificate for TFP from the Columbia University Center for Psychoanalytic Training and Research.[71]

Mentalization-based Treatment (MBT)

MBT integrates ideas from psychoanalytic theory, attachment theory,[72-74] and the neurosciences. Mentalizing is the ability to perceive the thoughts, beliefs, feelings, needs, desires, goals, purposes, and intentions of ourselves and others. The concept that deficits of self and others representations lead to the development of a personality disorder is borrowed from object-relations theory. However, MBT's main focus is on how mentalization of self and others builds the internal representational world, ultimately affecting interpersonal relationships. The adult's ability to accurately mentalize depends on the quality of early-life attachments.[59,72] Secure adult attachments reflect an early childhood where subjective experiences were adequately mirrored by a trusted adult.[59,72] A secure attachment leads to a genuine and sustained capacity to mentalize the self and others. Insecure attachment styles (e.g., avoidant-dismissive, anxious-resistant, or disorganized)[73,74] occur when early attachment figures are erratically congruent and incorrectly mirror the child's internal state and those of others.[42,43]

Under adverse life circumstances, an infant or child may have trouble accurately representing its own state (representing its self-state), or representing its caregiver's mental states as if this were its own mental state. A mentalizing impairment manifests as an insecure attachment style, leading to emotional dysregulation, loss of behavioral control, and the interpersonal difficulties frequently seen in patients with PDs. From the MBT viewpoint, it is the failure to accurately mentalize—to know one's own mind and those of others—that is the core deficit leading to the PDs. MBT, initially developed as a treatment for BPD, may be one of the few effective treatments for antisocial PD,[41] and likely has applications for the treatment of many other PDs.

The initial phase of MBT aims to engage the patient in the therapy by evaluating attachment style, mentalizing ability, and interpersonal functioning, providing psychoeducation about the PD and establishing a therapeutic contract. To evaluate attachment style, the MBT authors[72] strongly recommend the use of the Relationship Scales Questionnaire.[36]

The aim of the second phase is to enhance the patient's capacity for accurate mentalization, initially within the therapeutic relationship and subsequently in the patient's outside life. This leads to secure attachments, emotional stability, improved interpersonal relationships, and healthier life.

Mentalization-based Therapy and the Therapeutic Alliance

MBT, a psychoanalytic cousin, also views the therapeutic relationship as the crucial laboratory and essential vehicle to understand and resolve patient difficulties.

The basic therapeutic stance is "not knowing," meaning that the patient, better than the therapist, knows her or his own mind.[42] Therefore, MBT, as compared to TFP, views the therapist–patient relationship as essential and more egalitarian, needing warmth, acceptance, listening, and sharing. This establishes an environment different from TFP, which presumes patients will come to understand themselves with the aid of an expert who knows the patient's unconscious mind and will communicate this knowledge to the patient through interpretation. MBT therapists are ever curious about the subjective mind states of patients and therapists.[42,72] The MBT therapist's role is to both notice deficits in mentalization and use interventions that can restore the patient's capacity to mentalize. Interventions that can restore mentalizing capacity include maintaining the "not knowing stance," providing a secure attachment base, and promoting interpersonal engagement that is not too close nor too distant.

Mentalization-based Treatment and Countertransference

MBT accepts the views of the "classic" countertransference in which the therapist may have their own difficulties (unrelated to the patient) in mentalizing themselves or others, in ways which interfere with the patient's treatment. MBT asks therapists to "reflect" on their own deficits to mentalize and seek treatment, if needed, to overcome them.

MBT tends to avoid the use of the term "transference" and the concept of "totalistic countertransference," believing these concepts introduce confusion concerning what comes from the patient's past versus what is being experienced in the present (transference) and what feelings are transmitted from one mind to another (countertransference).[75] MBT prefers to focus on how therapist and patient co-create and influence the mental states of each other, and ultimately how therapist and patient view themselves and each other in the moment. The capacity to accurately mentalize and to sustain this ability within the therapeutic relationship becomes the template for how the patient can do this in the outside world. A change in the ability to accurately mentalize the self and others, when under stress, is the process that ultimately allows patients with PDs to develop a stronger identity, capacity for emotional and behavioral self-control, and meaningful and intimate interpersonal relationships.

A summary of MBT concepts, core strategies, therapeutic relationship, countertransference, and treatment goals is given in Table 6.2 (see p. 155). Interventions used by MBT therapists will be described in a later section. Review Chapter 9 for additional information and clinical illustrations of MBT practices.

MBT Training

Training for MBT typically is offered by experts in an introductory three-day course or one-month option, totaling 18 hours of seminars, with 21 hours of additional guided readings.[76-77] Ongoing weekly supervision by an MBT trainer, for one to two years, is offered for a fee. In addition, specialized training in MBT for the treatment of BPD, antisocial PD, adolescents, children, and groups are offered. Trainers use an MBT adherence scale to monitor the training. Trainings are offered by the Anna Freud Center[76] and McLean Hospital.[77]

Table 6.2. Mentalization-based Treatment

Key Concepts	Definition, Description, Use
Mentalization-based Theory of Personality Disorders	Psychological process of perceiving the thoughts, emotions, behaviors, and intentions of self/others. Genetics and early-life adversity leads to insecure attachments, deficits in mentalizing. which create emotional instability and interpersonal difficulties.
Attachment	Secure adult attachments reflect a childhood where subjective experiences were mirrored by a trusted adult leading to the capacity to accurately mentalize self/others. Insecure attachments (e.g., avoidant-dismissive, anxious-resistant, or disorganized) characterize all the PDs.
Mentalization Deficit: Psychic Equivalence	Deficit of rigid or concrete thinking paired with a definitive certainty that the person's position is accurate and correct (e.g., therapist is late, the patient is certain that the therapist hates him).
Mentalization Deficit: Pretend Mode	Occurs when a mental state is decoupled from reality; also called the "bullshit modes." The patient can't distinguish truth from the elaborations of truth (e.g., dreams, flashbacks, and paranoid delusions). These are in touch with reality (in some way) but are elaborated in ways unrelated to reality.
Mentalization Deficit: Teleological Mode	Deficit where actions and mental states are the same (e.g., if I think it, I must have done it).
Core Strategies	*Definitions, Description, Use*
Hyperactivation Strategies	Patient attaches intensely, too easily/quickly, inhibiting accurate judgments and trustworthiness of others. Intervene by decreasing the patient's urgency for closeness and foster a stable attachment to caring and helpful others.
Deactivation Strategies	Patient's emotional distancing leads to feeling insecure, negative self-representations, and increased levels of emptiness and distress. Foster a secure attachment.
Mixed Strategies	Alternating a hyperactive with deactivating strategy, or when there are attributes of both strategies that can be used at different times.
Therapeutic Relationship	*Definitions, Description, Use*
Therapeutic Stance	Maintain a stance of "not knowing" the mind of the patient. Step back from the therapist's empathy (to counteract the patient's hyperactive attachment strategy) when the patient is in distress to prevent an overly intense attachment; move closer when patient is distancing, using a deactivation strategy.
Therapist's Countertherapeutic Reactions	MBT believes the concept of totalistic countertransference confuses what comes from the patient or therapist. Therapists can temporarily lose their ability to mentalize the self or others, which corresponds to the patient's deficit in the capacity to mentalize. Therapists acknowledge classic countertransference and recommend self-reflection, supervision, or personal treatment, as needed.
Interventions or Techniques	See Table 6.8, p. 169
Treatment	*Definitions, Description, Use*
Individual treatment; partial hospital groups; inpatient	Individual 2x per week for 1–2 years. Partial hospital; intensive day treatment (weeks to month) both individual and/or in group.
Treatment Goals	Increase the patient's capacity to sustain mentalizing of self and others and to recover this capacity quickly if under stress. Accurate mentalizing leads to secure attachments, emotional stability, and improved interpersonal relationships and a healthier life.

Cognitive Therapy (CT)

CBT was originally designed as a short-term therapy, primarily for treatment of anxiety, phobias, obsessive-compulsive disorder, and depressive disorders. Gradually, CBT practitioners realized that this short-term treatment approach was not effective for patients with PDs at alleviating symptoms, changing behaviors, and improving functioning.[78] Treatment for PD from the CBT school is often called Cognitive Therapy (CT). Similar to other theories, CBT borrowed the PD concept from psychodynamic origins, emphasizing that the patient's particular beliefs about self and others are core features of all PDs. This realization led CBT to redirect its acute focus from automatic thoughts to core beliefs associated with the PDs, and to specify patients' varying beliefs for each of the PDs.[78] For example, the patient with NPD has a view of self as special and unique person, with others seen as less worthy or inferior. The narcissist's core belief is "because I am special, I am entitled to be admired, and deserve certain prerogatives and privileges." CT for the PDs describe a process where distorted and tenacious core beliefs about self/others are activated by current stressful events, leading to episodes of maladaptive thoughts, emotional dyscontrol, maladaptive behavior, and interpersonal difficulties.[79,80]

A core belief, also called "schema," involves more than an object relationship.[79] In addition to beliefs about oneself and ways of relating to others, a schema is a network of related memories, expectations, attitudes, thoughts, behaviors, feelings, and beliefs that determine a patient's worldview. Schemas developed in early life are modeled on attachments to caregivers and encoded during childhood. Dysfunctional working schemas vary for each of the PDs, and influence and create maladaptive adult coping styles, cognitions, feelings, and behaviors, leading to problematic relationships.

CT has a structured assessment phase[80] using the DSM-5, self-report measure of personality, discussion with informants, and typically administers a personality belief [81] and/or a schema questionnaire.[82] both borrowed from ST. The treatment phase is structured to limit patient TIBs, setting healthy treatment boundaries. CT remediates PD deficits through psychoeducation, teaching specific structured cognitive and behavioral skills.[79,80] Skills are designed to activate patients to examine, identify, and modify their core beliefs. Patients are given homework and are asked to practice these skills between sessions. Change in core beliefs and maladaptive coping leads to cognitive and behavioral changes that enable emotional control, self-sufficiency, and adaptive interpersonal relationships.

CT and the Therapeutic Alliance

The working alliance in CT is seen as a collaborative relationship, based on empiricism. It is a genuine relationship in the Rogerian sense, which is empathic and flexible, also permitting some limited personal disclosure.[79] The working alliance is the vehicle used to motivate patients to comply with treatment and to complete homework assignments, tasks, and practice skills.[80] The therapeutic relationship fosters treatment, but instead of change emerging through the relationship, it develops through education and the development of cognitive/behavioral skills. This view—that the therapeutic relationship is necessary but not essential to create change—came from the discovery that depression and anxiety could be treated with very little emphasis on the therapeutic relationship. It was discovered that CBT behavioral techniques such as hierarchical desensitization, flooding, and exposure response treatments were responsible for patient improvement. These interventions were not at all dependent on the relationship between therapist and patient.[78] However, as CBT began to focus on PD treatment, views that omit the power of the therapeutic relationship have been harder to maintain.

Aaron Beck realized that rigid inflexibility in style of patients with PDs made them less responsive to short-term CBT techniques. He framed the main problem for patients with PDs as a two-person, interpersonal, or relational problem.[78] With this conceptual shift, CT for PDs began to focus on the cognitive structures of information processing, learning schemas, and core beliefs, now considered responsible for the enduring dysfunctional patterns and overdeveloped maladaptive behavior seen in patients with PDs. Review Chapter 10 for more detailed information about CT for PDs.

CT and Management of Countertherapeutic Reactions

As the work with PDs developed, CBT therapists began to realize that patients with PDs, often refused to comply or rebelled against the directive approach.[79] They also recognized that patients with PDs were prone to misinterpret therapists' behaviors. Noncompliance and misunderstandings of therapist behavior typically led to poor outcomes. These realizations led to an acknowledgment that the quality of the therapeutic relationship did matter for the treatment of PDs.[79,80]

Beck and his earliest followers were distrustful and often hostile toward framing the relationship with patients based on transference and countertransference. Both these ideas were seen as inferential conjectures, not observed behaviors that could be tested.[78] This idea is understandable, because when it began, CBT was a new treatment approach, seeking to carve out its own niche, distinct from the dominant psychoanalytic approach.

Avoiding the term "countertransference," CT prefers to use the concept that "therapist-related thoughts and emotions,"[78] experienced and unmanaged in the therapeutic relationship, could result in treatment stalemates and failures.[79] CT offers the view that it is the patient's dysfunctional thoughts, emotions, behaviors, and schemas that are predominately responsible for activating disruptive equivalents in the therapist that can interfere with the progress of therapy. Beck suggested that these issues could be managed by therapists observing their own automatic thoughts, emotions, and behavior activated while working with their patients.

Judith Beck acknowledged that therapists treating patients with PDs may feel overwhelmed.[79] She has suggested that therapists need to identify their own dysfunctional reactions to their patients with PDs. Therapists should remain calm and non-defensive, and call out the patient's TIBs that obstruct treatment progress. She recommended that therapists set limits on patient behaviors and give feedback to the patient about their TIBs. She suggested that therapists need to recognize their own negative reactions to the patient by: monitoring their own thoughts, emotions, and behaviors; examining their level of empathy for the patient; developing realistic expectations for the treatment; and increasing their own self-care.[79] Supervision was always an option.

More recently, Morrey has also addressed management of difficulties in the CBT therapeutic relationship when treating patients with PDs.[83] She outlined a cognitive "interpersonal cycle," a worksheet used in supervision, to document the interactions of automatic thoughts, beliefs, feelings, and behaviors in both patient and therapist, and how they interact to produce a dysfunctional alliance.[84]

Some CBT authors have been more accepting of countertransference concepts, especially in longer treatments with patients who have PDs.[85,86] Prakso cautions that CBT clinicians should not deliberately provoke or ignore countertransference.[85] His focus is to recognize countertransference-induced schemas in therapists and that they can also occur with supervisors. He recommends discussions with colleagues and/or supervisors, so that countertransference won't interfere with treatment. [85]

Cartwright, also a CBT practitioner, recommends that CBT therapists not dismiss the concept of countertransference due to its origins, but rather investigate the potential applications of these concepts within cognitive frameworks.[87] She offers the following strategies to help CBT therapists coach themselves: self-talk; self-reflective practices; reflection with their supervisors; and practicing of the same relaxation techniques (breathing, calming, and mindfulness) that they teach their patients, to help them manage countertherapeutic reactions that may occur when treating patients with PDs.

A summary of CT concepts, core strategies, therapeutic relationship, countertransference, and treatment goals is described in Table 6.3, p. 158. Intervention used by CT

Table 6.3. Cognitive Therapy for Personality Disorders

Key Concepts	Definition, Description, Use
CT Concepts of PD	Genetics and early-life adverse experience lead to maladaptive automatic thoughts, persistent core beliefs about oneself and others, emotional dyscontrol, and interpersonal difficulties.
Specify the Patient's Problems	A detailed history determines which problems are treatable.
Current Situation	Describe how current life circumstances or situations elicit automatic thoughts, feelings, and maladaptive behaviors.
Describe Core Beliefs	Patients have specific core beliefs, developed in early childhood, (associated with each personality disorder) that form the templates for their views of self /others, which emerge as automatic thoughts in certain current situations.
Core Strategies	*Definitions, Description, Use*
Specify Treatment Goals	Set specific goal(s) and an agenda for each session.
Cognitive Restructuring	Identify negative thought patterns and reframe those thoughts so they're more positive and productive.
Restructure Core beliefs	Use core cognitive/behavioral interventions with the goal of changing self-view and improving interpersonal relationships.
Coping Strategies	Specify the patient coping strategies used to manage dysfunctional behaviors and core beliefs (e.g., core belief: "I am inadequate" –coping strategy – "I need others to help me").
Therapeutic Relationship	*Definitions, Description, Use*
Therapeutic Stance	Collaborative empiricism
Therapist's Countertherapeutic Reactions	CBT acknowledges therapist's problematic "therapy-related thoughts and emotions" which can result in treatment stalemates and/or failures in patients with PDs. Therapists need to identify their own dysfunctional reactions, remain calm, non-defensive, and call out patient's TIBs. Supervision is an option.
Interventions or Techniques	See Table 6.9, p. 170
Treatment	*Definitions, Description, Use*
Individual Outpatient Treatment	Individual weekly sessions; 20 sessions for 1 year.
Treatment Results	Change in core beliefs, maladaptive coping, leads to cognitive and behavioral changes fostering emotional control, self-sufficiency, and adaptive interpersonal relationships.

therapists will be described in a later section. Review Chapter 10 for additional information and clinical illustrations of CBT practices for the treatment of PDs.

CT Training

CT training begins with a recommended eight-hour course in CBT basics. This training is offered in a three-day workshop, for 18 hours, with ten additional 45-minute session for supervision. Therapy sessions are recorded and reviewed for two or three patients. Participants are required to submit cognitive conceptualization diagrams and score 44 or above on a CT rating scale. Courses are offered for a fee by the Beck Institute.[88]

Dialectical Behavior Therapy (DBT)

DBT is an evidence-based treatment that was developed for treatment of patients with BPD and applied to other PDs. It is a third-wave CBT treatment using dialectical philosophy, behavioral science, and mindfulness practice adopted from Buddhist traditions.[89,90] DBT biosocial theory conceptualizes that patients with PDs have pervasive difficulties with emotional regulation that can manifest with mercurial behavior. Dysregulation is characterized by high emotional vulnerability and deficits in the ability to modulate emotions, causing difficulties with relationships. Emotion dysregulation is derived from biological anomalies and results in emotional vulnerability; it is also derived from early-life relational history and adverse experiences, characterized as an invalidating environment. Other symptoms related to PDs are viewed as a consequence of dysregulated emotions. Patients with PDs have a prolonged emotional reactivity to both positive and negative stimuli and are very slow to return to their baseline functioning. DBT treatment targets include emotional regulation, distress tolerance, interpersonal effectiveness, and use of mindfulness techniques. DBT borrows other treatment techniques from CBT, such as chain analysis, diary cards, exposure response interventions, and cognitive rehearsal.

DBT establishes the treatment frame and contract by focusing on setting the boundaries between therapist and patient and minimizing TIBs. DBT's treatment frame and contract include: (1) the patient agreeing to one year of therapy, which may be renewed, if indicated, after one year; (2) the patient will be dropped from therapy if he or she misses four consecutive sessions; and (3) therapy is not unconditional; therapy will cease if the therapist feels unable to help the patient further, or if the patient pushes the therapist beyond his or her limits.[89] The patient is also instructed not to miss sessions due to low mood, feelings of hopelessness, or aversion to certain subjects. Prevention of suicidal and parasuicidal TIBs are early and primary treatment goals. Subsequently, DBT will focus on elimination or treatment for other TIBs including: (1) overt threats to the treatment[22] (i.e., financial difficulties, plans to move out of town); (2) addictions or eating disorders;[89] (3) requests to change treatment frequency;[89] (4) dishonesty or withholding information;[22] and (5) any other contract breaches such as presenting irrelevant material,[22] refusing to do homework or practice skills, arguing with the therapist.[89] Review Box 6.1, p. 141 for other components of setting the treatment frame.

DBT is designed to help patients assent to the dialectic of acceptance of who they are and the need to change, leading to the goal of developing a life that is worth living.

DBT and the Therapeutic Alliance

The DBT patient–therapist relationship is best described as a nonjudgmental coaching relationship, designed to facilitate behavioral change.[10] DBT focuses on the necessity of the therapeutic alliance, although not the primacy of the relationship as the main driver of change. Change is created through the therapist's use of modeling and operant and behavioral conditioning techniques. DBT recognizes that a warm, trusting relationship is important, and uses the relationship as a contingency (leverage) to facilitate patient compliance with skills training and behavioral change. DBT's main focus is to help the patient develop acceptance skills (mindfulness and distress tolerance) and change skills (emotional regulation and interpersonal effectiveness).[90]

DBT and Countertherapeutic Reactions

Similar to CT, the use of the term "countertransference" is mostly anathema to DBT practitioners, because they don't accept the "unconscious, intrapersonal attachment" and "relational dimensions" imbedded in this term. Instead, they emphasize that TIBs and related behaviors (SBIs, LIBs, QIBs) and therapy-destroying behaviors (e.g., violent or inappropriate sexual behavior; threatening the therapist) create countertherapeutic reaction in therapists.[23] These therapist treatment-interfering behaviors negatively impact the treatment.[23] DBT therapists continuously monitor their own intense or aversive reactions to patients, viewing these as clues to the patient's behavioral problem that must be solved.[23,89] DBT therapists frame their own negative emotions or mistakes directed at patients as indicating the patient is engaging in TIBs and that therapist's TIBs (Th-TIBs) have been activated by the patient.[23]

Addressing the Th-TIBs in a weekly consultation group is considered an essential part of DBT treatment.[89] The consultation group is composed of many DBT therapists who help each other frame new interventions and role play ways to set firm behavioral limits. The consultation group also encourages therapists to deal with their Th-TIBs using mindfulness practices before, during, and after each session.[23,89] Therapists are encouraged to mindfully observe, recognize, and respect their own clinical and personal limitations. The group also encourages all therapists: (1) to be non-defensive; (2) remind each other of the dialectic to accept their own mistakes and the need to change their own countertherapeutic behaviors; (3) communicate to their patients that the patient's behavior is worrisome or unacceptable; (4) strive to remain curious and willing to discuss their Th-TIBs with the patient; (6) explore the precipitants and consequences of the Th-TIB with the patient; (7) problem-solve; (8) use a pro and con list to find a solution; and (9) measure success of these efforts.[89] Ultimately, the consultation group is used to encourage therapists to set firmer limits on maladaptive patient behaviors and recognize their own limitations.

A summary of DBT concepts, core strategies, therapeutic relationship, therapist's countertherapeutic reactions, and treatment goals is described in Table 6.4 (see p. 161). Intervention used by DBT therapists will be described in a later section. Review Chapter 11 for additional information and illustrations of DBT clinical practices.

Table 6.4. Dialectical Behavioral Therapy

Key Concepts	Definition, Description, Use
DBT Concepts of PD	Biosocial theory of the etiology of PDs is that both biological abnormalities and adverse early-life experiences characterized by invalidation leads to emotional dysregulation and interpersonal difficulties.
Dialectics	Realities are interconnected and constructed as opposing forces (dialectics) that are continuously changing. Opposite views can exist simultaneously. The core dialectic: accept who they are, and simultaneously change their maladaptive behaviors.
Validation	Accept patients where they are, use empathic validation, being attentive to the patient, actively reflecting patients' thoughts, feelings, and interpretation of reality. Patients viewed as individuals of equal status. Assume that the patient's behavior serves a purpose.
Change	Change occurs after validation and is facilitated by use of classical and operant conditioning aided by cognitive strategies. Changing behavior includes acquiring skills, managing contingencies, correcting deficiencies in emotional and cognitive processes and interpersonal relationships.
Core Strategies	*Definitions, Description, Use*
Acceptance Skills Modules	Mindfulness and distress tolerance
Change Skill Modules	Emotional regulation and interpersonal effectiveness skills
Therapeutic Relationship	*Definitions, Description, Use*
Therapeutic Stance	Nonjudgmental coaching
Therapist's Countertherapeutic Reactions	Acknowledges therapist interfering behaviors (Th-IBs) These are therapist's difficulties in setting appropriate limits with their patients. Management of TH-IBs is crucial and are discussed in a weekly consultation group.
Interventions or Techniques	See Table 6.10, p. 170
Treatment	*Definitions, Description, Use*
Individual and Intensive Outpatient Treatment; Partial Hospitalization; Inpatient Care	DBT has three components: individual treatment, skills group, and consultation group, for a total of 3 hours per week. Intensive programs are offered daily for six months to a year.
Treatment Goals	Accept that realities are constructed as opposing forces that are continuously changing. Being accepted/validated is necessary to be able to accept the need to change. Practicing mindfulness, distress tolerance, emotional regulation, and interpersonal effectiveness aided by the use of contingency management, chain analysis, limit setting on TIBs/LIBs leads to the goal of having a life worth living.

DBT Training

Training for DBT is offered by experts and consists of 40 hours of training, supervision of three cases, and 12 months in a DBT consultation group. Training is offered for a fee. There are requirements to read the DBT manuals, do homework, and teach DBT skills to others. In addition, therapists are asked to learn and practice mindfulness skills for their own benefit, as well as offer this training to patients. There is a DBT exam. Fifteen hours

162   MULTI-THEORETICAL TREATMENTS OF PERSONALITY DISORDERS

of continuing education credits are required every two years to maintain certification. Certification is offered by DBT Linehan Board of Certifications.[91]

Schema Therapy (ST)

ST is a specialized, evidence-based treatment, eclectically based on cognitive, behavioral, and psychodynamic therapies (e.g., object-relations theory), borrowing concepts and interventions from attachment theory and experiential psychotherapies.[7] The goal of ST is to help patients find adaptive ways to meet their five universal emotional needs for (1) secure attachments; (2) autonomy, competence and a sense of identity; (3) freedom to express valid needs and emotions; (4) spontaneity and play; (4) realistic limits; and (5) self-control. The therapist reviews their patients' past, often traumatic early life, deficits in their caregivers, and their patients' resulting attachment style. This is done with empathic understanding and empathic confrontation to help patients to understand their specific needs, deficits, and benefits of change.

The ST perspective is that damaging early adverse life experiences (e.g., frustration of needs, abuse, neglect, excessive gratification, identification with destructive others, etc.) lead to the development of early maladaptive schemas (EMS).[7] The therapist identifies and facilitates change in one or more of 18 EMS. EMS are a set of memories, common emotions, body sensations, and cognitions that revolve around a childhood theme, such as abandonment, abuse/neglect, failure, rejection, and so on. When acute or chronic interpersonal or other emotional distress activates an EMS, specific habitual dysfunctional beliefs and maladaptive coping strategies from the past are also reactivated, and ultimately activate current dysfunctional emotions, thoughts, and behaviors. When EMS are activated, the patient has disturbed views of self and others, problematic interpersonal relationships, and ultimately dysfunctional lives.[7]

Therapists recognize and help the patient to modify one of three maladaptive coping styles.[7] These are:

1. *Fight/overcompensation*: Patients behave in the opposite way of their schema (e.g., an EMS of fear of abandonment leads the patient to developing quick intense, demanding, and unreliable attachments to others who are not well known).
2. *Flight/avoidance:* Patients deny or avoid awareness of one or more schemas (e.g., uses drugs, binge over-eating, or cutting themselves to distract themselves from their schema or belief that they are a failure, incompetent, or dependent).
3. *Surrender/freeze:* Patients cope by just accepting their schema is true and represents who they are (e.g., patients just accept that they are defective and must always feel ashamed).

ST therapists work to change and improve their patients' moment-to-moment coping styles and ways of being in the world that are characterized as "modes."[7,92] Maladaptive modes include: (1) child modes (e.g., vulnerable child, angry child, impulsive undisciplined child, and happy child); (2) dysfunctional coping modes (e.g., compliant surrender, the detached protector, and the over-compensator); and (3) dysfunctional parent modes (e.g., punitive parent and the demanding parent). ST therapists strive to help all patients function primarily in a healthy adult mode, which moderates, nurtures, heals the other modes, and enables optimal real-world functioning.

ST is structured with an assessment and education phase followed by a treatment phase. The assessment involves identification of dysfunctional life patterns, the early life origins of the EMS, and identification of coping styles and temperament leading to the case conceptualization.[7] Although not specifically specified, ST also addresses TIBs. Education is focused on describing the disorder and/or dysfunction and education of the patient about their case formulation. Treatment utilizes cognitive, behavioral, experiential, and psychodynamic interventions.[7,92]

ST limits TIBS, but is otherwise flexibly structured around presentation of new information, review of homework from the previous session, discussion with opportunity for questions and answers, experiential, cognitive, and behavioral work, and assignment of new homework. ST incorporates a wide array of borrowed cognitive, behavioral, experiential, and psychodynamic interventions designed to encourage the patient's development of new positive schemas, improve their real relationship with the therapist and their real-world interpersonal relationships, and develop functional lives.

ST and the Therapeutic Alliance

ST, similar to TFP and MBT, views the patient–therapist relationship as the essential relationship for motivating change. The therapeutic relationship is defined as "limited reparenting," in which corrective emotional parenting with a healthy therapist (adult) facilitates change.[7,92] ST therapists tailor their parental role to the temperament of the patient. They strive to meet the basic emotional needs of the patient by providing a secure attachment modeling autonomy, competence, and genuine self-expression. Therapists reveal their natural personalities (i.e., share their emotional responses and imperfections, make personal disclosures). Often, the therapist is spontaneous and playful, while also limiting TIBs and setting realistic goals.

Similar to CBT and DBT, ST also uses the vehicle of the therapeutic relationship to educate patients about their disorder and schemas. Rogerian views of the working alliance are in play (empathy, warmth, and genuineness), providing a holding environment where the patient feels safe and accepted, so that a strong emotional attachment to the therapist is developed. The ST therapist collaborates with the patient to develop a case formulation and achieve core therapeutic goals.

ST and Countertransference

The ST therapist intentionally asks the patient to share any negative feelings they may have toward the therapy, or the therapist, to prevent resistance to change or distance within the therapeutic relationship. The therapist acknowledges countertransference, utilizing problematic patient–therapist interactions that create feelings in the therapist to help the patient learn about their unconscious EMS.[86]

ST therapists must be able to distinguish their valid intuition about a patient's EMS from the triggering of their own schemas (classic countertransference reactions). Therapists are asked to learn about their own core schemas and to manage their own countertherapeutic schemas, coping styles, and modes from their past. To assess this, therapists are encouraged to ask themselves the following types of questions: (1) Are the patient's schemas clashing with mine? Are we triggering each other?; (2) Is there a mismatch between the patient's needs and my schema or coping style?; (3) Am I over-identifying with the patient because our schemas are similar?; (4) Are the patient's intense emotions or destructive behaviors triggering my avoidant behaviors?; (5) Has the patient triggered my dysfunctional parenting mode?; (6) Is my schema triggered when the patient fails to make progress?[7,86]

Similar to DBT, ST therapists manage their own countertherapeutic reactions with the patient by setting limits on either the patient's behavior or their own. Therapists set firm limits on the patient's suicidal or aggressive behavior, substance use, and so on. Therapists may also limit their own behaviors by disclosing less information, creating greater/lesser emotional distance with the patient, or taking more time off for self-care.

A summary of ST concepts, core strategies, therapeutic relationship, countertransference, and treatment goals is described in Table 6.5. Interventions used by ST therapists will be described in a later section. Review Chapter 12 for additional information and illustrations of ST clinical practices.

Table 6.5. Schema Therapy

Key Concepts	Definition, Description, Use
ST Concepts of PD	Genetics and early-life adverse experience lead to enduring schemas that are easily and perpetually activated by current stressors, leading to disturbed views of self and others and dysfunctional lives.
Patient Seek to Meet 5 Universal Emotional Needs	Focused on helping patient meet 5 core emotional needs. These include: (1) secure attachments; (2) autonomy, competence, and identity; (3) freedom to express valid needs and emotions; (4) spontaneity and play; and (5) realistic limits and self-control.
Early Maladaptive Schema	Schema questionnaire identifies 18 maladaptive schemas. Each of the PDs have different combinations of these schemas. For example, a patient with BPD may have three schemas: (1) mistrust, abused, deprivation; (2) abandoned abused; and (3) subjugation.
Coping Styles	Identify 1 of 3 coping styles. 1) Fight/overcompensation: patients behaves in the opposite way of the schema. 2) Flight/avoidance; deny or avoid awareness of the schema. 3) Surrender/ freeze: patients accept that their schema is true and that it represents who they are.
Schema Modes	Coping styles lead to a schema mode (a set of operative schemas) responsible for the patient's functioning. These include (1) *child modes* (e.g., vulnerable child, angry child, impulsive undisciplined child, happy child); (2) *maladaptive coping modes* (e.g., over-compensator, detached protector, compliant surrender); (3) *dysfunctional parent modes* (e.g., punitive critical or demanding parent). *Healthy adult mode* nurtures/protects, sets limits on the angry/impulsive child mode, moderates maladaptive coping and dysfunctional parent mode.
Core Strategies	*Definitions, Description, Use*
Develop a Case Formulation	Identify early maladaptive schemas, current modes, and current coping strategies.

(continued)

Table 6.5. Continued

Key Concepts	Definition, Description, Use
Improve Coping Strategies	EMS are activated by emotional distress or interpersonal problems which activates one of three coping styles: (1) *fight/ overcompensation* (e.g., patients behaves in the opposite way of the schema; (2) *flight/avoidance* (e.g., deny or avoid awareness of the schema; (3) *surrender/freeze* (e.g., patients just accept that their schema is true and that it represents who they are).
Change Schema Mode	Function, most of the time, in the healthy adult schema mode.
Therapeutic Relationship	*Definitions, Description, Use*
Therapeutic Stance	Limited reparenting: Therapist assumes a limited healthy parenting role to assist/modify the patient's coping strategies and modes of functioning, facilitating transfer of a healthy relationship within the therapy to the outside world.
Therapist's Countertransference	ST uses totalistic countertransference to understand events within the therapeutic relationship. Difficulty in the therapeutic relationship is a template for patients' experiences in their interpersonal relationships. ST recognizes classic countertransference and recommends awareness and modifications of one's own core schema which may be interfering with the treatment of patients.
Interventions or Techniques	See Table 6.11, p. 171
Treatment	*Definitions, Description, Use*
Individual and Intensive Outpatient Treatment; Partial Hospitalization	Individual treatment 1–2 hours per week with or without group for approximately 1 year.
Treatment Goals	Identify and label patient's modes, exploring the etiology of EMS, linking maladaptive modes to problems/symptoms; demonstrating the advantages of modifying or giving up a dysfunctional mode (especially maladaptive child modes), conducting dialogues between modes, moving the patient toward healthy adult mode. Generalizing the healthy adult modes to improve work/whole-life situation outside of therapy.

ST Training

Training for ST is offered by experts who teach ST theory, use of schema inventories, and provide demonstrations, case consultation, and supervision for a fee.[93] Participants attend 40 hours in an approved training program. They are required to use a ST case-conceptualization form and need to present their cases to an online special interest group. Twelve hours of continuing education credits in an individual or group setting is required every two years to maintain certification.

Good Psychiatric Management (GPM)

GPM is based on psychodynamic principles. It was the first EBP that demonstrated the essential effectiveness of case management as part of a core therapeutic strategy. GPM was developed by John Gunderson, from early origins as part of the American Psychiatric

Association's 2001 practice guidelines for the treatment of patients with BPD.[8] The name "good psychiatric management"[10] is derived from Winnicott's concept of "good enough mothering," meaning GPM is "good enough" treatment for patients with BPD. It developed into an evidence-based treatment, based on psychodynamic principles, after it was utilized as a control treatment in a large, single blind, multi-site trial of 180 patients with BPD, compared to DBT.[94,95] Suicidal patients with BPD were randomly assigned to receive either one year of DBT or GMP. Much to everyone's surprise, GMP did as well as DBT. Other indirect support for the efficacy of GPM comes from other treatment trials (supportive therapy and structured clinical management), where other generalist models did well compared to TFP and MBT, respectively.[96]

Two major advantages of GPM are its generalist approach to the treatment of patients with BPD and the fact that the treatment only requires one day of training to learn.[96]

GPM can be widely applied to a large group of patients with BPD, making a difficult disorder treatable by a large number of clinicians. The core treatment features of supportive psychotherapy, use of medications, treatment of comorbidities, and case management are well within the generalist provider's scope of regular outpatient psychiatric practice. This is a substantial public-health benefit inasmuch as other specialized PD treatments for BPD are not widely available in many communities. In addition, the practicality of one day of relatively inexpensive training makes it a commonsense alternative to all the other treatment modalities for the BPDs.[96]

GPM has a structured, though flexible, treatment frame, with an initial priority of managing suicidal TIBs. It begins with psychoeducation for patients with BPD. BPD is framed as "a problem with interpersonal hypersensitivity" caused by genetics and early life adverse/traumatic experiences. Patients learn about the potential for changes with GPM and comparisons of GPM with other specialized PD approaches. At its core, GPM is a structured, eclectic, pragmatic treatment, with the goals of helping patients find work and develop stable partnerships and meaningful interpersonal relationships. Case-management strategies are used to support the patient's activities of daily living (i.e., obtaining food and decent shelter, developing budgets, obtaining insurance, and assistance with a wide range of other activities supporting work and interpersonal connectedness). Comorbid treatment of medical, psychiatric, or addictive disorders is coordinated with referrals to community services. Psychopharmacology is used to treat symptoms of BPD and any comorbidities. Deliberate efforts are made to connect the patient's dysfunctional emotions, thoughts, and behaviors to interpersonal hypersensitivities and interpersonal and life stressors. Treatment duration and intensity is typically weekly but modified based on practical clinical considerations.

GPM and the Therapeutic Alliance

GPM's therapeutic stance is characterized as supportive within a psychodynamic frame.[10] The working alliance is based on a real dyadic yet professional relationship, with elements of transference in which the therapist may selectively disclose the impact that the patient has on the therapist as well as openly discussing the effect the patient has on others. The therapeutic alliance is similar to the DBT approach of patients accepting where they are in life, as well as the notion that certain behaviors need to change. Therapists rely heavily on listening, empathy, validation of the patient's painful experiences, and problem solving. There is a central focus on management of suicidal, homicidal, and other acting out behaviors as needed. The alliance is used to encourage patients and support the use of any and all interventions that foster the patient's building a stable, functional, and meaningful life.

GPM and Countertransference

GMP acknowledges that classic countertransference or therapist-generated countertransference can interfere with treatment; countertherapeutic reactions coming from the therapist's own life need to be monitored and managed by self-reflection and/or supervision.

Use of the therapist's totalistic countertransference is considered valuable and may be explored with the patient, but is not necessarily an essential part of the therapy.[10] If explored, it is used to help the patient understand how their relationship with the therapist may reflect their dysfunctional interpersonal relationships in the world.

A summary of GPM concepts, core strategies, therapeutic relationship, countertransference, and treatment goals is described in Table 6.6. Interventions used by GPM

Table 6.6. Good Psychiatric Management

Key Concept	Definition, Description, Use
Concepts of PD	Genetics and early-life adverse experience jointly lead to the development of PDs.
Core Problem	Patient with PDs present with emotional dysregulation and problematic interpersonal relationships which need repaired.
Develop a Meaningful Life	Focus on developing meaningful work and stable, helpful, and sustainable interpersonal relationships.
Core Strategies	Definitions, Description, Use
Psychoeducation	Educate the patient about their diagnosis and the importance of interpersonal hypersensitivity as a treatment focus.
Supportive/Psychodynamic Informed Treatment	Supportive interventions with some interpretations connecting interpersonal stressors and hypersensitivity as the primary causes of dysfunctional emotions, thoughts, and behaviors.
Focus on Life Outside of Therapy	Patients are focused on developing work, volunteer, or school activities, developing life partnerships, and/or sustaining meaningful interpersonal relationships.
Therapeutic Relationship	Definitions, Description, Use
Therapeutic Stance	Supportive and emphasizing that functioning in the outside world is most important.
Therapist's Countertransference	Recognizes both forms of countertransference and suggests supervision as an antidote if the therapist's reactions are interfering with the treatment of the patient.
Interventions Or Techniques	See Table 6.12, p. 171
Treatment	Definitions, Description, Use
Individual Outpatient Treatment;	Weekly session for as short or as long as it takes.
Treatment Goals	Decrease interpersonal hypersensitivity and stressors to foster the development of a functional life.

therapists will be described in a later section. Review Chapter 13 for additional information and illustrations of GPM clinical practices.

GPM Training

Training for GPM is the least intensive and the easiest to learn of all the EBPs for treatment of BPD. GPM was developed for the generalist mental health professional, so the one day of training does not require use of highly specialized techniques. An eight-hour course is offered in 12 modules. GPM training is also offered as a self-paced online course, for a fee. The training is offered by Harvard[97] or Mclean Hospital Gunderson Training Institute.[98]

Differences Among the Six EBPs for the Treatment of PDs

Theoretical orientation of the six EBPs are on a continuum from psychodynamic (TFP: psychodynamic, ego psychology, object relations, and attachment; and MBT: mentalization, object relations, attachment, neurosciences) to supportive (GPM: psychodynamic and case management) to eclectic (ST: psychodynamic, cognitive, behavioral, and experiential) to CT (more cognitive with some behavioral therapy) to DBT (more behavioral with some cognitive therapy). These differences in theory largely set the imprint for all the other differentiating features of their treatments. As expected, the core strategies for conceptualizing and guiding the treatment follow their theories. Review Tables 6.1 to 6.6 for details that can be used to compare and contrast these treatments along many dimensions.

The therapeutic stances of these EBPs vary and include technical neutrality (TFP), "not knowing the mind of the patient" (MBT), collaborative empiricism (CT), nonjudgmental coaching (DBT), limited reparenting (SF), and a supportive stance (GPM). All treatments agree that countertherapeutic reactions of therapists impact patient treatments, but each have different conceptions about this and varying approaches to managing them. TFP, MBT, ST, and GPM all utilize the concept of "classic countertransference" as work that therapists need to do so their own transferences don't interfere with the treatments of their patients. They also recognize totalistic countertransference as reflections of the patient's internal representations of self and others that become the patient's prototypes of interpersonal relationships in the real world. CT and DBT don't view countertransference or the subjective unconscious experiences of therapists as meaningful or useful clinically. They do emphasize the importance of countertherapeutic reactions caused by patients' (TIBs and Th-TBIs) that may impact the treatment. They resolve these problematic behaviors by setting limits on either the patient's and/or the therapist's behaviors.

A definition and explanation of many interventions offered by all six treatments are summarized in Tables 6.7 to 6.12 (see pp. 169–171). These are presented in separate tables to make it easier for clinicians with a single orientation to explore options for using interventions borrowed from other EBPs. These tables can be used to: (1) familiarize the reader with basics definitions of each intervention used in six EBPs for the treatment of PDs; (2) consider how one might apply these interventions to be therapeutically responsive to the needs of individual patients; (3) help clinicians in their efforts to determine for

Table 6.7. TFP Interventions

Self–Affect–Other (Object relations)	Self and other representation are linked by an affect (e.g., abused child–sadistic parent). Identify the dominant dyad; expect role reversal of self and other; identify object dyads that defend against each other.
Splitting	Images of self and other exist side-by-side without influencing each other. Self and Others are all good or all bad.
Projective Identification (PI)	Images of self and others are projected by the patient onto the therapist, followed by the patient's efforts to control the therapist as a way of unconsciously controlling their own feelings. Interpretation of PI reveals the templates for interpersonal relationship.
Enactments	Acting out between the patient and the therapist that symbolically and unconsciously represents different experiences of the self or other.
Confrontation	Presenting the patient with any discrepancies between their thoughts, emotions, or behaviors.
Clarification	Elaborating on something which is conscious to a broader understanding; make something observed more comprehensible.
Here and Now Interpretation	Connects the patient's conscious experiences with current experiences outside of awareness. Interpret dyads emerging in the therapeutic relationship and their relationship to current interpersonal relationships.
There and Then Interpretation	Connects aspect of the patient's current conscious experiences with early-life experiences. Interpret the link between dyads emerging in the therapeutic relationship to current outside relationships or to early-life attachment.

Table 6.8. MBT Interventions

Mentalizes Self and Others	Note when patient and therapist have either the capacity to mentalize self and others and when they lose this ability.
Empathic Clarification	Awareness of the mental state of self and others and being emotionally responsive to it.
Basic Interventions	• Provide a secure attachment. • Promote engagement that is not too close nor too distanced. • Look at things from multiple perspectives. • Acknowledge when you don't know. • Let patients know what you're thinking to permit them to examine their mentalizing of the therapist. • Acknowledge your own mentalizing failures and mistakes.
Challenge	Insert disruptive or irrelevant dialogue to break a non-mentalizing state.
Affect Focus	Share the therapist's subjective emotional sense of the current feelings within the therapeutic relationship at any given point in the session.
Contrary Move	Do the opposite of what the patient is doing. If the patient is "knowing," therapist presents as "unknowing"; if the patient is in self-reflection, focus on reflection about others; if the patient is creating emotional distance, create emotional closeness. If the patient is certain, present doubt.
Complex Intervention Mentalizing the Relationship	Validate the patient's experience within the therapeutic relationship; explore the therapist distortions; arrive at a mutual understanding; present alternative perspectives; monitor for new understandings.

Table 6.9. CT Interventions

Challenge Automatic Thought and Core Beliefs	Guid the discovery of emotions, somatic sensations, automatic thoughts, and core beliefs; use pro and con lists, imagery, and role plays to challenge thoughts and/or beliefs.
Change Dysfunctional Behaviors	Set specific and behavioral goals when patient has unrealistic expectations, goals that are too large or nonspecific, or if they avoid or deny core problems. Use journaling, activity scheduling, and behavioral experiments to challenge core beliefs.
Give Homework	Design and assign homework for practicing new skills and self-sufficiency, and tailor it to the individual; provide a rationale, detailed written assignments; use reminders and anticipate problems.
Use Exposure Techniques	Offer graded and immersive exposure to confront fear, phobias, and anxieties.
Use Relaxation Techniques	Teach the patient breathing, muscle relaxation, and guided imagery.
Role Playing	Problem-solving technique to improve communications, practice social skills and assertiveness.
Imagery	Help patients envision desirable long-term changes in the core beliefs designed to improve views of self and enhance interpersonal relationships.

Table 6.10. DBT Interventions

Acceptance Skills	*Mindfulness* Directing attention to the present moment, with an attitude of acceptance. Become aware of the emotional, reasonable, and wise minds, by nonjudgmentally observing, describing, and participating. *Distress Tolerance* Accept that pain/distress are part of life and can't be eliminated by addictions, eating disorders, etc. Skills to manage distress include: **STOP** skills (e.g., Stop, Take a step back, Observe, Proceed mindfully), pros and cons lists, distracting, self-soothing). IMPROVE skills are Imagery, Meaning, Prayer, Relaxing, One Thing, Vacation, and Encouragement of radical acceptance (total acceptance of reality).
Change Skills	*Emotional Regulation* Reduce emotional suffering by understanding, regulating, and decreasing unwanted emotions; decrease vulnerability to the emotional mind. *Interpersonal Effectiveness* 1) Core interpersonal skills: problem solving, social skills, and assertiveness; **DEAR MAN** skills (Describe, Express, Assert, Reinforce, Mindful, Appear confident, and Negotiate) to be used with specific interpersonal goals. 2) Learn to develop and maintain relationships (find friends and end destructive relationships). 3) Middle path: balance acceptance and change in relationships.
Contingency Management	Giving patients tangible rewards to reinforce positive behavioral change.
Chain Analysis	Assess all links in a chain of thoughts, emotions, behaviors, and sensations leading up to, during, and following a problematic behavior. Change any link by applying contingency management or by modeling behavioral skills which can lead to desirable outcomes.
Limit Setting	Set limits to decrease interfering behaviors (i.e., TIBs, LIBs, SIBs, QIBs).
Diary Card	Record emotions, drug and alcohol use, self-injury urges, suicidal ideation, and use of skills.

Table 6.11. ST Interventions

Schema Questionnaire	Identify 18 Early Maladaptive Schema
Cognitive Interventions	Challenge a schema, pro and cons of a coping styles, role-play a maladaptive mode (e.g., angry child mode) in a dialogue with healthy adult mode. Use flash cards which summarize problem or healthy responses. Construct a schema diary of healthy responses in the moment or in real-life situations.
Experiential Techniques	Use imagery to imagine and construct dialogs with people from the patient's childhood and current life who have reinforced their maladaptive schemas. Envision better parenting.
Dialogues	Use the empty chair technique, role-playing one side of a conflict speaking to the empty chair on the other side of the conflict and then switching chairs. Use to address two sides of ambivalence, to practice negotiating a difficult conversation with others or oneself, to practice resolving a problem or conflict.
Behavioral Pattern Breaking Interventions	Define problematic behaviors to change; identify triggering events; review pros and cons of a behavior; break maladaptive behaviors by rehearsing healthy behaviors.

themselves options of combining interventions from diverse modalities when struggling with patients who are not improving when using one therapeutic modality; (4) help researchers to determine for themselves if, how, and when they might combine interventions in various treatments as they search for new modalities or evidence of what is most effective for the wider range of patients with varying PDs.

Treatment goals across these six EBPs for PDs differ based on resolving the core problems as defined by each theory. Practical treatment recommendations vary by the intensity and frequency of sessions, setting in which they can be used, and recommended lengths of treatment.

Conclusion

This chapter describes how all six EBPs for PDs contend that there are genetic and early life adverse/traumatic environments that are responsible for the development of PDs. EBP for the treatment of PDs share six essential and common themes that include

Table 6.12. Unique Interventions GPM

Case Management	Providing aid in structuring the therapeutic environment (scheduling, completing homework, contacts with insurance or providers, establishing a budget). Provide basic needs (food, clothing, shelter); offer additional health-related services.
Using Adjunctive Modalities	Refer patient for group and/or family therapy, intensive outpatient or partial hospitalization program, alcoholics' anonymous, obtaining other addiction or eating disorder services.
Treating All Comorbid Conditions	Treat comorbid medical and psychiatric disorders; use medications to treat any comorbid psychiatric or addiction-related disorder.

Box 6.3　Resources for Patient, Families and Clinicians

- Oldham J, Morris LB. *The New Personality Self-portrait: Why You Think, Work, Love and Act the Way You Do*. New York, NY: Bantam; 2012.
- Feinstein RE: Transference focused psychotherapy for borderline personality disorder: clinical guide. *Am J of Psychiatry*. 2015; 172(6):589–590.
- Mentalization-based therapy. *Psychology Today*. https://www.psychologytoday.com/us/therapy-types/mentalization-based-therapy.
- Treating BPD with cognitive behavioral therapy. Very Well Mind. https://www.verywellmind.com/borderline-personality-disorder-therapy-425452.
- Dialectical behavioral therapy. Web MD.https://www.webmd.com/mental-health/dialectical-behavioral-therapy–1.
- What is schema therapy? Betterhelp. https://www.betterhelp.com/advice/therapy/what-is-schema-therapy/?utm_source=AdWords&utm_medium=-Search_PPC_c&utm_term=_b&utm_content=81347073590&network=g&-placement=&target=&matchtype=b&utm_campaign=6459244691&ad_type=text&adposition=&gclid=CjwKCAiAxeX_BRASEiwAc1QdkRbMJjE_U0iQHx0Pb5xI9G94S8GX96abnA5aJZW1ztlW5k6zP4QOZBoChXUQAvD_BwE.
- 2021 Good Psychiatric Management of BPD: Overview for NEABPD. NEABPD. https://www.borderlinepersonalitydisorder.org/wpcontent/uploads/2012/10/Palmer_NEABPD10_14_12a-1.pdf.

---

structuring the treatment, the need for therapist self-awareness, management of countertherapeutic reactions, the need to develop therapeutic responsiveness when treating different patients with different PDs, recognizing and repairing mistakes and therapeutic ruptures, and the need for therapists to get ongoing supervision and training.

Each of these six EBPs has different notions about the importance of the therapeutic alliance and suggests different ways to manage therapists' countertherapeutic reactions that are inevitable when treating patients with PDs. The chapter also defines the unique interventions used by the six EBPs. It is hoped that this information will be useful to clinicians and researchers. See Box 6.3 for additional resources for patients, families, and clinicians.

Conflict of Interest/Disclosure: The authors of this chapter have no financial conflicts and nothing to disclose.

References

1. Kernberg OF. *Borderline Conditions and Pathological Narcissism*. New York, NY: Jason Aronson; 1975.

2. Yeomans RF, Clarkin JF, Kernberg OF. *Transference-focused Psychotherapy for Borderline Personality Disorder: A Clinical Guide*. Arlington, VA: American Psychiatric Publishing; 2015.

3. Beck AT. *Cognitive Therapy and the Emotional Disorders*. New York NY: International University Press; 1976.

4. Beck, JS. *Cognitive Therapy; Basics and Beyond*. New York, NY: Guilford Press; 1995.

5. Bateman A, Fonagy P. The effectiveness of partial hospitalization in the treatment of borderline personality disorder; a randomized controlled trial. *Am J Psychiatry*. 1999;156:1563–1569.

6. Linehan MM, Armstrong HE, Suarez A, Allmon D, Heard HL. Cognitive behavioral treatment of chronically parasuicidal borderline patients. *Arch Gen Psychiatry*. 1991;48(12):1060–1064.

7. Young JE, Klosko JS, Weishaar ME. *Schema Therapy: A Practitioner's Guide*. New York, NY: Guilford Press; 2003.

8. American Psychiatric Association. Practice guideline for the treatment of patients with borderline personality disorder. *Am J Psychiatry*. 2001;158:1–52.

9. Gundersen JG, Links PA. *Borderline Personality Disorder: A Clinical Guide*. 2nd ed. Washington, DC: American Psychiatric Publishing; 2008.

10. Gundersen JG, Links PA. *Handbook of Good Psychiatric Management for Borderline Personality Disorder*. Washington, DC: American Psychiatric Press; 2014.

11. Levy KN, McMain S, Bateman A, Clouthier T. Treatment of borderline personality disorder. *Psychiatric Clinics*. 2018;41(4):711–728.

12. Levy KN, Clarkin JF, Yeomans FE, Scott LN, Wasserman RH, Kernberg OF. The mechanisms of change in the treatment of borderline personality disorder with transference focused psychotherapy. *J Clin Psychol*. 2006;62(4):481–501.

13. *Diagnostic and Statistical Manual of Mental Disorders* (DSM-5). Washington, DC: American Psychiatric Publishing; 2013.

14. Reichborn-Kjennerud T. The genetic epidemiology of personality disorders. *Dialogues Clin. Neurosci*. 2010; 12(1):103.

15. Perez-Rodriguez MM, Zaluda L, New AS. Biological advances in personality disorders. *Focus*. 2013;11(2):146–154.

16. Reichborn-Kjennerud T, Czajkowski N, Neale MC, et al. Major depression and dimensional representations of DSM-IV personality disorders: a population-based twin study. *Psychol Med*. 2010;40(09):1475–1484.

17. Rosenström T, Ystrom E, Torvik FA, Czajkowski NO, Gillespie NA, Aggen SH, Krueger RF, Kendler KS, Reichborn-Kjennerud T. Genetic and environmental structure of DSM-IV criteria for antisocial personality disorder: a twin study. *Behav Genet*. 2017;47(3):265–77.

18. Raine A, Lencz T, Bihrle S, LaCasse L, Colletti P. Reduced prefrontal gray matter volume and reduced autonomic activity in antisocial personality disorder. *Arch Gen Psychiatry*. 2000;57(2):119–127.

19. Raine A. Antisocial personality as a neurodevelopmental disorder. *Annu Rev Clin Psychol*. 2018;14:259–289.

20. Johnson JG, Cohen P, Brown J, Smailes EM, Bernstein DP. Childhood maltreatment increases risk for personality disorders during early adulthood. *Arch Gen Psychiatry*.1999; 56(7):600–606.

21. Johnson JG, Cohen P, Smailes EM, Skodol AE, Brown J, Oldham JM. Childhood verbal abuse and risk for personality disorders during adolescence and early adulthood. *Compr Psychiatry*. 2001;42(1):16–23.

22. Kernberg OF, Selzer MA, Koenigsberg HW, Carr AC, Appelbaum AH. *Psychodynamic Psychotherapy of Borderline Patients*. New York, NY: Basic Books; 1989.

23. Chapman AL, Rosenthal MZ. *Managing Therapy-interfering Behavior: Strategies from Dialectical Behavior Therapy.* Washington, DC: American Psychological Association; 2016.

24. Hayes JA, Gelso CJ, Goldberg S, Kivlighan DM. Countertransference management and effective psychotherapy: meta-analytic findings. *Psychotherapy.* 2018;55(4);496.

25. Gabbard GO. Countertransference: the emerging common ground. *Int J PsychoAnal.* 1995;76:475–485.

26. Trapnell PD, Campbell JD. Private self-consciousness and the five-factor model of personality: distinguishing rumination from reflection. *J Pers Soc Psychol.* 1999;76(2):284.

27. Kolden GG, Wang CC, Austin SB, Chang Y, Klein MH. Congruence/genuineness: a meta-analysis. *Psychotherapy.* 2018;55(4):424.

28. Nienhuis JB, Owen J, Valentine JC, et al. Therapeutic alliance, empathy, and genuineness in individual adult psychotherapy: a meta-analytic review. *Psychother Res.*2018;4;28(4):593–605

29. Kabat-Zinn J. Mindfulness-based interventions in context: past, present, and future. *Clin Psychol.* 2003;10(2):144–156.

30. Sng AA, Janca A. Mindfulness for personality disorders. *Curr Opin Psychiatry.* 2016;29(1):70–76.

31. Aggs C, Bambling M. Teaching mindfulness to psychotherapists in clinical practice: the mindful therapy programme. *Couns Psychother Res.* 2010;10(4):278–286.

32. Cohen JS, Miller LJ. Interpersonal mindfulness training for well-being: a pilot study with psychology graduate students. *Teach Coll Rec.* 2009;1111:2768–2774.

33. Greason PB, Cashwell CS. Mindfulness and counseling self-efficacy: the mediating role of attention and empathy. *Couns Educ Superv.* 2009;49(1):2–19.

34. Monsen JT, Eilertsen DE, Melgård T, Ødegård P. Affects and affect consciousness: initial experiences with the assessment of affect integration. *J Psychother Pract Res.*1996;5(3):238.

35. Fonagy P, Gergely G, Jurist EL, eds. *Affect Regulation, Mentalization and the Development of the Self.* New York, NY: Routledge; 2018.

36. Katznelson H. Reflective functioning: a review. *Clin Psychol Rev.* 2014;34(2):107–117.

37. Choi-Kain LW, Gunderson JG. Mentalization: ontogeny, assessment, and application in the treatment of borderline personality disorder. *Am J Psychiatry.* 2008;165(9):1127–1135.

38. Falkenström F, Solbakken OA, Möller C, Lech B, Sandell R, Holmqvist R. Reflective functioning, affect consciousness, and mindfulness: are these different functions? *Psychoanal Psychol.* 2014;31(1):26.

39. Fonagy P, Bateman A. Progress in the treatment of borderline personality disorder. *Brit J Psychiatry.* 2006;188(1):1–3.

40. Cologon J, Schweitzer RD, King R, Nolte T. Therapist reflective functioning, therapist attachment style and therapist effectiveness. *Admin Policy Ment Health.* 2017;1;44(5):614–625.

41. Bateman A, Bolton R, Fonagy P. Antisocial personality disorder: a mentalizing framework. *Focus.* 2013;11(2):178–186.

42. Allen JG, Fonagy P, Bateman AW. *Mentalizing in Clinical Practice.* Washington DC: American Psychiatric Publishing; 2008

43. Bateman A, Fonagy P. *Mentalization-based Treatment for Personality Disorders: A Practical Guide.* Oxford, UK: Oxford University Press; 2016.

44. Kernberg O. Notes on countertransference. *Am Psychoanal Assoc.*1965;13(1):38–56.

45. Gabbard GO, Wilkinson SM. *Management of Countertransference with Borderline Patients*. New York, NY: Jason Aronson; 2000.

46. Norcross JC, Wampold BE. A new therapy for each patient: evidence-based relationships and responsiveness. *J Clin Psychol*. 2018;74(11):329–341.

47. Paul GL. Strategy of outcome research in psychotherapy. *J Consul Psychol*. 1967;31(2):109.

48. Norcross JC, Wamploe BE. Evidence based psychotherapy responsiveness: the third task force. In: Norcross JC, Lambert MJ, eds. *Psychotherapy Relationships That Work, Volume 2: Evidence-Based Therapist Responsiveness*. 3rd ed. New York, NY: Oxford University Press; 2019:339.

49. Eubanks CF, Muran JC, Safran JD. Alliance ruptures and resolution. In Muran JC, Barber JP, eds. *The Therapeutic Alliance; An Evidence-based Approach to Practice and Training*. New York, NY: Guilford; 2010:74–94.

50. Colli A, Gentile D, Condino V, Lingiardi V. Assessing alliance ruptures and resolutions: reliability and validity of the Collaborative Interactions Scale-revised version. *Psychother Res*. 2019;29(3):279–292.

51. Tufekcioglu S, Muran JC, Safran JD, Winston A. Personality disorder and early therapeutic alliance in two time-limited therapies. *Psychother Res*. 2013;23(6):646–657.

52. Bordin ES. The generalizability of the psychoanalytic concept of the working alliance. *Psychol Psychother Theory Res Pract*. 1979;16:252–260.

53. Safran JD, Muran JC, Eubanks-Carter C. Repairing alliance ruptures. *Psychotherapy*. 2011;48(1):80.

54. Muran JC, Safran JD, Gorman BS, Samstag LW, Eubanks-Carter C, Winston A. The relationship of early alliance ruptures and their resolution to process and outcome in three time-limited psychotherapies for personality disorders. *Psychol Psychother*. 2009; 46(2):233.

55. Westra HA, Norouzian N. Using motivational interviewing to manage process markers of ambivalence and resistance in cognitive behavioral therapy. *Cognit Ther and Res*. 2018; 1;42(2):193–203.

56. Di Bartolomeo AA, Shukla S, Westra HA, Shekarak Ghashghaei N, Olson DA. Rolling with resistance: a client language analysis of deliberate practice in continuing education for psychotherapists. *Couns Psychother Res*. 2020 (advance online publication). https://doi.org/10.1002/capr.12335

57. Beutler LE, Harwood M, Michelson A, Song X, Holman J. Reactance and resistance level. In Norcross JC, ed. *Psychotherapy Relationships That Work; Evidenced-based Responsiveness*. 2nd ed. New York, NY: Oxford University Press; 2011:272–273.

58. Edwards CJ, Beutler LE, Someah K. Reactance level. In Norcross JC, Lambert MJ, eds. *Psychotherapy Relationships That Work, Volume 2: Evidence-based Therapist Responsiveness*. 3rd ed. New York, NY: Oxford University Press; 2019:188–211.

59. Bateman AW, Fonagy P. Mentalization-based treatment of borderline personality. In Widiger TA, ed. *The Oxford Handbook of Personality Disorders*. New York, NY: Oxford University Press; 2012:767–784.

60. Eubanks CF, Burckell LA, Goldfried MR. Clinical consensus strategies to repair ruptures in the therapeutic alliance. *J Psychother Integr*. 2018;28(1):60.

61. Feinstein RE. Descriptions and reflections on the cognitive apprenticeship model of psychotherapy training and supervision. *J Contemp Psychother*. 2021;51:155–164.

62. Watkins Jr CE. How does psychotherapy supervision work? Contributions of connection, conception, allegiance, alignment, and action. *J Psychother Integr*.2017;27(2):201.

63. Lambert MJ 2013. The efficacy and effectiveness of psychotherapy. In Lambert MJ, ed. *Bergin and Garfield's Handbook of Psychotherapy and Behavior Change*. 6th ed. New York, NY: Wiley; 2013:169–218.

64. Hill CE, Knox S. Training and supervision in psychotherapy. In Lambert MJ, ed. *Bergin and Garfield's Handbook of Psychotherapy and Behavior Change*. 6th ed. New York, NY: Wiley; 2013:169–218.

65. Yeomans FE, Levy KN, Caligor E. Transference-focused psychotherapy. *Psychotherapy*. 2013;50(3):449.

66. Stern BL, Yeomans F, Diamond D, Kernberg OF. Transference-focused psychotherapy for narcissistic personality In Ogrodniczuk JS, ed. *Understanding and Treating Pathological Narcissism*. Washington, DC: American Psychological Association; 2013: 235–252.

67. Racker, H. (1953). A contribution to the problem of countertransference. *Int J Psychoanal*. 1953:34: 313–324.

68. Racker, H. (1957). The meanings and uses of countertransference. The *Psychoanal Q*. 1957; 26(3):303–357.

69. Betan EJ, Westen D. Countertransference and personality pathology: development and clinical application of the countertransference questionnaire. In Levy RA, Ablon S. *Handbook of Evidence-based Psychodynamic Psychotherapy*. New York, NY: Springer; 2009:179–200.

70. Betan E, Heim, AK, Zittel Conklin C, Westen D. (2005). Countertransference phenomena and personality pathology in clinical practice: An empirical investigation. *Am J Psychiatry*. 2005;162(5):890–898.

71. Transference-focused psychotherapy training. Columbia University Center for Psychoanalytic Training and Research. https://www.psychoanalysis.columbia.edu/train/psychotherapy-programs/transference-focused-psychotherapy-program.

72. Bateman, AW, Fonagy PE. *Handbook of Mentalizing in Mental Health Practice*. Arlingtion, VA: American Psychiatric Publishing; 2012.

73. Ainsworth MD. The Bowlby-Ainsworth attachment theory. *Behav Brain Sci*.1978;1(3):436–438.

74. Bowlby J. The Bowlby-Ainsworth attachment theory. *Behav Brain Sci*.1979;2(4):637–638.

75. Barreto JF, Matos PM. Mentalizing countertransference? A model for research on the elaboration of countertransference experience in psychotherapy. *Clin Psychol Psychother*. 2018;25(3):427–439.

76. Mentalization-based treatment training. Anna Freud National Centre for Children and Families. https://www.annafreud.org/training/training-and-conferences-overview/online-training-live-and-self-directed-courses/mentalization-based-treatment-basic-training/.

77. Mentalization-based treatment. Mclean, Harvard Medical Affiliate. https://home.mcleanhospital.org/gpdi-mbtbasic?hsCtaTracking=7a74de0c-3878-4005-8dee-a5c13add4686%7Ce6918ea1-315b-48fe-8007-00c86c1ba5f4.

78. Beck AT, Freeman A, Associates. *Cognitive Therapy of Personality Disorders*. New York NY: Guilford Press; 1990.

79. Beck JS. *Cognitive Therapy for Challenging Problems: What To Do When the Basics Don't Work*. New York, NY: Guilford Press; 2005

80. Beck AT, Davis DD, Freeman A. *Cognitive Therapy of Personality Disorders*. 3rd ed. New York, NY: Guilford Press; 2015.

81. Arntz A, Dreessen L, Schouten E, Weertman A. Beliefs in personality disorders: a test with the personality disorder belief questionnaire. *Beh Res Ther*. 2004;42(10):1215–1225.

82. Young JE, Brown G. Young schema questionnaire-short form. Version 3. Psychological Assessment: 2005. https://opus.lib.uts.edu.au/bitstream/10453/123405/4/Phillips%20et%20al%20YSQ%20S3%2010.10.17.pdf.

83. Moorey, S. "Is it them or is it me?" Transference and countertransference in CBT. In Whittington A, Grey N. eds. *How to Become a More Effective CBT Therapist: Mastering Metacompetence in Clinical Practice*. Chichester, West Sussex, UK: Wiley; 2014:132–145.

84. Moorey S. The interpersonal cycle worksheet. Cognitive Connections. Posted 2013. https://cognitiveconnections.co.uk/wp-content/uploads/2014/01/Cognitive-Interpersonal-Cycle-Worksheets.pdf.

85. Prasko J, Diveky T, Grambal A, et al. (2010). Transference and countertransference in cognitive behavioral therapy. *Biomed Pap*. 2010;154(3):189–197.

86. Vyskocilova, J, Prasko J, Slepecky M, Kotianova A. Transference and countertransference in CBT and Schematherapy of personality disorders. *Eur Psychiatry*. 2015;30:144.

87. Cartwright, C. Transference, countertransference, and reflective practice in cognitive therapy. *Clin Psychol*. 2011;15(3):112–120.

88. Cognitive behavioral therapy for personality disorders. *Beck Institute*. https://psychwire.com/beck/cbt-essentialshttps://beckinstitute.org/workshop/cbt-for-personality-disorders/.

89. Linehan MM. *Cognitive-behavioral Treatment of Borderline Personality Disorder*. New York, NY: Guilford Press; 2018.

90. Linehan MM. *DBT Skills Training Manual*. 2nd ed. New York, NY: Guilford Press; 2015.

91. Dialectical Behavioral Therapy training. DBT: Linehan Board of Certifications. http://www.dbt-lbc.org/index.php?page=101133.

92. Arntz A, Van Genderen H, Drost J. *Schema Therapy for Borderline Personality Disorder*. 2nd ed. Hoboken, NJ: Wiley-Blackwell; 2021.

93. ISST certification in schema therapy. Schema Therapy Society. https://schematherapysociety.org/Certification.

94. McMain SF, Links PS, Gnam WH, et al. A randomized trial of dialectical behavior therapy versus general psychiatric management for borderline personality disorder. *Am J Psychiatry*. 2009;166(12):1365–1374.

95. McMain SF, Guimond T, Streiner DL, Cardish RJ, Links PS. Dialectical behavior therapy compared with general psychiatric management for borderline personality disorder: clinical outcomes and functioning over a 2-year follow-up. *Am J Psychiatry*. 2012;169(6):650–661.

96. Gunderson J, Masland S, Choi-Kain L. Good psychiatric management: a review. *Curr Opin Psychol*. 2018 Jun 1;21:127–131.

97. General psychiatric management. *Harvard University*. https://online-learning.harvard.edu/course/general-psychiatric-management-bpd?delta=0.

98. General psychiatric management. Gunderson Personality Disorders Institute. https://www.mcleanhospital.org/training/gunderson-institute.

7

Managing Patients with Personality Disorders in Medical Settings

Robert E. Feinstein

Key Points

- A personality style is the life-long habitual way of coping, which is manifested in how a patient feels, thinks, and behaves.
- Patients with a personality disorder appear rigid, extreme, and have maladaptive coping, which causes impairment in interpersonal, social, or occupational functioning.
- Patients suffering with a personality disorder are common in medical and psychiatric settings. Prevalence rates for personality disorders range from 9 percent in a community sample to 14.79 percent. 30.8 million Americans aged 18 years or older meet criteria for at least one personality disorder.
- DSM-5 describes personality traits of a patient as either Cluster A, odd and/or eccentric; Cluster B, dramatic, emotional, or erratic; or Cluster C, anxious or fearful. Once the cluster is identified, then one of 11 specific personality disorder categories may be diagnosed; see Table 7.1, p. 183.
- Clinicians can learn to use patient-originated countertransference as an aid to diagnosis; see Table 7.2, p. 185.
- A clinician's intense feeling, fantasies, or atypical medical behaviors directed toward a patient should lead all staff to suspect they are dealing with a patient who may have a personality disorder.
- Patients with personality disorders often display typical patient behaviors that affect their adherence to medical recommendations and the patient's utilization; see Table 7.3, p. 187.
- The three functional psychopathological levels of personality organization are neurotic, borderline, and psychotic levels of personality functioning. The assessment of reality testing, defense mechanisms, and object-relations or identity diffusion are the three factors which can be used for this classification; see Table 7.4, p. 189.
- The common coping styles and defense mechanism associated with each personality disorder are described in Table 7.5, p. 190.
- General management of a patient with a personality disorder begins with developing the clinician–patient alliance, using an informed shared decision-making focus for the medical encounter, and using general psychotherapeutic techniques.

> • There are 10 general intervention strategies that can be used to improve patient management; see Box 7.1, p. 195.
> • There are 12 positive coping styles that can be used to assist patients in improving their own adaptations to medical problems; see Box 7.2, p. 198.
> • Medication for a patient who has a personality disorder can be a useful adjuvant but is never the primary treatment. Prescribing for patients with personality disorders involves two main strategies: prescribing medication that targets specific personality traits, and also using medications to treating comorbid conditions.
> • There are specific interventions which can be used to manage patients with a specific personality disorder. This involves using clinician experiences of patient-generated countertransference reactions to aid in diagnosis, focusing on the patient's level of personality organization, being aware of common adherence and utilizations issues, and being empathic with patient's core fears and worldview. Using psychotherapeutic techniques to modify patient coping styles and interpret defenses can help medical practitioners optimize the medical care of these patients.

Note: This work is a revised version of a previously published chapter "Personality Traits and Disorders" in *Psychosomatic Medicine*. Philadelphia, PA: William and Wilkins, 2006, pages 843–865.

Introduction

Patients suffering with personality disorders can be difficult to manage and can elicit intense reactions in the clinician and medical staff who care for them. Kahana and Bibring[1] were among the first to describe managing personality types in a medical setting. Groves[2] wrote a famous article entitled "Taking Care of the Hateful Patient" in which he validated that clinician reactions to patient styles are both important to recognize and can be useful information for clinician and staff when trying to develop a management strategy. Patients with personality disorders have an unintentional ability to create problematic patient–clinician–staff relationships. This covert pressure, placed on the clinicians and staff, often affects how the medical team evaluates or diagnoses a patient and frequently affects clinician orders, laboratory tests, suggested treatments, and recommendations.

Prevalence rates for personality disorders range from 9 percent in a community sample[3] to 14.79 percent.[4] The National Epidemiologic Survey of Alcohol and Related Conditions[4] did the first national survey of 30.8 million Americans who were 18 years of age and older who met criteria for at least one personality disorder. These lifetime prevalence rates were approximately 7.9 percent obsessive-compulsive personality disorder, 4.4 percent paranoid personality disorder, 3.6 percent antisocial personality disorder, 3.1 percent schizoid personality, 2.4 percent avoidant personality disorder, 1.8 percent histrionic personality disorder, and 0.5 percent dependent personality disorder.[4]

Wave 2 of the National Epidemiologic Survey on Alcohol and Related Conditions revealed that the lifetime prevalence rate of borderline personality disorder was 5.9 percent, narcissistic personality disorder 6.2 percent, and schizotypal personality disorder 3.9 percent.[5]

In a primary care population, estimates are approximately 24 percent for all personality disorders combined.[6,7] It is common to encounter patients who meet criteria for more than one personality disorder.[6,7] Some patients have traits from several different personality disorders, yet do not meet criteria for any one disorder. These patients are often diagnosed with a mixed personality disorder.

Diagnostic rates of personality disorders increase dramatically in certain populations. For example, the rates of a comorbid personality disorder associated with other diagnoses are 28 percent in patients with alcohol disorders, 47 percent in patients with drug use disorders,[8] and 45.9 percent in patients with tendencies toward deliberate self-harm.[9] No data could be found concerning the prevalence of personality disorders on a consultation-liaison (C–L) service in a U.S. hospital. In Australia, using International Classification of Diseases diagnoses, 15 percent of patients referred to a C–L service had the diagnosis of a personality disorder.[10]

Patients with personality disorders often go unrecognized because they do not complain and often do not present with any overt symptoms. However, when interviewed, patients with personality disorders often will reveal interpersonal failures and describe multiple social and occupational dysfunctions. Most patients are recognized after an unpleasant or unexpected interpersonal interaction or are secondarily recognized by the complaints of spouses, family, friends, or others who have had more extended contact with the patient. Although many clinicians usually do not treat the underlying personality disorder, recognition and effective management of these difficult patients is routinely possible and often necessary in medical settings. The goal in the management of a patient with a personality disorder is to understand and manage them so that optimal medical care can be delivered. To assist clinicians, this chapter presents a personality disorder schema that can be used by clinicians and medical staff in hospitals, outpatient settings, psychiatric services, primary care, and integrated mental health settings for the diagnosis and management of these difficult patients.

Personality Styles or Personality Disorders

A personality style is the life-long habitual way of coping, which is manifested in how a patient feels, thinks, and behaves. Inborn personality styles are called *temperament*. Personality traits such as shyness or a high stimulus barrier are genetically acquired and can be observed at birth, and may be observed in a newborn nursery. Other personality traits that develop from the interaction with the environment are called *character*. Character traits, such as black-and-white thinking or depressive tendencies, can be environmentally acquired with genetic diathesis through early parent–child interactions. Every personality develops with enduring, unique, and evolving characteristics. Personality can be described generally according to a patient's feelings, thoughts, and behaviors, along with interpersonal, marital, family, or societal relationships. Personality can also be described according to various theories of personality development. For example, psychoanalytic theory has described personality, utilizing terms such as id, ego, adaptation to external reality, superego, ego ideal, affects, object-relations, self–object representations, self-perceptions/self-esteem, attachment, or relational characteristics A cognitive behavioral therapist may describe personality with terms such as perceptional organization, a set of core beliefs, a worldview, a schema, negative affects, irrational thoughts, maladaptive behaviors, a hierarchy of emotional needs, and a value system. The distinction between personality style and a personality disorder is a matter of degree. Personality styles tend to be stable over a lifetime but can be modified according to adaptive needs and by psychotherapy. Personality styles can become rigid, extreme, maladaptive, or damaging to self or others, and often cause functional impairment in interpersonal, social, or occupational functioning are called *personality disorders*. These disorders are more difficult to modify and may take life experiences and intensive long-term psychiatric/psychotherapeutic treatment assisted with pharmacotherapy to facilitate change. While everyone is unique, there seems to be a continuum of personality styles and disorders that are commonly encountered. Personality disorders can be easily recognized in the movies. These include the borderline personality disorder as portrayed by Glenn Close in Fatal Attraction, the narcissistic personality disorder played by Jack Nicholson in Carnal Knowledge or Tom Cruz in Top Gun, or the obsessive-compulsive personality disorder portrayed by Holly Hunter in Network News or Jack Lemon in the Odd Couple.

Diagnosis of Personality Disorders

Patients with personality disorders can be diagnosed utilizing a categorical or a dimensional approach. The categorical approach describes individuals as having clusters of associated traits, symptoms, or behaviors that form the discrete prototypes of personality. Categorical approaches have the advantage of colorfully describing and differentiating distinct personality styles and are easy for the clinician to use. The categorical classification system is the basis for the system used in the *Diagnostic and Statistical Manual of Mental Disorders, Fifth Edition* (DSM-5).[12] No longer used in the DSM-5, the DSM-IV-TR[11] encouraged clinicians to consider personality disorders in every patient as part of a multi-axial (Axis II) diagnostic system.

Rather than a categorical approach, many of the dimensional approaches describe facets of personality (traits) and rates them for presence, absence, and severity. There are 18 different personality dimensional models that are currently described in the literature.[13] One of the reasons for the extreme interest in dimensional models is that it seems likely that one or two individual personality traits, associated with each categorical diagnosis, may be responsible for producing most personality disorder dysfunction. If so, then it may be possible to design focal and shorter treatments that target specific traits of each personality disorder rather than trying to modify the whole personality. In the DSM-5, an appendix presents a hybrid model (functional dimensions and personality traits) based on personality functioning (self: identity and self-direction; and interpersonal functioning: empathy and intimacy) with specific pathological traits for each personality disorder.[12]

So how can a clinician or medical staff diagnose patients with personality disorders? It is most useful to combine the categorical and dimensional approaches. The DSM-5 has a dimensional component that begins with identifying the appropriate cluster of personality disorders. Each of these clusters broadly describes personality traits of the patient as either Cluster A, odd and/or eccentric; Cluster B, dramatic, emotional, or erratic; or Cluster C, anxious or fearful. Once the cluster or the dimension has been identified, then a specific personality disorder category may be diagnosed. The DSM-5 diagnostic schema for personality disorders is summarized in Table 7.1, p. 183. Since personalities are complicated, it is not unusual for a patient to meet criteria for two cluster diagnoses and more than one specific personality disorder diagnosis. The task of the clinician or medical staff is to pick up on the traits that are causing the most problems and develop an intervention strategy.

Table 7.1. Summary of Diagnostic and Statistical Manual-5: Personality Disorders

Cluster A (Odd, Eccentric)	Cluster B (Dramatic, Emotional)	Cluster C (Anxious, Fearful)
(1) Paranoid Expects exploitation/ harm; questions loyalty/ fidelity; bears grudges; easily feels slighted	(1) Antisocial Cruelty; problems with authority and unlawful behavior; dishonesty; irresponsibility; exploits others	(1) Dependent Indecisive; lacks initiative; submissive; helpless; dependent; fears abandonment
(2) Schizoid Loner; aloof; indifferent to praise or criticism; social anxiety; constricted affect	(2) Histrionic Overly emotional; seductive with sexual attention seeking; shallow/superficial	(2) Obsessive-compulsive Perfectionism; inflexibility; detail preoccupation; wishes to control others; stingy; over-conscientious; excessive morality or ethics
(3) Schizotypal Odd/eccentric; social anxiety; magical thinking; suspicious/ paranoid ideation	(3) Borderline Unstable intense relationships; self-destructive/suicidal; impulsive; affect instability; identity disturbances	(3) Avoidant Easily hurt; timid/fearful; social discomfort; avoids interpersonal interactions
	(4) Narcissistic Grandiose; inflated sense of self-importance; entitled; exploits others; lacks empathy; needs admiration; hypersensitive to criticism	
	From DSM-III-R: Self-defeating Suffers; self-sacrificing; defeats others; self-destructive; anhedonia; easily hurt	

Using a Clinician's Reactions or Countertransference to Diagnose a Personality Disorder

While DSM-5 categorical and dimensional approaches may be a useful aid to making a diagnosis, many clinicians and medical staff will clinically diagnose a patient by the reactions they feel and observe in themselves or in the staff taking care of the patient. There are two main sources for clinician reactions. Clinician-originated[14] reactions to a patient are feelings about the patient that emanate from the clinician's past life experiences, are reminiscent of relationships in the clinician's life, and reflect the interpersonal needs, professional choices, personal values, and biases of the clinician. This is also called clinician-generated countertransference. For example, a clinician might treat a patient as if the patient were his younger brother. He might yell at the patient for asking so many questions, or morally condemn the patient for being overweight.

The patient may provoke other reactions that may be felt by a clinician during doctor–patient interactions. These are called patient-originated clinician reactions.[14,15] We can identify a reaction in a clinician that originates from the patient when we observe that multiple doctors or staff feel similarly about the patient, even if they have not discussed the patient's case. For example, a patient who is frequently demanding and acting helpless may elicit feelings of hopelessness or helplessness in all of her healthcare professionals.

A clinician can learn to associate specific and characteristic caretaker reactions to specific DSM-5 diagnoses of personality disorders. For example, when the staff taking care of a medical patient is divided into two camps that either love or hate the patient, it is likely that the patient has a Cluster B diagnosis. This patient may also meet criteria for a borderline personality disorder. Diagnoses made by analyzing clinician reactions can give an experiential, deeper, and more complex picture of the personality dysfunction, which can lead to more specific and helpful interventions. Common patient-originated clinician reactions that are frequently associated with specific personality disorders are reviewed in Table 7.2, p. 185.

Patient-originated reactions can be either concordant or complementary.[16] Concordant clinician and staff reactions mean that the clinician feels the same as the patient. For example, the patient is depressed, and while interviewing the patient, the clinician also feels depressed. Complementary clinician reactions mean the clinician feels the opposite of the patient. For example, the patient is chronically suicidal, and the clinician is annoyed and feels homicidal toward the patient. Feeling what the patient feels (concordant) or feeling what the patient engenders in others (complementary) is helpful when trying to choose an issue that may require an intervention. Typical concordant or complementary patient-originated reactions elicited in the medical staff can be discovered when staff members become aware of their own intense feelings, uncharacteristic fantasies, or atypical medical behaviors that are elicited when they are working with patients who have personality disorders.

Intense Feelings

Intense emotions in the clinician or staff that are elicited through interpersonal interactions with the patient can include hate, fury, or frustration toward the patient. Alternatively, strong wishes to rescue a patient or give him or her exceptionally good care may also occur. Occasionally staff members may want to "adopt" a patient, feel love for a patient, or feel sexually aroused. These wishes may alternate with other wishes to avoid the patient, terminate the relationship, or transfer the patient to another service or colleague. In extreme cases, intense affects aroused in a medical staff member can lead him or her to commit damaging boundary violations. For example, a female patient on the gynecology service with a histrionic personality disorder was expressing suicidal thoughts to a male psychiatric resident during a consultation. A few days later, when the clinician did not hear from the patient as planned, he felt worried and panicked. He scheduled a home visit that he justified as a "safety check." Subsequently the couple became sexually involved to the detriment of all involved.

Clinician or Staff Fantasies

A clinician or staff member may also recognize that they are interacting with a difficult patient with a personality disorder by recognizing their own fantasies. Fantasies that are commonly generated in staff members by patients with personality disorders may include excessive worrying about a patient after normal work hours, dreaming about a patient, or experiencing exaggerated or intrusive, angry, sexual, or curious fantasies about the patient during personal times.

Table 7.2. Schema for Personality Disorder; Clinician Reactions, Worldview and Patient Fears

DSM-5 Classification	Clinician Reactions	Patient Worldview	Patient Fears
Paranoid	Fearful; sense of danger; mistrust; feeling accused, blamed, or threatened	Others are adversaries and are to blame; I am being examined; they are out to get me; I can't trust anyone	Exploitation; slights; betrayal; humiliation; physical intrusions from medical procedures
Schizoid	Detached or removed; wish to involve patient with others or to break through the isolation	I need space; I need to be alone; people are replaceable or unimportant	Emotional contact; warmth; intimacy; caring; intrusions or violations of privacy
Schizotypal	Detached; removed; "weird and alone" feelings; wish to involve others or to break through the isolation	Idiosyncratic, magical, or eccentric beliefs; I know what they're thinking/ feeling; premonitions	Emotional contact; warmth, caring; violation of privacy
Antisocial	Used, exploited or deceived; anger and a wish to uncover lies, punish, or imprison	People are there to be used and exploited; I come before all others	Boredom; loss of prestige, power, or esteem
Histrionic	Flattered, captivated, seduced, or aroused; flooded by emotions; depleted; wish to rescue	I need to impress, be admired/loved; I need to be taken care of, or helped	Loss of love, admiration, attention, or dependent care
Borderline	Feeling manipulated, angry, impotent, depleted, self-doubting; wish to rescue or get rid of the patient; guilty	I am very bad or very good; who am I?; I can't be alone	Separation, loss; emotional abandonment; not being loved and cared for; fluctuating self-esteem
Narcissistic	Devalued/overvalued; inferior/superior; fearful of patient's criticism or anger; wish to retaliate, devalue, or get rid of the patient	I am special; I am important; I come first; the world should revolve around me	Loss of prestige, image, power, or esteem
Avoidant	Frustrated because the patient often can't articulate fears; annoyed at the patient's weakness	I must avoid harm or be cautious, because I may get rejected, exposed, or be humiliated	Rejection; embarrassment in social situations; humiliation; exposure of inadequacies
Dependent	Depleted; annoyed at the patient's dependence; may deny the patient's reasonable needs	I am helpless without others; I can't make a decision; I need constant reassurance and care	Fears separation, independence, making decisions, and anger
Obsessive-compulsive	In a battle of control with negative reactions to patient stinginess; need for order; stubbornness; distanced from feelings; bored with details	People should do better and try harder; I must be perfect and make no errors or mistakes; details, not feelings, rule	Disorder, mistakes, imperfection; fears feelings, especially rage/ anger, anxiety, self-doubt, dependency
DSM-III-R: Self-defeating	Wish to rescue; sadistic fantasies that the patient will suffer and die; defeated; self-blame; self-doubt, or hopelessness and helplessness	I must suffer and sacrifice; I am a martyr; I should be punished	Loss of love; fears pleasure; fears recovery

Atypical Medical Behaviors by Clinicians and Staff Members

A physician, clinician, or staff member may also notice certain new medical behaviors with a specific patient that are not typical for their normal practice. These unusual behaviors should trigger self-examination by the physician, clinician, or medical staff, and consideration of the possibility that the patient may have a personality disorder. Frequently, patients with a personality disorder are capable of arousing unconscious reactions that lead to unusual new physician or medical staff behaviors. Common atypical medical behaviors aroused in the physician or medical staff may include the following: providing special nursing care, providing special food for a patient, ordering tests to placate a patient, and asking for more clinician attention for a patient. Physicians may find themselves ordering an unusual number of consults for a patient whose case does not seem to be medically complicated. The medical staff may suggest aggressive diagnostic testing or procedures when the yield of these tests is likely to be low. The staff may be considering heroic measures to save a patient that go way beyond those used in normal practice. Both physician and staff may find themselves repeatedly prolonging the time spent with a patient and/or family, or may offer free samples of drugs, lower the customary fees, offer free treatment, or develop a personal relationship with a patient. A physician, clinician, or other staff member who recognizes a provoked feeling experientially can learn to identify the subtype of personality disorders according to the feelings, fantasies, and atypical medical behaviors elicited. Most importantly, staff members that can recognize their unusual reactions will be better able to tolerate them and avert acting out their feelings with a patient. This will improve their medical decision making and patient care. A common psychiatric consultation is to help the medical staff understand and utilize their reactions to their patients for the benefit of all concerned. A list of common patient-originated clinician reactions that are associated with specific personality-disordered patients can be reviewed in Table 7.2, p. 185.

The Patient's Worldview and Patient Fears

The clinician or staff can apply principles of cognitive behavioral therapy (CBT) to greatly facilitate their management skills when working with personality-disordered patients and the staff members that treat them. The theory of CBT[17,18] is that patients have a worldview or a set of core beliefs and personality-specific fears that can be identified and directly influenced by conscious awareness. A patient's worldviews, and the fears that emanate from them, are exaggerated in intensity and idiosyncratic in their quality. These core beliefs and corresponding fears are rooted in a patient's basic personality organization. When an environmental stress occurs against the background of the patient's worldview, a reinforcing circular feedback loop ensues. A stressor, which is caused by an environmental or internal stress, interacts with the personality beliefs, and this triggers irrational thoughts. These "hot thoughts"[18] create irrational fears and negative moods or emotions that can lead to maladaptive behaviors and/or physical symptoms. Behaviors or symptoms can also feed back directly to confirm the patient's worldview and fears. Core beliefs and fears are readily activated in medical settings in which patients are sick and vulnerable. The capacity to delineate the distorted core beliefs and empathize with the patient's fears may allow physician, clinician, or staff to correct patient distortions. This can help the patient to improve the management of his or her feelings, thoughts, or behaviors. For example, a clinician saw a patient who was lonely and had no friends and was depressed. When asked why he had no friends, the patient responded "I don't make friends easily . . . I feel they judge me." The clinician identified the patient's "hot thought" as "I cannot make friends because I will be judged." He was also aware that this irrational thought is common in patients with avoidant personality disorders. In a CBT style, the clinician questioned "All friends will judge you?" and asked, "What is the evidence for and against this belief?" As the patient discussed this, he began to recognize that he was overstating his belief. The patient then said "Maybe I could find one nonjudgmental friend." Through the lens of this CBT formulation, a clinician can treat a problem directly or analyze the problem with the staff and suggest a range of cognitive interventions that may improve patient–staff relationships and the overall quality of medical care. The CBT worldview for each of the specific personality disorders is briefly described in Table 7.2, p. 185.

Patient Behaviors Affecting Adherence and Medical Utilization

Patients with personality disorders often display typical patient behaviors that affect their adherence to medical recommendations and the patient's utilization of medical and mental health services. A mental health clinician is in an ideal position to assist the medical staff in managing their expectations and in planning interventions geared toward optimizing the patient's medical care. For a detailed review of these issues for each personality disorder, see Table 7.3.

Table 7.3. Schema for Personality Disorders: Health Behaviors, Adherence, and Utilization

DSM-5 Classification	General Health Behaviors	Adherence	Utilization of Medical Services
Paranoid	Wariness, suspicion, mistrust, jealousy, self-sufficiency, counter-attacking, anger, violence	Adherence is difficult to obtain because the patient is suspicious of the need for compliance; problematic but may be easier when the patient is seeking relief from symptoms	Limited utilization, or as a condition for medical service utilization, the patient may seek detailed explanations or reasons for the diagnostic testing or the need for other services
Schizoid	Withdrawal; seeking isolation and privacy	May be difficult; will need reinforcement and monitoring; may need outreach services	Underutilization; outreach may help foster appropriate use of medical services
Schizotypal	Withdrawal; odd, autistic and/or magical behaviors/movements; seeks isolation and privacy	May be difficult; may need outreach, visiting nurse, or community resources, or case management services	Underutilization; may need outreach to gain reasonable and appropriate utilization of medical services

(continued)

Table 7.3. Continued

DSM-5 Classification	General Health Behaviors	Adherence	Utilization of Medical Services
Antisocial	Lies, deceit, and manipulation; violence; seeks secondary gain	May be resistant, problematic, or intolerant of the need for ongoing compliance requirements	May misuse medical resources for secondary gain
Histrionic	Dramatic; exhibitionism; expressiveness; impressionistic	Often dependent on others or inconsistent	May misuse or overutilize medical resources to gain attention from clinicians or medical staff
Borderline	Impulsive behaviors; suicidal actions; cutting; anger/violence; panic; anxiety; poor reality; stormy relationships	Inconsistent because adherence is easily influenced by emotional storms, interpersonal conflicts, or chaotic lifestyles	May misuse or overutilize for maladaptive behaviors such as suicidal or disruptive behaviors
Narcissistic	Self-aggrandizement; inflated/deflated self-image; entitled; devalues others; idealized; viciousness; envy; competitive	Can be problematic; intolerant of the need for ongoing compliance requirements	Feels entitled to use or may abuse medical services when needed
Avoidant	Avoidance; withdrawal; social timidity, caution, fear, anxiety	Diverted or delayed by avoidant behavior; adherence is guided by a wish to avoid disapproval of medical staff	Seeks medical services to secure approval or avoid criticism, not necessarily to seek the health benefits
Dependent	Unusually submissive; clinging, indecisive, childlike, needing to be taken care of	Dependent on others for medical supervision and easily overwhelmed by the demands of self-monitoring compliance	Underutilization when left to themselves, but may overutilize services when clinician or medical staff becomes the source of needed gratification
Obsessive-compulsive	Perfectionism, driven orderliness; logical, compulsive; controlling, critical; stubbornness/stinginess; workaholic; rational	Rigid and inflexibly follows the rules: disrupted or anxious if unexpected changes are required	Conflicted about utilization because fears of uncertainty may drive increased utilization, while fears of loss of control may decrease utilization
DSM-III-R: Self-defeating	Feels worse with good news; self-defeating, self-destructive	Dependent on others; may seek help, then reject help	Underutilization of medical services because they feel that they don't deserve them or that services won't help, or excessive utilization when they are treated badly

Psychopathological Level of Functioning

Kernberg[15,19] described a useful model for explaining the functional levels of personality organization. He described three functional psychopathological levels which include a psychotic personality organization (PPO), borderline personality organization (BPO), and neurotic personality organization (NPO). The psychoanalytic assessment of the psychopathological level of functioning is based on assessing: (1) reality testing/relation to reality; (2) use of major defensive styles; and (3) object-relations or identity diffusion. Review Table 7.4 for a detailed summary and description of these three psychopathological levels of functioning. Also see Chapter 2 for a broader discussion.

Patient Coping Styles and Defense Mechanisms

Using both a problem-solving and psychodynamic approach, a clinician can attempt to relieve a range of problems interfering with patients receiving optimal medical care. A problem-solving approach recognizes that patients have characteristic ways of dealing with the external environment, which are called coping styles. Common coping styles associated with each personality disorder are described in Table 7.5, p. 190.

In utilizing the psychodynamic approach, a clinician can also appreciate use of psychological processes known as defense mechanisms. Defense mechanisms can be either conscious (e.g., suppression) or unconscious (e.g., repression) and may be used by patients to resolve internal conflicts, manage moods, mediate external threats, and facilitate real world adaptations. By understanding the constellation of specific defenses and coping styles used with each personality disorder, a clinician may be able to utilize clarification, confrontation, and interpretation to modify the pathologic coping styles and defenses that are interfering with patient–clinician–staff alliances. Interpreting a patient's defenses and suggesting new problem-solving coping styles may enable the staff to provide the optimal or necessary medical care. For example, a patient with a borderline personality disorder felt hurt and abandoned by her physician's time off and accused the physician of not caring; she threatened suicide. By understanding the devaluing and acting-out defenses,

Table 7.4. Levels of Personality Organization

Psychotic Personality Organization (PPO)	Borderline Personality Organization (BPO)	Neurotic Personality Organization (NPO)
(1) Reality testing is lost: Psychosis, hallucination, delusions, inability to understand social context	(1) Reality testing: generally preserved; with stress, loss of sense of reality (e.g., dissociation, derealization, déjà vu depersonalization) rarely brief psychosis	(1) Reality testing intact
(2) Defenses: Denial, withdrawal, splitting and primitive defenses	(2) Defenses: splitting-centered over valued/devalued and primitive defenses	(2) Defenses: repression-centered and mature defenses
(3) Object-relations: chaotic or rapidly changing views of self and others	(3) Object-relations: Split and alternating views of self and others	(3) Object-relations; Stable complex integrated views of self and others

Table 7.5. Schema for Personality Disorders: Patient Coping Styles, Defenses, and Interventions

DSM-5	Level of Functioning	Patient Coping Styles and Defense Mechanisms	Interventions
Paranoid	PPO or BPO	*Coping Style* Guarded and protective of their autonomy, often with arrogant belief in their own superiority *Defenses* Projection: ascribe to others one's own impulses Projective identification: Project one's impulses plus control of others as a way to control one's own impulses. Denial: refusal to admit painful realities Splitting: Self and others are seen as all good or all bad	1. Empathize with patient's fear of being hurt; acknowledge complaints without arguing or ignoring 2. Openly and honestly explain medical illness 3. Correct reality distortions and unreasonable patient expectations 4. Gently question irrational thoughts, suggest more rational ones 5. Don't confront delusions 6. If the patient refuses care out of mistrust, rather than insist, ask if it's acceptable that you can disagree about the need for the test 7. Interpret projection (blame) and other defenses
Schizoid	PPO or BPO	*Coping Style* Inner world insulated from others *Defenses* Isolation of affect: thoughts stored without emotion Intellectualization: replace feelings with facts Denial and Splitting: see earlier Regression: revert to childlike thoughts, feelings, and behaviors	1. Empathize with the patient's need for both privacy and contact 2. Accept the patient's unsociability 3. Reduce the patient's isolation as tolerated 4. Neutrally impart medical information 5. Don't demand involvement or permit total withdrawal 6. Correct reality distortions and unreasonable patient expectations 7. Gently question irrational thoughts and suggest more rational ones 8. Interpret isolation and other defenses
Schizotypal	PPO or BPO	*Coping Style* Chaotic, disorganized *Defenses* Schizoid fantasy: retreat to idiosyncratic fantasy when faced with a painful experience Undoing; symbolic, magical action designed to reverse or cancel unacceptable thoughts or actions Regression, denial, and splitting: see earlier	1. Empathize with the patient's idiosyncratic style/ magical thinking and perceptions without directly confronting them 2. Recognize the need for privacy and contact 3. Accept the patient's unsociability and reduce the patient's isolation, as tolerated 4. Neutrally impart information 5. Don't demand involvement or permit total withdrawal 6. Correct reality distortions and unreasonable patient expectations 7. Gently question irrational thoughts and suggest more rational ones 8. Interpret regression and other defenses

Table 7.5. *Continued*

DSM-5	Level of Functioning	Patient Coping Styles and Defense Mechanisms	Interventions
Antisocial	BPO; PPO	*Coping Style* Seeks autonomy and freedom; seeks advantage or secondary gain *Defenses* Acting out: expressions in action behaviors rather than words or emotions	1. Empathize with patient's fear of exploitation and low self-esteem 2. Determine if you are being used for secondary gain; should you suspect dishonesty, verify symptoms and illness progression with others 3. Don't moralize; explain that deception results in your giving the patient poor care 4. Correct reality distortions and unreasonable patient expectations 5. Gently question irrational thoughts and suggest more rational ones 6. Interpret defenses
Histrionic	NPO or BPO PPO with Stress	*Coping Style* Self-centered, looking to be loved, emotion-driven, flirtatious and flighty *Defenses* Sexualization: functions or people are changed into sexual symbols to avoid anxieties Regression, acting out, and splitting: see earlier Dissociation: disrupted perceptions or sensations, consciousness, memory, or personal identity Somatization: physical symptoms caused by mental processes Repression: involuntary forgetting of painful memories, feelings, or experiences	1. Empathize with the patient's fear of losing love/care 2. Be friendly, not too reserved, not too warm 3. Discuss the patient's fears, reassure when possible 4. Use logic to counteract an emotional style of thinking 5. Set limits if patient regresses 6. Correct reality distortions and unreasonable patient expectations 7. Gently question irrational thoughts and suggest more rational ones 8. Interpret sexualization, regression, and other specific defenses
Borderline	BPO or PPO with stress: Best Functioning NPO	*Coping Style* Hostile dependency, chaotic lifestyle, and threatening, intimidating, or seeking intimacy/dependency or pseudo-autonomy *Defenses* Splitting, projection, projective identification, dissociation, regression, and acting out: see earlier Omnipotence: seeing self and others as all-powerful Idealization/devaluation: vacillating between seeing self or others as ideal and then deprecating/ devaluing self or others Mini-psychotic episodes	1. Empathize with patient's fear of abandonment/separation and plan for absences by arranging coverage 2. Express a wish to help and satisfy reasonable needs 3. Ask the patient to monitor impulsive behaviors with a diary 4. Set firm limits and do not punish 5. Correct reality distortions and unreasonable patient expectations 6. Gently question irrational thoughts and suggest more rational ones 7. Interpret splitting and other defenses 8. Negotiate emergency procedures in advance; if suicidal, the patient must go to the emergency room, if not safe; if the patient refuses emergency help when you offer, let the patient know in advance that this therapeutic breach may end the relationship

(continued)

Table 7.5. *Continued*

DSM-5	Level of Functioning	Patient Coping Styles and Defense Mechanisms	Interventions
Narcissistic	BPO or NPO	*Coping Style* Superiority and arrogance, self-aggrandizing, self-centered, self-protecting, demeaning, demanding, critical *Defenses* Splitting, projection, projective identification, acting out, denial, and regression: see earlier	1. Empathize with patient's vulnerability and low self-esteem 2. Don't mistake the patient's superior attitude for real confidence and don't confront entitlement 3. When you are devalued or attacked, acknowledge the patient's hurt and your mistakes and express your continued wish to help 4. If devaluing continues, offer a referral as an option, not as punishment 5. Correct reality distortions and unreasonable patient expectations 6. Gently question irrational thoughts and suggest more rational ones 7. Interpret splitting and other defenses
Avoidant	NPO or BPO	*Coping Style* Withdraw or escape, avoiding criticism *Defenses* Inhibition: restriction of thoughts, feelings, and behaviors to avoid shame, exposure to inadequacies, rejection, and humiliation Phobia: fears of objects, people, and/or situations, which are avoided to prevent anxiety Avoidance/withdrawal, regression, and somatization: see earlier	1. Empathize with patient's social fear, shame, shyness, and fears of revealing inadequacies, rejection, embarrassment, humiliation and anger 2. Help patient describe in details the feared situation 3. Encourage and support the need for the patient to gradually face their fears and stop the tendency to avoid; if this seems overwhelming, choose smaller fears to confront or refer 4. If frustrated or unclear about the nature of the fears, ask for detailed description of the problem 5. Gently elicit irrational thoughts and suggest more rational ones 6. Correct reality distortion 7. Interpret avoidance and other defenses
Dependent	NPO or BPO	*Coping Style* Passive, dependent, helpless *Defenses* Dependent: yearning for care, clinging, and needing direction Passive-aggressive: superficial compliance and passivity disguising stubbornness and anger Reaction Formation: unacceptable impulses expressed as the opposite Regression and Splitting: see earlier	1. Empathize with the patient's need for care 2. Frustrate total dependence 3. Be careful to avoid telling the patient what to do 4. Encourage independent thinking and action 5. Realize that what the patient says he or she wants is not necessarily what they need (e.g., caretaking) 6. Ask patient what it is about independence that is so frightening 7. Don't abandon or threaten termination, because some very dependent patients need regular clinician contact for life 8. Correct reality distortions and unreasonable patient expectations 9. Gently elicit irrational thoughts and suggest more rational ones 10. Interpret regression and other specific defenses

Table 7.5. *Continued*

DSM-5	Level of Functioning	Patient Coping Styles and Defense Mechanisms	Interventions
Obsessive-compulsive	NPO or BPO	*Coping Style* Inflexible, constricted, governed by rules and safety or security concern *Defenses* Isolation of affect, intellectualization, reaction formation, and undoing: see earlier Controlling: efforts to regulate objects or others to avoid anxiety Displacement: transfer of one's feelings from one person onto another Dependent: see earlier Inhibition: restricting thoughts, feelings, or behaviors for fear that unacceptable impulses will erupt and create anxiety or damage Phobias and repression: see earlier	1. Empathize with the patient's logical, detailed, unemotional style of thinking 2. If obsessive thoughts are interfering with medical care, ask about the patient's feelings 3. Don't struggle with the patient over control and critical judgments 4. Avoid abandoning the patient 5. Correct reality distortions and unreasonable patient expectations 6. Gently elicit irrational thoughts and suggest more rational ones 7. Interpret specific defenses
From DSM-III-R Self-Defeating	BPO or NPO	*Coping Style* Self-defeating and self-destructive *Defenses* Ambivalence: co-existence of opposing feelings Displacement, denial, projective identification reaction formation, passive-aggressive, and splitting: see earlier	1. Empathize with the patient's suffering 2. Acknowledge and appreciate the difficulty of the illness/treatments 3. Emphasize that recovery may be a slow steady process, the need for recovery can be presented as necessary to benefit others 4. Inquire about obvious self-destructive or self-defeating behaviors 5. Don't abandon 6. Correct reality distortions and unreasonable patient expectations 7. Gently elicit irrational thoughts and suggest more rational ones 8. Interpret specific defenses

a physician can begin to help this patient by not taking personally the patient's efforts to devalue or manipulate. The physician responded to this patient by empathizing with the patient's fears of abandonment. The formulation was that her suicidal threats were manipulative demands designed to prevent her physician from leaving. The physician clarified that the patient had a distorted belief that her time off was a personal abandonment. She added that time off does not really communicate anything about her ability or wish to medically care for her patient. She explained that she needs time off so she can refuel and be available to provide the patient's medical care over the long haul. The physician interpreted that the patient's suicidal threats were due to her anger at her doctor and were designed to try and prevent her physician from leaving. The patient sadly acknowledged this. She seemed reassured of her physician's return. The patient had a more realistic view of the limits of her doctor's availability. The patient was also informed about the medical treatment that was available to her when her doctor was off duty.

General Clinical Principles of Management and Intervention

Attending to the Working Alliance

A clinician can begin each patient encounter by listening, asking open-ended questions, and striving for an empathic connection with the patient. It is especially important to develop an alliance with those patients or family members that the clinician likes the least. Listening helps to establish the foundation of a therapeutic alliance based on trust, acceptance, and confidence. The working alliance is also fostered by the clinician's own self-awareness, an ability to acknowledge mistakes, and an awareness of his or her transference reactions. When possible, it is also helpful if the clinician can adapt to the patient's reasonable wishes or needs. Initial problems in a working alliance are often the first clue that the patient may have a personality disorder. As soon as the clinician becomes aware of any tension in the alliance, the clinician should help the patient to focus on issues in his or her present medical care. If the patient is able to express the problem clearly, the clinician should join with the patient in solving problems that will maximize the delivery of effective medical care. If the problem is primarily located in the clinician–patient relationship, then non-defensive reflective listening, clarifications, admitting mistakes, and expressing a wish to make things better are all often helpful. If the clinician believes there is a different problem affecting the alliance, the clinician can say "I believe that there is a different problem (and identify the problem; e.g., drinking) which is affecting my ability to help you get well and offer you the best medical care available. We need to think about this problem and come up with some solutions."

Focusing the Initial Interview

Patients with severe personality disorders often experience an inability to verbalize and/ or prioritize their most important medical concerns. Their perceptions of their conditions (and the staff who help them) are often distorted, because they are perceived through the lens of their characteristic worldview. For these patients, it is particularly important to strive for a mutually agreed upon medical focus. Short and long-term treatment goals can be considered. It is important to be consistent, reliable, and predictable in one's approach to medical problems. It is often helpful to use a process called *informed shared decision making*.[20] This takes time with the patient to discuss and negotiate the acute focus of medical care, short and long-term medical goals, strategies to achieve these goals, and specific timelines for accomplishing the prioritized medical plan.

Using Psychotherapeutic Techniques

In patients with personality disorders, a general medical approach may not be sufficient. After a brief period of immersion and listening to the patient's complaints, a clinician can respond with empathic responses that acknowledge the patient's fears (Table 7.2, see p. 185). If this is not helpful, the clinician can use general psychotherapeutic techniques. Uses of confrontation, clarification, or interpretation directed toward the current problem are best applied in the context of a good working alliance. A confrontation is not a battle, but instead is an observation made by the clinician, offered to a patient, that draws attention to contradictions in the patient's beliefs, thoughts, feelings, or behaviors. A clarification adds new information or perspective and elucidates misunderstandings, miscommunications, or other information that seems vague or confusing. The need for repeated clarifications occurs regularly with patients who have severe personality disorders. It is important to use clarifications before suggesting a new plan to correct a problem. Interpretations are integrating comments that link confrontations and clarifications with the patient's current problem that is interfering with medical care. Interpretations can be made about the immediate situation and may address the patient's core beliefs, irrational thoughts, fears, maladaptive behaviors, coping style, or defense mechanisms. Interpretations can also be directed at a difficulty in the medical staff–patient interaction, problems with patients coping with their disease, a patient's refusal of a necessary medical workup or treatment, or the patient's life circumstances. For example, an interpretation to a borderline patient with chronic pain might be: "I think you want relief from your pain. However, your refusal to adhere to my treatment recommendations makes relief from your pain unlikely (confrontation). You then get angry with me because your pain is not relieved, and so you do not keep your scheduled appointments (clarification). Instead of enlisting my help and using our services when the pain is overwhelming, you blame us for your pain and feel frustrated. Your anger helps you avoid dealing with the chronic reality of your condition (interpretation), which is that we can make your pain manageable but not cure it." Such interpretations take practice, but can powerfully restore a realistic and helpful doctor–patient relationship.

General Strategic Interventions

There are 10 strategic interventions that can generally be applied to all the personality disorders (see Box 7.1).

Box 7.1 General Intervention for Managing Personality Disorders

- Stabilize the external environment (attend to noise, privacy, light)
- Stabilize the internal environment (attend to basic needs, reality testing, give medication, if needed)
- Empathize with the patient's worldview
- Focus on improving the capacity to test reality
- Accept a patient's limitations
- Describe and confront unreasonable patient expectations and set limits
- Question irrational thoughts or behaviors related to care
- Discuss the patient's coping style and interpret defense mechanisms affecting care
- Use family support
- Use psychopharmacology as adjunctive treatment

Stabilize or Change the Patient's External Environment

Patients suffering with severe personality disorders will show fewer symptoms and a dramatic improvement in their acute emotional and behavioral functioning when the clinician obtains additional support from the environment. This may mean changing rooms, moving furniture, providing a television, bringing a clock or food, or even extending visiting hours for the patient. Other environmental interventions may include constant patient observations, having the nurse or nurse's aide spend more time with the patient, allowing additional telephone calls, and adding support from social services, volunteers, self-help support groups, and religious or psychiatric personnel. Calling the restraint team can be a very helpful intervention in an extreme crisis.

Stabilize the Patient's Internal Environment

Patients with personality disorders are often exquisitely sensitive and distressed by intolerable internal emotional states and desires. At a basic level, this often means attending to hunger, sleep deprivation, intoxication and withdrawal, necessary medical care, and basic creature comforts. Medication is often an essential part of the management strategy for stabilizing the patient's anxious, depressed, or agitated states. Low doses of antipsychotics and/or benzodiazepines are commonly used.

Empathize with the Patient's Worldview

All psychological interventions are dependent on a reasonable working alliance in which the patient feels understood by the medical team. Listening and reflecting on the problems identified by the patient while empathizing with their worldview can be extremely helpful. For example, a schizoid patient was refusing a needed colonoscopy. The clinician might empathize and try to intervene with this patient by saying, "I understand your need for privacy and space; hospitals are not the best places for this. Could we talk with you privately, for just a few minutes, about how a colonoscopy might help you? If this is all right, then we will leave you alone and return tomorrow to learn about your decision. Is that okay?"

Focus on Improving the Capacity to Test Reality

Patients with severe personality disorders can function at a psychotic, borderline, or neurotic personality level. Stressed patients with Clusters A and B personality disorders may transiently hear voices, hallucinate, have brief episodes of delusional thinking, or have other severe distortions in perceptions of reality (e.g., paranoia). This is not uncommon with paranoid, schizotypal, and borderline personality disorder, or other severely stressed patients who may be functioning at the PPO or BPO levels. If psychotic or other severe disturbances in reality are present, assess and treat them first. A stressed or medically ill patient can also present with a tenuous or disturbed relationship with reality. These states may include: a distorted sense of time; disturbances in the sense of reality, such as de-realization (watching your life as if it was a movie); depersonalization (not feeling a part of your own life); dramatic distortions of what has been said; transient misperceptions of real events that are interpreted according to core beliefs or irrational thoughts; or misunderstanding the clinician's or patient's role. They can also escalate to frank hallucinations or delusions. Such reality distortions are not usually dangerous, but they can lead to severe problems in doctor–staff–patient relationships if they are not recognized and treated. Verbalizing aloud the patient's illogical or distorted worldview can sometimes restore a more realistic assessment of reality. Further uncovering and clarifying the patient's irrational thoughts or fears and careful use of confrontation, clarification, and interpretation can be conjointly used to try to improve the patient's reality testing. If verbal techniques are not helpful, removing the patient from a stressful location (e.g., the emergency room) to a more supportive location (the floor) may be helpful. If needed, pharmacologic intervention such as the use of low doses of antipsychotic medications can also be extremely helpful.

Accepting the Patient's Limitations

By definition, patients with personality disorders are rigid in their approach to the world and limited in their capacity for social and occupational functioning. They do not seek or make changes quickly. Yet, they may seem reasonable enough at first impression that there is a temptation to try to change the patient. This typically leads to frustration for all concerned. Instead, it is better to accept their limited functioning. It may be helpful to focus on the patient's strengths and how things can be modified, instead of focusing on changing the patient.

Describe Unreasonable Expectations and Set Limits

Often patients with personality disorders have unreasonable expectations. For example, patients may expect a cure, demand the medical team's constant availability, or ask to be treated as special. They may want our help when they don't want to go to work; they may ask for excessive pain medication, or they may request multiple consultations with specialists when these are not required. It is extremely important to set limits on unreasonable requests. Effective limit setting involves first exploring why the patient feels that their particular expectations can or should be met. Then it involves a reasonable clinician response about both what can and cannot be done, while offering several options. The clinician can start with "What I can do is . . ." or "What I am unable to do is . . . for this reason." Ultimately, limit setting is about saying yes to any reasonable approximation of the patient's wishes or requests, and tactfully saying no to requests that are not practical or possible. A good rule for medical professionals is "Bend, don't break."

Questioning Irrational Thoughts or Behaviors

Patients often have irrational thoughts about their illness or the care they will receive, or they may misunderstand the clinician's efforts to communicate. One clinician said to a patient, "I think you will need a GI workup." The patient responded "I'm not a veteran, why would I need to go for a workup at a VA hospital?" Other less dramatic irrational thoughts include worries that "the medication will hurt or kill me," that getting an x-ray "will cause cancer," or that "donating blood can give you AIDS." The patient's irrational thoughts can be explored with the patient. For example, by asking "Why would we want to give you medication to hurt you?" or "What experiences have you had that make you concerned that an x-ray will cause cancer?"

In patients with BPO and NPO, these kinds of questions are typically clarifying and can reduce anxiety for many patients. In patients with PPO who are hallucinating or delusional, gentle exploration of a psychotic thought is also possible, but confronting delusional thought typically makes patients with PPO worse. Psychopharmacologic interventions with atypical or typical antipsychotics may also be helpful or required.

Discussing Coping Styles and Interpreting Defense Mechanisms

Discussing the patient's coping styles that are maladaptive and suggesting alternatives can be very effective. For example, a histrionic patient became panicked and emotionally distraught when she heard that she had a breast lump and possibly cancer. Accepting her emotional reaction first, it may be helpful to ask her, "Would it help to learn more about the diagnostic workup and the evaluation you will need for breast cancer? Did you know that breast lumps often turn out to be benign?" This coping style intervention says in effect "Your emotions may scare you, but perhaps more cognitive learning might calm you down." Pathological coping styles for each personality disorder can be reviewed in Table 7.5, p. 190, and common alternative positive coping styles are described in Box 7.2. Interpreting defenses requires the ability to recognize the defense and then to do the preparatory

---

Box 7.2 Coping Styles

- Action-oriented: taking an action to immediately rectify the problem
- Contemplative: quietly thinking over the problem before acting
- Controlling others: controlling other people's behaviors
- Centering: pausing and relaxing to gain control over one's emotions, thoughts, or behaviors
- Denial: can be adaptive, depending on the situation
- Emotional: using emotions such as tears, anger, or fear to help solve problems
- Help-seeking: asking others for help
- Informational: gathering information, then deciding
- Logical/rational: carefully reasoned, logical, deductive style
- Spiritual: asking for a higher power or for God's direction
- Trial and error: trying a random solution and if it fails, modifying it and trying again
- Wait and see: allowing time or circumstances to determine the outcome

confrontations and clarifications necessary before attempting to interpret the maladaptive defense.

Use Family Support

Families can help or hinder the management of a patient with a personality disorder. If the family is worsening the patient's symptoms, it may be best to exclude them from any intervention. If the family seems interested, then a three-part brief clinical assessment of the family can be done. This involves asking three questions: (1) Is the family willing to help? (2) Is the family available to participate in treatment and go to appointments with the patient? (3) Is the family competent or capable of facilitating treatment of the patient? If the family answers yes to all three, then a family approach can be pursued. If the family says no to any of these questions, or the clinician feels that the family is not capable of helping, then it may be wise to set up the treatment plan without the family's participation.

Psychopharmacology for Patients with Personality Disorders

Using medication for a patient who has a personality disorder can be a useful adjuvant but is never the primary treatment. Prescribing for patients with personality disorders is a complex process which involves two main strategies:

(1) Prescribe medications that target specific personality traits. For example: patients who have cognitive-perceptual symptoms or become psychotic (e.g., schizotypal or paranoid patients) or patients who become transiently psychotic (e.g., border-line patients) may benefit from adjuvant antipsychotic medications. Patients who are impulsive (e.g., antisocial, borderline, or histrionic patients) or are extremely obsessive/compulsive (e.g., patients with obsessive-compulsive personality disorders) may benefit from adjuvant selective serotonin reuptake inhibitors (SSRIs) or selective noradrenaline reuptake inhibitor (SNRIs). Patients with mood instability or affect dysregulation (e.g., Cluster B patients) may benefit from adjuvant mood stabilizers.

(2) Prescribe medications for the comorbidities that track with the personality disorders. For example, prescribe antidepressants for any patient with a personality disorder who has a comorbid depressive spectrum disorder. Prescribe a mood stabilizer or antipsychotic for patients suffering with comorbid bipolar disorder and a personality disorder (e.g., narcissistic patients). Review Chapter 15 for more detailed prescribing recommendations.

Specific Interventions for Each Personality Disorder

Each specific personality disorder may be managed using the overall approach outlined in Tables 7.1 to 7.5, pp. 183–190. This conceptual framework may make it possible to formulate some helpful interventions for the management of specific personality disorders in medical settings.

Paranoid Personality Disorder

Paranoid patients will have a basic mistrust of the clinician and may accuse or blame the doctor while fearing that he or she may be hurt, exploited, or invaded. Clinicians will typically have concordant patient-originated clinician reactions, and the clinician may feel fear, mistrust, or a sense of danger from the patient. Paranoid patients will tend to be isolative and will reject help except from a very small group of a trusted few. They will often react to suggestions for medical care with mistrust, excessive fault-finding, and sensitivity to criticism or hypervigilance. They may perceive slights and injustices, which they collect, remember, and will use as proof of the world's inequities. When invasive diagnostic or medical procedures are suggested or performed, the paranoid patient may react as if these procedures are personal attacks designed to undermine his or her freedom or power, or be denigrating. Paranoid patients can become threatening to medical staff. The paranoid patient may also experience panic and anxiety because unconsciously they misinterpret a procedure (such as drawing blood) as a bodily invasion or as a homosexual assault. Patients with paranoid personality disorder typically function at the level of a PPO. Clinically this appears as problems with reality testing, referential thinking, and exaggerated or unwarranted suspiciousness of others. Biological relatives of paranoid patients tend to have increased rates of schizophrenia.[12] Paranoid patients find it difficult to adhere to treatment recommendations and will underutilize medical care, or they will require detailed explanations of everything before they will even consider compliance with treatment recommendations. Their coping style is guarded and protective of their autonomy. They often appear arrogantly independent, and rely heavily on projection as their main defense. Using projection, they accuse the clinician of harms that reflect their own aggressive style of hurting or blaming others.

A clinician working with a paranoid patient needs to empathize with the patient's mistrustful and hypersensitive world view. The clinician should avoid arguing or attempting to reason the patient out of their paranoid perceptions. It is extremely important to gently use confrontations and clarifications to help correct the patient's distorted perceptions about his or her medical care and to set limits on unreasonable requests. Direct confrontation of an idea or reference has the paradoxical effect of making these patients more suspicious. Acknowledging that the patient's suspicion has an emotional reality can be helpful. Rather than confront mistrust or suspicions directly, acknowledge responsibility for any actions that the patient might have perceived as mistakes, for example, "I did not appreciate how it might scare you when I ordered that lab test." It may also help to openly express understanding and concern for the patient's rights. If there is a medical need for specialized testing, acknowledge the patient's suspiciousness and fears, describe openly and honestly the details of the procedures, the potential for pain, and the likely risks and benefits. If the patient still refuses to comply, do not use direct persuasion. Ask the patient "Is it alright with you if we have different opinions about what is medically indicated?" With the patient's consent to hearing a different opinion, openly discuss the medical necessity of the testing without trying to resolve the problem. At a future time, attempt a discussion of the patient's fears of complying with the necessary testing. It may take months for the paranoid patient to trust enough to consent to the appropriate treatment. Counter-projective statements can also diffuse the projections and distortions directed at the clinician. A counter-projective statement is one that helps the patient to access his or her feelings while focusing angry or suspicious feelings away from the clinician toward others who are not present. For example, a clinician harassed by an angry, suspicious, or blaming patient could use a counter-projective statement such as "You felt angry and scared when the lab technician drew your blood. You must be fearful of the results of these tests."

Schizoid and Schizotypal Personality

A schizoid and schizotypal patient may appear detached, withdrawn, aloof, unemotional, or may seek privacy. Schizoid patients may give the clinician the impression of being "loners." Schizotypal patients often create a sense that they are weird or strange because they may have odd autistic movements or reveal magical thinking. Clinicians commonly experience concordant reactions to both diagnoses, which may manifest as feeling uninvolved, detached, or disinterested in the patient. Alternatively, some clinicians experience complementary reactions, which manifest as a desire to break through the aloofness and finally get the patient talking and connected to others. At a superficial level, patients with these diagnoses may fear personal contact, emotional involvement, and invasion of their privacy. However, at the deepest levels, they may long for emotional contact that is not overwhelming and may seek a form of emotional connection in highly intellectual pursuits. They may react to suggestions for additional medical care with avoidance, withdrawal, apparent emotional detachment, or denial of the medical problem. Adherence to medical recommendations is often difficult to obtain. Consistent but short and infrequent contact often fosters the alliance. Upon discharge, reaching out to these patients, such as via infrequent but consistent appointment reminders, is often required to foster adherence and appropriate regular use of healthcare services.

Schizoid patients do not appear psychotic or idiosyncratic in their behavior. They often appear disengaged, have few social contacts, but can function at a borderline level of personality organization. However, when stressed by medical symptoms or illness, they may retreat to a psychotic level of functioning that may manifest as an extreme denial, withdrawal, or regression to childlike functioning. Schizoid patients may cope by insulating themselves from others or may use isolation, intellectualization, and denial as their main defenses to hide their emotions. Schizotypal patients more typically function at a psychotic level with impaired reality testing manifested by magical, odd, or psychotic modes of thinking. Schizotypal patients often cope by using a disorganized or chaotic style, and may use psychotic denial and regression to schizoid fantasy as their main defenses. They often appear severely idiosyncratic and withdrawn when stressed. Schizotypal personality disorder appears to confer a risk for the future development of schizophrenia, although most patients do not go on to develop overt schizophrenia.[12] Efforts to reach both schizotypal and schizoid patients are often perceived as intrusions into their privacy and may drive them away from the clinician. Patients with these disorders are often best approached gently, quietly, and with little expectation of establishing personal contact. It is generally helpful to accept their lack of sociability at a level that does not demand involvement or permit total withdrawal. Neutral or unemotional expressions of medical information are more likely to be heard and utilized.

Antisocial Personality Disorder

Patients with antisocial personality disorders can be superficially charming but are covertly trying to gain some advantage. They tend to exploit others for their own aims. They do fear they will become vulnerable, lose respect and admiration from others, or become easy prey to manipulation when they become ill. They expect to be exploited, demeaned, or humiliated. Like the narcissistic patient, they often have low self-esteem, excessive self-love, compensatory feelings of superiority, grandiosity, recklessness, emotional shallowness, and a lack of concern for others. Clinicians typically react with concordant reactions and may be fearful of being used, exploited, or deceived. Clinicians also feel complementary reactions, which can lead to anger, wishes to be free of the patient, to uncover lies, and to punish or imprison the patient. Antisocial patients often react to medical care with entitled demands for special treatment. When caught being dishonest, they may angrily attack or devalue the clinician. They may resort to a psychopathic coping style and act out by using manipulation, deception, lying, cheating, or stealing. They also use splitting as a major defense, which is why they may initially be liked and appear charming until their dishonesty is revealed. Antisocial patients function at the borderline level of personality organization, and their reality testing is intact. They can transiently lose reality testing when stressed by the potential of getting caught in their deceptive practices. This is typically manifested by impulsive actions that reveal severely impaired or even psychotic misjudgments. When they are receiving medical care for an illness, they may briefly adhere to clinician recommendations when they are ill. They will tend to underutilize medical services for legitimate illnesses and misuse medical services to get disability, housing, drugs, time off from work, or as protection from others who are angry at them. In the medical setting, when they have illnesses that require medical care, they function with many of the same characteristics as narcissistic personality disorder[21] and can be managed similarly (see section on narcissistic personality disorders). When they are not seriously ill, the clinician needs to be alert and anticipate the possibility that some patients may be covertly seeking secondary gain. It is important not to inadvertently collude with the patient's plans for secondary gain. For example, if the clinician thinks a patient's request for disability status is fraudulent or unwarranted, the patient should not be referred elsewhere for additional evaluations. If deception is suspected, the clinician can ask for verification of symptoms from other reliable sources. There is often dishonesty in a patient's communication in the form of withholding important information, partial truths, or outright lying, cheating, or stealing. If lying occurs, avoid moralizing, and grant the patient the reality that he or she has the power to fool all clinicians. The patient can be confronted with the notion that the main result of deception or giving false or inaccurate information is that the clinician is more likely to make poorly informed medical decisions, which will ultimately result in the patient receiving inadequate medical care. The clinician can explore with the patient why he needs to act so self-destructively. Patients may need to be reminded that the clinician's role is to help with medical problems and not to pass judgments or to help the patient obtain other benefits from the medical system.

Histrionic Personality Disorder

Patients with histrionic personality disorder have an emotionally expressive style, seek excessive attention, love, and are often dramatic. They fear they will not be loved, admired, or romantically pursued, and that they may lose the care that they dependently seek. Clinicians have varied reactions and may feel flattered, captivated, seduced, or sexually aroused by these patients. Alternatively, a clinician may feel overwhelmed by exaggerated or excessive emotions, embarrassed by the patient's flirtatious overtures, depleted by their superficial interpersonal needs, or angry at their superficial concerns. There are two different levels of this personality disorder.[15,21] Kernberg describes a "hysteric" who functions with a NPO with intact reality testing, defenses centered on repression, and stable and mature relations with others. The female hysteric has a flirtatious, clinging, childlike dependence within an intimate relationship, but can function at mature levels in social and work situations.[21] Male hysterics have similar psychological conflicts but may either appear as macho or effeminate.[21] The hysteric of either gender copes with the world in a self-centered and superficial way. Because they typically function well, they are often adherent to medical recommendations and utilize medical resources appropriately. If a hysteric becomes ill, he or she may react with a mild regression to a childlike, dependent, or clinging position. By contrast, the other type of patient with this disorder, the "histrionic" patient, functions with a BPO.[15,21] The patient can display transient losses of reality testing expressed as dramatic or overwhelming emotions. Their main coping style is flirtatiousness and/or sexualization of relationships. The histrionic patient uses defenses centered on splitting and regression. The histrionic patient is more self-centered and self-indulgent than the hysteric, having a pervasive childlike dependence that extends from intimate relationships into all aspects of social and occupational functioning. Female histrionics typically act flirtatious but may become indignant when a man shows sexual interest. Male histrionics also show the self-centered and dependent pattern, but additionally may be severely hypochondriacal or have antisocial features.[21] Histrionic patients of both sexes are erratic in their capacity for medical adherence and often overutilize medical services, because they sometimes overdramatize their medical complaints. They may react to medical care with regression, but unlike the hysteric patient, may use splitting defenses that cause them to perceive their doctor as either all good or all bad. In working with patients who are either hysteric or histrionic, a clinician needs to be friendly but not overly warm or too reserved. Hysteric patients often benefit from some limited gratification of their dependent wishes and a free discussion of their fears and emotions. They can often be reassured by information and an educational approach to their medical illness and are capable of expressing gratitude to the physician or clinician. In contrast, the intense dependency of histrionic patients is often made worse by satisfying the patient's needs. Offering excessive emotional care may make them greedy or more demanding. They may benefit from firm, kind, limit setting (especially to their sexual overtures). They can also benefit when the clinician uses logic to counteract their emotional style, discusses their irrational thoughts and expectations, and interprets splitting. These interventions may all be facilitated if there is a careful, limited gratification of their reasonable needs.

Borderline Personality Disorder

Borderline patients often develop hostile dependent relationships with their clinicians or the medical staff, and can be extremely demanding, clinging, helpless, self-destructive, or suicidal. Typical clinician reactions are a wish to rescue the patient or to get rid of the patient. Clinicians often feel manipulated, angry, depleted, exhausted, or self-doubting.

Borderline patients fear separation or abandonment. They may cope with threats of loss with panic, emotional instability, manipulation, anger, intimidation, or impulsiveness (suicidal, self-destructive, or violent outbursts). During periods of relative calm, their dependency can lead them to be adherent to medical recommendations, and they can use medical resources appropriately. However, this is easily interrupted by a chaotic and unstable lifestyle. Patients who are borderline are capable of stirring the healthcare system into frenzy and polarizing staff. They can be aggressive, devaluing, irritable, impulsive, and angry. They also can be dependent and clingy to their caretakers and may make entitled demands for special treatment when they get frustrated. They tend to relate to others by considering them all good or all bad, which significantly contributes to their dysfunctional lives and stormy interpersonal relationships. They function on the borderline level of personality organization where reality testing is typically intact. However, under stress, they may temporarily lose reality testing and manifest severe cognitive and perceptual distortions including episodes of dissociation, derealization, depersonalization, and perhaps brief mini-psychotic episodes. These intense disturbances are often brought on by affect storms, during intense interpersonal conflicts, or by substance abuse. During episodes of cognitive and perceptual distortions, they may readily misunderstand the clinician's intentions or instructions. These patients also have identity diffusion manifested by extreme fluctuations in self-perception, from the grandiose to an excessively harsh underestimation of their abilities. They also suffer from stormy and chaotic relationships with others. Their coping style in a healthcare setting is most commonly a hostile dependency. They rely heavily on splitting, projective identification, projection, and idealization and devaluing.

Office management of borderline patients involves an empathic understanding of their fears. These fears revolve around the threat to their security, or fears of separation and abandonment, and, secondarily, sensitivity to rejection and fears of humiliation. They require firm limit setting and clarity about what the clinician can realistically offer. When the clinician attempts to satisfy the patient's intense needs, it often results in an exhausted or angry clinician. This can be avoided by setting realistic limits, and correcting reality distortions or irrational ideas, while offering the patient several different ideas or options for more adaptive behaviors. Initial interventions should attempt to establish reality testing or to correct reality distortions. The use of adjunctive medication to manage these patients can be very helpful. The pharmacology should target cognitive-perceptual disturbances, affect dysregulation, or impulsivity. If reality testing is intact, the most helpful interventions can be aimed at decreasing the pathological splitting defenses by use of confrontation, clarification, and interpretations of the problematic situation.

Narcissistic Personality Disorders

Clinician reactions to the narcissistic patient are often very difficult to manage. The superior, critical, entitled, self-loving, arrogant attitude of these patients can be intimidating. When they are acting superior, they may elicit a complementary reaction in which the clinician feels devalued, inferior, or may fear the patient's anger or criticism. Alternatively, their lack of empathy and interpersonal exploitation can readily provoke a concordant reaction in the clinician such as anger and a wish to retaliate with harsh criticism or to belittle or get rid of the patient. The core fears of these patients are related to fragile self-esteem. They fear loss of power, potency, beauty, and fear they will be exploited if they are ever vulnerable. They cope with their low self-esteem by seeking power and control, and they often make unacknowledged demands for constant approval and praise from others. Any perceived insult to their grandiosity[15,21] makes them feel rejected, deflated, criticized, and frequently results in feelings of rage, shame, or humiliation. In a medical setting, a narcissistic patient can appear gracious or charming and is often experienced as a leader. If ill or in the patient role, they may challenge the authority of the medical staff and may denigrate staff or treat staff like servants. This belittling attitude tends to generate conflict and resentment in the medical staff. It is often difficult for a narcissistic patient to adhere to medical recommendations, because the need for medical care makes them feel weak and inferior, and brings home the loss of control of authority. Their need to be superior may lead them to underutilization of appropriate medical care or doctor-shopping for the "real expert." The narcissistic patients who are most difficult to manage function at the level of BPO. Their reality testing is typically intact, yet it can undergo severe distortions when they perceive slights, rejection, or competition from others with talent. Those narcissistic patients who have paranoid and antisocial features[21] have a worse prognosis. They often have a fragile identity that can swing from the grandiose to the worthless. They rely heavily on a coping style of superiority and arrogance, which is maintained by the use of the splitting defenses, which are designed to help them regulate self-esteem. The grandiose and superior self helps to defend them from feelings of extreme inadequacy, dependency, and vulnerability. When on the superior side of the split, a narcissistic patient may devalue, viciously attack, or degrade those around them. Alternatively, when feeling worthless, they may idealize and/or envy others who are, for the moment, seen as more powerful or successful. In this subservient position, their self-esteem plummets and they may present with depressive symptoms. Patients in this vulnerable state report a deep sense of worthlessness and may make deprecating and degrading self-attacks. Office management of the narcissistic patient requires that the clinician not mistake the patient's superior and entitled manner for genuine confidence. When being assaulted by a devaluing attack, it may help the clinician to see the attacking patient as a wounded child having a disruptive outburst. This may prevent retaliation from the clinician that would only escalate a worsening situation. Intervening in the face of a devaluing attack involves acknowledging that the patient feels hurt and that the patient also has a right to his or her opinions. If the patient can discuss his or her hurt feelings with a nonjudgmental and empathic clinician, the problem generally resolves, and a good clinician/staff–patient alliance is restored. If this is not possible, offer the patient (without malice, defensiveness, or apology) the right to seek another expert for consultation. This may help the patient to calm down and reconsider his or her position. In a long-term relationship with a narcissistic patient, the recurrent use of splitting can be interpreted. When the patient devalues the clinician, reminding the patient of their previous praise of the clinician can be helpful. The patient can be asked why he or she is feeling so critical and angry now. This may help elicit the patient's feelings of being hurt or vulnerable. When they admire or praise the clinician, preventively saying "I hope we can remember this for future visits if things don't go so smoothly" can be helpful. Other effective interventions include setting limits on the patient's entitlements, correcting irrational thoughts, and lowering expectations.

Dependent Personality Disorder

Patients with dependent personality disorder may be characterized by an exaggerated need for care or a need for direction from someone else. They feel helpless and inadequate when it comes to making even minor decisions such as what to wear or who should be their friends. They have a core belief that they cannot function alone, are completely incapable of taking care of themselves, and believe that they must have someone else to supply care and make decisions for them. Their major fear is that they will be helpless or overwhelmed. Although histrionic, borderline, and dependent personality-disordered patients are extremely dependent on others, they react very differently to the threat of loss of a significant other. The borderline patient becomes angry, enraged, or clinging, and the histrionic patient becomes dramatic and attention seeking, whereas the dependent patient becomes submissive and obsequious. Left to themselves, due to their generally passive nature, patients with dependent personality disorder are typically nonadherent to treatment recommendations and underutilize medical care. However, if they come to see their physicians, they are more likely to comply and take to heart what is recommended. Involving family or other key decision makers to oversee the patient's medical care is often the most effective intervention. Patients with a dependent personality disorder usually function at the neurotic or borderline level of personality organization. They have a passive or helpless style of copying and typically use defenses, which may include regression, passive-aggression, and reaction formation. Patients with dependent personality disorder are submissive and may assertively demand caretaking or cling to their caretakers. The extreme dependence of these patients can make clinicians feel annoyed, drained, or depleted. It is important to remember that dependent patient requests for more care often does not truly indicate what they need. They may need assistance in developing internal motivation and self-care plans. When ill, being in the sick role may be particularly gratifying to a dependent patient, and this secondary gain may delay recovery. To intervene with such a patient, the clinician must understand and empathize with the patient's need for caretaking, while at the same time encouraging and fostering independent thinking and actions. Since these patients often use medication, alcohol, food, and other means to satisfy their dependency needs, the clinician must be cautious in how these are used as part of a therapeutic plan. While it is important to frustrate total dependence, it is also important to avoid telling the patient what to do. Asking a dependent patient about their fears of more independence can be helpful. Correcting reality distortions, limiting unreasonable patient expectations, eliciting irrational thoughts, and suggesting more rational ones may also help. Interpretations of regression and other specific defenses may also help improve the patient's functioning in medical settings.

Obsessive-Compulsive Personality Disorder

Patients with obsessive-compulsive personality disorder (OCPD) are preoccupied with details, order, and control. Although their labels are similar, these patients differ in substantial ways from patients with obsessive-compulsive disorder (OCD). OCD patients have recurrent disturbing thoughts or obsessions that create marked subjective distress. They may also be driven to perform ritualistic or compulsive behaviors such as hand washing or checking and rechecking. These behaviors help them to manage, control, and distract themselves from intense anxiety. The core adaptive traits of patients with OCPD are orderliness, attention to detail, and an emphasis on rational thinking and logic. These traits are life-long patterns that many patients use adaptively in their professional lives. Patients with OCPD often view these traits as personal strengths. However, their attention to detail also leads them to a belief and/or worry that they must not make mistakes or that they must be perfect. They may interpret rules, regulations, and values rigidly and stubbornly. Patients with OCPD are often uncomfortable with feelings and emotional expression. They typically fear disorderliness, dirt, and angry emotions. The compulsive, critical, controlling, self-righteous side of their personalities often creates difficulty in their relationships with healthcare professionals and in relationships with their marital partners, coworkers, friends, or family. They can be stingy, orderly, and obstinate. Clinicians, who often have obsessive-compulsive personality traits themselves, may feel irritated and competitive with these patients over who wants to control the diagnostic workup or treatment plans. Patients with OCPD tend to be rigidly adherent to medical recommendations but may react strongly when treatment plans need to be clarified or modified. They tend to be ambivalent about utilizing medical care. Their anxiety, need for attention to details, and compulsiveness will tend to drive overutilization of medical services, whereas their need for certainty and control may keep them out of the office. Patients with OCPD usually function at the neurotic or borderline level of personality organization. The coping style, which predominates, is obsessing and being compulsive. Commonly used defense mechanisms include intellectualization, isolation, displacement, doing and undoing, and reaction formation. Using reaction formation, they may behave in a superficially deferential or obsequious manner to repress from themselves, and hide from others, their critical and self-righteous or angry feelings. These defenses are used against their anger and dependency needs, which are often consciously denied. Illness often represents a dangerous threat to the sense of self-control in patients with OCPD. The clinician should understand and empathize with this loss of self-control while at the same time helping the patient regain some control in the management of the problem. Struggles or conflicts with the patient over controlling tendencies should be avoided. Reality distortions, which may include excessive perfectionism, idealization of logic, and avoidance of feeling, can be gently elicited, explored, and worked through with the patient. Interpreting the anxiety underlying the obsessive-compulsive actions may enable the patient to be more centered and calm down.

Avoidant Personality Disorder

Patients with avoidant personality disorder are characterized by feelings of inadequacy and fears of criticism. They have low self-esteem and believe that they are inept and inadequate. They believe that others are critical and disapproving until proven otherwise. Although these patients crave human relationships and affection, their fear of being criticized, rejected, embarrassed, or hurt causes them to avoid social situations or meet new people. This shyness and avoidance protects them from their fears of being rejected or humiliated. In medical encounters, they fear revealing any aspects of themselves that may leave them vulnerable. Their timidity, hypersensitivity, and cautiousness can generate clinician feelings of either a wish to help the patient, or frustration or annoyance at the patient. Avoidant patients tend to be adherent to avoid criticism by their clinician, but tend to underutilize medical services. Patients with avoidant personality disorder tend to function at a neurotic level of personality organization. Most commonly they will use withdrawal as their major coping style and utilize defense mechanisms based on repression, which include inhibition, phobia, and isolation. Managing these patients is more effective when the clinician can recognize and empathize with the patient's social fears, including fear of the clinician. Patients may minimize symptoms or delay seeking help because they fear the clinician's criticism or because they feel unworthy or not important. The clinician should help the patient identify any specific fears revolving around the medical diagnostic or therapeutic plan. Irrational fears and thoughts can be gently corrected and alternative interpretations can be offered to the patient. Patients should be encouraged, with appropriate support, to face their fears as the best way of mastering them. If the clinician feels frustrated or annoyed, it is often helpful to encourage the patient to describe what he or she is finding most difficult about the current or proposed medical plan.

Self-Defeating Personality Disorder

Self-defeating patients are often suffering, depressed, self-sacrificing, and self-destructive. They repeatedly make bad choices that lead to failure or pain. This diagnostic category was eliminated from DSM because of gender bias (female) and an inability to get a general agreement about the diagnostic features. However, it is included in this chapter because patients who are self-defeating are ubiquitous and present difficult clinical problems for physician/clinicians and staff. A common reaction to a self-defeating patient is a wish to rescue them from their own self-destructiveness. Trying too vigorously to help these patients often results in a worsening of the patient's complaints and symptoms (e.g., hypochondria or multiple somatic complaints). This often leaves the clinician frustrated, angry, defeated, self-doubting, self-blaming, or hopeless. Alternatively, because they may reject help, these patients can arouse sadistic fantasies in the clinician such as a wish that the patient would suffer or die. Patients in this group are excessively dependent on love, support, and acceptance from others, and often have depressive symptoms. They cannot directly express their anger and may be harshly self-judgmental. They fear recovery, which to them means losing love and caring. Improvement of their medical condition often leads to the development of multiple new complaints that have no somatic basis. Patients with self-defeating traits may not adhere to treatment in an effort to not get well. They are typically ambivalent about the medical system, which they sometimes avoid. At other times they may seek a dependent attachment. Within this group, patients may function on either the neurotic or borderline level of personality organization. Neurotically functioning masochistic patients can make the clinician feel mildly guilty that they are causing the patient pain or suffering or are not adequately helping; the patient and clinician both suffer. However, these patients can often be helped and can express genuine gratitude toward the clinician. Borderline functioning masochistic patients are often passive-aggressive help-seeking rejecters, who can make their clinician feel both helpless and responsible for their suffering or self-destructiveness. Clinicians can manage these patients by empathizing with the patient's realistic medical suffering, symptoms or complaints from the illness. It should not be suggested that the patient's symptoms are psychological or that they will improve or be cured quickly. These optimistic predictions by the clinician may paradoxically increase the patient's symptoms, complaints, telephone calls, and office visits. Potential recovery can be presented as a likely but a distant reality. If the patient cannot permit or admit relief of the symptoms or suffering, he or she can be asked to speak less about their symptoms for the benefit of other family members.

Conclusion

Patients suffering with personality disorders are common in healthcare settings and contribute significantly to clinician's stress. Unexamined countertransference reactions and the absence of strategies for dealing with this difficult group of patients can often lead a clinician and the medical staff to provide suboptimal medical care. This chapter described a schema for managing personality disorders in a medical setting, which includes personality diagnosis, discussion about uses of countertransference, discovering the patient's belief systems, fears, coping styles, and defenses, predicting medical adherence and utilization to inform both general and specific interventions strategies designed for working with patients who have personality disorders. Review Box 7.3 for relevant resources for patients, families, and clinicians.

Conflict of Interest/Disclosure: The authors of this chapter have no financial conflicts and nothing to disclose.

Box 7.3 Resources for Patients, Families, and Clinicians

Patient and families

- The New Personality Self-Portrait: Map Your Personality. https://npsp25.com/
- Oldham J, Morris LB. *The New Personality Self-portrait: Why You Think, Work, Love and Act the Way You Do.* New York, NY: Bantam; 2012.
- National Alliance on Mental Illness. https://www.nami.org/About-Mental-Illness/Mental-Health-Conditions/Borderline-Personality-Disorder.
- American Psychiatric Association: Help with Personality Disorders. https://www.psychiatry.org/patients-families/personality-disorders
- National Institute of Mental Health. Borderline Personality Disorders. https://www.nimh.nih.gov/health/topics/borderline-personality-disorder/index.shtml

Clinicians

- The Personality Studies Institute. https://www.borderlinedisorders.com/.
- M.I.N.D. Clinic for Mood and Personality Disorders. https://www.columbiapsychiatry.org/research-clinics/m-i-n-d-clinic-mood-and-personality-disorders.
- Gunderson Personality Disorders Institute. https://www.mcleanhospital.org/training/gunderson-institute.
- Personality Disorder Assessment: Shedler-Westen Assessment Procedure. https://swapassessment.org.

References

1. Kahana RJ, Bibring GL. Personality types in medical management. In: Zinberg NE, ed. *Psychiatry and Medical Practice in a General Hospital*. Madison, CT: International Universities Press; 1964:108–123.

2. Groves JE. Taking care of the hateful patient. *N Engl J Med*. 1978; 298:883–887. doi:10.1056/nejm197804202981605

3. Samuels J, Eaton WW, Bienvenu OJ, Brown CH, Costa PT, Nestadt G. Prevalence and correlates of personality disorders in a community sample. *Br J Psychiatry*. 2002 June;180:536–542. doi: 10.1192/bjp.180.6.536

4. Grant BF, Stinson FS, Dawson DA, Chou SP, Ruan WJ. Co-occurrence of DSM-IV personality disorders in the United States: results from the National Epidemiologic Survey on Alcohol and Related Conditions. *Compr Psychiatry*. 2005; 46:1–5. doi: 10.1016/j.comppsych.2004.07.019

5. Stinson FS, Dawson DA, Goldstein RB, et al. Prevalence, correlates, disability, and co-morbidity of DSM-IV narcissistic personality disorder: results from the wave 2 national epidemiologic survey on alcohol and related conditions. *J Clin Psychiatry*. 2008; 69:1033. doi:10.4088/jcp.v69n0701

6. Moran P, Jenkins R, Tylee A, Blizard R, Mann A. The prevalence of personality disorder among UK primary care attenders. *Acta Psychiatr Scand*, 2000; 102:52–57. doi: 10.1034/j.1600-0447.2000.102001052.x

7. Gross R, Olfson M, Gameroff M, et al. Borderline personality disorder in primary care. *Arch Intern Med*. 2002; 162:53. doi: 10.1001/archinte.162.1.53

8. Grant BF, Stinson FS, Dawson DA, Chou SP, Ruan WJ, Pickering RP. Co-occurrence of 12-month alcohol and drug use disorders and personality disorders in the United States. *Arch Gen Psychiatry*. 2004; 61:361. doi: 10.1001/archinte.162.1.53

9. Haw C, Hawton K, Houston K, Townsend E. Psychiatric and personality disorders in deliberate self-harm patients. *Br J Psychiatry*. 2001; 178: 48–54. doi: 10.1192/bjp.178.1.48

10. Clarke DM, Smith GC. Consultation-liaison psychiatry in general medical units. *Aust N Z J Psychiatry*. 1995; 29:424–432. doi: 10.3109/00048679509064950

11. *Diagnostic and Statistical Manual of Mental Disorders: DSM-IV-TR*. Washington, DC: American Psychiatric Association; 2000.

12. *Diagnostic and Statistical Manual of Mental Disorders: DSM-5*. Washington, DC: American Psychiatric Association; 2013.

13. Widiger TA, Simonsen E. Alternative dimensional models of personality disorder: finding a common ground. *J Pers Disord*. 2005; 19:110–130. doi: 10.1521/pedi.19.2.110.62628

14. Beitman BD, Yue D. *Learning Psychotherapy: A Time-efficient, Research-based, and Outcome-measured Psychotherapy Training Program*. 2nd ed. New York, NY: Norton; 2004.

15. Kernberg, OF. *Borderline Conditions and Pathological Narcissism*. New York, NY: Rowman & Littlefield; 1985.

16. Racker, H. The meanings and uses of countertransference In: Arundale J, Bandler Bellman, D, eds. *Transference and Countertransference: A Unifying Focus of Psychoanalysis*. New York, NY: Routledge; 2018:127–173.

17. Beck AT, Davis DD, Freeman A, eds. *Cognitive Therapy of Personality Disorders*. New York, NY: Guilford; 2015.

18. Greenberger D, Padesky CA. *Mind Over Mood: Change How You Feel by Changing the Way You Think*. New York, NY: Guilford; 2015

19. Kernberg O. *Severe Personality Disorders: Psychotherapeutic Strategies*. New Haven, CT: Yale University Press; 1984.

20. Feinstein, RE. Prevention-oriented primary care: a collaborative model for office-based cardiovascular risk reduction. *Heart Dis.* 1999; 5:264–271. PMID: 11720633.

21. Kernberg O. *Aggression in Personality Disorders and Perversions*. New Haven, CT: Yale University Press; 1992.

8

Transference-focused Psychotherapy

Christopher Green and Frank Yeomans

Key Points

- Transference-focused psychotherapy (TFP) is an evidence-based treatment initially developed for the treatment of borderline personality disorder (BPD). It has been adapted for the treatment of other personality disorders, including narcissistic, histrionic, paranoid, dependent, and schizotypal personality disorders.
- TFP is a modified psychodynamic treatment based on ego psychology, object relations, and attachment theory.
- Internal representations of self and others are cognitive-affective units that are considered the building blocks of the psychological structure that develops in an individual's mind.
- Personality disorders result when the psychological structure of an individual's mind remains split. All-bad dyads (i.e., negative affect and representations) remain defensively *split off* from all-good ones, rather than having an *integrated* and varied array of nuanced and flexible dyads.
- All severe personality disorders have a borderline personality organization (BPO) which includes: (1) identity diffusion, (2) predominant use of spitting defense mechanisms, and 3) fragile reality testing.
- TFP's efficacy in patients with BPD has been demonstrated in three independent, international, randomized controlled trials.
- TFP first phase involves assessment, communication of the diagnosis, and establishment of the frame of treatment by means of the treatment contract.
- TFP second exploratory phase helps the patient gain awareness of the dyads (self-affect-other) that underlie their emotions and experiences and how these dyads play out in their therapy and life.
- The overarching strategy of TFP is to help the patient change from a split internal world to an integrated consolidated identity that involves complex, coherent, realistic experiences of self and others that allow for a stable life with the capacity for healthy interpersonal relationships.
- TFP tactics involve setting up and maintaining the treatment contract and frame and the conditions of treatment that allow therapy to take place.
- TFP prioritizes technical neutrality, countertransference, and the use of clarification, confrontation and interpretation focused on transference analysis

Introduction

Transference-focused psychotherapy (TFP) is an evidence-based treatment initially developed for the treatment of borderline personality disorder (BPD). It has been adapted for the treatment of other personality disorders, including narcissistic, histrionic, paranoid, dependent, and schizotypal personality disorders.[1,2,3] It can be useful in diverse applications, such as part of a general psychiatric assessment and medication management.[4,5,6] This chapter introduces the theory and practice of TFP illustrated with a clinical vignette. Ideally, it will stimulate the reader's interest to learn more about TFP and consider its use in clinical practice.

Theory of TFP

TFP provides both a model of the genesis and maintenance of personality pathology and a model for its treatment. Otto Kernberg and colleagues at the Weill Cornell Medical College developed TFP in response to the shortcomings of classical psychoanalysis as practiced in the mid-twentieth century in treating patients with BPD.[7] These patients often responded poorly to unstructured treatment that lacked sufficient delineation of goals, objectives, and an adequate treatment frame. This led Kernberg to modify some of the traditional psychoanalytic techniques and to strengthen the treatment frame when working with patients with BPD. The landmark Menninger study in 1972 provided initial evidence for the efficacy of this structured psychoanalytic model of therapy.[7]

"Transference," as part of the name TFP, refers to the psychological phenomenon in which an individual unconsciously transfers images from their internal world to a person in their present life. Transference is not limited to the treatment setting, but it is within the treatment setting that this phenomenon can be used therapeutically when patients transfer internalized experiences and beliefs from their early life to a treating therapist. These experiences include conscious and unconscious feelings, wishes, fantasies, impulses, and beliefs. These internalized images tend to be based on emotionally intense experiences and are organized in the mind into mental representations of the self in relation to another person, or "object relations." Object relations are relationship patterns, or dyads, that are fundamental in establishing a person's sense of self and of others and are therefore central to the patient's identity and personality.[8,9] In individuals with BPD, rigid and stereotyped internal images of self and others are activated in a way that interferes with an accurate understanding of interpersonal relationships. This can lead to repetitive maladaptive interactions (represented structurally by personality traits), contributing to profound psychological and functional difficulties in patients with personality disorders. However, when these maladaptive interactions manifest in therapy, the patient has an opportunity for therapeutic benefit by examining them with an empathic therapist.[10,11]

Kernberg took as the starting point for his model of personality pathology object- relations theory, derived in part from the work of Melanie Klein and Ronald Fairbairn.[12,13] Though influenced by the classic idea that symptoms come from conflicts between psychological drives and defenses, object-relations theory describes conflicts in terms of an individual's repertoire of internalized relationships between self and other (the two "objects" involved in a relationship). These internalized relationship patterns are referred to as "object-relations dyads" and are comprised of a specific image or representation of the self in relation to a specific representation of the other, linked by a strong affect.

These internal representations are instrumental in motivating feelings and behaviors in people. For instance, an adult might have a repertoire of internal dyads, and among these have a dyad in which he or she sees him or herself as a helpless child in relation to a hateful and withholding parent, with a corresponding affect of fear and anxiety. When current situations with authority figures trigger the experience of this dyad, the person might experience feelings (e.g., anxiety) and behaviors (e.g., submissiveness) that correspond to the internal dyad but not to the actual situation in the present moment. This could lead to chronic difficulties in life. A second example is a dyad in which the self is experienced as basking in the glow of a perfectly loving caretaker, with a corresponding effect of blissful wellbeing. As in the preceding example, this dyad might be triggered in a situation, such as a first date, in which it does not correspond to the objective reality.

Dyads are cognitive-affective units that are considered the building blocks of the psychological structure that develops in an individual's mind. They are internalized in the mind from birth on, based on emotionally intense experiences with caregivers of either an extreme positive/pleasurable nature or an extreme negative/painful nature. These experiences are posited to be part of every individual's development. The dyads are laid down as memory traces and are not exact replicas of lived experience but are images or representations of self or other that have been transformed by internal psychological forces: wishes, fears, fantasies, anxieties.[14]

In the first years of life, before the establishment of "object constancy,"[15] the dyads sort out into those of a totally positive ideal nature where needs are satisfied, imbued with loving feelings, and those that are totally negative where needs are frustrated, imbued with fearful and hateful feelings. This psychological organization is referred to as the "paranoid-schizoid" position. The paranoid-schizoid position is paranoid in that the aggression within the self is not consciously experienced as part of the self but is projected and perceived as outside of the self and coming from the frustrating other.[12] It is schizoid in that the organization is split into two disconnected segments, one with feelings of ideal caring and love and one comprised of feelings of maltreatment and aggression. These two components of the mind correspond to basic libidinal (loving and attachment-seeking) drives and aggressive (a mix of self-affirming and exploitative) drives. Conflicts between these two drives are at the root of much psychopathology.

In the course of normal psychological development between 18 and 36 months old, the individual's mental representations of both self and others move from narrow and extreme to become more complex, rich, and nuanced; that is, from a psychological structure that is split between all-positive and all-negative representations to a complex structure that integrates the full range of emotional potential in the images of self and others. This more mature organization, which continues to develop from age three on, adapts better to the challenges of life. It is sometimes referred to as the "depressive position" because: (1) the shift from two extreme views of self and other to a more nuanced, gray, "good enough" view entails the need to give up and mourn the idea that we can find perfection in self and/or others, and (2) the integration of the two extremes involves "taking back" the projected aggression and acknowledging, with painful guilt and remorse, that one harbors aggression and is capable of harming others.

In talking about this development model of the mind, what we are describing is also a structural model. From the latter point of view, and in keeping with the meaning of the term "psychodynamic" (the mind in motion), an individual who has developed the more complex integrated psychological structure can, under circumstances of external or internal stress, temporarily regress from the integrated to the split psychological mode. Kernberg's elaboration of object-relations theory links that theory to psychoanalytic ego psychology, in that internal objective relations dyads are seen as the building blocks of the more fully developed structures of the ego and superego. For example, one early internalized dyad might represent the self in relation to a critical punishing other ("You're bad for doing that!") while another dyad might involve praise ("What a good boy you are for doing that!"). Left unintegrated, these dyads result in a primitive and erratic internal sense of morality based on bad or good, punishment or praise. The integration of these and other dyads into a more complex system results in the more developed psychological structure of the superego.

An individual's repertoire of dyads in the mind is readily at hand to be activated as one goes through life. A given situation or event will trigger one of these dyads. The dyad then influences the individual's perception of the situation. The more split and less integrated the individual's psychological structure, the more the internal dyad will direct the patient's experience and behavior, even if the dyad does not correspond to the external reality. When the other person does not correspond to the object representation of the activated dyad, the interaction may be fraught with misunderstanding. In some cases, the individual may act in ways that induce the other to conform to the expected behavior through the process known as projective identification.

For example, a student with a long-standing, internalized dyad of helpless child (student)–critical parent (teacher) perceives his teacher as angrily attacking him when she corrects a mistake in his homework, when in fact, the teacher is trying to help him in good faith. In addition to affecting his perception of the outside world, the operant dyad could motivate the student to unconsciously provoke his teacher (via unconscious use of projective identification or enactments) to lose patience and thus become an uncharacteristically critical authority (parent) in reality, as well. In this latter case, the student: (1) unconsciously activates a dyad; (2) experiences himself as helpless; (3) imagines or believes that the teacher is critical (projection); and (4) influences the teacher in such a way that the teacher becomes critical in actuality and not just fantasy (identification with the student's projection). The defense of projective identification liberates the student from the unwanted feeling of being angry and critical himself, by evoking that feeling in the teacher instead.

Our view is that PDs result when the psychological structure of an individual's mind remains split. All-bad dyads (i.e., negative affect and representations) remain defensively *split off* from all-good ones, rather than having an *integrated* and varied array of nuanced and flexible dyads. This splitting is a key factor across severe PDs. The continuation of a split psychological structure into adulthood is seen in patients with borderline and narcissistic PDs. This split structure in PDs is attributable to a combination of factors, including genetics, temperament, child–parent mismatch, and early life trauma.[9,16]

In the previous example, the student could be overwhelmed with negative affect in the moment, feeling like a helpless child, then experiencing the reverse later when angrily denouncing the teacher, acting as a critical parent but without conscious awareness of this part. This oscillation between the two poles of a dyad (from self to other) is common in patients who use splitting, but often goes unnoticed by the patient who may continue to experience the self-representation of helpless criticized child, despite acting like the object representation of aggressive parental criticizer. In essence, the individual identifies with both poles of the dyadic relationship. Living out this repetitious dyad interferes with his experience of others and makes entering into deep and meaningful relationships very difficult. With a better-integrated view, learned during treatment, the student might be able to see the good and bad in the teacher and in himself, along with the different emotions that come with this.

Splitting is at the root of identity diffusion, a core characteristic of patients with severe PDs. Identity diffusion means a poor and fragmented sense of self and others, a chronic sense of emptiness, and difficulty in sustaining investment in work or relationships. These are common problems in patients with antisocial, borderline, histrionic, and narcissistic PDs. Furthermore, splitting and identity diffusion contribute to the dysregulated affect, unstable relationships, tendency to self-harm, and impulsivity seen in borderline personality disorder. It is hard to find stability in life if one's sense of self and others is oscillating and unstable.

Structural Models of PDs

The structural model of PDs[17] (based on level of personality organization) is distinguished from the more descriptive model found in the *Diagnostic and Statistical Manuals* (DSM) system.[18-22] The structural model posits that all severe PDs have a borderline personality organization (BPO) and share three common factors: (1) identity diffusion (e.g., primitive or split object relations); (2) predominance of primitive defense mechanisms (e.g., based on splitting); and (3) fragile reality testing when internal representations distort an accurate perception of external reality. This is a broader concept than the symptom-based DSM diagnosis of BPD. See Chapter 2 for more information on levels of personality organization. BPO includes patients described in the *Diagnostic and Statistical Manual of Mental Disorder* (DSM-5)[22] as antisocial, avoidant, dependent, histrionic, narcissistic, obsessive-compulsive, paranoid, schizoid, and schizotypal PDs, as well as BPD. This system of personality organization provides a more dimensional view of PDs in contrast to the more traditional categorical view based on symptoms and descriptive character traits.

The Alternative Model for Personality Disorders in Section III of the DSM-5[22] has commonalities with the personality organization viewpoint, as it also emphasizes self and other functioning. In terms of treatment considerations, this structural classification system calls for a treatment that puts emphasis on change at the level of psychological structure (e.g., movement and improvement from BPO structure to neurotic or a healthy personality organization.) Treatment focuses on the need to help the patient change from identity diffusion/identity fragmentation to a coherent and integrated identity.

Evidence for TFP

TFP's efficacy in patients with BPD has been demonstrated in three independent, international, randomized controlled trials. See Box 8.1, p. 218 for more information about the evidence base for TFP.

Box 8.1 Evidence for TFP

- TFP's efficacy in patients with BPD has been demonstrated in three independent, international, randomized controlled trials.[23-25]

Level of Evidence A
- A number of pre/post studies and a non-randomized, quasi-experimental comparison study demonstrate efficacy. [26-30]

Level of Evidence B
- In addition to fostering symptom change (e.g., decreased suicidality, depression, anxiety), TFP also is associated with change in psychosocial functioning and personality structure and functioning, including: improvement in reflective functioning; mentalization in attachment relationships; change in attachment security (from insecure to secure, disorganized to organized); and improvement in narrative coherence and personality organization.[31,32]
- In an fMRI study, functional changes achieved with TFP were found to correlate to brain changes.[33]

Key: Levels of Evidence; Strength of Recommendation Taxonomy (SORT)*
Level of Evidence A: Good quality patient-oriented evidence.
Level of Evidence B: Limited quality patient-oriented evidence
Level of Evidence C: Based on consensus, usual practice, opinion, disease-oriented evidence, or case series for studies of diagnosis
*Ebell MH, Siwek J, Weiss BD, Woolf SH, Susman J, Ewigman B, Bowman M. Simplifying the language of evidence to improve patient care. *J Fam Pract.* 2004 Feb 1;53(2):111–120.

Practice of TFP

In this section, we provide a broad overview of TFP treatment, not a comprehensive review, which is available elsewhere.[14,34] We offer several brief clinical vignettes to demonstrate the principles of this treatment.

The practice of TFP follows naturally from its theoretical base. TFP was developed to include two overlapping but somewhat distinct phases. The first phase involves assessment, communication of the diagnosis, and establishment of the frame of treatment by means of the treatment contract. As the treatment begins, the therapist sets limits that help the patient channel their acting-out behaviors into the treatment setting, where the painful affects that subtend the acting out can be experienced and understood. The affects are observed as they emerge in the patient's interaction with the therapist and in the patient's descriptions of their interactions with others outside of the therapy.

During the second, exploratory phase, TFP's goal is to help the patient gain awareness of the dyads that underlie their affects and experiences and how these dyads play out in their life as well as in the room with the therapist. Over time, with repeated use of the techniques of clarification, confrontation, and interpretation, the patient will gain a clearer awareness of experiences of self and other that originate in the self rather than in the outside world. The patient will be able to move from a set of narrow, rigid, extreme, and abruptly shifting views of self and others, to a more consolidated identity and a nuanced, realistic sense of self and other. Correspondingly, the patient will move from regular use of the defense mechanisms of splitting, omnipotent control, projection, and projective identification to more mature and more adaptive psychological defenses. As a result, he or she will develop more stable and deep relationships and experience fewer swings between emotional extremes. Both the patient's ability to navigate in the world and the quality of inner experience will have improved. TFP is designed to facilitate this transformation.

Assessment

The assessment phase is of vital importance. It can generally be done in two sessions, but may require more. When appropriate, collateral information or involvement from family members may be needed to get a complete picture of the patient. Some patients with poor functioning may have difficulty in describing their condition because of their personality disorder.

TFP process begins with a comprehensive psychiatric assessment, using a *structural interview* for this purpose.[17] This interview includes a standard history and mental status exam, but goes beyond these to provide an initial determination of a patient's level of personality organization or psychological structure. Is the patient's psychological structure integrated around a cohesive sense of self and others (e.g., neurotic or healthy personality organization), or is it split and fragmented, as in BPOs. The structural interview includes an assessment of the patient's identity, level of defenses, quality of object relations, moral values, and degree of aggression. The focus is on the differential diagnosis between DSM-5 BPD, other severe personality disorders, and other forms of psychopathology (e.g., to rule out bipolar illness or a psychotic pathology).

The TFP assessment begins with open-ended questioning, asking the patient to describe how they understand their past and present symptoms and problems, and their expectations of treatment. This serves multiple functions. It gives a sense of the patient's presenting complaint, whether they can tell a consistent and detailed story about themselves and their problems, and their ability to handle a cognitively demanding task.

Defenses

A preliminary assessment of a patient's go-to defenses can be determined during the initial interviews. As the interview progresses, the therapist does not shy away from inquiring about inconsistencies in a patient's narrative, clarifying ambiguous statements, and may even consider floating trial interpretations. It is expected that this will increase a patient's anxiety as internal conflicts (e.g., between wishes for dependency and fears thereof) are touched, and defenses against them are mobilized where they can be seen in the "here and now" of the interview. While everyone uses a variety of defenses, the key distinction to make is whether the patient predominately uses the splitting-based defenses characteristic of BPO (most pathological), neurotic repression-based defenses, or mature defenses (healthiest).

The structural interview includes descriptions of both the patient and important others, how the patient experiences the interviewer in the here-and-now context of the interview, and inquiry about any inconsistencies noted. While this approach may increase a patient's anxiety and is therefore inadvisable for psychotic individuals, it is useful in the assessment of patients with normal, neurotic, or BPOs. From this interview, the therapist can understand the patient's relation to reality, use of defenses, object relations, aggression, and level of moral functioning.

Identity Diffusion

The evaluator will ask the patient to describe themselves and at least one other significant person. This can give insight into whether the patient's world is populated by relatively shallow, polarized, or diffuse representations—or more rich, coherent, and complex ones. For instance, someone with a low level of BPO might describe their best friend simply as "nice" or as someone who likes music, without being able to paint much more of a portrait, even with the therapist's further prompting. This situates an individual's level of personality functioning on a spectrum from normal to mild neurotic (subsyndromal) organization to high, mid, or low levels of BPO.

Object Relations

The quality of object relations, which is related to interpersonal functioning, is also assessed. Here the basic question is: to what degree is the patient able to sustain relationships that are mutual and flexible and, in the case of romantic ones, combine sexual with emotional intimacy? A related inquiry would seek to determine whether the individual can sustain a strong level of investment in their work or other interests. Individuals organized at the neurotic level of personality organization, in contrast to those at the borderline level, have an integrated self. Conflicts in neurotic individuals have to do with difficulty comfortably integrating one aspect of psychological life, usually either sexual or aggressive feelings, into their sense of self. Therefore, a neurotic individual may have a stable marriage but with an inhibition with regard to experiencing full sexual pleasure without guilt. In contrast, individuals at the borderline level of organization have difficulty establishing harmonious and stable relations with others because those relations are complicated by the impact of internal mental representations that interfere with getting to know others in depth. Relationships tend to be marked by ongoing conflicts and abrupt interruptions.

Reality Testing

Assuming that overt psychotic processes (e.g., schizophrenia, a psychotic mood disorder, or substance intoxication) have been ruled out, more subtle deficits in reality testing, stemming from a personality disorder, should be assessed. For example, an aspiring novelist with BPO and narcissistic traits may have a grandiose belief that his next book will definitely be a bestseller and plan on this to finance his therapy. If he is unable to reflect on the possibility that it may not be a bestseller when challenged by the interviewer, this would imply impaired reality testing without the total loss of reality testing seen in psychosis. This flaw in reality testing introduces an added complication, as an inability to pay for treatment jeopardizes the therapy.

Aggression

Aggression is addressed during the contracting phase.[35] This assessment includes determining how aggression is controlled or how impulses are deployed, as well as self- or other-directedness of aggression. The degree of aggression informs the overall view of the personality. For instance, frequent cutting episodes might indicate significant aggression directed at the self and poor impulse control. Such forms of acting out are a means of discharging uncomfortable emotional states. The treatment frame will involve parameters to limit such acting out with the double goal of protecting the patient and of making the uncomfortable emotional states more available for psychological exploration.

Moral Values/Superego Function

Finally, one needs to determine the level of the patient's internal *moral system*. Patients with PDs generally present with a continuum from, at best, rigidity in moral functioning, to a complete lack of moral principles. Increasing levels of antisocial traits (indicated by unremorseful lying, stealing, or assault) are associated with the need for more structure in the treatment frame and have a poorer prognosis; in some cases, antisocial personality disorder may be a contraindication to therapy.

Communication of Diagnosis, Treatment Contracting, and the Therapeutic Frame

Communication of the Diagnosis

It is increasingly clear that good clinical practice includes a discussion of the diagnostic impression with the patient.[14,16,36] It is both clinically beneficial and ethical to tell the patient one's findings, discuss the various treatment options, and finally obtain informed consent for the treatment.

The discussion of diagnosis establishes a common understanding that the treatment of a PD includes a focus on psychological exploration. A description of BPD in layman's terms can both simplify what can be a confusing concept and serve to remove any stigma attached to the terms. It may be helpful to describe that BPD involves difficulties in four areas: (1) intense and rapidly shifting emotions; (2) conflictual and unstable interpersonal relations; (3) the discharge or avoidance of emotions by means of acting-out behaviors; and (4) an underlying problem in one's sense of self. One exception to full discussion of diagnosis may be for some narcissistic patients who might have a particularly negative reaction to the widely stigmatized term "narcissistic." Nonetheless, even in this case, it is important to relate the symptoms and functional problems the patient is experiencing to the patient's psychological processes. For example, in speaking with a patient with narcissistic personality disorder whose presenting symptom is depression, the therapist might say: "Your depression may be related to the impact of an extreme and rigid image of what you should be or would have to be to feel at all good about yourself." This lays the groundwork for a shared understanding between patient and therapist that the cause of the patient's problems is driven by the structure of their personality.

After giving the diagnosis and putting it into the context of the patient's current difficulties, the therapist should discuss the various possible treatment approaches, such as mentalization-based Therapy (MBT), cognitive behavioral therapy (CBT) for PDs, dialectical behavior therapy (DBT), Schemas Therapy (ST), or good psychiatric management (GPM). Review Chapters 5 and 6 for more information about these treatments.

TFP is a challenging treatment but is believed to offer the possibility of the most significant change in the patient's subjective sense of self and level of functioning.[36] Studies have established the evidence base for TFP (see Box 8.1, p. 218) as a treatment that helps both with the symptoms of BPD and with the psychological processes of reflective function, attachment security, and coherence of the patient's narrative.[23,24,32] While these studies involved cases that went on for a year, in clinical practice TFP usually extends to longer periods.

The Treatment Contracting and the Therapeutic Frame

If TFP is the agreed-upon approach, the treatment can progress to the contracting phase where the frame of the therapy is established and various expectations and contingencies are agreed upon. In order to be able to do the work of therapy, both patient and therapist need a viable working environment. This environment is established by setting up the treatment contract that follows the discussion of diagnosis.[14,34,37] Patient and therapist agree to the basic conditions of treatment and to how they will address any patient behaviors, such as self-harm, eating disorders, or substance abuse, that pose obstacles to carrying out the treatment. The basic conditions include regular session times, consistent attendance, and adherence to an exploratory model of treatment. TFP was developed as a twice-weekly individual therapy. Certain healthcare systems limit the session frequency to once-weekly, and research is being planned to study this frequency.

With regard to the conduct of therapy, the patient's role is to say whatever comes to mind that may have some bearing on current problems as these relate to the core problems that brought the patient to treatment. The therapist's role is to listen and interpret in ways that might help further understanding. An additional implicit role of the therapist is to tolerate and "contain" the intense affects that emerge from the patients. This part of the therapist's role involves management of countertransference reactions, which will be discussed. It should also be made clear that the therapist's role does not involve giving advice, problem solving, or coaching. This is because we can help the patient grow more and achieve maximal autonomy if we do not fill in for functions that they have the potential to fulfill.

Many patients with severe PDs, such as those with BPD, engage in various forms of acting out. Acting out can be in discreet actions such as self-harm, substance abuse, eating disordered behaviors, unsafe sexual practices, or in more chronic attitudes and behaviors, such as negligence at work. These behaviors have a destructive impact both on the patient's life and on the therapy, in that a focus on crises makes it more difficult to do deeper psychological exploration. The therapist explains that the patient can choose an alternate treatment that would address crises as they occur and take the form of case management, or the patient can choose the type of therapy offered by TFP that involves the effort to understand the underlying factors that contribute to those behaviors and to the patient's inability to achieve satisfaction in life. Agreeing upon a plan about how these behaviors will be addressed during the contracting phase can help avoid having these behaviors intrude into the therapy, and generally leads to a decrease in and eventual end to these behaviors. For example, a crisis plan might be that a patient who is worried about acting on suicidal thoughts should call 911 or go to the emergency department.[6,14,38]

An underlying concept is that the therapist provides therapy but not emergency interventions, which are provided by other parts of the psychiatric system. If encouraged to access emergency services if needed, most patients find that they have a measure of control that may be surprising. In addition, acting-out behaviors often diminish when the therapist is not directly involved in dealing with them. Finally, the careful agreement about the conditions of treatment is seen as part of building the therapeutic alliance.[38]

Patients with PDs often have difficulty remaining in treatment, especially if the work of psychotherapy challenges their standard ways of thinking and behaving, as TFP often does. An agreement about what the patient will do in response to experiencing distress helps limit the patient's turning to acting-out behaviors to manage or discharge the distress. Once the contract is established and the treatment has begun, if the patient deviates from the treatment frame established by the contract, the therapist brings this to the patient's attention and explores what they might learn from the deviation. For example, how might a patient who is regularly late for sessions be managed? With one patient, that behavior might represent ambivalence about being in therapy, and the treatment would benefit from discussion of that ambivalence rather than continuing to express it in action. In another case, the patient may be enacting an internal dyad in which the caretaker is seen as neglectful and the lateness may unconsciously create a scenario to see if the therapist will address the lateness or will react in the anticipated negligent way. This is an example of a deviation from the frame, an enactment of part of the patient's personality structure—the experience of self as neglected. Discussion of such deviations from the frame can advance understanding of the patient's internal world. In rare cases, a patient's repeated deviations from the treatment conditions make it impossible to carry out the therapy. The therapist points out that the patient is not allowing the work to be done and, if the situation continues, the therapy will need to end due to patient non-adherence.

An important part of the contract particular to TFP is that the patient is required to have some sort of meaningful structured activity (e.g., studies, volunteer work, or employment) and social engagements outside of the therapy. This is important for several reasons. To use the language of behavioral therapy, this helps leverage "behavioral activation," increasing the patient's engagement in the world, challenging the patient's assumptions, and providing a testing ground for insights gained in therapy. Furthermore, this requirement addresses, head-on, the patient's difficulties and conflicts about making long-term investments throughout life. This part of the contract is in keeping with establishing clear goals of therapy.[34] The goal of increasing understanding alone is not sufficient for a successful treatment, since TFP is also geared to help patients improve their functioning and satisfaction in life. Therefore, the patient is asked to bring something specific, such as being able to hold a job or establish an intimate relation to the therapy. Eventual achievement of these concrete personal goals would be the external manifestation of deeper psychological change in the form of identity consolidation.

Therapy Strategies, Tactics, and Techniques

The TFP manuals[14,34] organize the use of psychodynamic ideas by guiding the therapist to think at three levels when carrying out therapy: strategies, tactics, and techniques.

Strategies

The overarching strategy of TFP is to help the patient change from a split internal world to an integrated one with a consolidated identity that involves complex, coherent, realistic experiences of self and others that allow for a stable life with the capacity for healthy interpersonal relationships. This change begins by exploring the transference and is generalized to other relationships in the patient's life. To achieve this overall strategy, the therapist must learn to think in terms of the more specific strategies involved in the process. These include: (1) identifying, or naming, the internal dyad guiding the patient's experience of the therapist at any given moment; (2) helping the patient see that, in an unconscious way, the patient identifies with the object representation within the dyad as well as the self-representation; and (3) helping the patient become simultaneously aware of the emotional extremes which are experienced sequentially without being able to connect them.

The first specific strategy listed is to *name the dyad*. This involves reflecting on the experience in the session in order to understand and increase the patient's awareness of the internal representations of self and other that emerge in the relation to the therapist, as in other relations, and help the patient reflect on these experiences. It is important for the therapist to both "name the actors" and describe the affect associated with the experience. For example, "It seems as though when I don't respond immediately after you say something, you begin to feel a combination of disappointment and anger. One possibility behind these feelings is an idea that I'm neglectful and haven't been paying attention to you. In that case, you experience me as a 'pretend caretaker' who doesn't really care for you, and you experience yourself as a person suffering from my neglect and my lack of genuine concern."

The second specific strategy is to be alert to *role reversals within the dyad*. This helps the patient begin to see parts of themselves that they tend to project and only see in others. The phenomenon of role reversals was previously described in the example of the student's experience of and behavior toward his professor. Bringing attention to role reversals is an important way of helping the patient become aware of, and then manage and integrate, parts of the patient's internal world that are split off from awareness in the "paranoid-schizoid" organization. Most typically, the patient is not aware of aggressive affects, as these are felt to be unacceptable as part of the self and are generally projected onto others. Helping a patient gain awareness of their feelings does not make him or her a "bad" person, as the patient fears. Instead, it helps the patient integrate the aggressive feelings, an innate part of the human psyche but which the patient found unacceptable because, in the split psychological organization, the experience of *any* aggressive feelings would make the patient feel *totally* aggressive and bad. This way of thinking implies that one is either *all good* or *all bad*, a frame of mind that does not correspond to the reality of human life or the world. Splitting creates endless difficulty in adapting to the world. This attitude was expressed by a young woman patient who said, "I'd rather be dead than think I have *anything* in common with that abusive father of mine." This intolerance of any inkling of her aggressive feelings, which in her mind would make her *totally* aggressive, made it difficult to for her to accept any angry or aggressive feelings that might fall within the range of average human experience.

It is interesting that a patient can act out aggression, toward self or others, without any conscience awareness of the aggression. For example, a patient described throwing books at her husband because he forgot her birthday. In telling this story, she spoke of her husband as the "bad one" and described her throwing the books as her defending herself against his lack of love; she could not see any aggression in her actions. An analogous situation came up in therapy when the same patient told her therapist that she had come to session with a gun in her purse. When the therapist, attending to safety concerns, told her that guns were not allowed in his office, the patient became enraged that the therapist did not trust her enough to realize that she made up the story. She did not see any aggression in her making up the gun story in the first place; nor did she recognize herself as threating to use the gun on herself or him. The therapist's task was to tactfully bring to her attention her aggressive and angry emotions and to help her realize that her aggressive feelings are a normal part of human experience; the problem is not feeling angry or aggressive, but rather it can be a problem if one acts aggressively or destructively. At one point, the therapist said; "If you have these feelings without being aware of them, they control you. However, if you are aware of them, you can control your angry feelings."

The third specific strategy of TFP is to bring the patient's awareness to the radically different and extreme ways in which they can experience the same person, including the therapist. That is, this strategy is to directly address the internal split. The goal is to help the patient understand what motivates and maintains this separation of extreme feeling states. For example, a patient told his therapist in one session that she was the best therapist on earth and that he was lucky to have her. The next week, he called her stupid, dishonest, and corrupt. Patients in whom splitting is a primary defense mechanism experience each one of these states without remembering the other. What the patient feels in the moment *is his reality*. The therapist, acting as historian of the relationship and offering an invitation to reflect on an apparent contradiction (also called a confrontation), wondered with the patient about how to understand these two vastly different and opposing feelings states. Work at this level takes time, since the patient is likely to say "I was an idiot when I thought you were a good therapist." However, the therapist can help the patient understand two things: (1) it is very difficult and painful to accept that the therapist the patient sees as so perfectly good also has flaws and imperfections; and (2) it is difficult to acknowledge any aggression the patient feels; when negative aggressive feelings arise, it can feel better to project the emotion and see all the "badness" in the other. These insights and integration of self and other representations correspond to a shift from the paranoid-schizoid position to the depressive position.

Early on in the course of therapy, affects may be especially intense as patients are prone to splitting and sometimes engage in idealization/devaluation or experience paranoid feelings in relation to the therapist. It is important to explore these affects. In other words, the initial transference may be quite extreme, and the patient may experience the transference as the only possible reality. For example, if the therapist looks at the clock, the patient might think it can *only* mean that he does not like her and wants to get rid of her. However, application of techniques that will be described can lead to putting the patient's powerful affective experience of the therapist into words, helping the patient reflect on initial "automatic" reactions that may be distorted by internal representations.

Tactics

Review the "Treatment Contracting and the Therapeutic Frame" section for many tactics commonly used in TFP. As the treatment moves forward, additional tactics are used by the therapist to help the patient prioritize the most important material when multiple themes or issues are present in a session.

Techniques

Monitoring the Patient's Communications

How does the therapist fully understand what "actors" are involved in the current therapeutic interaction? The therapist does this by monitoring three levels, or channels, of informational communication. While TFP is indeed a "talk therapy," in addition to the verbal mode of communication, TFP prioritizes and utilizes two other forms of patient communication: (1) the patient's nonverbal behaviors and attitudes, and (2) countertransference (the therapist's internal emotional response to the patient). Observing nonverbal communication, including the patient's body language, facial expressions, and actions, can reveal a great deal about the patient. Since the patient's underlying psychological structure is split, different parts of the patient's internal experience may be expressed by the different channels of communication. Is their affect congruent with the content of what they are saying? For example, a patient may be saying that he is having thoughts of killing himself while looking at the therapist with a provocative smile; a patient may be saying that a situation with a boyfriend does not concern her in the least while clenching her fists and speaking with a rising tension.

In order to fully appreciate what is going on in the patient's mind, the therapist must be attuned to all three levels of communication and their own experience in the session to get a sense of what internal representations are activated in session. This is where therapeutic neutrality and countertransference come into play.

Therapeutic Neutrality

Therapeutic neutrality is a frame of mind that the therapist adopts when listening to the patient and feeling their experiences in session. It should be emphasized that, before entering into any interpretative work per se, the therapist must be able to contain the intense affects that the patient may bring to the session; that is, experience the patient's affects without avoiding them or overtly reacting. Therapeutic neutrality helps in this effort. Neutrality is not a matter of the therapist striving to be a blank slate or coldly aloof. Rather, the therapist should stay out of the fray of whatever operant dyad the patient has activated while recognizing the as-if quality of the transference.

It is especially important that the therapist remain neutral in relation to the components of the internal conflicts the patient is experiencing. The therapist does not take sides with one part of the psychological conflict, and instead needs to stay neutral toward both sides of a currently activated dyad. For example, a patient was experiencing a conflict between one side of her mind which was pressuring her to stay in school while the other side of her mind was rebelling against this pressure. One way patients escape from this kind of internal conflict is to project one part of the conflict onto another person. This patient did this by seeing the pressure to stay in school as coming from her therapist rather than from within herself. In this example, if the therapist had sided with one part of the patient's internal conflict by saying "You should stay in school" or sided with the other side of the conflict ("You should leave school if that would make you feel better"), the therapist would have participated in the externalization of an internal psychological conflict. The therapist taking sides in any way diminishes the possibility of the patient resolving the conflict within herself.

While the TFP therapist generally maintains a position of therapeutic neutrality, neutrality may need to be temporarily set aside when an emergency cannot be resolved through understanding and interpretation. Should a therapist have to temporarily suspend neutrality during a crisis, once the crisis is over, neutrality can be restored to enable exploration of the meaning and need for this temporary deviation.

Countertransference

Countertransference, or how the therapist experiences himself in relation to the patient, helps the therapist understand the patient's self and other representations which are communicated via the dyad activated in session. The simplest form of countertransference is *concordant countertransference*,[39] in which the therapist is in empathy with what the patient is consciously feeling (e.g., the patient and therapist both feel sorrow). The second, more complex, form of countertransference is *complementary countertransference* (e.g., the patient and therapist feel opposite emotions). This corresponds to the defense mechanism of projective identification. In projective identification, the patient manages to subtly provoke feelings in the therapist that the patient may be unable to accept in himself and attempts to control the therapist's behavior as a way to manage his own feelings. For example, a patient who is not comfortable with aggressive feelings may repeatedly frustrate the therapist in ways which provoke countertransference anger in the therapist. The patient, "sensing" the therapist's anger, asks "Are you angry with me?" In this case, the therapist can become aware of the projected unconscious angry part of the patient's internal world that, at the moment, is beyond the patient's awareness. The therapist can then use this countertransference information to help the patient understand her defenses against feeling her own anger. The therapist should become aware of and monitor their countertransference in parallel with the other modes of communication. In this way, countertransference can be used to understand the patient's internal world of self and object representations and can minimize countertherapeutic enactments with the patient. Countertransference can be helpful in augmenting the therapist's understanding and guiding interventions, but is not typically directly communicated to the patient. To extend the simple example above, the therapist would not say "I'm angry" but rather suggest "There does seem to be something going on involving anger here. It might help to think about where it's coming from," and then go on to review the interaction and how the patient's actions might have a provocative quality related to anger.

Clarification, Confrontation, and Interpretations

How do we interpret to create meaning in TFP? Generally, we do not do this as a declaration or pronouncement of understanding. We use a process of increasing the patient's awareness and understanding of their mind by repeated application of the three steps: clarification, confrontation, and interpretation. In the process of TFP, these steps can overlap and complement one another.

Clarification involves asking the patient to fill in any gaps of information, clarify precisely what the patient is saying, or clear up any miscommunications or incomplete understandings. It is a request for clarification from the patient rather than the therapist offering the patient clarification. It is a way to assess the extent and limitations of the patient's awareness and is intended to help the patient clarify their own ambiguities or intentions. Confusing or missing information is frequently found in discourse with patients who have not yet achieved an integrated identity. For instance, gaps in a patient's narrative may serve to maintain a certain role in a dyad or avoid what would be painful awareness of the identification with the other side of the dyad. The patient who felt her throwing books at her husband was solely an expression of her feeling unloved, was denying that her action was aggressive. Asking this patient to clarify her reasons for throwing books may permit her to recognize her anger.

Confrontation goes beyond clarification by asking the patient about what seem to be contradictions or inconsistencies in what the patient is presenting, whether in verbal or nonverbal behavior. Confrontation is not a hostile challenge to the patient. Rather it is an invitation for the patient, presented by the therapist with curiosity and interest, to reflect on an inconsistency in the patient's thoughts, feelings, and behaviors, and to see what can be learned from this. The information obtained from clarification and confrontation supplies the material for interpretation.

An interpretation takes what one has learned from clarifications and confrontation and combines this information with our understanding of mental processes and defenses. Interpretations present the patient with a hypothesis of the meaning, explanation, motivation, or reason for a particular experience or behavior. This may result in the patient gaining an incremental insight about something confusing or unconscious, or may provide an opportunity to derive the meaning of a symptom or an acting-out behavior. A useful guide to interpretation is to focus on interpreting what is affectively dominant at the moment, as this will likely be most salient and explain more of the patient's experience.[14,34] In addition, it is generally most effective to work from surface-to-depth; for example, identifying the actor in the dyad or a defense being used before interpreting the emotion or impulse being defended against. An interpretation that includes reference to a patient's nonverbal communication and the therapist's countertransference (anger in this case) might be: "You seem very anxious and fearful, as though I could be, or am, threatening to you in some way. I wonder if part of your anxiety has to do with concern about your possible angry feelings that are scary to think about or experience."

Transference Analysis

Consistent transference analysis is a core aspect of TFP treatment. This is the most significant challenge to therapists who tend to focus on the content of the patient's verbal communication rather than on the patient–therapist interaction. The emphasis on transference analysis is based on the idea that an individual's personality pathology and structure will emerge more in the *way* the patient is interacting with the therapist than from the content of *what* they are saying. For example, a man in his late 60s presented for help with chronic depression and suicidal ideation. Even though he had all the apparent elements of a successful career, family, and life, his depression continued for years during a prior supportive psychodynamic therapy and medication trials. In initiating TFP, the therapist's diagnostic impression was of narcissistic personality disorder at a borderline level of psychological organization. After the establishment of the treatment frame, the patient began, as instructed, to say what came to mind. In the first three therapy sessions, the patient's discourse consisted of telling stories about his "exotic" upbringing in another country. The therapist noted that her countertransference was to feel entertained. She also realized that, based on what the patient was saying, she had no idea that the patient was struggling with any psychiatric problems. With this in mind, she intervened at the level of transference analysis by saying: "I'm wondering about something. You've come here because of serious problems with depression and suicidal thoughts, and yet what you're telling me seems very far from these issues. I'm wondering how we can understand this." In reflecting together, the therapist helped the patient realized that his "default position" was to feel the need to entertain others because of a deep-seated and unconscious belief, based on a dyad, that no one would be interested in him for "who he is." This exploration led to the typical work with a narcissistic-borderline level patient of getting to know his core sense of self as inadequate and defective, and seeing how the patient attempts to avoid this feeling by promoting a "pumped up" image of himself. Work had to be done to help him integrate these split images of himself, integrating his inflated, demanding, and ideal self-image with an image of himself as inadequate and not worthy of interest. Integrating these split images to a healthier view of himself allowed him to ultimately accept himself as human, with abilities and imperfections.

With ongoing transference analysis, therapy evolves as the patient changes.[14,34] A patient such as this narcissistic man can move from the paranoid-schizoid position to the depressive position and develop a more realistic understanding of the rich complexity and limitations of himself and others. He may use more mature defenses, have a greater ability to regulate his affect, and ultimately develop a more integrated personality. As therapy progresses, sessions become calmer, allowing for the possibility to explore deeper aspects of the patient's conflicts. Missed opportunities in life or mistakes in the past related to the patient's earlier pathology are reflected upon and mourned in a way that allows the patient to deal with regrets and move forward. The change to a more integrated identity is accompanied by symptom improvement, a more realistically positive sense of self and others, and a new ability to build a better more functional life.

Brief Clinical Case

Ann, a 30-year-old single woman, sought help for: (1) recurrent depressive mood with suicidal ideation; (2) periodic self-injury in the form of cutting; (3) a history of substance abuse, including heroin, with current periodic alcohol and cocaine abuse; (4) difficulty finding a relation that would lead to marriage and family; and (5) low work functioning in relation to her level of intelligence and potential.

Ann grew up in a socioeconomically deprived family. Her intelligence was recognized in the public school system and, with support from her teachers, she received a scholarship to a good college. She was performing well in college but dropped out after a year. She took various low-level jobs before applying to another college where she was accepted. After a year, she dropped out of college again. She repeated this pattern two more times over the ensuing years. She also had begun therapy twice before in her 20s but dropped out of each treatment after a few months.

At the age of 30, she was employed at a low-level job when she decided to enter therapy.

Ann was involved in a years-long relationship with a boyfriend who did not want to commit to a monogamous relationship, marriage, and family. Staying in this relationship revealed her masochistic dependency.

Dr. T's structural interview led to a diagnosis of mid-range BPD based on the presence of identity diffusion, a predominance of use of primitive defense mechanisms, and a significant degree of self-injury. She did not show the type of intense aggression or antisocial features that would have put her in the low level of the BPD range. Dr. T discussed her diagnosis of BPD, framing his description in layman's terms as he reviewed her difficulties in four areas: (1) she had difficulty with intense and rapidly shifting emotions (life as an "emotional roller coaster"); (2) she had difficulty with relationships, which tended to be chaotic and conflictual; (3) she displayed self-harm that were attempts to deal with overwhelming emotions; (4) and, at the core of the disorder, she lacked a clear and coherent self that would provide a foundation and a sense of order and meaning in life.

Dr. T discussed the goals and conditions of treatment. Ann's goals were: (1) improvement in her mood; (2) stopping self-harming behaviors; (3) sobriety; (4) establishing a more satisfying intimate relationship; and (5) developing a better work experience.

In the contracting phase, the description of patient and therapist roles were discussed. Other elements of the treatment contract that were discussed included: (1) making her best effort to stay in touch with and communicate her difficult emotions rather than discharge them in self-harm; (2) committing to sobriety with the help of a 12-step program; and (3) taking steps to improve her work situation. In relation to work, Ann said she had thoughts of taking evening courses at a community college. They agreed that she would enroll in two evening courses. Dr. T kept the goal of achieving a healthy intimate relationship in mind. However, he did not set up a specific treatment goal of ending her current unsatisfying relationship, since change in the area of intimate relations generally takes place as the patient's self-understanding increases.

The first five months of therapy went generally well. Ann attended sessions and spoke of her difficulties, her wishes, and her frustrations. Ann discussed periodic frustration with Dr. T. She complained at times that he "just sat there" while at other times she told him he was the best therapist she had ever had, and expressed pleasure and satisfaction with what seemed like progress. In essence, she alternated between experiencing him as negligent or as exceptionally helpful, in ways that seemed extreme and contradictory. It emerged that her most frequent experience of herself in the therapy was as "one of Dr. T's patients," with the feeling that he had no genuine interest in her and just "did his job." Another experience of her emerged more clearly when Dr. T felt an intense countertransference pressure to perform well for her, experiencing in his countertransference an intense split off part of herself.

Ann's progress included staying sober with the exception of a couple of slips. The meaning of these slips was explored. It emerged that one motivation for Ann's slips was to elicit Dr. T's response; would he bring up the question of her adherence to attending the 12-step meetings? Would he show concern for her wellbeing? In other words, she anticipated a neglectful response from him. Ann also drank to avoid feeling under pressure in certain situations. In addition to mostly staying sober, another manifestation of her progress was Ann's attending her evening classes. She reported that she was doing well but expressed some frustration that she was not the "star" student in her class.

Five months into the treatment, a crisis arose. Ann began a session by saying "I'm dropping out of school and dropping out of therapy! I'm sick and tired of all this pressure you're putting on me." Dr. T's initial countertransference was to feel like a concerned parent, and he felt the urge to say: "Don't do that. You've been doing well in both areas and you shouldn't give up now." However, he reflected on this countertransference, keeping in mind the concepts of therapeutic neutrality and the frame of treatment. It seemed to him that Ann was externalizing her conflict. She felt an inordinate amount of internal self-pressure which she was experiencing as coming from Dr. T. With this understanding, Dr. T began his intervention by remembering part of the therapy frame, specifically, the discussion of treatment goals. He reminded Ann:

"I'm thinking about your comment that you're sick and tired of the pressure that I'm putting on you. When I look back on our initial discussions about beginning therapy, it seems to me that it was your idea to take the evening courses."

Ann a bit uneasily: "Well . . . Yes . . . ."

Dr. T: "So it's interesting that now you feel that you have to get away from me, and from your classes, to be free of this overwhelming pressure. The question is, where is the pressure coming from? Right now, you feel it's from me. But I wonder if it might come from somewhere in you. As you say, you could leave me and leave school, but I'm not sure you'd get away from the pressure. I suspect you'd begin to feel it again . . . that it's a pressure you place on yourself. Avoiding that pressure could be one reason you've used drugs—to get away from that feeling. So . . . you could leave therapy but, if you are putting pressure on yourself, it might be better to stay here and try to get to know the 'pressure' part of you and figure out what to do with it. This might be a better option than trying to escape pressure by leaving therapy, leaving school, or using drugs."

This interaction helped shed light on a dyad; the relentlessly harsh task-master/judge who can never be satisfied, and the suffering and exhausted victim. Ann's dyad was related to many of her difficulties in life. This awareness helped Ann recognize that the pressure she experienced as external was within her. This allowed her to stay in therapy and to continue to work on this and related problems.

In reviewing this case, we see that what first emerged fully in the therapy was a persecutory part of Ann's internal world that she tended to see or project into others. As the therapy progressed, evidence emerged that revealed the idealized segment of her internal world: it was not enough to be good. Ann lived with the unspoken idea that one can be perfect. Her belief that others "had it all together" in an ideal way was intimately linked to her attacks on and rejection of herself and to her attacks on Dr. T, and others, when she perceived flaws in them. It is important to be aware that the "all good" ideal segment of her internal world was as pathological as the "all bad" persecutory side. The ideal self is pathological because it is unattainable, and as unrealistic as is the "all bad" self-image. Patients with BPD often set out in pursuit of perfection and become depressed and destructive when they fail to achieve it. By the end of Ann's therapy, she realized that she could get satisfaction from her studies and work even if she was not a star. She realized that she could find love with a man who did not pump himself up in a grandiose macho way, but instead offered her a genuine commitment even if he disappointed her at times. The latter awareness helped her leave the relationship in which she was masochistically submitting to a narcissistic man and move on to a mutually gratifying relationship.

Conclusion

TFP offers a unique approach to treating patients with personality disorders. A TFP treatment starts with an assessment of the patient that includes addressing the patient's chief complaint, symptoms, and PD diagnosis, but also assesses the personality structure and determines the patient's level of functioning. The discussion of the treatment contract, or agreement, establishes the therapeutic frame. A certain paradox may be seen in the frame, which allows for the active empowerment of the provider and patient (instead of helplessness) while also setting strict requirements for treatment. The treatment

---

Box 8.2 Resource for Patients, Families, and Clinicians

- The International Society for TFP (ISTFP). http://istfp.org. This website has information about training opportunities and lists TFP resources in many different countries.
- Transference-Focused Psychotherapy-New York (TFP-NY). http://tfpny.com. This website coordinates information about TFP across North America.
- An introductory book: Yeomans FE, Clarkin JC, Kernberg OF. *A Primer on Transference-Focused Psychotherapy for Borderline Patients*. Northvale, NJ: Jason Aronson; 2002

---

frame provides a stable environment to help the provider and patient weather the affective storms and chaotic life of the patient.

With the treatment frame in place, the therapy proceeds to immersion in the patient's experience (engendering the therapist's empathy, reflection, and understanding), with the eventual goal of helping the patient's internal experience evolve from the fragmentation of the "paranoid-schizoid position" to the integrated and coherent identity that characterizes the "depressive position."

Evidence suggests that TFP can lead to structural personality change, including improvements in reflective functioning/mentalization, attachment security, and the coherence of the patient's narrative.[27] This evidence is significant with regard to clinical considerations and also supports the therapy's hypothesized mechanism of action: the shift from an unintegrated to an integrated sense of self and others, and its beneficial impact on affect tolerance and the capacity to reflect.

In addition to its use as a manualized long-term individual therapy, the principles and techniques of TFP can be used separately as tools to inform a wide array of clinical encounters and settings, including general practice, psychopharmacology, consultation-liaison, emergency, and inpatient psychiatry.[6,4,16]

Those tools include: (1) the need to consider a diagnosis of personality disorder or personality disorder traits in assessing patients in all psychiatric settings; (2) the need to establish a clear and adequate treatment frame for all types of clinical situations; and (3) the benefit of understanding every clinical encounter through the lens of the patient's internal experience of self and other as a way of maximizing empathy and effective communication in every clinical encounter. Review resources for patient, families, and clinicians in Box 8.2.

Conflict of Interest/Disclosure: The authors of this chapter have no financial conflicts and nothing to disclose.

References

1. Kernberg OF. Therapeutic implications of transference structures in various personality pathologies. *J Am Psychoanal Assoc*. 2019;67(6):951–986. doi:10.1177/0003065119898190

2. Caligor E, Clarkin JF, Yeomans FE. Transference-focused psychotherapy for borderline and narcissistic personality disorders. In: Kealy D, Ogrodniczuk JS, eds. *Contemporary*

Psychodynamic Psychotherapy. New York, NY: Academic Press; 2019:149–161. doi:10.1016/B978-0-12-813373-6.00010-6

3. Diamond D, Yeomans FE, Kernberg OF, Stern BL. *Transference-focused Psychotherapy for Narcissistic Pathology.* London: Guilford: 2021.

4. Zerbo E, Cohen S, Bielska W, Caligor E. Transference-focused psychotherapy in the general psychiatry residency: a useful and applicable model for residents in acute clinical settings. *Psychodyn Psychiatry.* 2013;41(1):163–181. doi:10.1521/pdps.2013.41.1.163

5. Hersh RG. A psychodynamic approach for the general psychiatrist: using transference-focused psychotherapy principles in acute care settings. *Psychiatr Clin North Am.* 2018;41(2):225–235. doi:10.1016/j.psc.2018.01.006

6. Hersh R. Augmenting psychiatric risk management: practical applications of transference-focused psychotherapy (TFP) principles. *Psychodyn Psychiatry.* 2019;47(4):441–468. doi:10.1521/pdps.2019.47.4.441

7. Kernberg OF, Burnstein ED, Coyne L, Appelbaum A, Horwith L, Voth H. Psychotherapy and psychoanalysis: final report of the Menninger Foundation's psychotherapy research project. *Bull Menninger Clin.* 1972;36:1–275. PMID: 5030799.

8. Joseph B. Transference: the total situation. *Int J Psychoanal.* 1985;66(4):447–454.

9. Kernberg OF. Therapeutic implications of transference structures in various personality pathologies. *J Am Psychoanal Assoc.* 2019;67(6):951–986. doi:10.1177/0003065119898190

10. Høglend P, Bøgwald K-P, Amlo S, et al. Transference interpretations in dynamic psycho-therapy: do they really yield sustained effects? *Am J Psychiatry.* 2008;165(6):763–771. doi:10.1176/appi.ajp.2008.07061028

11. Clarkin JF, Cain NM, Lenzenweger MF. Advances in transference-focused psychotherapy derived from the study of borderline personality disorder: clinical insights with a focus on mechanism. *Curr Opin Psychol.* 2018;21:80–85. doi:10.1016/j.copsyc.2017.09.008

12. Klein M. Notes on some schizoid mechanisms. *Int J Psychoanal.*1946;27:99–110.

13. Fairbairn WRD. Synopsis of an object-relations theory of the personality. *Int J Psychoanal.* 1963;44(2):224–225.

14. Yeomans FE, Clarkin JF, Kernberg OF. *Transference-focused Psychotherapy for Borderline Personality Disorder: A Clinical Guide.* Washington, DC: American Psychiatric Publishing; 2015:xv, 411.

15. Piaget, J. *The Construction of Reality in the Child.* Cook M, trans. New York, NY: Basic Books; 1954.

16. Hersh R, Caligor E, Yeomans F. Transference-focused psychotherapy (TFP) principles in work with the families of patients with severe personality disorders. In: Hersh RG, Caligor E, Yeomans, FE, eds. *Fundamentals of Transference Focused Psychotherapy.* Cham, Switzerland: Springer; 2016:91–120. doi:10.1007/978-3-319-44091-0_4.

17. Kernberg OF. *Severe Personality Disorders: Psychotherapeutic Strategies.* New Haven, CT: Yale University Press; 1986:xiv, 381.

18. *Diagnostic and Statistical Manual of Mental Disorders.* 3rd ed. Washington DC: American Psychiatric Association; 1980.

19. American Psychiatric Association. *Diagnostic and Statistical Manual of Mental Disorders.* 3rd ed., rev. Washington DC: American Psychiatric Association; 1987.

20. *Diagnostic and Statistical Manual of Mental Disorders.* 4th ed. Washington DC: American Psychiatric Association; 1994.

21. *Diagnostic and Statistical Manual of Mental Disorders.* 4th ed, rev. Washington DC: American Psychiatric Association; 2000.

22. *Diagnostic and Statistical Manual of Mental Disorders.* 5th ed. Washington DC: American Psychiatric Association; 2013.

23. Clarkin JF, Levy KN, Lenzenweger MF, Kernberg OF. Evaluating three treatments for borderline personality disorder: a multiwave study. *Am J Psychiatry.* 2007;164(6):922–928. doi:10.1176/ajp.2007.164.6.922

24. Doering S, Hörz S, Rentrop M, et al. Transference-focused psychotherapy v. treatment by community psychotherapists for borderline personality disorder: randomised controlled trial. *Br J Psychiatry.* 2010;196(5):389–395. doi:10.1192/bjp.bp.109.070177

25. Giesen-Bloo J, van Dyck R, Spinhoven P, et al. Outpatient psychotherapy for borderline personality disorder: randomized trial of schema-focused therapy vs. transference-focused psychotherapy. *Arch Gen Psychiatry.* 2006; 63(6):649–658. doi: 10.1001/archpsyc.63.6.649

26. Clarkin JF, Foelsch PA, Levy KN, Hull JW, Delaney JC, Kernberg OF. The development of a psychodynamic treatment for patients with borderline personality disorders: A preliminary study of behavioral change. *J Person Disord.* 2001;15: 487–495. doi: 10.1521/pedi.15.6.487.19190

27. Clarkin JF, & Levy KN. A psychodynamic treatment for severe personality disorders: Issues in treatment development. *Psychoanal Inq.* 2003;23(2):248–267. doi: 10.1080/07351692309349033

28. Cuevas P, Camacho J, Mejia R, Rosario I, Parres R, Mendoza J, López D. Cambios en la psicopatologia del trastorno limitrofe de la personalidad, en los pacientes tratados con la psicoterapia psicodinamica. *Salud Mental.* 2000;23(6):1–11.

29. López D, Cuevas P, Gomez A, Mendoza J. Psicoterapia focalizada en la transferencia parael trastorno limite de la personalidad. Un estudio per el pacientes femininas. *Salud Mental* 2004;27(4):44–54.

30. Fischer-Kern M, Doering S, Taubner S, et al. Transference-focused psychotherapy for borderline personality disorder: change in reflective function. *Br J Psychiatry.* 2015;207:173–174. doi: 10.1192/bjp.bp.113.143842

31. Levy KN, Diamond D, Clarkin JF, Kernberg OF. Changes in attachment, reflective function, and object representation in transference focused psychotherapy for borderline personality disorder. *J Consult Clin Psychol.* 2006 Dec;74(6):1027–1040. doi:10.1037/0022-006X.74.6.1027

32. Levy KN, Meehan KB, Kelly KM, et al. Change in attachment patterns and reflective function in a randomized control trial of transference-focused psychotherapy for borderline personality disorder. *J Consult Clin Psychol.* 2006;74(6):1027–1040. doi:10.1037/0022-006X.74.6.1027

33. Perez D, Vago D, Pan H, et al. Frontolimbic neural circuit changes in emotional processing and inhibitory control associated with clinical improvement following transference-focused psychotherapy in borderline personality disorder. *Psychiatry Clin Neurosci.* 2015;70:51–61. doi:10.1111/pcn.12357

34. Caligor E, Kernberg OF, Clarkin JF, Yeomans FE. *Psychodynamic Therapy for Personality Pathology: Treating Self and Interpersonal Functioning.* Washington DC: American Psychiatric Association Publishing; 2018.

35. Kernberg OF. *Treatment of Severe Personality Disorders: Resolution of Aggression and Recovery of Eroticism*. Washington DC: American Psychiatric Association Publishing; 2018.

36. Gunderson JG, Fruzzetti A, Unruh B, Choi-Kain L. Competing theories of borderline personality disorder. *J Pers Disord*. 2018;32(2):148–167. doi:10.1521/pedi.2018.32.2.148

37. Radcliffe J, Yeomans F. Transference-focused psychotherapy for patients with personality disorders: overview and case example with a focus on the use of contracting. *Br J Psychother*. 2019;35(1):4–23. doi:10.1111/bjp.12421

38. Yeomans FE, Gutfreund J, Selzer MA, Clarkin JF, Hull JW, Smith TE. Factors related to dropouts by borderline patients: treatment contract and therapeutic alliance. *J Psychother Pract Res*.1994;3(1):16–24. PMID: 22700170.

39. Racker H. The meanings and uses of countertransference. *Psychoanal Q*. 1957;26:303–357.

9

Mentalization-based Treatment

Robert P. Drozek and Jonathan T. Henry

Key Points

- *Mentalization* refers to the fundamental psychological capacity to "read," access, and reflect on mental states (e.g., thoughts, emotions, desires, attitudes) in oneself and other people.
- Personality disorders can be understood in terms of global and context-dependent deficits in the person's ability to mentalize.
- Mentalization-based Treatment (MBT) is an evidence-based treatment for borderline personality disorder, with emerging research supporting its utility for antisocial personality disorder and adolescent self-injury.
- As a treatment, MBT works to strengthen patients' ability to initiate and maintain mentalizing under circumstances of emotional and interpersonal stress.
- MBT's therapeutic stance is active, inquisitive, and non-authoritative; techniques include empathic validation, elaboration of affect, careful sharing of one's own perspective, and exploration of interpersonal patterns in the therapeutic relationship.

Introduction

Mentalization-based treatment (MBT) is a leading psychosocial treatment for personality disorders (PDs).[1] MBT is second only to dialectical behavior therapy (DBT) in empirical support for treating borderline personality disorder (BPD),[2,3] with research supporting its utility in treating patients with antisocial personality disorder (ASPD) as well.[4] The term "mentalization" refers to the fundamental psychological capacity to "read," access, and reflect on mental states (e.g., thoughts, emotions, desires, beliefs, attitudes) in oneself and other people. As a psychotherapeutic treatment, MBT works to strengthen patients' ability to initiate and maintain mentalizing under circumstances of emotional and interpersonal stress, resulting in increased stability in patients' emotions, relationships, behaviors, and overall sense of self.[5]

The construct of mentalization was originally formulated by Peter Fonagy in psychoanalytic terms in 1989.[6] Fonagy then collaborated with Anthony Bateman to manualize and research MBT in the United Kingdom in the 1990s, publishing the first randomized controlled trial in 1999.[7] Since that time, MBT has emerged as a widely used treatment for PDs, with expanded applications in the treatment of trauma, eating disorders, depression, substance use disorders, and psychosis.[5] In this chapter, we review MBT's theory of PDs, as well as the broad principles and techniques employed in the treatment. We close with a detailed case example illustrating MBT's therapeutic strategies.

Mentalization and Personality Disorders

MBT conceptualizes PDs in terms of global and context-dependent disruptions in the capacity to mentalize, that is, to reflect in a flexible and adaptive way on mental states in oneself and others. To understand the shape of these disruptions in patients with PDs, it is important to consider what *healthy* mentalizing looks like, outside the context of psychopathology. Construed most broadly, mentalization can be oriented toward ourselves and toward other people. Within that dimension, mentalizing tends to focus on three basic areas: the *content* of mental states (the "what"); the *context* of mental states (the "why"); and the *process* of how we relate to those states (the "how"; see Box 9.1).

When we are mentalizing about content, we are interested in the "what" of the mind: the specific thoughts, beliefs, emotions, needs, desires, feelings, attitudes, self-concepts, values, and personality traits that are continuously unfolding inside of ourselves and other people. When mentalizing about context, we move beyond considering "what" people are feeling to reflect on the *relationship* between those mental states and other facets of experience: history, current life circumstances, behaviors, and other psychological processes. Mentalizing can also be approached from the perspective of *process,* that is, *how* the person relates to those different facets of mind: flexibly versus rigidly, psychologically versus concretely, and authentically versus disconnectedly.

Box 9.1 What Does Good Mentalizing Look Like?

Content (the "what")
- Observing and accessing mental states in ourselves: our own thoughts, emotions, desires, beliefs, and attitudes
- "Reading" and considering mental states in others: other people's thoughts, emotions, desires, beliefs, and attitudes

Context (the "why")
- Reflecting on the reciprocal relationship between mental states and various contextual factors in ourselves and others: history; current situation; other psychological processes (e.g., other thoughts, emotions, desires, etc.); specific behaviors; and broader interpersonal patterns

Process (the "how")
- Flexible and tentative consideration of mental states in ourselves and others
- Internal, psychologically elaborated reflection on experience
- Curious, engaged experience of our own mental states
- Attentive, empathic experience of others' mental states

Synthesizing aspects of attachment theory, psychoanalysis, and contemporary developmental psychology, MBT suggests that the capacity to mentalize develops within the context of attachment relationships in which caregivers are optimally attuned to the emotional experiences of the developing child.[8] When caregivers mirror the child's emotional states, that mirroring corresponds sufficiently with the child's primary affects, while also clearly referring to the *child's* emotions, rather than simply expressing the caregivers' own feelings at the time. As these mirroring processes are internalized by the child, the child acquires the capacity to mentally *represent* their own subjective states, which serves as the foundation for the development of a sense of self: "Unconsciously and pervasively, with her behavior the caregiver ascribes a mental state to the child that is ultimately perceived by the child and internalized, permitting the development of a core sense of mental selfhood."[8(p286)]

When the caregiver is unable to adaptively mirror the child's emotional states (e.g., if mirroring does not cohere with the child's primary emotions, or if there is insufficient distinction between the caregiver's emotions and the child's emotions), the child internalizes an image of the *caregiver's* emotions rather than their own, never developing the robust capacity to represent their own subjective states. These processes serve as the precursors for the development of PDs (see Box 9.2). Especially in emotionally intense attachment relationships, individuals with PDs can struggle to "hold onto" their ability to mentalize. They can become confused and overwhelmed by their own feeling states, and they can ignore or misread the mind states of others. They can fail to understand what might be leading them to feel what they are feeling, or to recognize their own role in contributing to the interpersonal processes that make them feel so distressed. And they can alternate between rigid and concrete forms of thinking (what MBT refers to as "psychic equivalence" and "teleological" modes, respectively) and dissociated, emotionally disconnected forms of experience (which MBT calls "pretend" mode).[1]

These problems with mentalizing take a unique shape depending on the personality disorder in question. In BPD, patients can struggle to understand and reflect on their own minds, leading them to be excessively focused on *other people's* minds in order to feel like they have a full sense of existence. Patients with BPD are often rigidly invested in the idea that they are "bad" or "worthless," and they are vulnerable to reflexively assuming that others are victimizing them or treating them cruelly. In ASPD, patients tend to experience the world in more concrete and "visible" terms, exhibiting less curiosity about their own feelings and desires. While these patients can accurately perceive

---

Box 9.2 Mentalization and Personality Disorders

- Healthy mentalizing involves attentiveness to three domains: content (the "what"); context (the "why"); and process (the "how).
- The capacity to mentalize develops within the context of attachment relationships in which caregivers are optimally attuned to the emotional experiences of the developing child.
- PDs can be understood in terms of global and context-dependent deficits in a person's ability to mentalize.
- Specific PDs are associated with characteristic difficulties in the domains of mentalizing.

other people's mind states, they struggle to empathize with others, especially when focused on attaining some tangible or power-oriented goal. In narcissistic personality disorder (NPD), patients rigidly endorse particular valued self-concepts, basing their sense of self-esteem on "extrinsic" factors such as success, attractiveness, and other people's positive opinions of them. They can struggle with accessing and representing more vulnerable subjective states in themselves (e.g., insecurity, shame, desires for attention), also often disregarding and dismissing other people's independent viewpoints and desires.[9]

Evidence for Mentalization-based Treatment

MBT is second only to DBT in the robustness of its evidence base for personality disorder treatment.[3] The first randomized controlled trial of MBT allocated 38 patients with BPD to either 18 months of partial hospitalization or treatment as usual.[7] The partial hospitalization involved once weekly individual MBT, thrice weekly MBT group therapy, once weekly psychodrama group, and a weekly community meeting. Treatment as usual involved outpatient psychiatry visits, with inpatient and partial hospitalization as necessary but without formal ongoing psychotherapy. The results were dramatic, with significant reductions in suicide attempts and self-injury, improved depressive symptoms, fewer inpatient hospitalization days, and better social and interpersonal functioning for patients receiving MBT. Subsequent follow-up eight years after randomization revealed lasting improvements in suicidality, rates of remission from BPD symptomatology, time spent in other psychiatric treatment, psychiatric polypharmacy, global function, and vocational status.[10]

In a subsequent study, 134 patients with BPD were randomly allocated to either outpatient MBT or structured clinical management, an active control condition.[11] Outpatient MBT consisted of once weekly individual MBT and once weekly group MBT for 18 months; structured clinical management also offered individual and group therapy but focused on case management, advocacy support, and problem solving. Both groups showed considerable improvement in the composite outcome of suicidal behavior, severe self-injury, and hospitalization. However, the MBT group showed a greater magnitude of improvement at the end of the treatment period. Eight years after randomization, a significantly higher proportion of patients receiving MBT remained free of suicide attempts, self-injury, and psychiatric hospitalization, although only 66 percent of the MBT participants and 56 percent of the control group could be contacted at year eight, limiting the strength of this evidence.[12] Subgroup analysis demonstrated that patients with BPD and comorbid ASPD benefited from MBT as well, demonstrating reductions in measures of anger, hostility, and paranoia.[4]

MBT was adapted for an adolescent population (MBT-A), which involved one year of once weekly individual and once monthly family therapy.[13] Study authors randomized 80 adolescents with a history of self-harm to either MBT-A or treatment as usual, a nonmanualized condition whereby patients were referred to qualified community providers for individual counseling, family therapy, and/or medication management. Once again, MBT reduced occurrences of self-harm as well as severity of depressive symptoms compared to the control group. Statistical analysis revealed that the benefit of MBT was likely mediated by improved mentalizing and reduced attachment avoidance.

Other randomized trials of MBT for the treatment of BPD have faced challenges. One study comparing outpatient MBT to supportive psychotherapy found improvement in both groups but few differences between treatments; notably, the study did not include systematic adherence monitoring.[14] Another study adapting MBT for eating disorders (MBT-ED) in patients with BPD symptoms suffered high dropout.[15] A multi-site randomized trial for BPD found MBT in a day hospital setting was not superior to specialist treatment as usual; however, both treatments were effective, and MBT was delivered by newly set-up services while specialist treatment as usual was delivered by well-established services.[16] One randomized study adding MBT to concurrent treatment of BPD and substance use disorder treatment found no significant outcome differences, but most of the therapists did not show sufficient adherence to MBT.[17] Adding a primarily group-based MBT intervention (MBT-G) for adolescents with BPD symptoms to treatment as usual did not demonstrate significant differences between treatments.[18] Overall, trials indicate that MBT improves BPD-related outcomes. Whether or not differences are detected between MBT and control groups may in part depend on the degree to which control groups implement other evidence-based BPD treatments, as specialist BPD treatments may be similarly effective.[3]

The Cochrane collaboration recently reviewed the efficacy of psychosocial treatments for BPD, including seven randomized trials of MBT.[3] The authors conclude that despite methodologic flaws in some studies, MBT is likely effective at reducing suicidality, self-harm, and depressive symptoms in patients with BPD (Level of Evidence = 2). Further research is needed to assess MBT's efficacy in treating ASPD[4] and its promise in treating symptoms of NPD.[9] See Box 9.3 for a summary of the evidence for MBT.

Box 9.3 Evidence for Mentalization-based Treatment

- Meta-analysis: 7 RCT[3] Level B
- RTC: partial hospitalization versus treatment as usual.[7] Level A
- RCT: outpatient MBT or structured clinical management, an active control condition.[11] Level A
- RCT: 8-year follow-up[11] limited response rate.[12] Level B
- RCT: MBT-Adolescence: MBT versus treatment as usual. Weekly individual and monthly family.[13] Level A
- RCT: MBT versus supportive psychotherapy.[14] Level B
- RCT: MBT-Eating Disorders and BPD symptoms.[15]
- RCT: MBT for BPD versus specialist treatment (equivalent) Day Hospital.[16]
- RCT: MBT for antisocial personality disorder. Level C
- Opinion: MBT for narcissistic personality disorder. Level C

Key: Levels of Evidence; Strength of recommendation taxonomy (SORT)*
Level of Evidence A: Good quality patient-oriented evidence.
Level of Evidence B: Limited quality patient-oriented evidence
Level of Evidence C: Based on consensus, usual practice, opinion, disease-oriented evidence, or case series for studies of diagnosis.
*Ebell MH, Siwek J, Weiss BD, Woolf SH, Susman J, Ewigman B, Bowman M. Simplifying the language of evidence to improve patient care. *J Fam Pract.* 2004 Feb 1;53(2):111–120.

Indications for Treatment

MBT is an effective treatment for patients with BPD, especially patients with depression, suicidality, self-injurious behavior, frequent inpatient hospitalizations, and significant challenges with social, interpersonal, and vocational functioning.[7,10,11] MBT may be useful for individuals with BPD and more severe psychopathology, for example patients who meet diagnostic criteria for multiple PDs and a greater number of other psychiatric diagnoses.[19] In particular, MBT might benefit patients with comorbid BPD and ASPD, including those who struggle with anger issues, hostility, paranoia, self-harm, and suicidality.[4] In addition, MBT has efficacy for adolescents who struggle with depressed mood and self-harming behaviors.[13]

Existing research includes both men and women, suggesting that MBT is helpful for both genders. Given MBT's low dropout rates ranging from 2 percent to 15 percent, it could be a good fit for patients who struggle with treatment adherence and follow-through.[20] MBT developers Bateman and Fonagy have recently suggested, "At a clinical level, patients with marked interpersonal problems who have a personality disorder rooted in mentalizing vulnerability and attachment problems may benefit from MBT."[20(p2901)] (See Box 9.4 for a summary of the indications for MBT.)

Box 9.4 Indications for Mentalization-based Treatment

- MBT is an evidence-based treatment for borderline personality disorder, including patients with depression, suicidality, self-injurious behavior, frequent inpatient hospitalizations, and significant challenges in social, interpersonal, and vocational functioning.
- MBT is more effective than treatment-as-usual for patients with more severe psychopathology, including patients with comorbid borderline and antisocial PDs.
- MBT has utility for both men and women.
- MBT is possibly helpful for adolescents with depression and self-injury, as well as patients who struggle with treatment adherence.

Treatment Approach

MBT has been implemented in partial hospitalization programs,[7,21,22] outpatient treatment,[4,11,19] and group-based protocols.[23-25] On an outpatient basis, individual MBT is often delivered in conjunction with group MBT, although the model allows for a flexible adaptation to a variety of therapeutic contexts, including stand-alone individual therapy in outpatient psychiatry clinics or in the private practice setting. Here we will review the structure, therapeutic stance, and clinical techniques involved in the provision of individual MBT to patients with PDs. This will illustrate MBT's fundamental therapeutic principles, which tend to cut across diverse delivery formats (see Box 9.5, p. 243).

Box 9.5 Therapeutic Approach of MBT

Structure and format
- Diagnosis-giving
- Informed consent
- Safety-planning
- Collaborative development of a written MBT formulation, including problem areas and goals for treatment

Therapeutic stance
- "Not-knowing"
- Active structuring of sessions
- Management of patients' arousal

Clinical interventions
- Content-based (e.g., empathic validation, clarification, affect elaboration)
- Context-based (e.g., contextualization of affect)
- Process-based (e.g., identifying areas of non-mentalizing, attempting to stimulate mentalizing and deeper reflection)

Mentalizing the therapeutic relationship
- Directing the session focus toward the relational issue
- Affect elaboration and empathic validation of the patient's experience
- Therapist assumption of responsibility
- Addressing problems in mentalizing
- Inviting reflection on new understanding

Structure and Format of the Treatment

The treatment begins by therapists assessing for and delivering the diagnosis of personality disorder, and then discussing with patients how these challenges are understood and addressed from a mentalizing viewpoint. The evidence base for MBT is reviewed, and patients make an informed decision about whether they would like to proceed into a structured treatment. If so, therapists work with patients to complete important preparatory work common to many therapies for PDs: developing a safety plan, identifying potential barriers to treatment, and considering strategies to address these challenges when they arise. In more formal MBT, patients attend the 8–12 session introductory psycho-educational group known as MBT-I, where the key constructs of mentalizing and PDs are introduced to patients in a group format.[1] In an outpatient or private practice setting, therapists can coordinate with ancillary treaters (e.g., psychopharmacologist, case manager, group therapist) to discuss the plan to initiate MBT and to prepare for continuity and comprehensiveness of care throughout the course of the treatment.

With these introductory steps completed, the treatment proceeds into the more explicit "mentalizing" phase, where therapist and patient collaborate to develop a written "mentalization-based formulation" of the patient's strengths and challenges in mentalizing. This formulation includes general information included in most psychosocial assessments (e.g., functional challenges, goals for treatment, descriptions of important relationships), with a specific emphasis on patients' unique difficulties with mentalizing, and especially how those difficulties play out in their relationships with others. The aim of the formulation is to provide something of a "snapshot" of the therapist's understanding of the patient at the outset of the treatment, in a humble and non-authoritative manner that is consistent with the spirit of MBT (see the section, Therapeutic Stance). The therapist revises the formulation based on the patient's feedback, ultimately working toward a collaborative agreement about the goals for treatment. Treatment proceeds by focusing on the problem areas identified in the formulation, with therapist and patient working together to address these areas through a shared focus on mentalization.

There is no single formula for MBT formulations, and there is significant variability in the shape these formulations take across different MBT therapists and across different patients. While formulations can be written in either third- or second-person (e.g., "he/she/they" vs. "you"), they tend to be written to and *for* the patient, avoiding extensive jargon and using the patient's own language as much as possible. Employing the description reviewed earlier, we have found it useful to focus on strengths and weaknesses in mentalizing in the areas of content, context, and process. A sample MBT formulation for a patient named Lucas, whose treatment we will discuss in greater detail later in the chapter, illustrates this approach.

Mentalization-based Formulation of Lucas

Lucas is a 35-year-old man entering individual therapy to address difficulties with emotional instability, low self-esteem, and feelings of insecurity and jealousy in his relationship with his wife. Lucas struggles with intense worry that his wife is either going to abandon him or be unfaithful to him; he becomes highly emotional, requests constant reassurances from his wife that she will never leave him, and on one occasion, read her text messages without permission. This has resulted in significant interpersonal conflict with his wife, after which Lucas will fantasize about suicide is order to calm himself. Lucas' goal is to improve stability in his marriage, which he understands will require him to learn how to improve his self-esteem, reduce his insecurity, and manage his jealousy without trying to control his wife.

Mentalizing Strengths
When not beset by jealous feelings, Lucas appears adept at "reading" the emotional states of others, and he often experiences significant empathy for friends, family members, and others with whom he is not romantically involved. He is acutely aware of issues of power and control when he observes the interactions of others. He easily accesses and names his own feelings of jealousy and anger when triggered, as well as joy and pleasure in the absence of triggers.

Triggers for Emotional Dysregulation
Lucas reports intense jealousy when imagining that his wife has even thought about another man. He notes these feelings and behaviors have reliably occurred in his prior

romantic relationships. Since childhood, he has felt extremely uncomfortable whenever he is alone, signaling long-standing insecure attachments. He experiences feelings of abandonment during the brief periods of his adult life when he is not in a romantic relationship, resolving only with the next romance.

Challenges with Mentalizing

Content of Mentalizing. In moments of emotional intensity, Lucas can become extremely confused about what he is feeling, struggling to "put words on" his different emotional states. He is quick to assume that his wife does not love him anymore, finding it difficult to remember and trust those moments when she expresses her feelings of commitment to him.

Context of Mentalizing. Lucas is not easily able to determine the antecedents of emotional dysregulation; as he understands it, feelings of jealousy seem to occur "out of nowhere," making them difficult to anticipate and manage.

Process of Mentalizing. Lucas often rigidly believes his wife is being unfaithful to him, despite limited evidence. Conversely, he can become very focused on scant evidence, believing strongly, for example, that his wife wants to sleep with a male coworker simply because she is having a conversation with him. In these moments of jealousy, Lucas often struggles to empathize with his wife's emotions and desires, especially her potential feelings of discomfort in response to his suspicious and controlling behaviors.

Implications for the Present Treatment

If Lucas becomes emotionally invested in the therapy, he may begin to fear that the therapist is going to reject or abandon him, quietly gathering evidence to support this belief. This has apparently played out in past treatment relationships, leading Lucas to preemptively terminate therapy in order to avoid potential abandonment. Therefore, it will be important for Lucas and his therapist to preemptively address these challenges, with Lucas working to communicate his concerns as they arise, and the therapist explicitly inquiring about how Lucas is feeling if he appears to be more anxious or withdrawn.

Therapeutic Stance

MBT's therapeutic approach has been referred to as the "not-knowing" stance: "a sense that mental states are opaque, and that the therapist can have no more idea of what is in the patient's mind than the patient and, in fact, probably will have a lot less."[1(p186)] From the perspective of MBT, it is impossible to ever fully know the contents of another person's mind, or even the contents of one's own mind. This leads to a position of relative humility, where therapists eschew "interpretations" and authoritative declarations about the meaning and content of patients' experiences. Instead, therapists approach the therapeutic interaction with a sense of curiosity and tentativeness, attempting to stimulate a process of mutual reflection in which both parties are seeking to understand mental states (e.g., thoughts, emotions, desires) in themselves and the other person. MBT practitioners avoid definitive and confident language about mental states (*"You clearly feel . . ."*; *"The reason why you did this is . . ."*), instead asking questions about patients' experiences (*"How did you end up feeling when you learned you did not get the job?"*; *"What do you think was so upsetting to you in that interaction?"*), and offering marked qualifications about their own ideas and impressions (*"It sounds like that made you feel . . ."*; *"I am gathering that . . ."*; *"From my perspective . . ."*; *"I am wondering if . . ."*).

MBT's therapeutic stance is also highly active, existing somewhere "midway" between cognitive-behavioral therapy and traditional psychoanalysis. Whereas therapists working psychodynamically are often less "active" in their clinical approach (e.g., allowing extended silences, rarely setting agendas for sessions, offering interpretations and observations largely in response to patients' material), MBT therapists are more active and engaged in their therapeutic approach: asking open- and closed-ended questions (*"What was that like for you, when your boyfriend started criticizing you?"; "In the past, I know that you felt quite insecure at work . . . could any of that be coming up for you now?"*); directing attention to specific aspects of patients' narratives (*"Could we go back for a moment, and could you tell me a bit more about how that argument with your mother unfolded?"*); and structuring sessions based on patients' formulations and treatment goals (*"What would you like to put on the agenda today?"; "Personally, I have been curious about where things stand with your urges to self-injure, and I was wondering if we could check-in on that"*). However, whereas cognitive-behavioral therapists are active in their provision of didactic content (e.g., highlighting cognitive distortions, teaching skills to address problem areas, assigning homework), MBT therapists are primarily active from an exploratory standpoint, that is, by doggedly directing therapeutic attention to the topic of mental states in self and others.

MBT therapists are also especially attentive to patients' degree of emotional activation in the present moment. The MBT model proposes that, for patients with PDs, the ability to mentalize is inversely related to their level of affective arousal.[26] Therapists work to help patients remain at something of a "sweet spot" of emotional intensity: emotionally activated enough to be engaged in the interaction, but not so excited or overwhelmed that it becomes too challenging for them to hold on to their reflective capacities. MBT practitioners are thus continuously monitoring patients' emotional states, in relation to the narrative content under discussion but also in response to the therapists' own participation in the therapeutic dialogue. As patients start to move into more intense emotional terrain, therapists are prepared to employ a range of strategies to "cool things down" in the interchange. These include empathic validation (*"I think it is really understandable this would all be so upsetting to you. You were really looking forward to spending the weekend with your wife, and you had no idea her brother was going to visit"*), which helps patients to feel more "seen" by the therapist; asking more cognitively oriented questions (*"What do you make of her comment to you in that discussion?"*), which allows patients to temporarily shift focus away from the emotionally charged content; and assuming responsibility for one's own role in the patient's emotional disruption (*"I'm worried that I came across as a bit critical back there, and I really didn't mean to . . ."*), which helps patients feel less blamed and criticized by the therapist. In all of these ways, MBT therapists work to titrate patients' level of emotional arousal, creating an interpersonal climate that is optimally conducive to adaptive mentalizing.

Clinical Interventions

Individual MBT sessions start with the therapist collaboratively working with patients to "set an agenda" for the session, based on patients' broader treatment goals as well as recent events or issues that are occupying the patient. As patients discuss these topics, therapists have one primary task: to ask questions and make comments in order to stimulate patients' mentalization, that is, their capacity to reflect on mental states in a flexible, authentic, and adaptive manner. MBT therapists attempt to tailor their interventions to patients' mentalizing abilities in the present moment, without allowing their own mentalizing to "outpace" patients' current levels of reflection. To do this most effectively, therapists tend to approach the therapeutic dialogue in somewhat of a stepwise manner: first helping patients to represent the *content* of mental states in themselves and others; then working with patients to elaborate the *context* of these states; and finally attempting to address any challenges in the *process* of mentalizing that have emerged through the therapeutic dialogue. We will consider these steps in turn.

Content-based Interventions

Content-based interventions include empathic validation, clarification, and affect elaboration. These interventions help patients to increasingly identify and represent "what" they are feeling, which over time leads to an increased sense of identity and self-coherence: who they are as people, and what really matters to them. *Empathic validation* refers to the therapist's marked, contingent, and supportive reflection of the patients' experiences. Whenever patients are speaking, they are giving voice to some experience of themselves and others. Rather than try to evaluate, comment on, or change that impression, MBT therapists attempt to "put words on" their own understanding of how patients experience their worlds. This validation is *marked* in that it maintains a distinction between the therapist's mind and the patient's mind (*"It sounds like you were feeling . . ."*). It is *contingent* in that it attempts to "match" or "correspond" to the patient's subjective impression in the present moment (*"You see him as a really bad person, and you don't want to have anything to do with him anymore"*). And it is *supportive* in that it affirms that it is reasonable and understandable for the patient to experience the situation in this particular way (*"No wonder this was so devastating for you. You thought this relationship was going to last forever"*). If patients themselves are explicitly articulating their emotions as they speak, MBT therapists tend to include the affects in question in their empathic reflections (*"You seem to feel quite angry with him, but also a little bit hurt"*). However, when patients are more cognitively or externally focused in their narratives, therapists still begin by reflecting these narratives as expressed (*"You really disagree with her"*; *"You suspect that he has a lot of psychiatric issues, and he really needs treatment"*), proceeding to employ affect elaboration techniques in order to help patients' further represent their own emotional states in these scenarios.

Clarification involves requesting information about the external details or "facts" of a situation, from the patient's perspective (*"What did you actually say to your mother in that text you sent her?"*; *"Could you take me back to that morning when you ended up cutting . . . what did you do when you woke up that day?"*). Because the instability associated with PDs is so influenced by environmental factors, all of MBT's more "advanced" technical strategies (e.g., affect elaboration, affect contextualization, process-oriented techniques) are predicated on therapists and patients having a clear picture of the relational and situational contexts in which patients' challenges unfold. *Affect elaboration* is a broad family of strategies employed to help patients represent, expand, and deepen their experience of their emotional states. This involves explicitly asking about patients' emotions and desires (*"What do you think you were feeling in that conversation?"*; *"Do you have a sense of how you are wanting your mother to respond to you?"*); inviting further elaboration of previously expressed emotional states (*"Could you say more about this feeling of sadness?"*; *"What was that like for you, to be so angry at your friend?"*); trying to expand the range of patients' emotions (*"What else came up for you when he said that to you?"*;

"In addition to being angry with her, are you in touch with anything you might be wanting from her right now?"); and encouraging reflection about patients' sense of self and identity (*"When you received that feedback, how did that make you feel about yourself?"*; *"You mentioned 'hating yourself' in that moment . . . could you say more about that feeling?"*).

These content-based interventions gradually allow patients to express a broader range of experiences in the therapeutic dialogue, inspiring a more diverse and nuanced set of emotions and desires, a clearer picture of their own actions and interpersonal patterns, and a more comprehensive picture of their environments, relationships, and interactions with others. Once all of these processes are "on the table," MBT therapists can employ *context-based* interventions.

Context-based Interventions

Context-based interventions are techniques geared toward stimulating patients' reflection about the relationship between their mental states and the broader context of their experiences. Examples include inviting patients to reflect on the relationship between their mental states and the environmental/interpersonal factors elicited through clarification (*"You mentioned you have been feeling more anxious and irritable, now that you are about to start working again. How do you understand the connection between these things?"*); to consider the possible connection between different emotions elicited through emotional elaboration (*"When he did not text you back, you initially felt quite afraid, but then you quickly became angry at him. What is your sense of that shift?"*); and to regard the link between these emotions and patients' subsequent behavior patterns (*"So it sounds like you felt quite hurt by your father's comment, and then you got really quiet and stopped talking to him. How did the hurt lead to the withdrawal?"*). These techniques are organized in what MBT calls a "mentalizing functional analysis," which is especially useful in exploring patients' challenges with maladaptive behavior patterns, including self-injury and interpersonal conflict.[1(pp227–233)] As patients are able to mentalize in these ways, they begin to experience a greater sense of agency in their lives: they enjoy a sense of continuity across time; understand how they influence and are influenced by their environments; and are able to increasingly recognize and regulate their own emotions and behaviors in their relationships.

Process-based Interventions

As therapists implement these techniques, they will begin to notice patients' forms of non-mentalizing discussed earlier: rigid thinking (e.g., *"I am worthless and unlovable"*; *"He is a bad person and just wants to harm me"*; *"Your opinion of me determines my value"*); concrete thinking (*"I need to take this action in order to feel better"*; *"If you do not relate to me in a certain way, that means you do not care about me"*; *"My value depends on my possession of specific visible factors: attractiveness, success, effective performance, etc."*); and psychological disconnection (e.g., intellectualization, dissociation from one's emotions, lack of interest in others' minds, decreased empathy). These processes often overlap with challenges in mentalizing identified in patients' mentalization-based formulations we have discussed, and so patients will already have some level of awareness of these processes and how they relate to their personal goals for treatment.

In response to patients' difficulties with rigidity and concreteness, therapists begin by empathically validating the experience in question (*"So when he did not text you back, it felt completely devastating to you: He clearly does not love you anymore"*). Therapists invite patients to reflect on their process of arriving at that perspective (*"Help me understand how you got there, that your boyfriend no longer loves you"*), also exploring the impact of these forms of stuckness on patients (*"What did that do to you, to believe that this relationship was finally over?"*). Throughout these explorations, therapists intentionally avoid "challenging" patients' viewpoints at the level of verbal content. However, as patients consider their *relationship* to their own perspectives (e.g., how they arrived at the perspective, how their certainty impacts them), they implicitly start to relate to their experience as a mental state, rather than a veridical reflection of "reality."

At some point in these discussions, patients often give voice to some more nuanced representation of their experience. Therapists privately "hold onto" these moments, returning to them at a later stage of the discussion to gently invite further elaboration (*"Earlier you mentioned, 'Perhaps I was over-reacting to all of this.' What were you getting at that there?"*). Once patients have elaborated a broader range of their own feelings and viewpoints about a situation, therapists are also free to share their own perspective, albeit in a marked and tentative way that does not assert any special authority about "the truth" of the situation (*"I know you are quite confident that he was trying to send you a message by not texting you back, but I just keep wondering if there could be other things going on for him"*; *"You've mentioned in the past that you can sometimes feel a bit sensitive to criticism . . . could that ever be relevant to this situation at all?"*). The aim of all of these interventions is not to "correct" the patient's viewpoint by bringing it into alignment with some predetermined vision of reality, but rather "to enhance the patient's mentalizing by broadening the patient's perspectives on an event."[20(p2900)] As patients are able to reflect more broadly within the sessions, these forms of reflection tend to generalize to emotionally charged experiences outside of sessions, resulting in the various forms of functional improvement (e.g., increased emotional stability, decreased suicidality and self-injury, improved vocational functioning) demonstrated in the research on MBT.[12]

Different therapeutic strategies are employed when patients are more *disconnected* from themselves and others. Rather than encouraging more "reflection" and "consideration" in these moments, MBT therapists work to help patients access their own emotions more fully, while also reckoning with the reality of mental states in other people. Along these lines, techniques include shifting the focus away from abstractions to something more specific and reality-based (*"This sounds really important. Could you share about a recent example of this?"*); asking questions about patients' emotional states in the present moment (*"Could you try to put words on what emotions you are feeling right now, as you are sitting here in this office?"*; *"Could you look inward a bit here: What do you think you are most wanting from me right now, as we talk about this situation?"*); and explicitly "naming" the form of disconnection patients are exhibiting (*"You seem to be 'in your head' quite a bit today, and it is difficult for me to get a clear sense of what you are feeling"*; *"You are talking a lot about your wife's daily activities, but you don't seem to be focusing much on her emotional states"*).

When these more cautious methods have proven ineffective, MBT recommends employing a *challenge*, understood as a surprising, irreverent, often provocative comment that has the effect of "waking patients up" to more authentically access their own emotional states, or to consider the mental states of the therapist. As an intervention, challenge is somewhat difficult to prescribe, since the most effective challenges are conducted in a manner that is unique to the relationship in question.[1(pp257-269)] All therapeutic dyads have characteristic relational processes that are unfolding continuously, which are usually only implicit and unarticulated in customary interactions: therapist and patient say typical things to each other; speak in a certain tone of voice; hold a specific body posture; and so on. Challenges tend to transgress or violate these implicit norms, in a manner that is surprising and mildly disruptive for the patient without being cruel or traumatic.

Consider, for example, a patient who talks extensively about feeling irritated toward others, rejecting the therapist's regular attempts to inquire about how *other people* might be feeling in these situations: "Why do I care how they're feeling?" Especially stymied and exasperated one day, the therapist responded, "Sometimes I wonder if they think you're kind of being a jerk to them." This stopped the patient in his tracks: "Wait, why would they think that *I* was being the jerk?" The therapist countered, "That's a very good question. What do you think about that?" This led the patient to start considering this reflexive tendency to dismiss and reject the perspectives of others, a long-standing pattern that had caused significant interpersonal disruptions in his life. This example illustrates the central characteristics of a challenge: an unexpected communication (e.g., the therapist's mildly aggressive perspective) that violates an implicit relational norm (e.g., of the therapist encouraging the patient to consider others' perspectives), which briefly "shocks" the patient into authentically considering the mind states of themselves or others (e.g., the therapist's opinion that the patient might be playing a role in her or his own interpersonal challenges), thus opening up the pathways for reflective consideration of the topic in question.

Mentalizing the Therapeutic Relationship

For patients with PDs, the ability to mentalize is indirectly related to the activation of their attachment systems. When PD patients are emotionally aroused, or when they feel like they are at risk for rejection or criticism from others, they tend to experience the challenges with mentalizing (e.g., rigidity, concreteness, disconnection) that precipitate their functional challenges. This point informs the foundational importance of the therapeutic relationship in MBT. Because this relationship inevitably triggers patients' intense emotions and attachment needs, patients' characteristic challenges in mentalizing inevitably manifest themselves and impact the relational processes unfolding between them and their therapists. As patients are able to notice these processes in the here and now, and to adaptively reflect on relevant mental states in themselves and the therapist, they gradually internalize such processes and become able to notice and reflect on them in their interpersonal relationships.

Common indicators for mentalizing the therapeutic relationship include an interpersonal disruption between therapist and patient; a sense of "stuckness" in the therapy; the therapist persistently experiencing some subjective state that is likely relevant to the patient's interpersonal patterns outside of therapy (e.g., feelings of frustration and anger, desire to argue with or "punish" the patient, a sense of boredom or disconnection); the patient explicitly referring to the therapist or the treatment itself; or the appearance of one of the interpersonal patterns identified in the formulation.[1(p277)] While traditional psychodynamic approaches often construe these processes as examples of "transference" and "countertransference" experiences, MBT tends to steer clear of language that blurs the distinction between the past and the present (e.g., transference, enactment) or between the therapist's mind and the patient's mind (e.g., projective identification, countertransference).[1(pp275–276)] Rather, because our primary aim in MBT is to encourage the patient's reflection about mental states, we view these processes as an opportunity for patients to mentalize each person's distinct experience of the current interpersonal process, "to think about the relationship they are in at the current moment."[1(p275)]

The process of mentalizing the relationship in MBT synthesizes many of the principles already outlined in this chapter. The therapist proceeds by actively directing the session focus toward the relational issue in question (*"You mentioned that you have been feeling angry with me since our last appointment. Is that something that we could talk about a bit more?"*); employing affect elaboration techniques to help patients articulate their experience of the situation (*"Could you take me back to that moment and say a bit about what that was like for you?"*; *"What emotions came up for you when I said that?"*; *"Do you have a sense of what you might have been wanting from me at that moment?"*); and utilizing empathic validation techniques to supportively validate patients' experience of the relational issue (*"I see, so not only were you frustrated with me, but you felt hurt by me, like I wasn't really focusing on how hard you have been working in the treatment, and in your life overall"*).

Rather than presume that patients' perceptions of the scenario are determined strictly by their pathology, MBT sees all interpersonal interaction as essentially bidirectional and co-created, in that therapists are always influencing how patients perceive the therapeutic relationship. Once patients' experiences have been sufficiently elaborated and validated, MBT therapists proceed to explicitly assume responsibility for their part in the relational process in question. For example, in the case of the patient who was upset at her therapist for not being sufficiently validating in the previous session, the therapist might say, "Now that we've talked it through a bit, I can understand why you found our last session so upsetting. I think that I was quite focused on exploring your thoughts and feelings in that argument with your boyfriend, but I missed that you were actually feeling quite proud of yourself, and you were wanting me to validate how well you had handled yourself in the argument. It makes a lot of sense that this would have been so hurtful to you, and also why it made you angry."

Usually by this point in the process, some difficulty in mentalizing has emerged in the patients' narratives. Patients might be "missing" an important mental state in themselves or others *(content-related problems)*; they might be failing to consider some relevant aspect of the situation in question *(context-related problems)*; or they could be rigidly attached to a particular viewpoint of themselves or others *(process-related problems)*. Privately taking note of the challenge in mentalizing, therapists proceed to employ the specific interventions that are tailored to the specific mentalizing problem.

In the previous example, the therapist began to suspect that the patient might have been experiencing the therapeutic interaction in an overly concrete or visible fashion. Consistent with MBT's interventions for concrete/teleological thinking (see the section, Clinical Interventions), the therapist invited the patient to share about how she arrived at her perspective.

Therapist: Help me understand how you got there, this sense that I was not appreciating your successes. *[Inviting further elaboration]*

Patient: Of course you weren't proud of me. You never said anything about that. You just kept asking questions about my feelings.

Therapist: I see, so since I didn't explicitly *say* that I was proud of you, and since I was talking about some other thing, it seemed clear to you that I was not impressed with how you handled yourself in the argument. *[Empathic summary of patient's perspective]*

Patient: Well, I guess you could have felt proud but not said it, but that's not the point. You should have been more supportive of me that day.

Therapist: Perhaps you're right, and I'm very open to thinking about that with you. But I don't want to lose something you just said. Even though I didn't say I was proud of you, I might have felt it? *[Inviting reflection about an area of possible nuance]*

Patient: I mean, of course. People don't always say what they're feeling, and I guess I didn't really know what you were thinking.

Therapist: I am really glad that you're noticing this. I should say that I actually felt like I *was* quite impressed with how you handled yourself in the argument. It sounds like you were really able to consider your boyfriend's perspective while holding on to your own viewpoint of the situation, which I know has been challenging for you in the past. At the time, it didn't occur to me to communicate that to you explicitly. To be honest, I don't think I was really aware that you were wanting this from me. *[Sharing the therapist's own feelings and experience of the interaction]*

Patient: Well, I didn't want to actually say anything about it. It's kind of embarrassing to ask for compliments from somebody, especially your therapist. It makes me feel kind of needy, like I'm a child.

In this interchange, after exploring the patient's experience of the relational disruption, the therapist also communicated personal emotions and perceptions of the interaction in question. This is a frequently utilized technique in relational mentalizing, the aim of which is to help patients work toward a more expansive view of the current relationship: to understand how the therapist is experiencing them, to recognize the differences between their perspective and the therapist's perspective, and ultimately "to recognize his/her part in creating those states."[1(p282)]

At this point in the session, the patient had arrived at a broader, more elaborated perspective on the disruption in the treatment relationship: a recognition that the therapist might have had feelings that were not expressed at the time, as well as a recognition that her own self-judgments (i.e., about her desires for attention) might have inhibited her from communicating her wishes to the therapist. The final step of mentalizing the relationship thus involves inviting further reflection on the "new understanding" that has emerged throughout this process.[1(p278–281)] The therapist asks questions aimed at placing this understanding in a broader emotional context for the patient: *"What about expressing your feelings makes you feel like you are being 'needy,' or acting like a child?"*; *"Does this pattern feel relevant to other areas of your life?"*; *"What would have to be different for you to feel like you could express these feelings here?"* By reflecting on these issues from the perspective of their lives more generally, patients gradually construct *meta-representations* of themselves as thinking and feeling agents in interactions with other thinking and feeling agents, which over time can lead to greater reflectiveness and flexibility in interpersonal relationships.

Case Study: Lucas

To illustrate MBT's therapeutic principles, we return to Lucas, the patient who was introduced in the section "Structure and Format of the Treatment." At the outset of treatment, the therapist utilized the approaches we've already outlined: delivering the diagnosis of BPD; providing psycho-education about the diagnosis and treatment through the framework of mentalizing; developing a written safety plan; delivering the MBT formulation; and collaboratively agreeing to commence treatment to address Lucas' difficulties with emotional and interpersonal instability in his relationship with his wife.

Consistent with these goals, the therapist and Lucas directed their attention to Lucas' difficulties with insecurity and jealousy. Utilizing techniques of empathic validation and affect elaboration, the therapist worked with Lucas to develop a shared understanding of his sense of urgency and desperation to preempt infidelity. Clarification revealed that Lucas's wife had never been unfaithful, nor had he experienced this in past relationships. As such, his jealousy defied simple explanation. Employing affect elaboration strategies, the therapist explored with Lucas his broader feelings of insecurity that were generated in his relationship with his wife. Lucas shared his opinion that his wife was in a "different league" from him in terms of attractiveness. He described her as "the most beautiful woman I have ever seen," while he saw himself as "average, at best." He had a good career, and he knew he was intelligent, but he secretly harbored the belief that his wife was only with him out of pity: "I know that she loves me, but I don't really think she is attracted to me. I feel like, once she finds out that she can do better, she is going to leave me." This new recognition helped to explain why Lucas felt so threatened when his wife interacted with other men.

Having gotten a great deal of mental content "on the table," the therapist began to utilize more context-based interventions. Lucas described a recent situation where, on one of their planned date nights, his wife shared she was extremely tired and wanted to go to bed early rather than spend time with him. Lucas responded by becoming angry and storming out of the house, then driving around in his car, crying, and listening to their wedding song on repeat. In session, the therapist worked with Lucas to conduct a "mentalizing functional analysis" of this interaction. Lucas initially viewed his anger as flowing directly from getting "ignored," but he slowly pieced together that indeed he felt hurt and rejected just prior to becoming angry. The therapist invited Lucas to consider the possible relationship between these different feeling states: "How did you go from feeling hurt and rejected to feeling so angry, and then leaving the house?" This led to a period of several sessions where Lucas began to reflect on his tendency to quickly "switch" from his more vulnerable emotional states (e.g., insecurity, hurt, rejection) to these more angry states: "I just can't stand it when I feel like she is rejecting me. I feel powerless and weak, like there is nothing I can do to stop it. But then when I get angry and push her away, I feel like I finally have some control, like I'm not going to lose myself to her." As Lucas recognized these "switch points" in himself, he became increasingly able to slow down when he felt rejected by his wife, and to reflect on a wider range of his emotions (e.g., love, insecurity, fear, anger, desire for closeness), without reflexively jumping to anger and withdrawal in order to make himself feel more stable.

Having gained a greater ability to consider his own feelings in situations of conflict, Lucas began to mentalize his wife as well, and to spontaneously reflect on the impact that his reactiveness was having on her. However, he would still periodically enter sessions rigidly convinced that his wife was not attracted to him and was going to leave him. In these moments, the therapist employed more process-based interventions, focusing on how Lucas transitioned so quickly from feeling safe and connected with his wife to feeling so anxious and mistrustful. Lucas ultimately arrived at a broader perspective about the way that his mentalizing could turn "on and off" under different circumstances: "I think when I am feeling more confident in myself, I am less likely to become suspicious of her. But then when I have had a bad day and I am feeling insecure, I end up getting a lot more paranoid." Lucas began to refer to these paranoid states as his "detective mode," and he and the therapist worked to consider the mental processes involved in this "detective mode": what emotions and circumstances triggered it; how it impacted him as well as his wife; and the ways in which he became narrowly focused on *certain* facts in these moments, and less connected to other aspects of the scenario (e.g., his wife's expressed love for him) that might be equally important.

As Lucas became increasingly able to mentalize in these ways, he reported notable improvements in the problems that led him to seek treatment: decreased feelings of jealousy; fewer arguments with his wife; and an improved ability to spend time by himself without feeling intense panic and anxiety. In session one day, Lucas was describing a recent conversation with his wife about purchasing their first home together. His wife was extremely excited about this, but he was worried about moving forward due to financial concerns. In the midst of this session, Lucas became quiet, withdrawn, and seemingly distracted. The therapist called attention to this shift, and Lucas explained that he was feeling upset by the therapist's questions. Applying techniques involved in "mentalizing the therapeutic relationship," the therapist invited Lucas to share more about these feelings, and what was upsetting him specifically. Lucas expressed that he felt like the therapist was asking lots of questions about his wife's feelings and desires, without showing much interest in how *he* was feeling about their interaction: "Sometimes I feel like you are 'taking her side' whenever we have a fight, that you care more about her than you do about me."

The therapist worked to empathically validate Lucas's experience here, also assuming responsibility for his role in this interchange: "I am really grateful that you are bringing this to my attention, and sharing your feeling here. I think that you are right: I was asking more questions about your wife's feelings than your feelings. I can understand why that would be hurtful to you, and also how you might start to worry that I care more about her experience than yours. I would only add that, from my perspective, I was feeling *quite* interested in hearing about what this was bringing up for you, especially since I know you have been really worried about your finances lately. In terms of my questions about your wife, I know that you have had the goal of 'staying connected' to how your wife is feeling in more heated discussions, so I had thought that was what you were wanting to focus on in this situation."

Lucas felt a bit sheepish in response to this, because he had forgotten that he had set that as his goal: "I just automatically assumed that there was something else behind your questions. I guess that I can sometimes get into 'detective mode' in my relationship with you as well. . . ." This led Lucas and the therapist to start exploring how Lucas's feelings of insecurity and jealousy can manifest themselves in his other relationships: with his coworkers, in his friendships, and in his family relationships.

During these later stages of therapy, Lucas became more consistently able to consider his wife's point of view and to catch himself before going into "detective mode," in his marriage and in his relationships more broadly. Lucas's wife observed significant differences in Lucas's overall level of stability, leading her to feel much closer and more connected to him. Lucas expressed notable changes not just in their relationship, but in his manner of feeling about himself: "I can still get insecure sometimes, but I feel more able to just *talk* about my feelings, without attacking the other person or trying to push them away. I just feel so much more stable in myself now. Like even if the other person rejects me, I'm going to be able to handle it, and it's not going to destroy me. For the first time in my life, I feel like there's some part of me that is not just controlled by other people. It has been a long time coming, and it is a huge relief."

Conclusion

In this chapter, we have offered a broad introduction to the theory, practice, and evidence base of mentalization-based treatment (MBT). We explored the construct of mentalizing, its relevance to PDs, and the specific techniques involved in an MBT treatment. Broadly speaking, MBT works to strengthen the resilience of patients' capacity to reflect on mental states in themselves and others. Throughout the course of the treatment, patients gradually develop an improved ability to "hold onto" their minds in situations of emotional and interpersonal unrest, resulting in improvement in many of the functional challenges prompting them to seek treatment. Over time, this can lead to significant developments in patients' sense of self and identity. Patients increasingly understand what they are feeling and why they are feeling it; they learn to access those feelings in a deeper way; and they gain the ability to flexibly reflect on beliefs states (e.g., about themselves, about others) that have caused them significant pain throughout their lives. At the same time, patients gain an increased ability to understand and empathize with *other people's* mental states, thus opening up new pathways for connection, mutuality, and meaning in their relationships with others. See Box 9.6 for further information about the theory, practice, and training of MBT.

Conflict of Interest/Disclosure: The authors of this chapter have no financial conflicts and nothing to disclose.

Box 9.6 Resources for Patients, Families, and Clinicians

- Anna Freud Centre in London. For comprehensive information about MBT training, supervision, and publications, visit the MBT page of this site. https://www.annafreud.org/training/mentalization-based-treatment-training/.
- Gunderson Personality Disorders Institute at McLean Hospital. Learn about MBT training and online supervision offered in the United States. https://www.mcleanhospital.org/training/gunderson-institute.
- Bateman, A, Fonagy, F. *Mentalization-based Treatment for Personality Disorders: A Practical Guide.* Oxford, UK: Oxford University Press; 2016. For the most comprehensive presentation of the theory and technical principles of MBT, consider purchasing the main MBT treatment manual.
- Anna Freud Centre YouTube channel. View videos illustrating the clinical practice of MBT. https://www.youtube.com/watch?v = OHw2QumRPrQ.

References

1. Bateman A, Fonagy P. *Mentalization-based Treatment for Personality Disorders: A Practical Guide*. Oxford, UK: Oxford University Press; 2016.

2. Oud M, Arntz A, Hermens ML, Verhoef R, Kendall T. Specialized psychotherapies for adults with borderline personality disorder: a systematic review and meta-analysis. *Aust N Z J Psychiatry*. 2018;52(10):949–961.

3. Storebø OJ, Stoffers-Winterling JM, Völlm BA, et al. Psychological therapies for people with borderline personality disorder. *Cochrane Database Syst Rev*. 2020(5). https://doi.org//10.1002/14651858.CD012955.pub2.

4. Bateman A, O'Connell J, Lorenzini N, Gardner T, Fonagy P. A randomised controlled trial of mentalization-based treatment versus structured clinical management for patients with co-morbid borderline personality disorder and antisocial personality disorder. *BMC Psychiatry*. 2016;16:304.

5. Bateman A, Fonagy P, eds. *Handbook of Mentalizing in Mental Health Practice*. 2nd ed. Washington, DC: American Psychiatric Association; 2019.

6. Fonagy P. On tolerating mental states: Theory of mind in borderline personality. *Bulletin of the Anna Freud Centre*. 1989;12(2):91–115.

7. Bateman A, Fonagy P. Effectiveness of partial hospitalization in the treatment of borderline personality disorder: a randomized controlled trial. *Am J Psychiatry*. 1999;156(10):1563–1569.

8. Fonagy P, Gergely G, Jurist EL. *Affect Regulation, Mentalization and the Development of the Self*. London, UK: Routledge; 2018.

9. Drozek RP, Unruh BT. Mentalization-based treatment for pathological narcissism. *J Personal Disord*. 2020;34:177–203.

10. Bateman A, Fonagy P. Eight-year follow-up of patients treated for borderline personality disorder: mentalization-based treatment versus treatment as usual. *Am J Psychiatry*. 2008;165(5):631–638.

11. Bateman A, Fonagy P. Randomized controlled trial of outpatient mentalization-based treatment versus structured clinical management for borderline personality disorder. *Am J Psychiatry*. 2009;166(12):1355–1364.

12. Bateman A, Constantinou MP, Fonagy P, Holzer S. Eight-year prospective follow-up of mentalization-based treatment versus structured clinical management for people with borderline personality disorder. *J Personal Disord*. 2020 Jun.

13. Rossouw TI, Fonagy P. Mentalization-based treatment for self-harm in adolescents: a randomized controlled trial. *J Am Acad Child Adolesc Psychiatry*. 2012;51(12):1304–1313.

14. Jørgensen CR, Freund C, Bøye R, Jordet H, Andersen D, Kjølbye M. Outcome of mentalization-based and supportive psychotherapy in patients with borderline personality disorder: a randomized trial. *Acta Psychiatr Scand*. 2013;127(4):305–317.

15. Robinson P, Hellier J, Barrett B, et al. The NOURISHED randomised controlled trial comparing mentalisation-based treatment for eating disorders (MBT-ED) with specialist supportive clinical management (SSCM-ED) for patients with eating disorders and symptoms of borderline personality disorder. *Trials*. 2016;17(1):549.

16. Laurenssen E, Luyten P, Kikkert MJ, et al. Day hospital mentalization-based treatment versus specialist treatment as usual in patients with borderline personality disorder: randomized controlled trial. *Psychol Med.* 2018;48(15):2522–2529.

17. Philips B, Wennberg P, Konradsson P, Franck J. Mentalization-based treatment for concurrent borderline personality disorder and substance use disorder: a randomized controlled feasibility study. *Eur Addict Res.* 2018;24(1):1–8.

18. Beck E, Bo S, Jørgensen MS, et al. Mentalization-based treatment in groups for adolescents with borderline personality disorder: a randomized controlled trial. *J Child Psychol Psychiatry.* 2020;61(5):594–604.

19. Bateman A, Fonagy P. Impact of clinical severity on outcomes of mentalisation-based treatment for borderline personality disorder. *Br J Psychiatry.* 2013;203(3):221–227.

20. Bateman AW, Fonagy P. Mentalization-based treatment. In: Sadock BJ, Sadock VA, Ruiz P, eds. *Kaplan & Sadock's Comprehensive Textbook of Psychiatry.* 10th ed. Philadelphia, PA: Wolters Kluwer; 2017:2894–2904.

21. Bales DL, Timman R, Andrea H, Busschbach JJ, Verheul R, Kamphuis JH. Effectiveness of day hospital mentalization-based treatment for patients with severe borderline personality disorder: a matched control study. *Clin Psychol Psychother.* 2015;22(5):409–417.

22. Bales D, van Beek N, Smits M, et al. Treatment outcome of 18-month, day hospital mentalization-based treatment (MBT) in patients with severe borderline personality disorder in the Netherlands. *J Personal Disord.* 2012;26(4):568–582.

23. Griffiths H, Duffy F, Duffy L, et al. Efficacy of mentalization-based group therapy for adolescents: the results of a pilot randomised controlled trial. *BMC Psychiatry.* 2019;19(1):167.

24. Bo S, Bateman A, Kongerslev MT. Mentalization-based group therapy for adolescents with avoidant personality disorder: adaptations and findings from a practice-based pilot evaluation. *J Infant Child Adolesc Psychother.* 2019;18(3):249–262.

25. Bo S, Sharp C, Beck E, Pedersen J, Gondan M, Simonsen E. First empirical evaluation of outcomes for mentalization-based group therapy for adolescents with BPD. *Personal Disord.* 2017;8(4):396.

26. Fonagy P, Bateman A. The development of borderline personality disorder—a mentalizing model. *J Personal Disord.* 2008;22(1):4–21.

10
Cognitive-behavioral Therapy

Matthew W. Southward, Stephen A. Semcho, and Shannon Sauer-Zavala

---

Key Points

- Cognitive-behavioral therapy (CBT) for personality disorders is based on the theory that the way people think about stressful situations influences their emotional, behavioral, and physiological responses to those situations.
- There are relatively few randomized controlled trials of CBT for personality disorders, which limits our ability to draw strong conclusions regarding these effects. However, CBT is relatively efficacious, especially for treating symptom clusters that are associated with a variety of personality disorders.
- CBT is a relatively structured, time-limited intervention that involves the completion of between-session skills practice.
- CBT applies cognitive restructuring, the downward arrow technique, behavioral experiments, activity scheduling, imagery, and mindfulness techniques to address difficulties associated with personality disorders.
- Delivered once weekly for up to a year, CBT targets core cognitive schemas of patients with personality disorders that persist beyond acute episodes of psychiatric impairment using cognitive, behavioral, and experiential skills.
- Manual assisted cognitive therapy (MACT) is a six-week, guided, self-help adjunctive treatment that teaches cognitive, behavioral, and relapse prevention strategies for depressive symptoms and self-harming behaviors and substance use.
- The Unified Protocol for Transdiagnostic Treatment of Emotional Disorders (UP) is a 12–16 week treatment that teaches patients pre-specified mindfulness and cognitive skills in addition to emotional exposures to reduce avoidance of emotional experiences.
- CBT, MACT, and the UP are each relatively efficacious in the treatment of some features of several personality disorders.

Theoretical Principles of Cognitive-behavioral Therapy for Personality Disorders

Cognitive-behavioral therapy (CBT) is based on a theory relating events in a person's life, their thoughts stemming from these events, and their further emotional, behavioral, and physiological responses.[1] These factors form the general architecture of cognitive-behavioral theory. In this theory, an event (e.g., a breakup, being fired, or a negative memory) prompts automatic thoughts about oneself, other people, and/or the world at large. These thoughts and interpretations induce or co-occur with emotional reactions, physiological changes, and/or urges to behave in certain ways. Given the accessibility of thoughts to evaluation and manipulation, and their central role in the unfolding of a person's experiences, CBT emphasizes cognitions in the maintenance and treatment of personality disorders. Because personality disorders are characteristic patterns of thinking, feeling, and behaving, CBT is designed to help patients understand and challenge their patterns of thinking to adopt more adaptive behaviors that can help shape both emotions and, with repeated practice, personality itself. CBT includes specific techniques within this architectural framework to address patients' thoughts, behaviors, and emotions. In this chapter, we introduce CBT for personality disorders as a principle-driven treatment based on the CBT theory, including examples of several specific techniques that CBT providers can use with patients with personality disorders. We also review two specific manualized versions of CBT that have been applied to patients with personality disorders.

CBT is a relatively structured, time-limited treatment designed to teach patients skills to challenge maladaptive patterns of thinking and behaving.[1] Common structural components of CBT include: (1) goal-setting at the start of treatment to establish a mutually agreed-upon set of observable goals with clear methods to assess progress on these goals throughout treatment; (2) agenda-setting at the start of each session to establish a mutually agreed-upon set of topics the patient and therapist will explore together during the session; and (3) skill practice by the patient, both in session and between sessions, tailored to the patient's goals in treatment. CBT sessions involve a review of: (1) how the patient used different therapy skills in response to stressors since the previous session; and (2) how the patient is progressing toward her/his goals (e.g., changes in target symptoms, feedback from others on the quality of the patient's relationships, or functional outcomes attained).

CBT applies cognitive and behavioral skills to address maladaptive thinking and actions. Cognitive skills may include cognitive restructuring or reappraisal (e.g., thinking about a stressful situation from multiple perspectives), downward arrow techniques (e.g., unearthing the core belief underlying the initial automatic thought), and imaginal exposures (in which a patient imagines themselves in a difficult situation responding more effectively or taking other perspectives in that situation). Behavioral skills may include behavioral experiments or emotional exposures to test whether an initial negative thought or prediction is true, planning activities more in line with a patient's values, and role-playing exercises to help a patient practice new skills or responses in session. Although these skills form the bedrock of CBT interventions, CBT is a principle-based treatment framework rather than a step-by-step treatment manual. This means that CBT providers may implement techniques drawn from other treatments or traditions to elicit cognitive or behavioral change. These techniques may include mindfulness and acceptance practices, dialogues between a patient and their younger self, and values identification and clarification.

The combination of these techniques may be especially useful for patients with personality disorders after they've recovered from acute psychological distress.[1] Patients without a personality disorder often seek treatment for an episodic experience of psychopathology (e.g., a depressive episode or a heightened period of generalized anxiety). Patients experiencing these episodes of relatively acute distress are often motivated to try many of these primary cognitive and behavioral skills that are, in turn, reinforced by the reductions in their distress that result from using these skills. Patients with personality disorders will likely be similarly motivated to try these skills and see similar benefits. However, even though the acute distress may be resolved using these skills, the longer-standing patterns of maladaptive cognitions and behaviors characteristic of personality disorders remains. Thus, supplementing the traditional repertoire of CBT techniques with those drawn from other traditions, while retaining a focus on targeting maladaptive cognitions and behaviors, may contribute to the efficacy of CBT for personality disorders.

Empirical Evidence for CBT for Personality Disorders

Relatively few randomized controlled trials (RCTs) of CBT for personality disorders have been conducted, limiting our ability to draw strong conclusions regarding its effects. Those that have been conducted provide some evidence that CBT is relatively efficacious for personality disorders.[2] CBT provided over one year to patients with borderline personality disorder (BPD) has been shown to lead to fewer suicide attempts than treatment-as-usual (TAU),[3] as well as less hopelessness, impulsivity, and dropouts as compared to Rogerian supportive counseling.[4] At two-year follow-up, CBT for BPD has also shown longer-term benefits than supportive counseling and TAU, with patients in CBT reporting less anxiety, distress, and fewer dysfunctional cognitions than those in TAU,[3] and lower symptom severity than those in supportive counseling.[4] Similarly, group CBT for avoidant personality disorder (AVPD) that allows patients to practice and receive feedback on their interpersonal behaviors with others, *regardless* of structured skill instruction, has also led to reductions in anxiety, depression, and shyness.[5–7] In contrast, individual CBT for AVPD that incorporates *structured* cognitive and behavioral skill instruction delivered over six months has led to greater reductions in anxiety, behavioral avoidance, and dysfunctional beliefs compared to brief dynamic therapy.[8] CBT for obsessive-compulsive personality disorder (OCPD) delivered weekly for one year has also led to clinically significant reductions in depressive and OCPD symptoms.[9] Some evidence suggests CBT may be more efficacious than interpersonal psychotherapy (IPT) at treating depression for people with AVPD[10,11] or those with more personality disorder features of any type.[12] However CBT may be less efficacious than IPT at treating depression in OCPD.[10] More recent research has failed to replicate both of these effects.[13,14] Finally, CBT for antisocial personality disorder (ASPD) did not demonstrate an advantage in reducing anger, negative beliefs about others, or verbal and physical aggression relative to TAU.[15] See Box 10.1, p. 262 for a summary of the effectiveness of CBT for the treatment of PDs.

Indications for CBT

Many parts of the theory and interventions used by dialectical behavior therapy (DBT) and Schema Therapy (ST) were borrowed from CBT. However, CBT as a stand-alone treatment for personality disorder is relatively less studied than other evidence-based treatments for PDs. CBT for the PDs has no definitive indications or contraindications for the treatment. Manual assisted cognitive therapy (MACT), reviewed in a later section, is weakly indicated for all personality disorders and is

---

Box 10.1 Level of Evidence for the Effectiveness of CBT for Personality Disorders

---

CBT for Personality Disorders

- Eight high-quality RCTs have been conducted. These studies have found mixed evidence that CBT leads to changes in acute distress or personality disorder outcomes. Across all personality disorders, the strength of recommendation for CBT for personality disorders is Level B.
- For BPD and AVPD, the strength of evidence is also Level B.
- For OCPD and ASPD, the strength of evidence is Level C.

Manual Assisted Cognitive Therapy (MACT)

- Three high-quality, but small, RCTs have been conducted. These studies suggest MACT leads to decreases in depressive symptoms and the frequency of self-harming behaviors.
- One larger RCT failed to find a benefit of MACT: Level C.
- The strength of recommendation for MACT for reducing depressive symptoms and the frequency of self-harm behaviors in Cluster B personality disorders with or without comorbid substance use is therefore Level B.

Unified Protocol for Transdiagnostic Treatment of Emotional Disorders (UP)

- Four single-case experimental design studies have been conducted. These studies have consistently reported that the UP leads to reductions of BPD features and, in one study, remission from BPD for the majority of patients. Level B.
- The strength of recommendation for the UP in reducing BPD features is therefore Level B.

Key: Levels of Evidence; Strength of recommendation taxonomy (SORT)*
Level of Evidence A: Good quality patient-oriented evidence.
Level of Evidence B: Limited quality patient-oriented evidence
Level of Evidence C: Based on consensus, usual practice, opinion, disease-oriented evidence, or case series for studies of diagnosis
*Ebell MH, Siwek J, Weiss BD, Woolf SH, Susman J, Ewigman B, Bowman M. Simplifying the language of evidence to improve patient care. *J Fam Pract*. 2004 Feb 1;53(2):111–120.

---

indicated to treat some aspects of self-harm and substance use in patients with BPD. The Unified Protocol for Transdiagnostic Treatment of Emotional Disorders (UP), also reviewed in a later section, is indicated to treat symptoms of BPD and some of the common features associated with many personality disorders including emotional dysregulation, depression, and anxiety. It has not yet been validated as a specific treatment for any particular personality disorder with the exception that it is weakly indicated for avoidant, obsessive-compulsive, and antisocial personality disorders.

CBT Techniques

CBT techniques which can be used when working with patients who have PDs include working with cognitive schemas and conditional assumptions, identifying core beliefs using the downward arrow technique, identifying maladaptive behaviors and devising behavioral experiments, activity scheduling, using imagery, and mindfulness.

Cognitive Schemas and Conditional Assumptions

In a CBT framework, personality disorders develop and are maintained through the activation of core cognitive schemas, a theory shared with schema therapy.[1] Schemas are networks of thoughts, beliefs, expectations, and attitudes about oneself, others, and the world. For example, a schema may revolve around the core belief that "I'm a bad person." This core belief serves as the focal point of the schema, such that all other thoughts, attitudes, and expectations reflect an aspect of the belief or are interpreted in light of it. For instance, a person may endorse conditional assumptions around this core belief such as, "If anyone tries to get to know me, they won't like me," or "If I have any negative thoughts about my children, I'm unfit to be their parent." These assumptions are conditional in that they are predicated on certain situations unfolding (e.g., a person trying to get to know them; having any negative thoughts about one's children). These examples also demonstrate the overgeneralized nature of such conditional assumptions and the pervasive thoughts which are characteristic of personality disorders. Whereas anyone might hold relatively limited conditional assumptions (e.g., "If someone from the opposite political party tries to get to know me, they probably won't like me"), people with personality disorders tend to apply these assumptions regardless of contextual feedback. Because cognitive schemas influence how people interpret the world around them and the likelihood of engaging in different behaviors, one of the first steps in CBT for personality disorders is identifying these schemas.

Clinical Vignette: Cognitive Schema of a Woman with Borderline Personality Disorder

Daniela is a 40-year-old Hispanic woman presenting with BPD. Over the first few sessions, her therapist asks questions to identify and better understand her cognitive schemas.

Therapist: You mentioned having a hard time trusting people. Does that come up with most people or with certain people or certain situations in particular? [clarifying whether this is a core belief or a conditional assumption]

Daniela: At this point in my life, it's most people, even if I think I know them well.

Therapist: I see. When you say "at this point in your life," does that mean this belief is more recent or has it often been true about you? [inquiring about longer-standing patterns of beliefs]

Daniela: It's been true as long as I can remember. I guess I should tell you, I was sexually abused growing.

Therapist: I'm so sorry to hear that, and thank you for telling me. I know it's not always comfortable to bring up experiences like that, especially with someone new. May I ask who perpetuated the abuse? [validating patient's willingness to discuss a difficult subject; inquiring further to understand the abuse]

Daniela: It was a babysitter. My parents didn't do anything about it even after I tried to tell them.

Therapist: Goodness, well I can see how you would have learned to be mistrustful of other people if this abuse was happening to you and your own parents didn't attempt to stop it, despite you telling them it was happening. [clearly making the connection between patient's developmental experience and core belief; normalizing patient's belief in the context of their developmental experience]

When you feel like you can't trust someone, what do you do? [inquiring about the connection between a core belief and maladaptive behaviors]

Daniela: I usually just shut down. I get lightheaded and I can't think straight. I just want the interaction to be over.

Therapist: I hear you. So when you're feeling mistrustful of others, many times you'll feel lightheaded and have a hard time concentrating to the point that you just shut down in the hopes the interaction will end soon. Is that right? [validating by communicating understanding; restating patient's response to ensure therapist's understanding]

Daniela: Yes.

Therapist: I appreciate you walking me through this. I think this really highlights the core beliefs and cognitive schemas we were talking about earlier. Is it fair to say you have a core belief that "Other people cannot be trusted" and that, when this belief is activated around someone else, certain behaviors also get activated like shutting down, feeling lightheaded, and having a hard time focusing?

In this exchange, the therapist identifies and labels the patient's core belief ("other people cannot be trusted"), explores whether this belief is conditional on any particular people, and clearly connects this belief with avoidant or maladaptive behaviors that may be limiting for the patient. Throughout the exchange, the therapist is validating and normalizing the patient's experience and checking in with her to ensure that she/he is correctly understanding the patient. Validating, normalizing, and checking in all contribute to strengthening the therapeutic alliance with the patient by communicating understanding, respect, and trust. This may be particularly helpful with this patient and when working with patients with personality disorders more broadly.

Identifying Core Beliefs: Downward Arrow Technique

A patient's core beliefs can be identified by use of a clinical inquiry called the downward arrow technique. With this technique, providers first identify a patient's automatic thought. Someone with histrionic personality disorder (HPD), for instance, may notice distress around the automatic thought, "The bartender was talking more to my friend than me." A CBT provider would use the downward arrow technique to probe the meaning of this thought for the patient to progressively uncover the patient's core belief. CBT providers use questions such as: "If that thought was true, what would it mean about you?"; "Why does this thought matter to you?"; and "What would happen if this thought was true?" A patient with HPD may respond that this automatic thought means that her/his friend is more attractive or interesting to others. When the therapist probes further, the patient may indicate that having more attractive or interesting friends would mean the patient cannot be the center of attention and that is intolerable. If the therapist probes further with the downward arrow questions and the patient is unable to generate further meanings, this suggests that they may have identified one of the patient's core beliefs.

In a CBT or schema-focused framework, core beliefs are pervasive thoughts a person holds about themselves, other people, or the world more broadly. Core beliefs are relatively independent of the context, unlike conditional assumptions. The patient with HPD expressed the core belief, "It is intolerable not to be the center of attention." If the therapist probed this thought further with a patient with dependent personality disorder (DPD), that patient may express the core belief that "I'm helpless without others' attention and care." If the therapist probed the thought further with a patient with narcissistic personality disorder, this patient may respond with the core belief that "I deserve others' attention." Patients' core beliefs may be more specifically characteristic of their personality disorder (see Table 10.1 for examples). It's important to communicate to patients with personality disorders that all people hold core beliefs. Doing so normalizes patients' experiences and may help them be more open to exploring their beliefs. The CBT provider's goal is to collaboratively explore and address any core beliefs that may be maladaptive for the patient and their goals. Providers may use the examples in Table 10.1 as indicators of core beliefs of patients with specific personality disorder presentations.

Table 10.1. Personality Disorders and Characteristic Core Belief(s)

Personality Disorder	Characteristic Core Belief(s)
Antisocial	Others are there to be exploited. It's not my responsibility if people's feelings get hurt. Don't be a sucker—take what's yours.
Avoidant	I am inadequate. I am defective. I am unlikable. I don't fit in. People don't care about me. People will reject or criticize me.
Borderline	I am inherently unacceptable. My emotional pain will never stop. There will be nobody to care for me. I am bad/evil and deserve punishment.
Dependent	I am incapable. The world is a dangerous place. I'm vulnerable to others' wishes.
Histrionic	I should be the center of attention. It is awful if other people ignore me. I must entertain and impress people.
Narcissistic	I am inferior and alone. I am rare and special. I am different and superior. Others should recognize how special I am.
Obsessive-compulsive	I must avoid mistakes at all costs. There is one right response to each situation. Mistakes are intolerable. Any deviation from what is right is automatically wrong.
Paranoid	Others are out to get me. Everyone only looks out for themselves.
Schizoid	I don't need anyone else. I prefer to be left alone. The world is uncaring.
Schizotypal	I am different, unique, gifted.

Clinical Vignette: Avoidant Personality Disorder

Jackson is a 25-year-old African-American man who meets criteria for AVPD. He raises some distressing thoughts he was having since the previous session.

Jackson: I was going to reach out to friends to hang out this week, but I thought, "What's the point?"

Therapist: I know you've mentioned similar reactions when we've discussed reaching out to friends before. This might be a great situation to use the downward arrow method to see if there are any core beliefs going on behind the scenes of that thought. Would you be willing to work it through with me?

Jackson: Sure.

Therapist: Great. Can you tell me why it's pointless to reach out to friends?

Jackson: Well, they haven't been responding lately, so I don't see why they'd start now.

Therapist: I know there can be many reasons why people don't respond. Are there any reasons that feel particularly true to you when you think about their lack of response?

Jackson: I mean, I don't think they like me. I'm not that great to be around, especially when I'm like this.

Therapist: When these thoughts emerge, do you think there's something about you that makes you not great to be around?

Jackson: I feel like I'm a downer, I'm awkward and don't know what to say, and whenever people start to get close to me, that's when relationships end. I think I'm just fundamentally unlikable.

Therapist: It sounds like that might be the core belief here: "I'm fundamentally unlikable."

The therapist follows up each comment by the patient with questions designed to elicit the meaning behind each of the patient's thoughts. In this case, the therapist focused on what meaning the patient's thoughts had regarding himself, although they may have chosen to focus on the meaning of the patient's thoughts regarding other people's trustworthiness. Throughout this exchange, the therapist is explicitly labeling the steps. They highlight that it may be useful to explore core beliefs based on what the patient said. They suggest the downward arrow method as a promising technique to structure the exploration, and they label the final thought as a potential core belief. Clearly labeling each step and connecting them to the patient's experiences are thought to provide the most useful structure for patients with personality disorders to organize and understand their thoughts and core beliefs.

To challenge the core beliefs of patients with personality disorders, CBT providers can utilize thought records. Thought records can be especially useful when working with patients with personality disorders, because they provide a clear and straightforward structure for patients. In its most basic form, a thought record consists of two columns: one for automatic thoughts and one for alternative responses. In this case, automatic thoughts (e.g., "What's the point in hanging out with friends?") would be replaced with a core belief (e.g., "I'm fundamentally unlikeable"). To complete the thought record as it applies to core beliefs, patients would list their core belief(s) in the first column. In the second column, patients would ask themselves various questions to explore whether the core belief is accurate and/or effective for them. Jackson's therapist may ask him, "Think of someone who's fundamentally unlikeable. What are they like?" He may reply that they are characterized by dishonesty, bad intentions toward others, and disagreeable behaviors. Then the therapist may ask, "How accurately do those traits describe you?" If

Box 10.2 Questions to Develop Alternative Responses to Core Beliefs

- What evidence do I have that this belief is true?
- What evidence do I have that this belief is false?
- Am I assuming something about someone else, or have they explicitly expressed this?
- How often does this situation actually occur?
- What would it look like if someone was _____? What characterizes this type of person? What would they be doing/saying/thinking?
- How well does this description actually match my behaviors/words/thoughts?
- How would I know for sure if this belief was true or false?
- What are all the factors involved in these situations? How much of these situations am I responsible for? Are others responsible for?
- How well does this belief align with my values?
- What's the worst case scenario of this belief?
- How can I cope effectively with that worst case scenario?

Jackson does not honestly think those traits describe him well, his therapist would ask "What traits would describe you more accurately instead?" Jackson would write these traits down in the alternative response column. Further questions providers may use are listed in Box 10.2.

Providers can work through a thought record with their patient in session, and encourage patients to hold onto and continue adding alternative responses to it throughout their work together. Core beliefs and cognitive schemas have presumably developed through repeated reinforcement over a long period of time. By keeping thought records about these core beliefs handy, patients have a list of readymade responses they can use to challenge the maladaptive belief. Doing so makes alternative responses more accessible and easier to think of, which can in turn enhance how true they feel.

Clinical Vignette: Obsessive-Compulsive Personality Disorder
Bernadette is a 32-year-old White woman diagnosed with OCPD.

Therapist: What you just said sounds like it might be a core belief: "I must avoid mistakes at all cost." To address these beliefs, we can systematically evaluate how accurate and helpful they are using what's called a thought record. Thought records help us write out our thought process so we can take a step back from it and see whether our core belief is the whole story. Would it be okay if we practiced using one with that core belief?

Bernadette: Okay.

Therapist: Great! So in the first column, under Core Belief, we can write "I must avoid mistakes at all cost." Now, in the second column, under Alternative Responses, we want to think about all the evidence around this belief. First off, why is it bad to experience mistakes?

Bernadette: It means I'm worthless. Like if I can't even do the simplest things right, what value do I really have?

Therapist: Let's think that through! Who is someone you really value or you think is a valuable person?

Bernadette: My coworker, Jasmine, really stands out to me.

Therapist: What is it about her that you really value?

Bernadette: She's really good at what she does but is down to earth. She's constantly winning these employee-of-the-month awards but she will always make time to answer questions or mentor younger folks. She's also just a genuinely nice person.

Therapist: Has she made any mistakes?

Bernadette: I guess so. I remember her saying she really goofed on the numbers behind a big project from her division and had to work some serious overtime to fix it.

Therapist: So, even though she makes mistakes, she's still a valuable person?

Bernadette: Hmm, she is. Those mistakes don't define her in my mind, especially because she's been able to address them.

Therapist: Have you been able to fix mistakes you've faced?

Bernadette: Some of them! But I definitely have so many regrets.

Therapist: And it seems plausible that Jasmine might have done things differently, too, if she had the chance, but that doesn't define her value as a person. Is that fair?

Bernadette: Yeah, I guess so.

Therapist: Maybe one alternative response to write down is "Even people I value and admire make mistakes, and those mistakes don't define them?"

In this example, the therapist is using Socratic questioning to elicit examples, thoughts, and reactions from the patient to examine if the patient's core belief (i.e., "I must avoid mistakes at all costs") really is the whole story. Because the patient says this core belief indicates something about her inherent value, the therapist begins the line of inquiry by asking for the patient's definition of what it means to be valuable. The therapist asks for an example of someone in the patient's life to bring this definition to life. Then the therapist connects the value of this person to the patient's core belief around making mistakes to explore if mistakes negate a person's value. The patient's responses were rich and multifaceted. The therapist may have instead decided to explore how frequently people (e.g., the coworker, the patient) make mistakes, whether the patient actually knows how often other people make mistakes, and how bad the consequences are for people who make mistakes. The therapist would encourage the patient to write down any alternative responses generated by these questions on the thought record, to carry the thought record with her, and review it or add to it throughout their work together to enhance the accessibility of the alternative responses. By practicing identifying automatic thoughts and core beliefs in session, CBT providers hope to model for patients how to catch these thoughts and beliefs in real life. By writing down alternative responses that patients can take with them after session, providers intend for patients to more easily bring them to mind between sessions. This process is designed to weaken patients' beliefs in their initial automatic thoughts and core beliefs so that they can more accurately evaluate their experiences of themselves, others, and the world around them.

Identifying Maladaptive Behaviors and Devising Behavioral Experiments

Patients with personality disorders often present with a mix of over- and underdeveloped behaviors. Overdeveloped behaviors are those that a patient uses frequently, regardless of context, whereas underdeveloped behaviors are those that a patient rarely uses. Overdeveloped behaviors used by patients with personality disorders may be effective in the moment and are likely maladaptive in the long run. These behaviors may include under-engagement strategies (e.g., suppression, dissociation, avoidance) or over-engagement strategies (e.g., yelling, excessively seeking reassurance, overly sexualized behaviors). Underdeveloped behaviors are those that are more likely to enhance patients' functioning in the long run, whether or not they are effective at improving the short-term situation patients face. These behaviors may include cognitive reappraisal, acceptance, problem-solving, distraction, and relationship-enhancing behaviors such as complimenting others, initiating plans, and asserting one's needs. In addition to probing for patients' schemas and beliefs, CBT providers also inquire into patients' behavioral repertoires to better understand how they respond to stressful situations. Assessing and targeting patients' behavioral repertoires is a technique shared between CBT and DBT.

Clinical Vignette: Identifying Maladaptive Behaviors

Therapist: What kinds of things do you do when you're with your friends? [open-ended question to allow patient to explore the full range of his repertoires]

Jackson: I'm a pretty quiet guy to begin with, so I don't usually say too much. It also takes me a long time to respond to people because I'm trying to think through whether something I say will sound stupid.

Therapist: Oh, that's helpful to know. Do you mean you take a long time to respond to people in the moment or when they invite you? [clarifying patient's repertoire]

Jackson: Both.

Therapist: Thank you for clarifying that. Are there any other things you do too much in these situations? [prompting for further examples of behaviors]

Jackson: I think I space out, because I can't remember a lot of what people say. This makes me freeze up when they're talking to me and I just start sweating like crazy.

Therapist: Thank you for describing that. These are excellent examples for social situations. What kinds of behaviors come up at work? [exploring other areas of the patient's life]

Jackson: As you know, most of my work is by myself. When I do have to have a meeting, I get so nervous beforehand. I'm convinced I'm going to do something embarrassing so I try to show up right before the meeting and leave the moment it's over.

Therapist: Oh, I see. It sounds like you put off responding in social situations and try to limit how much you're noticed in work situations. It also sounds like these situations do make you feel very uncomfortable to the point of sweating, having a hard time focusing, and even spacing out. Are those the main responses? [consolidating patient's report and checking that the therapist understands]

Jackson: Yeah, as far as I can think of.

Here, the therapist provides a framework in which to explore the patient's over- and underdeveloped behaviors. The therapist begins by asking open-ended questions to allow the patient to highlight behaviors that stand out to him as particularly noteworthy, relevant, or interfering. Because the therapist does not know what behaviors will be most important to the patient, this open-ended exploration provides initial information about how the patient views his behaviors. As they continue, the therapist continues to ask relatively open-ended questions but frames these questions in terms of specific contexts to provide more comprehensive coverage of areas of the patient's life. The therapist does this by explicitly asking about both over- and underdeveloped behaviors as well as by asking if the same behaviors elicited in social settings arise in a work context. Given that personality disorders may present with similar expressions across contexts, Jackson's similar overdeveloped avoidant behaviors in social and work settings (i.e., being quiet, taking time to respond in the moment, and to social invitations) make sense. Jackson also identifies underdeveloped avoidant behaviors, such as limiting how much he's noticed and, implicitly, engaging in few relationship-enhancing behaviors. At the same time, different contexts may provide different affordances or be paired with unique associations that elicit different responses from patients. Thus, it is important to comprehensively assess the domains of a patient's life to identify their over- and underdeveloped behaviors.

Because these behaviors may be reinforcing in the moment,[16] patients have likely developed beliefs about these strategies. Patients may believe that these strategies are ultimately useful for them, that other strategies they use less frequently would not be effective, or that they are simply unable to use any other strategies. CBT providers can address these beliefs by designing behavioral experiments with their patients. Behavioral experiments build on alternative responses from patients' thought records. Sometimes, alternative responses don't feel as true to patients because they have not tried out different behaviors enough, and so do not have the lived experience of the consequences of those behaviors to draw from like they do with overdeveloped behaviors. Behavioral experiments are thus designed by the therapist and patient to practice different behaviors and allow the patient to experience what consequences actually result.

After exploring alternative responses, CBT providers may ask patients how they can get more information about their core belief and test it. Such tests often involve replacing overdeveloped behaviors with underdeveloped ones. For instance, patients with ASPD who assumes coworkers don't mind when they cancel at the last minute (overdeveloped behavior) might be encouraged to ask coworkers what they think (underdeveloped behavior). Patients with DPD may practice making a relatively small daily decision for themselves without input (underdeveloped behavior) and notice whether any negative consequences arise. Patients with paranoid personality disorder may resist the urge to keep their blinds shut (overdeveloped behavior) by opening them to facilitate acting as if they were not being followed (underdeveloped behavior). Patients are encouraged to treat these as tests; that is, they are not asked to commit to these behaviors for the rest of their lives. Instead, CBT providers encourage patients to give these experiments the best chance to succeed so they can learn what new consequences result.

Activity Scheduling

Given that personality disorders involve characteristic patterns of behaviors, it can be useful to assess a patient's activities in a given week and replace certain activities that contribute to dysfunctional behaviors related to the core schemas. Once these schemas are agreed upon, the provider may ask the patient to record what they do, every hour of each day, from one session to the next, and mark situations in which dysfunctional aspects of their core belief arose. At the next session, providers and patients can review this record to identify activities that co-occur with dysfunctional aspects of their core beliefs, to explore if specific aspects of these activities can be modified to decrease the impacts of the dysfunctional aspects of their core beliefs. Finally, providers can work with the patient to plan different activities that are less likely to activate these dysfunctional core beliefs, or to use different behaviors that can actively challenge these beliefs. The goal of activity scheduling, a technique implemented in DBT for accumulating short-term positive emotions, is not to distract from or avoid experiencing core beliefs, but rather to increase the range of experiences patients have in their lives so they have a wider variety of information from which to draw on when cultivating alternative responses.

Clinical Vignette: Activity Scheduling

Marcus is a 45-year-old mixed-race veteran who presents with paranoid personality disorder (PPD).

Therapist: Would you be willing to review your activity log? Are there any particular days that stand out when you noticed feeling more suspicious of others?

Marcus: Wednesday and Thursday I had to go to the VA for a doctor's appointment and couldn't shake the feelings.

Therapist: Great job identifying those days. Let's look at it together. So you went to the VA from 9–11am on Wednesday and Thursday, and I see your ratings of suspiciousness started to go up even in the hour before you left and for a couple hours after. What were you doing or thinking about during those hours?

Marcus: Before I left, I kept thinking how I was being hung out to dry by the people at the VA and that these appointments wouldn't get me anywhere. After the appointments, I was watching YouTube videos to try to relax and they kept advertising these insider accounts of the tricks people use at the VA to keep all the patients in check, which sent my suspiciousness through the roof.

Therapist: I think watching those might make anyone feel more suspicious! It sounds like both the thinking about the appointment beforehand and the videos afterwards really contributed to feelings of suspiciousness. Because you have a couple appointments again next week, what different behaviors could we plan to use in those time slots to maybe combat the suspiciousness?

Marcus: Hmm, maybe beforehand I could do one of my workouts to focus my mind on exercising and not the appointment. Then afterwards, instead of watching videos, I could go for a walk or, even better, I could plan to get lunch with some of my friends there! That always helps to take my mind off things for a bit.

Therapist: Perfect! Let's write those down in those timeslots in a fresh activity log here so you remember them.

Imagery

Guided imagery, a technique shared with schema therapy, may be a useful in-session experiential-behavioral technique for patients whose schemas relate to specific memories or who are unwilling to practice behavioral experiments. The goal of guided imagery is to reshape patients' schemas by allowing them to fully experience the emotions associated with difficult memories, observe new details about the memory, and learn that they can successfully cope with the memory. To practice guided imagery, CBT providers will first explain the rationale for bringing a difficult memory to mind. They will explain that their role is to remain neutral and reserved during the imagery exercise to allow the patient to fully experience it. The provider will request the patient to provide a rating of distress from 0 (none at all) to 10 (the most distress imaginable) throughout the exercise to ensure the patient is able to tolerate the exercise. If the patient is willing to proceed, they will ask that the patient close their eyes and, when they are ready, begin to recall out loud the difficult memory. The provider may prompt the patient for details or ask for the next event in the memory as they see fit. However, providers refrain from giving much feedback until the end of the exercise, at which point they may provide warmth and validation to reinforce the patient for completing the difficult exercise.

Patients may be under-engaged or over-engaged during guided imagery exercises. Under-engagement means patients do not feel the strong emotions the memory typically evokes. This may be because patients are using cognitive strategies to remain distant from the memory or because they have sufficiently habituated to the memory over time without realizing it. To troubleshoot under-engagement, providers would first assess the patient's experience during the exercise. They may ask the patient to describe more details of the memory before fully imagining it again. Finally, providers can ask the patient to provide these details, further sensory and emotional details, and slow the pace of the description down so that the patient can fully feel each aspect of the difficult memory.

Over-engagement means patients feel the emotions of the memory so strongly that they interfere with patients' ability to engage with the memory. Over-engagement may be expressed as uncontrollable crying, dissociation, or a panic attack. To troubleshoot over-engagement, the provider may ask the patient to repeat the exercise so as not to reinforce avoidance. They may modify the situation slightly, either by providing some more indicators of warmth and safety than normal (in the case of crying or a panic attack) or asking the patient to physically stand up and balance on one leg or hold something in balance (in the case of dissociation) to better ground them during the exercise. After a successful imagery exercise in which the patient's distress level drops, the provider should debrief with the patient about what they gained from the experience. If they developed any further alternative responses to their core belief, these should be documented on their thought record.

Clinical Vignette: Imagery

Therapist: Thanks for being willing to do this imagery exercise, Marcus. Like we talked about, one of the ways that emotions like suspiciousness get maintained is by us trying to suppress memories that bring up suspiciousness or by dwelling on them, only focusing on aspects of the situation that line up with that emotion. What we want to do is give you practice intentionally bringing these memories to mind to help you get used to them and explore other details within them that may not make you feel as suspicious. Do you have questions about that so far?

Marcus: No, that sounds like what we discussed before.

Therapist: Good. So what I'd like you to do is call to mind the memory of your meeting with the doctor at the VA when she told you your benefits would be cut. I want you to describe it to me moment by moment from when you were called into the meeting to when you left. Tell me what emotions you were feeling, what thoughts you noticed, what behaviors you used or wanted to use, and how your body felt physically at each point in the meeting. I'll ask you to rate your distress as we go through it from 0 (no distress at all) to 10 (the most distress you've ever felt). I'll also try to stay quiet and neutral until we're done so you can more fully experience it. Are you ready to get started?

Marcus: Ready as I'll ever be.
Therapist: Thank you. Could you rate your distress now before we start?
Marcus: I'm at a 6.
Therapist: Thanks. Go ahead and start.

Mindfulness

Mindfulness and acceptance-based strategies are being increasingly incorporated into cognitive-behavioral treatments for a variety of disorders, including personality disorders.[17] The core principles of mindfulness are: (1) a focus on the present moment; (2) in a way that is nonjudgmental, open, and accepting of one's experience as it unfolds. Mindfulness is often applied to help patients disengage from maladaptive cognitive and behavioral processes without directly challenging the content of these responses. Given that patients with personality disorders have more strongly developed patterns of maladaptive cognitive and behavioral processes, mindfulness may be an effective alternative to directly challenging patients' thoughts and behaviors. Mindfulness techniques are also implemented in DBT in many forms, including What Skills, How Skills, and Wise Mind.

CBT providers may use formal meditation recordings with their patients to practice guiding their attention to different aspects of experience (e.g., physical sensations, emotions, thoughts, behavioral urges) with intention.[17] Patients may also benefit from more informal mindfulness practices, such as pausing in the middle of a session and asking the patient to nonjudgmentally notice and describe their experience. This can be a particularly grounding exercise when a patient experiences higher distress, as a way to tolerate it without avoiding the experience. Providers may also ask patients to rephrase certain descriptions in a less judgmental way, and compare their emotional responses to draw out the contrast between the immediate emotional effects of judgmental versus nonjudgmental language.

Clinical Vignette: Mindfulness

Therapist: We could talk about mindfulness all day, but often it's much easier to understand if we actually practice it. Would you be willing to do an exercise now?
Marcus: Sure thing.
Therapist: Great. I know you mentioned watching some YouTube videos that prompted feelings of suspicion. Do you remember any of them?
Marcus: I think so. I could at least pull them up.
Therapist: Excellent. Let's do that and I want to watch just 2 minutes of one of them. I'll do this with you. I want us both to practice being fully present in the moment by focusing our attention on our experience of the video. That means noticing any thoughts, judgments, emotions, and physical sensations that come up while we're watching it. If we notice our minds wandering to other topics, gently guide them back to the experience of the video. Would you be willing to try that?
Marcus: I am.
Therapist: What did you notice while we watched that? What thoughts, emotions, and sensations came up for you?
Marcus: It was easy to focus at first because I get really wrapped up in this stuff. But then I thought about how I was only focusing on the video and not my experience of the

video. So I tried to check in with what I was thinking and feeling. I noticed some excitement at the thought of finding out the secret in the video. That excitement got my heart rate up just a little bit and, you might've noticed, my leg started shaking. I also noticed some thoughts that I couldn't even trust you as I felt the suspicion rise. It was helpful to take a little step back and observe those experiences instead of getting fully caught up in them. I bet I would believe them much more strongly if we weren't doing this mindfulness exercise.

Therapist: Thank you for being willing to share that and target those aspects of your experience.

The Alliance and In-session Behaviors

The therapeutic alliance may be especially important when working with patients with personality disorders, given that the interpersonal difficulties that characterize personality disorders will likely arise in session. CBT providers must be even more attentive to the nuances of patients' and their own emotional reactions in and between sessions. Providers should not be afraid to name the patient's emotional reactions nonjudgmentally in session, or ask about them with genuine curiosity, to help patients and themselves better understand how patients are receiving session material. The alliance can be extremely useful as a corrective emotional experience for patients as a model of new interpersonal behaviors and as motivation to remain in treatment. Thus, being willing to devote session time to checking in with patients about their impression of the alliance is often time well spent.

To strengthen the alliance, CBT providers are encouraged to spend more time learning about their patient's developmental history, which demonstrates care and investment in the patient, than they might when working with patients without a personality disorder. Whenever a patient demonstrates an effective behavior, clear and appropriate reinforcement is ideal. Given that many patients with personality disorders experience shame in response to positive feedback, providers should inquire about how their reinforcement is received by their patients to find a response style that is actually reinforcing for each patient and contributes to his/her growth. Such effective behaviors may even, or especially, include negative feedback expressed to the provider. Patients with personality disorders may have less experience giving appropriate negative feedback, or have a history of being punished when giving feedback, so reinforcing more adaptive behaviors can enhance the bond with the patient. Genuine self-disclosure is another tool CBT providers may use to strengthen the alliance. Targeted and intentional self-disclosure can engender trust with the patient, especially if others in their lives only inconsistently provide such genuine responses. Finally, liberal use of validation may be warranted and particularly effective for patients with personality disorders.[18]

Validation may take many forms, including paying attention to patients, restating patients' comments to communicate that they are being understood, and normalizing patients' responses. Normalizing patients' responses can be especially useful, as patients with personality disorders often receive feedback that their responses are incorrect. Providers may instead communicate that patients' emotional responses, thoughts, or behaviors make sense in a given situation, either because of their personal developmental history or because anyone would likely respond the way they did.

When difficulties in the alliance arise, CBT providers can apply a cognitive lens to the alliance rupture to investigate the beliefs underlying both parties' responses. Providers should be attentive to their own biases that may develop in and between sessions. The most salient example occurs when providers have a negative emotional reaction to seeing a certain patient on their schedule for the day. In addition to seeking consultation to productively address these reactions, providers may assess their own automatic thoughts in these moments. They may complete their own thought record and explore whether the automatic thoughts they notice in response to their patient are connected with any core beliefs about their patient or the providers' own ability to help. When investigating patients' responses to an in-session rupture, providers may ask how the patients saw the interaction, what they heard from the provider, and what it made them think of, in addition to the emotions elicited by it. The provider can always validate the patient's emotional response. Then, if the provider agrees with the patient's assessment, they may repair by apologizing and problem-solving a solution together. If the provider disagrees and has a hypothesis about the patients' unstated cognitive schema, they may explain their thought process to reach a mutual understanding. Either way, providers are encouraged to be fully open to patients' negative feedback, as the behaviors that brought patients to treatment often tend to elicit punishing or invalidating responses from other people.

Specific Manualized CBT for Personality Disorders

CBT is a principle-based, individual-treatment approach to personality disorders. However, more structured treatments for personality disorders have been developed that either incorporate CBT principles, include a group component, or both. These treatments, including DBT and schema-focused therapy, can be reviewed in dedicated Chapters 11 and 12 respectively. However, two structured approaches to individual CBT for personality disorders have also been developed: manual assisted cognitive therapy (MACT), and the Unified Protocol for Transdiagnostic Treatment of Emotional Disorders (UP). We will review each of these approaches in turn.

Manual Assisted Cognitive Therapy

MACT is a brief, manualized, six-session cognitively oriented intervention initially designed to treat patients who engage in repeated, deliberate self-harm.[19] MACT focuses on specific symptoms or behaviors often seen in patients with personality disorders, although it is not a specific treatment for personality disorders. It can be used for patients with BPD, AVPD, and PPD. The MACT workbook contains six chapters which teach patients to use problem-solving (e.g., behavioral chain analysis, pros and cons of self-harming behaviors), cognitive approaches (e.g., awareness and monitoring of thoughts and emotions), and relapse prevention strategies (e.g., education about substance use, coping strategies to avoid future self-harm). Patients complete worksheets within corresponding MACT chapter, with the support of the therapist, who assists patients in selecting specific antecedents and behavioral goals relevant to reducing future self-harm.[19]

Empirical Evidence for MACT for Personality Disorders

MACT was originally designed to treat self-harming behaviors and substance use. Since then, it has been tested among patients with BPD and, to a lesser extent, those with AVPD or PPD.[20] Three RCTs of MACT have been conducted to date. Compared to TAU, MACT led to greater reductions in the frequency of self-harm and depressive symptoms and was more cost-effective in a sample of 32 patients with BPD.[19] Compared to no treatment, MACT demonstrated reductions in the frequency and severity of self-harm among 30 patients with BPD who were already engaged in treatment.[21] Compared to TAU, MACT led to significant improvements in depression, anxiety, and suicidal ideation among 20 patients with BPD, AVPD, or PPD and comorbid substance use.[20] Taken together, these results suggest that MACT is an efficacious, cost-effective intervention for patients with personality disorders with or without comorbid substance use. However, in a large multi-site RCT of 480 patients with a variety of disorders, similar proportions of patients in MACT reported any self-harm as those in TAU, although patients in MACT reported less frequent use of self-harm behaviors.[22] Of note, MACT contributed to reduced overall healthcare costs for patients with personality disorders except those with BPD, for whom MACT led to increased healthcare costs. These results thus provide inconsistent evidence regarding self-harm behaviors and cost effectiveness for patients with personality disorders.

MACT includes several elements from CBT, such as cognitive restructuring, psychoeducation, problem-solving, and relapse prevention.[2] However, MACT is typically delivered in two to six individual sessions as opposed to 15 to 50 sessions of CBT.[2,19] This brevity results from MACT's focus on identifying and reducing specific, discrete self-harm behaviors, rather than the broader scope of dysfunctional cognitions that define CBT. MACT is specifically focused on the use of crisis survival skills, such as acute distress tolerance, to reduce antecedents and frequency of self-harm behaviors. One particular antecedent targeted in MACT is alcohol and substance abuse. MACT teaches patients skills to analyze and abstain from using alcohol and other substances to reduce the likelihood they will subsequently use self-harm behaviors to manage difficult emotions that may arise during substance use.

Due to the differences between MACT and CBT, providers who wish to utilize MACT should consider several specific points of emphasis. Because MACT is designed for patients to take the lead in working through the materials, providers may assume more of a supporting role than they might in traditional CBT. Specifically, a MACT provider may answer patients' questions, provide additional background information on relevant chapters, or help patients process their own responses to the worksheets that they have completed. On the other hand, a MACT provider may need to be more direct in some cases. This may include providing direct psychoeducation on alcohol and substance use, deliberately elucidating pros and cons of certain patient behaviors, and suggesting specific behaviors that will be targets of intervention. MACT providers would also likely benefit from additional background knowledge regarding alcohol and substance misuse and deliberate self-harm behaviors. Higher therapist competence in MACT was associated with greater reductions in depression scores, but not self-harm, among patients exhibiting self-injurious behaviors,[23] suggesting that competence is relevant for some, but not all, patient outcomes.

Finally, treatment adherence may be a struggle for many who participate in MACT.[24] In one study, patients achieved significant clinical outcomes despite attending fewer than half of the total sessions on average, possibly suggesting that the initial components of MACT that focus on behavioral chain analyses of self-harming behaviors, advantages and disadvantages of self-harm, problem-solving behaviors, and self-monitoring of cognitive and emotional responses may be more impactful for patients than the later sessions that focus on distress tolerance, substance use, and relapse prevention.[24] In another large multi-site trial, 38 percent of patients did not even attend one session.[22] Providers delivering MACT should work to ensure fidelity, competence, and adherence to maximize the benefits for patients.

Unified Protocol for Transdiagnostic Treatment of Emotional Disorders

The Unified Protocol (UP) for Transdiagnostic Treatment of Emotional Disorders[17] is an individual cognitive-behavioral intervention developed to address a range of psychological disorders characterized by aversive reactions to frequently occurring negative emotions.[26] These negative emotions, in turn, lead to efforts to escape, suppress, or otherwise avoid emotional experiences.[27] The goal of the UP is to extinguish distress in response to strong emotions by teaching patients a range of cognitive, behavioral, and mindfulness skills that increase patients' tolerance of emotions. Developing tolerance of emotions may be particularly relevant for patients with personality disorders, because chronic emotion regulation difficulties may contribute to the interpersonal, cognitive, and behavioral dysfunction characteristic of several personality disorders. Compared to extant treatments for personality disorders, the UP is relatively brief, as it is generally administered across 16–20 once-weekly outpatient sessions.[17]

Empirical Evidence for the UP for Personality Disorders

BPD is the personality disorder most strongly characterized by functional processes (i.e., aversive, avoidant responses to frequently occurring negative emotions).[28] Because of this, the UP has primarily been studied in the context of BPD. Specially, four single case experiments have been conducted on three samples of patients with BPD. First, in a multiple baseline design with eight participants, Lopez and colleagues[29] found that five patients no longer met criteria for BPD following treatment with the UP, and six patients no longer met BPD criteria after one-month follow-up. Further, five patients scored below clinical cutoffs in depression at post-treatment, and six scored below clinical cutoffs at one-month follow-up.[30] In contrast, seven patients scored below clinical cutoffs in anxiety at post-treatment but only three retained these gains at one-month follow-up.[30] In a third single case experiment, three of five patients with BPD reported large reductions in BPD features, anxiety and depressive symptoms, and emotion dysregulation.[31] Finally, in a study conducted in Iran, all patients with BPD and comorbid disorders reported some reductions in emotion dysregulation and BPD features from baseline to post-treatment and/or one-month follow-up.[32] This pattern of results suggests that the UP may be a useful approach for some, but not all, patients with BPD.

The UP may be especially appropriate for the many patients with less severe symptoms of BPD, because these patients may offer an opportunity to directly treat core functional processes (i.e., aversive, avoidant responses to emotions) using the exposure-based elements of the UP. These patients may more readily benefit from therapeutic techniques aimed at building emotional tolerance, whereas those with recurrent high-risk behaviors (i.e., suicidal actions, serious substance misuse) may require crisis survival skills (i.e., distraction) that are counter to the goals of the UP, yet necessary for patient safety.

Clinical Principles and Applications of the UP to Personality Disorders.
A detailed account of each skill included in the UP has been described elsewhere.[33]
However, aspects of each module that are particularly relevant to BPD symptoms are
highlighted and described. The Understanding Emotions module provides psychoeducation regarding the functional, adaptive nature of a range of emotions (anger, anxiety,
sadness, joy), which are broken down into three components (cognitions, behaviors, and
physical sensations). This module may be particularly useful for patients with BPD, as
they are likely to view their emotions as problematic, criticism-eliciting events rather
than normal, adaptive experiences due to chronic invalidation by others in their lives.[34]
Furthermore, people with BPD often engage in avoidance-oriented behaviors[35] and
may benefit from learning how these activities provide short-term relief at the cost of
increased discomfort in emotional situations in the future.

The Mindful Emotion Awareness module introduces the concept of present-focused
and nonjudgmental attention. Mindfulness training may be an especially useful
skill, given that judgmental responses to emotional experience are common in BPD.
Mindfulness practices in the UP include formal, guided meditation scripts and in vivo
practices. The formal meditation scripts allow patients to practice nonjudgmental attention to their thoughts, emotions, and physical sensations while being guided by a recording. The in vivo mindfulness practices allow patients to pause in their daily lives
and nonjudgmentally observe their thoughts, emotions, and physical sensations before
deciding on an effective course of action.

The Cognitive Flexibility module teaches patients to engage in cognitive restructuring to address maladaptive thoughts and the downward arrow technique to identify
and challenge core schemas. The emphasis in this module is on developing flexibility in
one's thinking; specifically, patients are encouraged to generate as many other possible
interpretations of emotion-eliciting situations and schemas as possible. This approach
to cognitive restructuring is particularly well-suited to patients with BPD who may have
frequently been accused of distorting or misperceiving situations by significant others,
and may respond poorly to a therapist pointing out "irrational" thoughts.[34]

The Countering Emotional Behaviors module provides skills for addressing avoidance and escape behaviors that may maintain or exacerbate emotional disorder symptoms. This module involves identifying behaviors that promote avoidance of emotional
experiences and practicing alternative behaviors that allow the patient to stay in touch
with these experiences to learn that they can handle them. Therapists and patients collaboratively identify naturally occurring emotional experiences. Collaboratively, they
build an exposure hierarchy to identify which experiences are most important for the
patient to stay in touch with and practice. For patients with BPD who struggle with interpersonal difficulties, an example may be identifying the urge to give one's partner the
"cold shoulder" after the partner forgets to take out the trash. Patients may practice an
alternative behavior of approaching their partner with warm and curious-seeming interpersonal behaviors (e.g., gentle tone, asking questions, making requests, no demands)
to politely but firmly ask their partner to take out the trash. Although potentially uncomfortable in the moment, this behavior allows the patient to learn how to approach an
interpersonal disagreement.

Treatment culminates with the Confronting Physical Sensations module in which
patients engage in activities that elicit strong emotions and remain in those situations
long enough to learn that they can tolerate these emotions. Example activities include
breathing through a thin straw to mimic difficulties breathing, spinning in a chair to

elicit dizziness and/or nausea, and staring at oneself in a mirror before quickly looking away to elicit disorientation. These activities are personalized to the physical sensations the patient has the most difficulty tolerating. By practicing each exercise for at least 30 seconds on multiple days, patients can learn that they do not need to use maladaptive behaviors (e.g., self-harm, substance use) to avoid these uncomfortable feelings. As already indicated, these exercises may be most effective for patients with BPD who are relatively less severe and able to tolerate such exposures without dissociation or marked increases in suicidality.

Many of these techniques used in the UP are shared with DBT. For instance, the Understanding Emotions module of the UP covers similar content as the Understanding and Labeling Emotions skill in DBT; the Mindful Emotion Awareness module of the UP covers similar content as the Mindfulness module in DBT; the Cognitive Flexibility module of the UP covers similar content as the Checking the Facts skill in DBT; and part of the Countering Emotional Behaviors module of the UP covers similar content as the Opposite to Emotion Action skill in DBT. The primary differences in content between these treatments is the UP's focus on directly exposing patients to difficult emotions. Establishing a hierarchy and conducting emotional exposures in the Countering Emotional Behaviors module and implementing the Confronting Physical Sensations module of the UP are distinct from DBT in that they require patients to experience difficult emotional and physical sensations directly. These skills are not prohibited in DBT; however, they are not explicitly included in the treatment. DBT teaches patients skills to manage difficult and intense negative emotions, rather than confronting and resolving them. These discrepancies likely result from the development of the two treatments: DBT was designed to treat self-harming behaviors, which requires more safety and management skills, whereas the UP was designed to treat a range of anxiety and related disorders, for which the most effective techniques include emotional exposure exercises.

Conclusion

CBT for personality disorders encompasses a wide range of techniques stemming from the hypothesized role of cognitive schemas in driving and maintaining the chronic emotional, behavioral, and physiological responses characteristic of personality disorders. Keeping these schemas in mind, probing for their activation, and testing alternative explanations, all while attending to the patient–therapist alliance, are the key principles of conducting CBT with patients with personality disorders. These principles help ground the use of techniques from other experiential or third-wave traditions in a CBT framework. Providers may choose from at least three modes of CBT, depending on the patient's presenting problem and availability for treatment. MACT may be most appropriate for patients with self-harming behaviors who are self-motivated but cannot complete more than six sessions. The UP may be most appropriate for patients with BPD who can tolerate emotional exposures and participate in up to 20 sessions. CBT more broadly may be appropriate for any patient with a personality disorder who can attend longer-term treatment. Although more research is needed on the efficacy of CBT for personality disorders, these preliminary results are encouraging for these impairing conditions. Review Box 10.3, p. 280 for CBT resources for patient, families, and clinicians.

Conflict of Interest/Disclosure: The authors of this chapter have no financial conflicts and nothing to disclose.

Box 10.3 Resources for Patients, Families, and Clinician

- Beck Institute for CBT on what is CBT. https://beckinstitute.org.
- Beck Institute for CBT on Personality Disorders. https://beckinstitute.org/%D1%81ondition/personality-disorders/.
- American Psychiatric Association on Personality Disorders. https://www.psychiatry.org/patients-families/personality-disorders/what-are-personality-disorders.
- The Mayo Clinic on CBT. https://www.mayoclinic.org/tests-procedures/cognitive-behavioral-therapy/about/pac-20384610.
- Wood J. *The Cognitive-behavioral Therapy Workbook for Personality Disorders: A Step-by-Step Program.* Oakland, CA; New Harbinger Publication; 2010.
- Barlow DH, Sauer-Zavala S, Farchione TJ, et al. *Unified Protocol for Transdiagnostic Treatment of Emotional Disorders: Workbook.* 2nd ed. New York: Oxford University Press; 2018.
- Find a CBT therapist. https://www.findcbt.org/FAT/.
- Find a UP therapist. http://www.unifiedprotocol.com/Patient-Resources/Find-a-UP-Certified-therapist/70/.

References

1. Beck AT, Davis DD, Freeman A, eds. *Cognitive Therapy of Personality Disorders.* 3rd ed. New York, NY: Guilford Press; 2015.

2. Matusiewicz AK, Hopwood CJ, Banducci AN, Lejuez CW. The effectiveness of cognitive behavioral therapy for personality disorders. *Psychiatr Clin North Am.* 2010; 33(3): 657–685. doi:10.1016/j.psc.2010.04.007

3. Palmer S, Davidson K, Tyrer P, et al. The cost-effectiveness of cognitive behavior therapy for borderline personality disorder: results from the BOSCOT trial. *J Pers Disord.* 2006; 20(5): 466–481. doi:10.1521/pedi.2006.20.5.466

4. Cottraux J, Note ID, Boutitie F, et al. Cognitive therapy versus Rogerian supportive therapy in borderline personality disorder. Two-year follow-up of a controlled pilot study. *Psychother Psychosom.* 2009; 78(5): 307–316. doi:10.1159/000229769

5. Alden L. Short-term structured treatment for avoidant personality disorder. *J Consult Clin Psychol.* 1989; 57(6): 756–764. doi:10.1037//0022-006x.57.6.756

6. Stravynski A, Belisle M, Marcouiller M, Lavallée YJ, Elie R. The treatment of avoidant personality disorder by social skills training in the clinic or in real-life settings. *Can J Psychiatry.* 1994; 39(8): 377–383. doi:10.1177/070674379403900805

7. Stravynski A, Marks I, Yule W. Social skills problems in neurotic outpatients. Social skills training with and without cognitive modification. *Arch Gen Psychiatry.* 1982; 39(12): 1378–1385. doi:10.1001/archpsyc.1982.04290120014003

8. Emmelkamp PM, Benner A, Kuipers A, Feiertag GA, Koster HC, van Apeldoorn FJ. Comparison of brief dynamic and cognitive-behavioural therapies in avoidant personality disorder. *Br J Psychiatry.* 2006; 189: 60–64. doi:10.1192/bjp.bp.105.012153

9. Strauss JL, Hayes AM, Johnson SL, et al. Early alliance, alliance ruptures, and symptom change in a nonrandomized trial of cognitive therapy for avoidant and obsessive-compulsive personality disorders. *J Consult Clin Psychol.* 2006; 74(2): 337–345. doi:10.1037/0022-006X.74.2.337

10. Barber JP, Muenz LR. The role of avoidance and obsessiveness in matching patients to cognitive and interpersonal psychotherapy: empirical findings from the treatment for depression collaborative research program. *J Consult Clin Psychol.* 1996; 64(5): 951–958. doi:10.1037//0022-006x.64.5.951

11. Joyce PR, McKenzie JM, Carter JD, et al. Temperament, character and personality disorders as predictors of response to interpersonal psychotherapy and cognitive-behavioural therapy for depression. *Br J Psychiatry.* 2007; 190: 503–508. doi:10.1192/bjp.bp.106.024737

12. Carter JD, Luty SE, McKenzie JM, Mulder RT, Frampton CM, Joyce PR. Patient predictors of response to cognitive behaviour therapy and interpersonal psychotherapy in a randomised clinical trial for depression. *J Affect Disord.* 2011; 128(3): 252–261. doi:10.1016/j.jad.2010.07.002

13. McBride C, Atkinson L, Quilty LC, Bagby RM. Attachment as moderator of treatment outcome in major depression: a randomized control trial of interpersonal psychotherapy versus cognitive behavior therapy. *J Consult Clin Psychol.* 2006; 74(6): 1041–1054. doi:10.1037/0022-006X.74.6.1041

14. Huibers MJ, Cohen ZD, Lemmens LH, et al. Predicting optimal outcomes in cognitive therapy or interpersonal psychotherapy for depressed individuals using the personalized advantage index approach [published correction appears in PLoS One. 2016;11(2):e0148835]. *PLoS One.* 2015;10(11):e0140771. doi:10.1371/journal.pone.0140771

15. Davidson KM, Tyrer P, Tata P, et al. Cognitive behaviour therapy for violent men with antisocial personality disorder in the community: an exploratory randomized controlled trial. *Psychol Med.* 2009; 39(4): 569–577. doi:10.1017/S0033291708004066

16. Southward MW, Semcho SA, Stumpp NE, MacLean DL, Sauer-Zavala S. A day in the life of borderline personality disorder: a preliminary analysis of within-day emotion generation and regulation. *J Psychopathol Behav Assess.* 2020;42(4):702–713. doi:10.1007/s10862-020-09836-1

17. Barlow DH, Farchione T, Sauer-Zavala S, et al. *Unified Protocol for Transdiagnostic Treatment of Emotional Disorders: Therapist Guide.* 2nd ed. New York, NY: Guilford Press; 2018.

18. Benitez C, Southward MW, Altenburger EM, Howard KP, Cheavens JS. The within-person effects of validation and invalidation on in-session changes in affect. *Personal Disord.* 2019; 10(5): 406–415. doi:10.1037/per0000331

19. Evans K, Tyrer P, Catalan J, et al. Manual-assisted cognitive-behaviour therapy (MACT): a randomized controlled trial of a brief intervention with bibliotherapy in the treatment of recurrent deliberate self-harm. *Psychol Med.* 1999; 29(1): 19–25. doi:10.1017/s003329179800765x

20. Davidson KM, Brown TM, James V, Kirk J, Richardson J. Manual-assisted cognitive therapy for self-harm in personality disorder and substance misuse: a feasibility trial. *Psychiatr Bull.* 2014; 38(3): 108–111. doi:10.1192/pb.bp.113.043109

21. Weinberg I, Gunderson JG, Hennen J, Cutter CJ Jr. Manual assisted cognitive treatment for deliberate self-harm in borderline personality disorder patients. *J Pers Disord.* 2006; 20(5): 482–492. doi:10.1521/pedi.2006.20.5.482

22. Tyrer P, Tom B, Byford S, et al. Differential effects of manual assisted cognitive behavior therapy in the treatment of recurrent deliberate self-harm and personality disturbance: the POPMACT study. *J Pers Disord.* 2004; 18(1): 102–116. doi:10.1521/pedi.18.1.102.32770

23. Davidson K, Scott J, Schmidt U, Tata P, Thornton S, Tyrer P. Therapist competence and clinical outcome in the Prevention of Parasuicide by Manual Assisted Cognitive Behaviour Therapy trial: the POPMACT study. *Psychol Med.* 2004; 34(5): 855–863. doi:10.1017/s0033291703001855

24. Morey LC, Lowmaster SE, Hopwood CJ. A pilot study of Manual-Assisted Cognitive Therapy with a Therapeutic Assessment augmentation for borderline personality disorder. *Psychiatry Res.* 2010; 178(3): 531–535. doi:10.1016/j.psychres.2010.04.055

25. MacLeod AK, Tata P, Evans K, et al. Recovery of positive future thinking within a high-risk parasuicide group: results from a pilot randomized controlled trial. *Br J Clin Psychol.* 1998; 37(4): 371–379. doi:10.1111/j.2044-8260.1998.tb01394.x

26. Cassiello-Robbins C, Southward MW, Tirpak JW, Sauer-Zavala S. A systematic review of Unified Protocol applications with adult populations: Facilitating widespread dissemination via adaptability. *Clin Psychol Rev.* 2020; 78: 101852. doi:10.1016/j.cpr.2020.101852

27. Barlow DH, Sauer-Zavala S, Carl JR, Bullis JR, Ellard KK. The nature, diagnosis, and treatment of neuroticism: back to the future. *Clin Psychol Sci.* 2014; 2(3): 344–365. doi:10.1177/2167702613505532

28. Sauer-Zavala S, Barlow DH. The case for borderline personality disorder as an emotional disorder: Implications for treatment. *Clin Psychol (New York).* 2014; 21(2): 118–138. doi:10.1111/cpsp.12063

29. Lopez ME, Thorp SR, Dekker M, et al. (2019). The unified protocol for anxiety and depression with comorbid borderline personality disorder: a single case design clinical series. *Cogn Behav Ther.* 2019; 12: E37. doi:10.1017/S1754470X19000254

30. Lopez ME, Stoddard JA, Noorollah A, et al. Examining the efficacy of the Unified Protocol for Transdiagnostic Treatment of Emotional Disorders in the treatment of individuals with borderline personality disorder. *Cogn Behav Pract.* 2015; 22(4): 522–533. doi:10.1016/j.cbpra.2014.06.006

31. Sauer-Zavala S, Bentley KH, Wilner JG. Transdiagnostic treatment of borderline personality disorder and comorbid disorders: a clinical replication series. *J Pers Disord.* 2016; 30(1): 35–51. doi:10.1521/pedi_2015_29_179

32. Mohammadi F, Bakhtiari M, Arani AM, Dolatshahi B, Habibi M. (2018). The applicability and efficacy of transdiagnostic cognitive behavior therapy on reducing signs and symptoms of borderline personality disorder with co-occurring emotional disorders: a pilot study. *Iran J Psychiatry Behav Sci.* 2018; 12(1): e9697. doi:10.5812/ijpbs.9697

33. Payne LA, Ellard KK, Farchione TJ, Fairholme CP, Barlow DH. Emotional disorders: a unified transdiagnostic protocol. In Barlow DH, ed. *Clinical Handbook of Psychological Disorders: A Step-by-Step Treatment Manual.* New York, NY: Guilford; 2014:237–274.

34. Linehan MM. *Cognitive-behavioral Treatment of Borderline Personality Disorder.* New York, NY: Guilford Press; 1993.

35. Southward MW, Cheavens JS. Quality or quantity? A multistudy analysis of emotion regulation skills deficits associated with borderline personality disorder. *Personal Disord.* 2020; 11(1): 24–35. doi:10.1037/per0000357

11
Dialectical Behavior Therapy

Sheila E. Crowell, Parisa R. Kaliush, Robert D. Vlisides-Henry, and Nicolette Molina

Key Points

- At its core, dialectical behavior therapy (DBT) is a behavioral therapy uniquely integrating Zen (i.e., mindfulness) and acceptance and change principles for the treatment of patients with personality disorders and other conditions.
- DBT was designed to shape maladaptive behavior and help distressed individuals act toward goals using classical conditioning, operant learning, and modeling.
- DBT clinicians adhere to three central principles of dialectic philosophy, including wholeness, polarity, and continuous change.
- DBT is an effective evidence-based treatment developed initially for borderline personality disorder, but recently expanded to treat other personality disorders and conditions.
- There is an extensive evidence base for DBT, and researchers continue to evaluate modifications and adaptations of the model.
- DBT involves weekly individual treatment for clients, weekly skills group, and weekly consultation group for therapists.
- Phone coaching is used when a client is in need of skills coaching, and as a way to learn and practice interpersonal and relationship skills with the therapist.
- DBT teaches four skills modules: mindfulness, distress tolerance, emotion regulation, and interpersonal effectiveness.
- A primary function of individual therapy is to enhance client motivation by linking proximal behavior change to more distal goals. Therapists seek to understand what would make the client's life worth living.
- The DBT pre-treatment contract explains the nature of therapy and commitment required to benefit from DBT.
- The DBT contract is a written document negotiated between therapist and client during the first three–four weeks of treatment.
- The "House of DBT" is an allegory used to teach clients about the four stages of DBT, which include: improving behavioral control and increasing skills use (Stage 1), improving emotional regulation and experiencing (Stage 2), bolstering overall quality of life through developing fulfilling relationships (Stage 3), and improving capacity for joy (Stage 4).

- Chain analysis is the primary insight tool of DBT. It functions to slow down the events leading to a problematic behavior so that the client can more clearly see their patterns of thinking, feeling, and acting.
- Solutions analysis teaches clients that when faced with a problem, they can either solve it, change their emotional response, tolerate or accept it, or do nothing and potentially make it worse.
- DBT is a philosophically rich, multi-stage treatment that can take months or years for a therapist to learn.
- DBT is most effective when delivered by adherent practitioners who have received comprehensive training and are adherent to the treatment model.

Introduction

Dialectical behavior therapy (DBT) is an evidence-based psychotherapy developed by Marsha Linehan to treat complex patients who are self-injuring, suicidal, or who have borderline personality disorder (BPD).[1] The premise, structure, and philosophy were detailed initially in a series of manuscripts,[2,3] which were foundational to the treatment manual and skills training book that outlined core tenets of the therapy.[4-6] DBT is a third-wave cognitive behavioral therapy (CBT) that is principle-based and philosophically rich; it is specifically founded on principles of behaviorism and enriched through the philosophy of dialectics. It is now among the most empirically supported and widely disseminated psychotherapies.[7]

Since its initial development for those with BPD and/or chronic self-injurious thoughts and behaviors (SITBs), DBT has been extended to help those struggling with many complex clinical conditions, such as post-traumatic stress disorder, mood and anxiety disorders, substance abuse, eating disorders, and other personality disorders (PDs).[8-13] DBT is now recognized as an effective psychotherapy for adolescents and adults with clinical struggles characterized by emotion dysregulation, impulsivity, interpersonal difficulties, and chronic unrelenting suffering.[14-16] The rich history of DBT is described in Marsha's (Dr Linehan requested we refer to her as Marsha) memoir, where she recounts her own painful struggle with SITBs as a young woman, her commitment to healing, and, ultimately, her vow to help others out of a "hell" that she knew personally.[17]

Adherent DBT practitioners form a community of mental health professionals who are devoted to the lifesaving mission of suicide prevention. Importantly, the concept of suicide prevention in DBT diverges from the status quo in the field, favoring the time-intensive work of guiding patients toward their "life worth living" rather than frequent, short-term hospitalizations. DBT practitioners also conceptualize psychopathology more broadly than the dominant biomedical perspective. While not disregarding biological contributors to psychiatric disorders, DBT therapists view many current problems as stemming from skills deficits that can be remedied through new learning. Relatedly, "wise mind" is the first skill taught in DBT classes because effective DBT is only possible when therapists and patients collaborate as equals, each bringing their own wisdom to the task of transforming patients' lives.

To become a DBT therapist, a mental health professional must devote six months toward initial intensive study, commit to a consultation team for the duration of their

DBT work, and engage in ongoing learning and personal growth (e.g., through daily mindfulness practice). Together, team members serve as individual therapists and skills coaches, and function as a support network for patients and one another. Overall, DBT is a flexible, adaptive, and constantly evolving treatment based upon the latest clinical trials and practice-based evidence. However, it cannot be applied partially or haphazardly. The success of DBT has led many independent practitioners to incorporate elements of DBT into their work without the support or structure of the full model. Many medical centers have invested only partially in DBT, resulting in small rogue teams of highly dedicated and overworked clinicians who often are viewed skeptically within the broader system. Adherent practitioners know that DBT is not always effective, but partial DBT can be harmful, sometimes leaving patients and their loved ones unwilling to try again.

In this chapter, we provide a brief overview of DBT for patients with PDs for readers who are not familiar with this form of psychotherapy. This overview will provide sufficient coverage to become conversant in the model and, ideally, inspire further learning. For more experienced DBT practitioners, this chapter includes some of our "lessons learned" in the practice of treating PDs. This is consistent with the narrative tradition in the broader DBT community, a practice that has advanced the therapy and improved patient outcomes. We primarily outline evidence for DBT as a treatment for PDs and identify limitations and future directions for the field. We argue that DBT is one of the most effective interventions for patients with PDs and other complex clinical problems *if* it is applied consistently and adherently with the support of a consultation team.

About Dialectical Behavior Therapy

DBT emerged through a process of trial and error. Initially, Marsha (Dr Linehan requested we refer to her as Marsha) sought to apply standard cognitive-behavioral techniques with patients who were chronically suicidal and often carried a diagnosis of BPD. To her surprise, they reacted negatively to the many change-focused techniques of CBT, which they described as excruciatingly invalidating. Thus, Marsha piloted Rogerian techniques, emphasizing congruence, unconditional positive regard, empathy, and a nonjudgmental stance. However, patients also expressed dissatisfaction with acceptance-based approaches, which invalidated their urgent need to change unbearable life circumstances. Faced with this paradox, Marsha's approach evolved into a rapid "dance" between acceptance and change. Her therapy became dialectical, a method derived from a philosophy where "truth" is discovered iteratively through a synthesis of seemingly opposing dialectics; the primary dialectical tension was acceptance-based approaches versus change-based strategies. What resulted was a structured therapy integrating behavioral science and acceptance-based approaches with a dialectical style.

Etiological Model

The biosocial theory is the guiding etiological model in DBT.[4,18] Although initially developed to explain the emergence and maintenance of BPD symptoms, DBT practitioners now apply the biosocial theory to many distinct psychiatric diagnoses. The core premise of the biosocial theory is that severe emotion dysregulation emerges when a biologically vulnerable child is reared within a chronically invalidating environment. The biosocial theory is founded on the principle that day-to-day transactions between child, caregiver(s), and other social/environmental forces gradually reinforce ineffective behaviors while simultaneously punishing effective strategies. Thus, neither parent nor child can reliably get their needs met, and the child fails to develop more skillful strategies for managing distress, navigating relationship conflict, maintaining focus, and regulating emotions. This model is intended to be "judgment-free" in that no family member is blamed. This nonjudgmental stance is central to DBT case formulations.

A biosocial formulation identifies specific characteristics of the client that may have increased their vulnerability to psychopathology. For example, as a young child they may have been more behaviorally impulsive, difficult to soothe, or more emotionally reactive, sensitive, intense, or labile than other children. This likely represents a partially heritable diathesis toward BPD that, alone, is not a sufficient explanation for the development of adult BPD. Such children require specific parenting strategies from a very early age. A biosocial formulation acknowledges that an additional factor contributing to the development of PDs is a "poor fit" with the environment, which the client experiences as invalidating. There are numerous invalidating environments that DBT clients describe. At one extreme, clients describe chronic abuse, neglect, sexual exploitation, loss of a parent, exposure to substance use, caregiver instability, or other negative experiences that severely compromised their upbringing. At another extreme, many clients describe a stable and fairly typical upbringing, yet one where they always felt inadequate, out of place, or like the "problem child" in the family. In many cases, clients describe invalidating environments outside of their family of origin, such as bullying at school, sexual assault by a peer or trusted adult, exposure to racism, homophobia, transphobia, or other experiences of abuse, trauma, or rejection. It is unclear whether experiences of invalidation differ based upon PD diagnosis. However, there are likely differences in the heritable vulnerabilities for different PDs. For example, those with Cluster B PDs are more likely to be emotionally under-inhibited, whereas those with Cluster C PDs may be more emotionally over-inhibited. Either extreme could increase the likelihood of invalidation. Understanding the client's unique experiences of emotional invalidation is a key element of DBT case formulation. Review Box 11.1 for some lessons learned for describing the biosocial theory to a patient.

Box 11.1   Lessons Learned in Practice: Using Metaphors

DBT therapists often use metaphors to describe the biosocial theory in a nonjudgmental manner. For example, an emotionally sensitive person with a personality disorder can be described as having a large emotional range, much like coloring with the emotional equivalent of a "128-pack of crayons." Other friends and family members, in contrast, have emotional experiences that are more like the eight or 16-pack of crayons. Both experiences are valid, and yet could be contributing to misunderstandings in relationships. A skilled DBT therapist uses metaphor strategically to promote rapid learning of key therapy concepts.

Assumptions of DBT

The DBT model has several explicit assumptions, or beliefs, that guide therapists' and clients' collaborative work:

1. Patients with PDs are doing the best they can *and* they need to do better, try harder, and be more motivated to change.
2. Patients may not have caused all of their problems, but they have to solve them anyway.
3. The lives of those with a PD in DBT are unbearable as they are currently being lived.
4. Patients must learn new behaviors in all relevant contexts.
5. Patients cannot fail in therapy.
6. Therapists need support.

These assumptions are designed to be provocative, deliberately challenging therapists and clients to think about their work collaboratively and dialectically. Initially, many clients struggle with the first assumption, that they are both doing their best and need to improve. Skilled therapists use this first assumption to highlight the many ways in which life presents seemingly opposing sentiments that can be conceptualized as "both/and" rather than "either/or" statements. Typically, the assumptions of DBT are presented as one of the first components of the DBT contract, presented early in pre-treatment (see Stages of Treatment). See Box 11.2 for information on presenting the DBT contract with a patient.

Functions and Modes of Treatment

There are five functions of comprehensive DBT: (1) improve client motivation to change; (2) enhance client capabilities; (3) facilitate generalization of client capabilities to their natural environments; (4) enhance therapist motivation and capabilities to treat clients effectively; and (5) help structure the environment to bolster client and therapist capabilities. All five functions must be met in order to practice comprehensive DBT. There are five modes, or treatment components, designed to address these functions (see Figure 11.1, p. 288).

Box 11.2 Lessons Learned in Practice: DBT Contract

The DBT contract is a written document negotiated between therapist and client during the first three to four weeks of treatment. This contract serves to detail a shared understanding of the treatment model, therapist and client expectations, DBT and agency policies, and a treatment timeline. Although many elements of the contract do not change, client and therapist often edit some elements, such as phone coaching hours. The therapist may agree to extend their typical hours if the client commits to call only when they are willing to use skills, and to call crisis numbers for times of willfulness or imminent risk. The therapist may ask their clients to practice calling crisis numbers before agreeing to edit their contract.

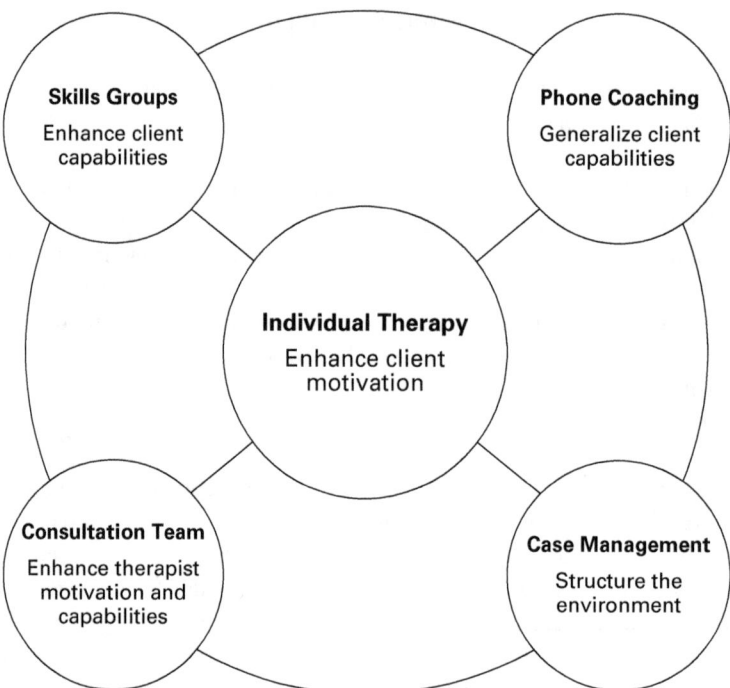

Figure 11.1. The Five Modes of DBT

Individual Therapy

The first mode of treatment is individual psychotherapy for patients with PD. Weekly (or occasionally twice weekly) therapy supports the function of improving client motivation to change and serves as the hub for all other treatment modes. Individual therapists achieve this function by building strong and genuine relationships with their clients and by skillfully balancing acceptance, change, commitment, and didactic strategies. They guide clients in replacing problematic behaviors with those that are more effective and help clients reduce factors that interfere with building a life worth living. Individual DBT therapists strive to keep sessions limited to once per week. Exceptions to this rule are made to support faster or more effective progress through treatment (e.g., a second exposure therapy session might be scheduled weekly for clients with OCD). It is important that additional sessions are not scheduled due to crisis or, if they are, this reinforcer of additional therapist contact is linked explicitly to practicing effective behaviors (e.g., the client has been using skills to reduce risk and needs additional support to bolster skills use). Therapists are especially attuned to not offering extra sessions for those with dependent PD traits, or fewer sessions for those with avoidant PD traits.

Through individual psychotherapy, clients are introduced to a weekly tracking sheet, or diary card. The diary card allows clients to record their daily emotions, thoughts, urges, behaviors, and skills used, providing a highly detailed road map toward individualized treatment targets. Diary cards focusing on life-threatening behaviors are commonly used in patients with self-harming or suicidal behaviors. For PD patients with different life-threatening behaviors (e.g., substance use, restrictive eating), those will be tracked instead. The diary card is developed collaboratively early in pre-treatment and is

---

Box 11.3 Lessons Learned in Practice: Client Goals and Treatment Targets

---

A primary function of individual therapy is to enhance client motivation by linking proximal behavior change to more distal goals (e.g., reducing alcohol use now may contribute to greater relationship satisfaction in the long term). Therapists seek to understand the key elements that would make the client's life worth living. Problem behaviors that interfere with those goals are tracked on the diary card and strategically targeted in session, focusing on life-threatening and therapy-interfering behaviors first, rather than the "problem of the week." Targeting life-threatening behaviors first is a non-negotiable element of DBT therapy, even though those problems are often a "solution for the client while being a problem for the therapist." If a client is unwilling to target life-threatening behaviors, they may be referred to a higher level of care.

---

targeted toward the client's treatment goals. For example, a client with avoidant PD may decide to work on the goal of more frequent social interactions. The therapist would add this to the diary card and also clearly tie the client's goal to the interpersonal effectiveness skills taught in DBT group. See Box 11.3 for information about linking client goals to DBT treatment targets, and a related lesson.

Skills Training Groups

Weekly skills classes support the function of enhancing client capabilities to solve problems, such as difficulties with mindfulness, distress tolerance, emotion regulation, and interpersonal effectiveness. Weekly skills training groups last about two hours and are an optimal setting for structured skills acquisition. Unlike process-oriented psychotherapy groups, DBT classes are primarily didactic. The first hour of group is devoted to a brief mindfulness activity, review of prior week skills practice, and a short break. The second hour is devoted to new skills teaching and assigning homework for the upcoming week. Classes are typically co-taught by two leaders who rotate the roles of homework review and teaching new content. Some DBT groups include reviewing the back half of the diary card, which tracks weekly skills use. For adolescent clients, there are adolescent-only and adolescent-and-family (i.e., parents included) class options. Because there is no clear evidence for or against including parents, most DBT practices elect the model that works best for their setting and clientele (e.g., inpatient settings typically do not include parents, whereas outpatient practices typically do). The function of skills classes is to teach skills (i.e., "to get the content in"), whereas the individual therapist is responsible for skills generalization in daily life, typically via phone coaching.

Phone Coaching

Phone coaching supports the function of generalizing client capabilities to their natural environments. This treatment mode is arguably one of the most critical (and misunderstood) components of DBT, and differentiates it from other evidence-based interventions. Given the complexity and severity of most DBT clients' lives and behaviors, this treatment mode is vital for helping clients learn to apply skills in vivo. Clients and their individual therapists engage in phone coaching via text messaging and phone calls. Phone coaching is most effective when used for clear and specific reasons, such as asking for validation, requesting assistance with skills use, or providing updates on life events and/or skills usage.

Although clients are welcome to seek support during a crisis, it is not the role of the DBT therapist to replicate crisis services, such as local suicide hotlines. Indeed, it is important that therapists are careful not to reinforce ineffective client behaviors: for example, by responding more quickly or warmly in response to crisis behaviors. This is the rationale behind the DBT "24-hour rule." Clients are asked to call the therapist *before* a crisis to seek strategies for avoiding problem behaviors. If they engage in self-harm or other life-threatening behaviors, the client is required to wait 24 hours before phone coaching is resumed. For patients with PDs, the 24-hour rule helps to increase predictability in the relationship, support independent skills use, and minimize the chance that crisis behaviors will be inadvertently reinforced through increased therapist contact. It is important for therapists and clients to have pre-established plans for what clients should do during the 24-hour period (e.g., crisis prevention plans) if the crisis continues or worsens.

Phone coaching is intended to be brief, structured, and within therapists' pre-established limits. For instance, therapists may discuss with their clients during pretreatment that they will not respond to phone coaching calls or text messages between 8:00 PM and 8:00 AM, and then work with their clients to formulate a plan if phone coaching is anticipated to be necessary between those hours. Once phone coaching is established, contacting therapists too frequently or infrequently may be considered a therapy-interfering behavior. The nature of these therapy-interfering behaviors may differ by diagnosis. For example, calling or texting repeatedly for reassurance would be considered a therapy-interfering behavior for a client with OCPD but might be briefly encouraged for a client with avoidant personality disorder. Phone coaching can provide many opportunities for clients and therapists to discuss therapy-interfering behaviors (see Box 11.4). In the early stages of therapy, scheduled phone coaching may be

---

Box 11.4 Lessons Learned in Practice: Making Phone Coaching Effective

Although the primary function of phone coaching is to generalize skills, it also allows clients to learn and practice valuable interpersonal skills. For example, therapists' coaching hours are described as "limits" (i.e., natural bounds on their capacity to coach, such as needs for sleep or family time) rather than "boundaries" (i.e., arbitrary rules related to power differentials). When limits are tested, therapists and clients can discuss therapy-interfering behaviors, such as whether the therapist needs to practice flexibility, the client needs to practice respecting the therapist's schedule, or both. Modeling the safeguarding of limits is valuable for clients with PDs, who often struggle to protect limits in their own lives.

needed to help clients and therapists become more comfortable and effective with this treatment mode.

Consultation Team

A consultation team supports the function of enhancing therapist motivation and capabilities to treat clients effectively. DBT can be incredibly challenging work, and a weekly or biweekly consultation team is where therapists support each other in becoming more skillful, knowledgeable, capable, compassionate, and DBT-adherent. Standard consultation team roles include an administrative team leader, who sees clients on the team and whose role typically does not rotate. The other three roles typically rotate weekly or monthly and include: (1) a meeting leader, who runs the meeting agenda; (2) a meeting observer, who highlights—oftentimes by ringing a mindfulness bell—when team members demonstrate non-mindfulness or judgmental language; and (3) a note-taker, who records the problems and solutions that were discussed during the meeting.

There are four characteristics of a DBT consultation team that differentiate it from other evidence-based treatment consultations. First, a DBT consultation team is a community of therapists treating a community of clients. In other words, individual therapists treat not only their individual clients, but support the care of every client on the DBT team. If one therapist's client dies by suicide, then all team members acknowledge that they have lost a client to suicide. Therapists commit to practice DBT adherently and treat clients as effectively as possible. Second, whereas most mental health consultation teams focus on clients' behaviors, DBT consultation team focuses on client and therapist behaviors: It is "therapy for the therapists." Team members use DBT principles, such as problem identification, solution generation, validation, and commitment strategies to guide each other in improving their motivation and capabilities. If a therapist feels frustrated or betrayed by their client's engaging in life-threatening behaviors, they may request validation from their team members as well as strategies for staying mindful and effective in the therapy room. Team members acknowledge that working with clients who have PDs can be both challenging and rewarding. Importantly, therapists can use team discussions to monitor whether they have inadvertently fallen into a problematic interpersonal interaction pattern with their client, such as invalidating a client with BPD, setting low expectations for a client with dependent PD, not challenging the behaviors of a client with antisocial personality disorder, or repeatedly praising a client with narcissistic PD.

A third related and unique characteristic of a DBT consultation team is therapist vulnerability. DBT therapists are encouraged to show more vulnerability in this team setting than in any other healthcare team setting, and more experienced members may model this culture of compassion, support, and vulnerability for newer staff members and trainees. Finally, a DBT consultation team is unique in its emphasis on dialectics. In true DBT fashion, team members acknowledge polarizations in their ideas and opinions and seek synthesis. Even if team members polarize toward one perspective together, they are encouraged to pause and ask, "What perspectives are we missing?" A DBT consultation team begins with a brief mindfulness activity followed by a reading of one or more team agreements. These agreements acknowledge the dialectical nature of the therapy, the importance of not serving as a go-between for client communications, the need for therapists to observe (and stretch) their own limits, a focus on flexibility over consistency, a call to be deeply empathic, and an acknowledgment of our inherent fallibility as therapists and humans.

Case Management

Case management is the final treatment mode, and serves to structure the therapeutic environment in order to bolster client and therapist capabilities. This role often is managed by a team social worker or administrative support person. The case manager may support the client and team by facilitating ease of scheduling, obtaining signed releases of information for the therapist to connect with other professionals, letting clients know about group homework when they miss group, and serving as an interface between the team and other administrators in the system. DBT clients often have complicated treatment histories and may be involved with other healthcare providers, such as medical doctors, psychiatrists, and social workers, or parole officers and legal representatives. DBT therapists can serve in a case-management role by being the hub of treatment across these different services, because it is in the clients' best interests to have consistent treatment goals. However, in an effort to promote effective interpersonal communication, enhance client autonomy, and not treat their clients as fragile, DBT therapists are strongly encouraged to not serve as intermediaries between these professionals and their clients, but to guide their clients in playing active roles in their own case management.

Stages of Therapy

DBT often is described as a skills-based intensive treatment. In reality, it is a four-stage treatment with unique stage-based treatment targets. The DBT four-stage model affords a great deal of flexibility to clinicians working with highly complex and dysregulated individuals. Like many evidence-based treatments (EBTs), DBT stages (comparable to EBT "modules") are organized and curated to each client's needs and goals. Many clients complete DBT in 6–12 months, proceeding from pre-treatment to Stage 1. Other clients progress through every DBT stage, which can take two years or longer. Although we present DBT's stages and substages as if they are linear and sequential, each can have substantial overlap with one another, shift in order, and even be skipped entirely.[19] The "House of DBT" is used as an allegory to explain the four stages of DBT to clients. Each stage directly tackles a problem central to the client's lived experience. Each stage has as an overarching treatment goal, with specific targets. See Box 11.5, p. 293 and Figure 11.2, p. 293 for more information about the stages of DBT.

Pre-treatment Commitment

Pre-treatment, or commitment, occurs prior to beginning Stage 1. This phase lasts anywhere from two to six sessions. It begins by orienting the client to the biosocial model and building a therapeutic alliance; it ends when the therapist and client agree to sign the DBT contract. Although not formally a treatment stage, pre-treatment is a critical component of the intervention. The primary goals of this phase are to: (1) build trust between therapist and client; (2) orient the client to the structure and goals of DBT; (3) obtain a

Box 11.5 Lessons Learned in Practice: The House of DBT

The "House of DBT" is an allegory used to teach clients about the four stages of DBT (see Figure 11.2). "Right now, your life is unbearable as it is currently being lived. It's like you are trapped in the basement of a house and the floor is on fire. Unfortunately, the only way out is a hot metal ladder, but you have no shoes and no gloves. Your friends and family have heard you in the basement calling for help and have tried to lift you out. Yet, even when they succeed, you inevitably fall back into the basement because you didn't climb out on your own. The basement is Stage 1 of DBT and the ladder is all the skills you will learn. My job is to help you get up to the main floor of the house by staying on the ladder, even when it is incredibly hard. Once you get to the main floor, we will work on Stage 2 processing of trauma and other emotional experiences, which will involve many new challenges before you can climb to the next level. When you climb to Stage 3, we will work on any other remaining problems, such as depression, anxiety, or relationship problems. Most people decide that they are done with therapy after completing the first three stages. However, some people decide that they want to achieve their highest purpose. For those people, we work on climbing up to the roof of the house and reaching for the stars."

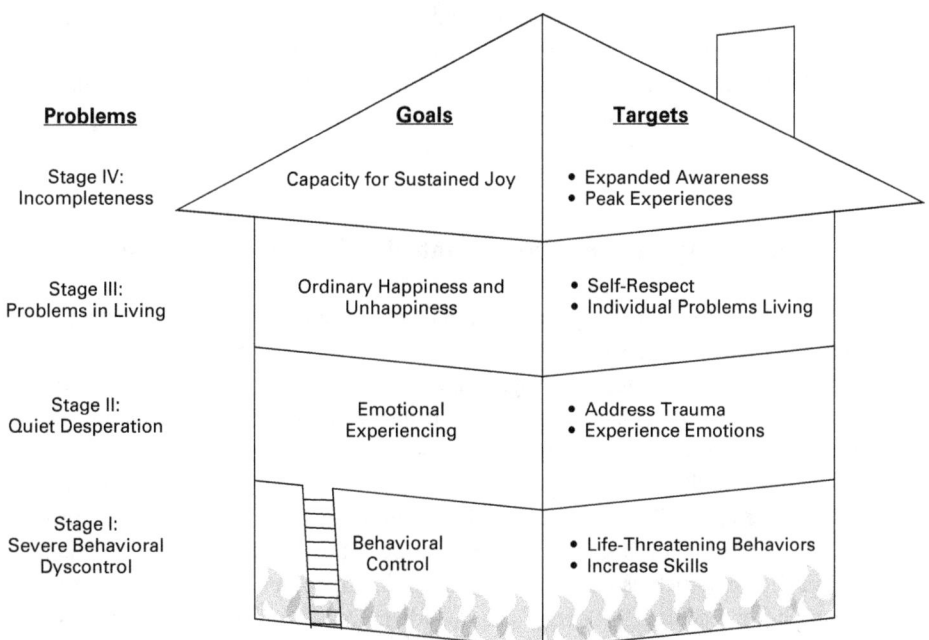

Figure 11.2. The House of DBT Depicting the Four Stages of Treatment

> ### Box 11.6 Lessons Learned in Practice: The DBT Contract
>
> Effective orientation to DBT begins with the DBT contract, which outlines the philosophy of DBT, key policies, therapist and client agreements, and commitments for both therapist and client. Once signed, the contract serves as a reminder of the client's wise-minded decision to commit fully to DBT. It can be reviewed in therapy when progress is slow or when conflict emerges. Occasionally, the DBT team may decide to sign the contract on behalf of the client. This is done when the client is an optimal fit for DBT but needs to learn new skills and begin phone coaching before being able to make a wise-minded agreement. This is communicated to the client as the team's sign of faith that they and the therapist are moving in the right direction and that DBT is a good fit.

commitment from the client to stop, or at least target, life-threatening or other problem behaviors; (4) identify the client's "life worth living" goals; and (5) begin skills group and phone coaching.

Pre-treatment represents a balancing act for therapist and client. When done well, it sets a solid foundation for the duration of the six-month contract. However, the client's crisis behaviors do not stop during this stage. It is important to establish an agenda each session that balances the therapist's need to orient the client to DBT with the client's need to get help with current crises, all while cultivating a warm and predictable therapeutic environment that inspires mutual motivation. The specific content of pre-treatment varies depending upon the client's diagnoses, goals, and presenting problems. For example, clients with BPD may require emphasis on interpersonal conflict and suicide ideation, while clients with avoidant personality disorder may require emphasis on trust-building and therapy-interfering avoidant behaviors. Pre-treatment helps shape client behaviors in session in order to increase therapist motivation to continue working with the client. Adherent DBT therapists know that even just one hour of orientation can save months of shaping, making pre-treatment one of the most important DBT phases. Pre-treatment is where the DBT contract is signed; see Box 11.6.

Stage 1: Improve Behavioral Control and Increase Skills Use

The primary treatment targets in Stage 1 DBT are to improve behavioral control and increase skills use. Each session follows a structured format beginning with diary card review, which establishes the session agenda. Given their critical role in agenda setting, clients must complete diary cards prior to or during the first 10 minutes of session. Then, clients and therapists collaboratively establish their agenda, loosely following this order: (1) self-injurious or life-threatening behaviors (SIBs); (2) therapy-interfering behaviors (of client or therapist; TIBs); (3) quality-of-life-interfering behaviors (e.g., daily problems; QIBs); and (4) skills acquisition (see Treatment Targets). TIBs can include fairly common behaviors, such as arriving late to session, not completing the diary card, or misuse of phone coaching. TIBs may also include more concerning behaviors, such as threatening the therapist, bringing a weapon to clinic, or developing a private (e.g., romantic or business) relationship with another group member. SIBs and TIBs are the highest targets in DBT because they are behaviors that could potentially cause harm to the therapy relationship or end the client's ability to remain in DBT.

These treatment targets also serve as a guiding framework for progress through Stage 1. Although all targets are fair game for the content of each session, therapists should be careful to not move consistently onto TIBs if the client has not shown steady progress in reducing SIBs. In many ways, each DBT target can be conceptualized as its own EBT, lasting several weeks to months until problem behaviors are reduced to near-zero levels and skillful behaviors are consistent. During Stage 1, clients participate in one round of weekly skills classes, which lasts approximately six months. Although Stage 1 DBT can be completed in six months, there is more empirical support for 12 months' duration.[20] Many clients graduate from DBT after completing Stage 1 and do not need further treatment.

Stage 2: Improve Emotional Regulation and Experiencing

Stage 2 DBT can be completed sequentially or concurrently with Stage 1 treatments,[21] and typically begins after clients achieve sufficient behavioral control over SIBs, address TIBs, and reliably complete diary cards and skills homework. This stage aims to enhance and improve emotional experiencing among clients after they consistently demonstrate effective emotion regulation. For clients who meet (or nearly meet) criteria for PTSD, Stage 2 may focus on trauma processing, most often using prolonged exposure (PE). In fact, DBT-PE, developed by Dr. Melanie Harned, represents an integrated protocol for combining DBT Stages 1 and 2.[22] DBT clinicians may choose to implement cognitive-processing therapy or other evidence-based trauma treatments. For clients without trauma histories, Stage 2 therapy often centers around processing strong emotions (e.g., anger, guilt) and reducing behavioral avoidance, commonly with traditional CBT protocols or acceptance and commitment therapy (ACT).[23] Similar to Stage 1, many clients graduate treatment after completing Stage 2. However, many clients need to revisit Stage 1 elements periodically after trauma processing, and this protocol is included in DBT-PE treatment.[24]

Stages 3 and 4: Bolstering Overall Quality of Life and Improving Capacity for Joy

These higher-level DBT stages focus on continuing to help clients solidify and generalize DBT skills, bolstering their overall quality of life and improving their capacity for joy. Clients in these stages learn more traditional cognitive-behavioral and acceptance-based therapeutic skills for managing psychopathology and distress (e.g., depression, anxiety), thus reducing risk of relapse into problem behaviors. Additionally, Stages 3 and 4 continue to cultivate regular mindfulness practice. Stage 3 focuses on improving clients' life through goal attainment and developing meaningful and fulfilling relationships. Stage 4 focuses on improving capacity for joy. These clients work to create meaning and feel connected to the world around them. This final Stage 4 of DBT corresponds with the peak of Maslow's hierarchy of needs.[25] Clients in Stage 4 consider their place in the world through self-actualization and reflect on how to achieve their greatest potential within their life worth living.

Treatment Targets

DBT functions to align client motivations and behaviors with their life worth living by implementing a hierarchy of treatment targets that address goal-interfering problem behaviors. Each week, behaviors and crises are addressed in individual therapy in the order of highest priority treatment target. Although treatment targets are structured hierarchically, DBT therapists may address them flexibly.

Self-harm and Life-threatening Behaviors

The highest priority treatment target is self-injury and life-threatening behaviors. DBT therapists often describe this target to clients with warmth and irreverence, explaining that "no treatment can be effective if you are not alive." Life-threatening behaviors include suicidal behaviors such as suicide ideation, preparations for death, or suicide attempts, non-suicidal self-injury, high-risk substance use, disordered eating behaviors that are medically concerning, and other high-lethality behaviors such as substance use, violence, or eating disorders.

Therapy-interfering Behaviors (TIBs)

This treatment target entails client or therapist behaviors that interfere with effective treatment. These behaviors are addressed openly and nonjudgmentally in individual or group therapy sessions. TIBs may include missing sessions, arriving late, not doing homework between sessions, not engaging with treatment goals, misusing phone coaching, or other behaviors that damage the therapeutic relationship. Therapist TIBs could include becoming non-dialectical, missing or arriving late to sessions, pushing for treatment goals that the client is unwilling to agree to, saying things in session that have a hurtful impact (even if the intent was not hurtful), or other behaviors that rupture trust and/or disrupt progress.

Quality-of-life Interfering Behaviors (QIBS)

The third treatment target addresses behaviors that interfere with clients' quality of life. These behaviors may limit their motivation in treatment and for building a life worth living. QIBS may include mental health crises (e.g., substance use, depression, post-traumatic stress), financial crises, and problems at home.

Skills Acquisition

The fourth treatment target involves improving clients' behavioral skills. Skills acquisition occurs primarily during skills group, where clients learn skills that can replace problematic, goal-interfering behaviors. These skills include mindfulness, interpersonal effectiveness, emotion regulation, and distress-tolerance techniques.

Dialectics and Dialectical Dilemmas (i.e., Secondary Targets)

The heart of DBT is, indeed, dialectics. The philosophy of dialectics offers a flexible foundation from which to treat clients who present with complicated life experiences and clinical symptoms. According to this treatment philosophy, reality is made up of nearly constant contradictory and polarizing forces, and change occurs only through tension and synthesis of these polarities. DBT clinicians adhere to three central principles of this philosophy: wholeness, polarity, and continuous change.[4] The principle of "wholeness" emphasizes the entirety of a situation over individual parts. The biosocial theory, for instance, outlines that BPD traits arise from transactions between person and environment over time; no single element of a dynamic system is at "fault." The principle of "polarity" highlights that reality is never in perfect balance. Rather, it comprises seemingly opposing forces, each offering their own truth to a situation, and a new, ultimate truth can arise from the integration, or synthesis, of these opposing forces. Of course, synthesis leads to a new set of polarities and the process continues, which relates to the third principle of "continuous change." The interconnected and polarized qualities of life that are explained by the first two principles generate a wholeness that is in a constant state of change. DBT clinicians guide their clients in accepting constant change and harnessing it to move toward a life worth living.

The primary dialectic in DBT is that between acceptance and change, which relates directly to Marsha's trial-and-error process of balancing change-focused CBT techniques with acceptance-based approaches when developing DBT (see Figure 11.3). DBT clinicians explain and model for their clients that moving toward a life worth living involves constantly dancing between acceptance and change. Clinicians and clients accept the reality of clients' life circumstances *and* practice skills in order to change ineffective behavior patterns. They enter treatment together with one of several assumptions that people are doing the best they can, given their resources, *and* people need to do better, try harder, and be more motivated for change. Broadly, the mindfulness and distress-tolerance skills are thought of as acceptance-based, meaning that these skills teach clients to accept and

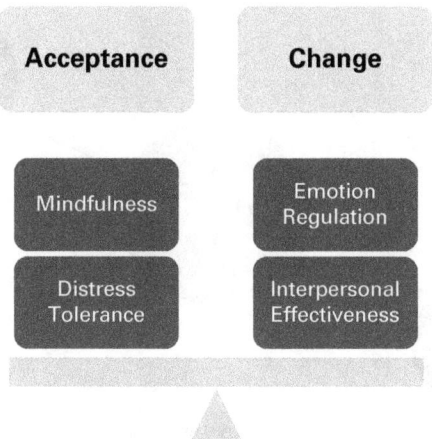

Figure 11.3. The Four Broad Skills of DBT, Conceptualized as Acceptance or Change-Based

gain clarity into their experiences. Change-based skills, emotion regulation, and inter-personal effectiveness help clients learn how to alter their behavior. Skilled DBT thera-pists move quickly between acceptance and change strategies, attempting to balance the two as depicted in Figure 11.3.

Dialectical Dilemmas

Under the overarching dialectic of acceptance and change, Marsha identified three ad-ditional dialectical dilemmas that describe common behavioral patterns exhibited by DBT clients. These dilemmas are depicted in Figure 11.4 (with respective poles). For example, one dialectical dilemma is the tension between emotional vulnerability and self-invalidation. In general, active passivity, emotional vulnerability, and unrelenting crises are capture as under-controlled behaviors. In contrast, inhibited grieving, self-invalidation, and apparent competence represent over-controlled behaviors. A dialec-tical synthesis sits at the middle of each dilemma.

The first of these dilemmas is that between emotional vulnerability and self-invalidation, the second between active passivity and apparent competence, and the third between unrelenting crisis and inhibited grieving. These dialectical dilemmas are also referred to as secondary treatment targets. These secondary treatment targets tend to emerge regardless of PD and are not always predictable based upon diagnosis. For example, one might hypothesize that those with BPD would polarize more toward un-relenting crisis with fewer instances of inhibited grieving. However, many BPD clients with a significant trauma history engage predominantly in behaviors consistent with in-hibited grieving with few observable crisis behaviors. Synthesizing the polarities of these dilemmas is a guiding force in Stage 1 treatment.

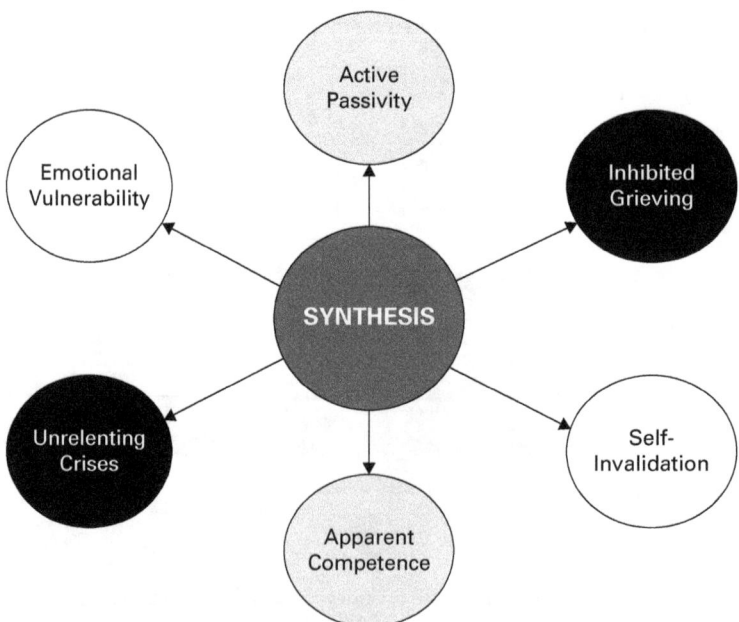

Figure 11.4. The Dialectical Dilemmas of DBT

Emotional Vulnerability and Self-invalidation

This first dialectical dilemma aligns with the biosocial model in that it reflects clients' vacillating experiences with extreme emotional sensitivity and socially influenced self-invalidation of these emotional experiences. In terms of emotional vulnerability, clients may be likened to burn-wound victims. To burn victims, even the slightest breath of air on their skin can be torturous. Many DBT clients, especially those with BPD, experience a similar level of excruciating pain with even the slightest touch to their emotions; like burn-wound care, which entails cleaning the wound directly, treatment with these clients entails working directly with their emotions. Clients may oscillate between anger and bitterness in response to this pain, and hopelessness and fragility, behaving as though they must be protected at all costs from any emotional experiences.

In some ways, the emotional vulnerability that is experienced on one side of this dialectical dilemma can be safer than what is experienced on the other side: self-invalidation. Whereas anger, hopelessness, and other forms of emotional vulnerability may be expressed overtly by clients, self-invalidation can more easily go undetected by clinicians. Oftentimes, clients' self-invalidating practices are pernicious and even more extreme than the forms of invalidation that they experienced in their environments. This can be especially true for clients with avoidant or dependent PD. On this side of the dialectic, clients may oscillate between intense self-loathing, whereby they view themselves as broken, damaged, or at fault for their emotional vulnerability, and unrealistic perfectionism, which stems from their environments oversimplifying what it takes to solve their problems. Self-invalidation may present as clients denying or suppressing emotional experiences.

Active Passivity and Apparent Competence.

This second dialectical dilemma pertains to DBT clients' help-seeking communication. In terms of active passivity, clients may exhibit both demanding and willful help-seeking behaviors, as well as helplessness that is reinforced intermittently by others offering assistance. Active passivity is one of the primary reasons why individuals with BPD are labeled negatively as "manipulative" by non-DBT practitioners. This judgment implies volition and conscious awareness of help-seeking behaviors, which often is far from the truth among these clients.

Similar to self-invalidation, apparent competence has the potential to be quite dangerous. Whereas clinicians may feel pulled to assist their clients in the face of active passivity, they may assume that their clients are doing well when there is apparent competence and consequently missed critical signs of distress. Apparent competence typically presents when clients fear ridicule or criticism in response to asking for help, or when others assume that they should be capable of coping with their problems, which can be especially common among those with avoidant PD or OCPD. It may be detected when clients are unable to generalize skillful behaviors across contexts, or when their internal experiences clearly do not match what they outwardly express. Clinicians must take extra care to monitor apparent competence because it often arises when clients are most distressed.

Unrelenting Crises and Inhibited Grieving

This third dialectical dilemma attends to clients' experiences with trauma and experiential avoidance. Unrelenting crises may result from: (1) common life situations that morph into crises due to clients' lack of resources and support; (2) devastating life events;

or (3) crisis-generating behaviors, such as impulsivity, emotion dysregulation, and self-injurious behaviors. In reality, all three of these factors likely interact with each other over time to facilitate this dilemma. Although these behaviors often occur in BPD, they are also quite common among those with other PDs and merit close attention regardless of diagnosis.

Inhibited grieving presents when clients avoid painful emotions that are associated with traumatic experiences and loss. DBT clients may have lost their childhoods, their innocence, family members or friends, their sense of self, or love from another. Clients' avoidant behaviors range from those that are more passive, such as dissociation, to those that are more active, such as binge drinking. DBT clinicians must go beyond helping their clients experience emotions and help them tolerate and live with their pain and grief. Again, these struggles are common across all PDs but can be especially common among those with Cluster B PDs and paranoid PD. Addressing inhibited grieving among DBT clients can be quite challenging because oftentimes, through self-invalidating practices, they convince themselves that they should not have had what they lost in the first place. Also, some clients may fear that they cannot recover from grief once they allow themselves to experience it.

Behaviorism, Chain Analysis, and Solution Analysis

At its core, DBT is a behavioral therapy. Although it uniquely integrates Zen and acceptance principles, it was designed first and foremost to shape maladaptive behavior and help distressed individuals act toward goals.[26] Classical conditioning, operant learning, and modeling sit at the heart of DBT.[27] Behaviorism maintains that mammalian brains are wired to associate stimuli and consequences. In anticipation of a consequence, humans can be classically conditioned to respond a certain way. Operant learning refers to when a behavior is shaped by its rewarding or punishing consequences; that is, rewarding outcomes make a behavior more likely to occur, and punishing consequences do the opposite. Modeling refers to learning through observation. All three types of learning are used by DBT clinicians to understand and treat client problems. DBT assumes that virtually everything humans do can be understood behaviorally, making it essential for clinicians to understand the rich nuances underlying behaviorism. These and other behavioral strategies are employed in DBT.[28]

Behaviorism

Behavioral theory provides a means for DBT clinicians to conceptualize client problems through concrete, observed mechanisms. Factors that lead to, mitigate, and maintain psychopathology can be understood through behavioral models. Furthermore, behavioral case formulation aids clinicians in discerning the most effective strategies for helping clients meet their goals and reduce distress. DBT clinicians are encouraged to discuss case formulations with their clients in order to bolster clients' insights regarding their behavioral patterns. As a result, clients and therapists work collaboratively on generalizable behavioral learning concepts to produce lasting change. Clients also are taught several skills designed to help them analyze and problem-solve their own behaviors.

Chain Analysis

Chain analysis is one of the most useful tools employed by DBT therapists. Chain analyses help clients and therapists detect patterns and sequences that lead to problematic behaviors, which can be any targets deemed relevant to treatment.[4] The most common example is an instance of self-harm or heightened suicidality. However, for a client with OCPD, the problem behavior might be an episode of perfectionistic reordering of objects around the home or office, which facilitated avoidance of a potentially stressful event.[29] Once the problem behavior is identified and described, often with assistance from the client's diary card, the therapist can guide the client through a chain analysis, diving into *what* led to the problem behavior (i.e., "chains") and *why* each element of the chain led to the next (i.e., "links"). Clients may need to be prompted for additional details, such as their thoughts, physiology, behaviors, and emotions.

Figure 11.5 highlights the DBT chain-analysis process. Clients and therapists take a collaborative discovery approach, and view chain analyses like detectives. As a team, they identify a target behavior that warrants a chain analysis. They then discuss vulnerability factors, links, precipitating events, and short- and long-term consequences. This process helps clients better understand their own patterns of thinking and behaving.

This "detective" work allows therapists and clients to develop deeper understanding of what caused a problem behavior. Through repeated chain analyses, higher-order patterns become clearer. This level of detail is essential for clients to recognize micro- and macro-level behaviors that lead to problems and distress. With a strong therapeutic alliance, established goals, and highly specific chains and links, behavior can be more easily altered. As such, the ultimate goals of chain analyses are to help clients develop insight into their own behavior patterns, and for clinicians to teach concrete strategies for altering behavior. See Box 11.7, p. 302 on chain analysis.

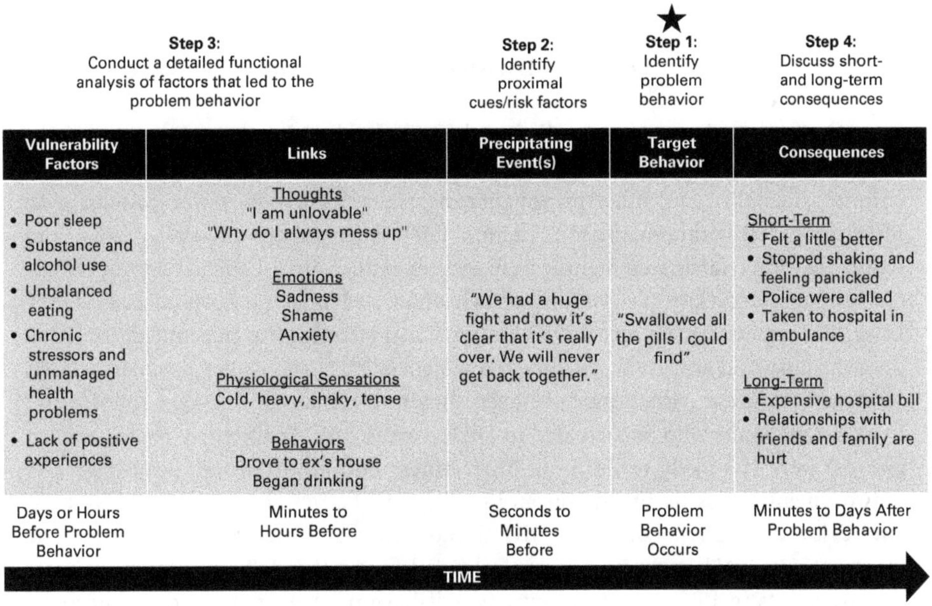

Step 3: Conduct a detailed functional analysis of factors that led to the problem behavior		Step 2: Identify proximal cues/risk factors	★ Step 1: Identify problem behavior	Step 4: Discuss short- and long-term consequences
Vulnerability Factors	**Links**	**Precipitating Event(s)**	**Target Behavior**	**Consequences**
• Poor sleep • Substance and alcohol use • Unbalanced eating • Chronic stressors and unmanaged health problems • Lack of positive experiences	Thoughts "I am unlovable" "Why do I always mess up" Emotions Sadness Shame Anxiety Physiological Sensations Cold, heavy, shaky, tense Behaviors Drove to ex's house Began drinking	"We had a huge fight and now it's clear that it's really over. We will never get back together."	"Swallowed all the pills I could find"	Short-Term • Felt a little better • Stopped shaking and feeling panicked • Police were called • Taken to hospital in ambulance Long-Term • Expensive hospital bill • Relationships with friends and family are hurt
Days or Hours Before Problem Behavior	Minutes to Hours Before	Seconds to Minutes Before	Problem Behavior Occurs	Minutes to Days After Problem Behavior

TIME →

Figure 11.5. Visual Depiction of a Chain Analysis

Box 11.7 Lessons Learned in Practice: Chain Analysis

Chain analysis is the primary insight tool of DBT. It functions to slow down the events leading to a problem behavior such that the client can see more clearly their patterns of thinking, feeling, and acting. Early in therapy, chain analysis also functions as a mild punisher of ineffective behaviors; clients often want the therapist to provide validation or immediate guidance for how to cope in the wake of a crisis rather than reliving the crisis event in excruciating detail. Both functions, insight and punishment, serve to reduce the frequency of life-threatening behaviors over time.

Solution Analyses

After completing chain analyses, therapists and clients work collaboratively toward alternative behaviors, developing solution analyses. Clients are taught that when faced with a problem, they can either solve it, change their emotional response, tolerate or accept it, or do nothing (and potentially make it worse). It is important for clients to embody the dialectical philosophy when considering possible solutions in order to avoid black-and-white thinking.[27]

Over the course of numerous chain and solution analyses, therapists can use behavioral strategies to shape clients' behaviors and help them develop skills related to distress tolerance, emotion regulation, interpersonal effectiveness, and mindfulness. Over time, clients tend to become effective at completing chain and solution analyses on their own. Teaching clients to use behaviorism to analyze and shape their own behaviors better equips them to achieve their goals, cope with stressors, and minimize negative consequences.

Evidence for DBT and Treatment of Personality Disorders

Since the first randomized controlled trial (RCT) led by Marsha in the early 1990s,[1] DBT has accrued significant empirical support for treating individuals with BPD, chronic suicidality, and other personality disorders.[30] Early RCTs for patients with BPD compared comprehensive 12-month DBT to treatment-as-usual (TAU), and found that DBT facilitated significantly greater reductions in suicide attempts, suicidal thoughts, severity of self-injurious behaviors, and inpatient hospitalizations.[31-35] Later RCTs continued to reveal DBT's unmatched effectiveness in reducing emotion dysregulation and anxiety,[36] self-directed violence,[16,37,38] and use of psychiatric crisis services.[37-39] These reductions have been shown to remain at one-year follow-up.[39] In addition, adults who participated in DBT (versus TAU or activities-based support groups) were less likely to drop out of treatment and reported significantly greater improvements in skills utilization and quality of life.[36,40] Finally, a recent systematic review of 75 RCTs compared DBT to more than 16 different psychotherapeutic interventions, TAU, and wait-list controls, and found that DBT resulted in greater improvements in BPD symptom severity, self-harming behaviors, and psychosocial functioning.[30] Overall, this immense body of literature supports DBT as a feasible and effective intervention for individuals who have been stigmatized and mislabeled as untreatable.

In addition to demonstrating DBT's efficacy in reducing life-threatening and treatment-interfering behaviors and improving quality of life, these RCTs unmasked the substantial amount of resources that are needed to implement comprehensive DBT. Treatment centers may attempt to offset limited resources by implementing "partial DBT." For example, they might offer only skills training classes with no individual psychotherapy or consultation team; this strategy can be harmful to patients and their families if mislabeled as DBT.[41] Fortunately, there is growing evidence in support of a variety of DBT interventions that can address treatment centers' inabilities to execute comprehensive DBT. For instance, DBT that is shorter in duration (i.e., approximately six months) has demonstrated similar improvements to that of standard treatment length.[40,42,43] Also, studies have explored DBT with and without skills training groups,[26] and although participants reported more reasons for living and less suicide thoughts and attempts across all treatment variations, interventions with skills training groups yielded faster reductions in anxiety and depressive symptoms and lower frequencies of non-suicidal self-injury during treatment.

Mounting evidence supports the efficacy of DBT for other populations and psychiatric conditions, such as working with adolescents and those with substance use disorders (SUD). For instance, Marsha and her colleagues adapted DBT for individuals with comorbid BPD and SUD and found that DBT facilitated significant reductions in substance use.[32] These findings were replicated by a number of other research groups.[44-47] DBT-A, a version of DBT adapted for adolescent populations, has prompted reductions in depression, self-injury, time hospitalized, interpersonal sensitivity, suicidal ideation, and physical aggression.[48-54]

DBT also has demonstrated cross-cultural efficacy. RCTs in Spain, Norway, Great Britain, Australia, and the Netherlands found that DBT was more effective than TAU.[16,40,55-57] In addition, research groups in Germany, Ireland, the Netherlands, Canada, Italy, and Taiwan found that DBT promoted significant reductions in anxiety, hopelessness, depression, self-injurious behaviors, and severity of BPD symptoms.[58-64] Review Box 11.8, p. 304 for a breakdown of the most robust evidence for DBT.

Conclusions: Limitations of DBT and Future Directions

DBT is a philosophically rich and effective EBT for treating many PDs, emotion dysregulation, and risky behaviors transdiagnostically. It has saved the lives of clients, many of whom were stigmatized or previously viewed as untreatable. However, there are still many limitations to DBT and areas for future research. It is a time-intensive and often quite costly treatment, typically lasting at least 12 months and often longer in practice. Although one could argue that 12 months is short relative to a lifetime of suffering, researchers are continuing to test whether six-month protocols are similarly effective. A full DBT treatment also can be expensive. For reasons that are unjustifiable, many third-party payers do not reimburse skills groups. This often leads agencies to lower skills group costs, which strains agency resources and can lead them to abandon DBT altogether. When large agencies give up on DBT, private and self-pay practices become the only option for clients. DBT also requires a significant amount of learning, especially in the weekly skills classes. Thus, in our experience, clients who have recently

Box 11.8 Level of Evidence for the Effectiveness of DBT

12-month DBT

- Nine high-quality RCTs have been conducted.[1,26,32–34,37,56,62]
- These studies report significant reductions in self-harm, suicide ideation, substance use, depression, hopelessness, and hospitalizations.
- Five non-RCTs found improvements in emotion regulation skills and reductions in impulsivity, substance use, anxiety, depression, hopelessness, suicide attempt, and hospitalizations.[39,45,48,58–59]
- The strength of recommendation for 12-month DBT for borderline personality disorder (BPD) with or without comorbid substance use is Level of Evidence A.

6-month DBT

- Two small high-quality RCTs have been conducted.[31,40]
- Results of RCTs found reductions in self-harm, suicide ideation, depression, hopelessness, and hospitalizations.
- Three non-RCTs reported reductions in self-harm, suicide ideation, depression, hopelessness, and target behaviors.[38,43,55]
- The strength of recommendation for 6-month DBT for BPD is Level of Evidence B.

DBT Skills Training Only (DBT-ST)

- Five RCTs have been conducted with DBT-ST of varying lengths (2–12 months).[26,36,47,63–64]
- Results from those studies prompted improvements in distress tolerance, emotion regulation, and reductions in alcohol use, self-harm, suicide attempt, and depression.
- Two non-RCTs found improvements in emotion regulation, and reductions in suicide attempts, depression, and consecutive days of abstinence from alcohol.[46,60]
- The strength of recommendation for DBT-ST for BPD with or without comorbid substance use is Level of Evidence B.

DBT Cross-culturally

- Nine high-quality RCTs with DBT of varying lengths (5–12 months) found reductions in impulsivity, self-harm, suicide ideation, hospitalizations, posttraumatic stress disorder symptom severity, and improvements in distress tolerance, emotion regulation, anger, and quality of life.[16,37,40,51,56–57,62–64]
- Five non-RCTs with DBT of varying lengths (5-week to 12-month) found reductions in suicide ideation, depression, hopelessness, anxiety, and borderline symptoms.[55,59–61]

- RCTs were conducted in Spain, Norway, Great Britain, Australia, and the Netherlands and non-RCTs were conducted in Germany, Ireland, Canada, Italy, Taiwan, and the Netherlands.
- The strength of recommendation for DBT for BPD when implemented in other cultures is Level of Evidence A.

Note: There is evidence for DBT for Adolescents (DBT-A), but studies have not used personality disorders as a focus.
Key: Levels of Evidence; Strength of recommendation taxonomy (SORT).*
Level of Evidence A: Good quality patient-oriented evidence.
Level of Evidence B: Limited quality patient-oriented evidence.
Level of Evidence C: Based on consensus, usual practice, opinion, disease-oriented evidence, or case series for studies of diagnosis.
*Ebell MH, Siwek J, Weiss BD, Woolf SH, Susman J, Ewigman B, Bowman M. Simplifying the language of evidence to improve patient care. *J Fam Pract.* 2004 Feb 1;53(2):111–120.

completed electroconvulsive shock therapy or engage in high levels of substance use (i.e., use leading to blackouts) often need 12 months of skills classes due to slower progress in the first round of treatment.

Relative to other EBTs, DBT is among the most well-researched therapies. However, even more research is needed on component analyses (e.g., identifying which components are necessary), cultural adaptations, use in young adolescents and children, and specific multi-diagnostic populations.[11,45,52] For example, our team has faced challenges when suicidal clients with OCD/OCPD reassurance-seeking behaviors use phone coaching primarily for validation and intermittently for crisis-related coaching. The therapist has to be particularly attentive to supporting the client with skills generalization and crisis reduction, while not inadvertently reinforcing OCD symptoms. Similarly, the interface between PTSD and other diagnoses (e.g., BPD, substance use, mood disorders), continues to be a challenge for DBT therapists in daily practice.

Both DBT and DBT-PE have clear criteria for moving between behavioral control and increasing skills use (Stage 1) and recovering from trauma (Stage 2);[4,21] yet, it is often difficult for clients and therapists to be sure that those criteria have been met, even with regular assessments. Many times, the difficulty of trauma treatment leads to a resurgence of behavioral dyscontrol (Stage 1). In practice, many therapists are confronted with the difficult decision of whether to pause trauma treatment to revisit skills, or whether such a pause constitutes avoidance and increases the risk that the client will fear restarting trauma work.

Impressively, DBT has translated well from RCTs to community practice. This is likely because DBT has always been targeted toward complex, high-risk, multi-diagnostic clients, such as those who often are excluded from other RCTs. One challenge described by many DBT practitioners is identifying an end date for treatment, given that an advantage of RCTs is a clearly defined endpoint. In practice, this is much more difficult due to strong bonds between therapists and clients and the capacity for DBT to stretch (i.e., across the four stages) in order to address new client goals. Regular assessment (i.e., approximately every six months) is critical for helping clients and therapists ensure that growth and progress are continuing. Assessment is also critical for those who are considering adaptations to DBT. Common adaptations in practice include: "skills only," which typically involves skills in the absence of any other DBT component; "CBT-plus," which, allows clients in other EBTs to join a skills group; and a shortened or compressed DBT sometimes happens in inpatient or residential settings. Although these adaptations may be effective, we strongly recommend that therapists provide informed consent about the ways in which DBT has been modified and the potential downsides of receiving a partial dose of the treatment.

In sum, DBT is one of the most effective, well-researched, and lifesaving therapies for the treatment of personality disorders and other complex patient groups. However, it is not a therapy for the faint-of-heart. As Marsha Linehan has often said, DBT therapists go "where angels fear to tread."[65] The work of DBT is both terrifying and thrilling for therapists and their clients, resulting in strong bonds as they collaboratively confront clients' life-threatening behaviors. Through their work, nearly all DBT therapists lose a client to suicide, drug overdose, or an eating disorder. However, they do not face this loss alone. The treatment team, other clients in skills group, and a vast international community of DBT clinicians provide a support network for each individual therapist, allowing them to continue their meaningful work of saving lives. Review resources for patients, families, and patients in Box 11.9.

Conflict of Interest/Disclosure: The authors of this chapter have no financial conflicts and nothing to disclose.

Box 11.9 Resources for Patients, Families, and Clinicians

- Behavioral Tech: A Linehan Institute Training Company. https://behavioral-tech.org/.
  - Resources for patients and families. https://behavioraltech.org/resources/resources-for-clients-families/.
  - Resources for clinicians. https://behavioraltech.org/resources/resources-for-providers/.

Recommended reading for clinicians

- Pryor K. *Don't Shoot the Dog: The New Art of Teaching and Training*. Reprint ed. New York, NY: Simon & Schuster; 2019.
- Ramnerö J., Törneke N, *The ABCs of Human Behavior: Behavioral Principles for the Practicing Clinician*. Oakland, CA: Context Press; 2008.
- Miller AL, Rathus, JH, Linehan, MM. *Dialectical Behavior Therapy with Suicidal Adolescents*. New York, NY: Guilford Press; 2017.

Recommended reading for patients, families, and clinicians

- Aitken R. *Taking the Path of Zen*. New York, NY: Northpoint Press; 1982.
- Kabat-Zinn J. *Mindfulness for Beginners: Reclaiming the Present Moment— And Your Life*. Louisville, CO: Sounds True; 2012.
- Van Gelder K. *The Buddha and the Borderline: My Recovery from Borderline Personality Disorder through Dialectical Behavior Therapy, Buddhism, and Online Dating*. Oakland, CA: New Harbinger; 2010.
- Porr V. *Overcoming Borderline Personality Disorder: A Family Guide for Healing and Change*. New York, NY: Oxford University Press; 2010.

References

1. Linehan MM. Cognitive-behavioral treatment of chronically parasuicidal borderline patients. *Arch Gen Psychiatry.* 1991; 48(12): 1060–1064. doi:10.1001/archpsyc.1991.01810360024003

2. Linehan MM, Wagner AW, Cox G. *Parasuicide History Interview: Comprehensive Assessment of Parasuicidal Behavior.* Seattle, WA: University of Washington; 1989.

3. Linehan MM. *Dialectical Behavior Therapy for Treatment of Parasuicidal Women: Treatment Manual.* Seattle, WA: University of Washington; 1984.

4. Linehan MM. *Cognitive-behavioral Treatment of Borderline Personality Disorder.* New York, NY: Guilford Press; 1993.

5. Linehan MM. *Skills Training Manual for Treating Borderline Personality Disorder.* New York, NY: Guilford Press; 1993.

6. Linehan MM. *DBT Skills Training Manual.* 2nd ed. New York, NY: Guilford Press; 2015.

7. Hayes SC, Follette VM, Linehan MM. *Mindfulness and Acceptance: Expanding the Cognitive-behavioral Tradition.* New York, NY: Guilford Press; 2004.

8. Bohus M, Dyer AS, Priebe K, et al. Dialectical behavior therapy for post-traumatic stress disorder after childhood sexual abuse in patients with and without borderline personality disorder: a randomized controlled trial. *Psychother Psychosom.* 2013; 82(4): 221–233. doi:10.1159/000348451

9. Rosenthal ZM, Lynch TR, Linehan MM. Dialectical behavior therapy for individuals with borderline personality disorder and substance use disorders. In: Frances RJ, Miller SI, Mack AH, ed. *Clinical Textbook of Addictive Disorders.* 3rd ed. New York, NY: Guilford Press; 2005: 615–636.

10. Dulit RA, Fyer MR, Haas GL, Sullivan T, Frances AJ. Substance use in borderline personality disorder. *Am J Psychiatry.* 1990; 147(8): 1002–1007. doi:10.1176/ajp.147.8.1002

11. Harley R, Sprich S, Safren S, Jacobo M, Fava M. Adaptation of dialectical behavior therapy skills training group for treatment-resistant depression. *J Nerv Ment Dis.* 2008; 196(2): 136–143. doi:10.1097/NMD.0b013e318162aa3f

12. Hill DM, Craighead LW, Safer DL. Appetite-focused dialectical behavior therapy for the treatment of binge eating with purging: a preliminary trial. *Int J Eat Disord.* 2011; 44(3): 249–261. doi:10.1002/eat.20812

13. Safer DL, Jo B. Outcome from a randomized controlled trial of group therapy for binge eating disorder: comparing dialectical behavior therapy adapted for binge eating to an active comparison group therapy. *Behav Ther.* 2010; 41: 106–120. doi:10.1016/j.beth.2009.01.006

14. Fleischhaker C, Böhme R, Sixt B, Brück C, Schneider C, Schulz E. Dialectical behavioral therapy for adolescents (DBT-A): a clinical trial for patients with suicidal and self-injurious behavior and borderline symptoms with a one-year follow-up. *Child Adolesc Psychiatry Ment Health.* 2011; 5:3. doi:10.1186/1753-2000-5-3

15. James AC, Winmill L, Anderson C, Alfoadari K. A preliminary study of an extension of a community dialectic behaviour therapy (DBT) programme to adolescents in the looked after care system. *Child Adolesc Ment Health.* 2011; 16(1): 9–13. doi:10.1111/j.1475-3588.2010.00571.x

16. Mehlum L, Tørmoen AJ, Ramberg M, et al. Dialectical behavior therapy for adolescents with repeated suicidal and self-harming behavior: a randomized trial. *J Am Acad Child Adolesc Psychiatry.* 2014; 53(10): 1082–1091. doi:10.1016/j.jaac.2014.07.003

17. Linehan MM. *Building a Life Worth Living: A Memoir.* New York, NY: Random House; 2020.

18. Crowell SE, Beauchaine TP, Linehan MM. A biosocial developmental model of borderline personality: elaborating and extending Linehan's theory. *Psychol Bull.* 2009; 35(3): 495–510. doi:10.1037/a0015616

19. Crowell SE, Rith KA. Dialectical behavior therapy. In: Tinsley HEA, Lease SH, Griffin Wiersma NS, ed. *Contemporary Theory and Practice in Counseling and Psychotherapy.* Thousand Oaks, CA: SAGE Publications; 2015: 201–230.

20. McMain SF, Chapman AL, Kuo JR, et al. The effectiveness of 6 versus 12-months of dialectical behaviour therapy for borderline personality disorder: the feasibility of a shorter treatment and evaluating responses (FASTER) trial protocol. *BMC Psychiatry.* 2018; 18(1): 230. doi:10.1186/s12888-018-1802-z

21. Harned MS, Chapman AL, Dexter-Mazza ET, Murray A, Comtois KA, Linehan MM. Treating co-occurring Axis I disorders in recurrently suicidal women with borderline personality disorder: a 2-year randomized trial of dialectical behavior therapy versus community treatment by experts. *J Consult Clin Psychol.* 2008; 76(6): 1068–1075. doi:10.1037/a0014044

22. Harned MS, Korslund KE, Linehan MM. A pilot randomized controlled trial of dialectical behavior therapy with and without the dialectical behavior therapy prolonged exposure protocol for suicidal and self-injuring women with borderline personality disorder and PTSD. *Behav Res Ther.* 2014; 55: 7–17. doi:10.1016/j.brat.2014.01.008

23. Luoma JB, Hayes SC, Walser RD. *Learning ACT: An Acceptance and Commitment Therapy Skills-training Manual for Therapists.* Oakland, CA: New Harbinger; 2007.

24. Harned M. What is DBT PE? Treating PTSD. Published 2018. https://dbtpe.org/treatment-overview.

25. Maslow, A. A theory of human motivation. *Psychol Rev.* 1943; 50: 370–396.

26. Linehan MM, Wilks CR. The course and evolution of dialectical behavior therapy. *Am J Psychother.* 2015; 69(2):97–110. doi:10.1176/appi.psychotherapy.2015.69.2.97

27. Wagner AW, Linehan MM. Applications of dialectical behavior therapy to posttraumatic stress disorder and related problems. In: Follette VC, Ruzek JI, eds. *Cognitive-behavioral Therapies for Trauma.* 2nd ed. New York, NY: Guilford; 2006: 117–145.

28. Staddon JE, Cerutti DT. Operant conditioning. *Ann Rev Psychol.* 2003; 54: 115–144. doi:10.1146/annurev.psych.54.101601.145124

29. Miller TW, Kraus RF. Modified dialectical behavior therapy and problem solving for obsessive-compulsive personality disorder. *J Contemp Psychother.* 2007; 37: 79–85.

30. Storebø OJ, Stoffers-Winterling JM, Völlm BA, et al. Psychological therapies for people with borderline personality disorder. *Cochrane Database Syst Rev.* 2020;5. doi:10.1002/14651858. CD012955.

31. Koons CR, Robins CJ, Tweed JL, et al. Efficacy of dialectical behavior therapy in women veterans with borderline personality disorder. *Behav Ther.* 2001; 32(2): 371–390. doi:10.1016/s0005-7894(01)80009-5

32. Linehan MM, Schmidt H, Dimeff LA, Craft JC, Kanter J, Comtois KA. Dialectical behavior therapy for patients with borderline personality disorder and drug-dependence. *Am J Addict.* 1999; 8(4): 279–292. doi:10.1080/105504999305686

33. Linehan MM, Dimeff LA, Reynolds SK, et al. Dialectical behavior therapy versus comprehensive validation therapy plus 12-step for the treatment of opioid dependent women meeting criteria for borderline personality disorder. *Drug Alcohol Depend.* 2002; 67(1): 13–26. doi:10.1016/s0376-8716(02)00011-x

34. Linehan MM, Comtois KA, Murray AM, et al. Two-year randomized controlled trial and follow-up of dialectical behavior therapy vs. therapy by experts for suicidal behaviors and borderline personality disorder. *Arch Gen Psychiatry.* 2006; 63(7): 757. doi:10.1001/archpsyc.63.7.757

35. Turner RM. Naturalistic evaluation of dialectical behavior therapy-oriented treatment for borderline personality disorder. *Cogn Behav Pract.* 2000; 7(4): 413–419. doi:10.1016/s1077-7229(00)80052-8

36. Neacsiu AD, Eberle JW, Kramer R, Wiesmann T, Linehan MM. Dialectical behavior therapy skills for transdiagnostic emotion dysregulation: a pilot randomized controlled trial. *Behav Res Ther.* 2014; 59: 40–51. doi:10.1016/j.brat.2014.05.005

37. Feigenbaum JD, Fonagy P, Pilling S, Jones A, Wildgoose A, Bebbington PE. A real-world study of the effectiveness of DBT in the UK National Health Service. *Br J Clin Psychol.* 2011; 51(2): 121–141. doi:10.1111/j.20448260.2011.02017.x

38. Pasieczny N, Connor J. The effectiveness of dialectical behaviour therapy in routine public mental health settings: an Australian controlled trial. *Behav Res Ther.* 2011; 49(1): 4–10. doi:10.1016/j.brat.2010.09.006

39. Coyle TN, Shaver JA, Linehan MM. On the potential for iatrogenic effects of psychiatric crisis services: the example of dialectical behavior therapy for adult women with borderline personality disorder. *J Consult Clin Psychol.* 2018; 86(2): 116–124. doi:10.1037/ccp0000275

40. Carter GL, Willcox CH, Lewin TJ, Conrad AM, Bendit N. Hunter DBT project: randomized controlled trial of dialectical behaviour therapy in women with borderline personality disorder. *Aust N Z J Psychiatry.* 2010; 44(2): 162–173. doi:10.3109/00048670903393621

41. Koerner K, Dimeff LA. Overview of dialectical behavior therapy. In: Dimeff LA, Koerner K, eds. *Dialectical Behavior Therapy in Clinical Practice: Applications Across Disorders and Settings.* New York, NY: Guilford Press; 2007: 1–18.

42. McMain SF, Guimond T, Barnhart R, Habinski L, Streiner DL. A randomized trial of brief dialectical behaviour therapy skills training in suicidal patients suffering from borderline disorder. *Acta Psychiatr Scand.* 2017; 135(2): 138–148. doi:10.1111/acps.12664

43. Stanley B, Brodsky B, Nelson JD, Dulit R. Brief dialectical behavior therapy (DBT-B) for suicidal behavior and non-suicidal self injury. *Arch Suicide Res.* 2007; 11(4): 337–341. doi:10.1080/13811110701542069

44. Axelrod SR, Perepletchikova F, Holtzman K, Sinha R. Emotion regulation and substance use frequency in women with substance dependence and borderline personality disorder receiving dialectical behavior therapy. *Am J Drug Alcohol Abuse.* 2011; 37(1): 37–42. doi:10.3109/00952990.2010.535582

45. Beckstead DJ, Lambert MJ, DuBose AP, Linehan M. Dialectical behavior therapy with American Indian/Alaska Native adolescents diagnosed with substance use disorders: combining an evidence based treatment with cultural, traditional, and spiritual beliefs. *Addict Behav.* 2015; 51: 84–87. doi:10.1016/j.addbeh.2015.07.018

46. Cavicchioli M, Movalli M, Vassena G, Ramella P, Prudenziati F, Maffei C. The therapeutic role of emotion regulation and coping strategies during a stand-alone DBT skills training program for alcohol use disorder and concurrent substance use disorders. *Addict Behav.* 2019; 98:106035. doi:10.1016/j.addbeh.2019.106035

47. Wilks CR, Lungu A, Ang SY, Matsumiya B, Yin Q, Linehan MM. A randomized controlled trial of an internet delivered dialectical behavior therapy skills training for suicidal and heavy episodic drinkers. *J Affect Disord.* 2018; 232: 219–228. doi:10.1016/j.jad.2018.02.053

48. Goldstein TR, Fersch-Podrat RK, Rivera M, et al. Dialectical behavior therapy for adolescents with bipolar disorder: results from a pilot randomized trial. *J Child Adolesc Psychopharmacol*. 2015; 25(2): 140–149. doi:10.1089/cap.2013.0145

49. Lenz AS, Conte GD. Efficacy of dialectical behavior therapy for adolescents in a partial hospitalization program. *J Couns Dev*. 2018; 96(1): 15–26. doi:10.1002/jcad.12174

50. McCauley E, Berk MS, Asarnow JR, et al. Efficacy of dialectical behavior therapy for adolescents at high risk for suicide: a randomized clinical trial. *JAMA Psychiatry*. 2018; 75(8): 777–785. doi:10.1001/jamapsychiatry.2018.1109

51. Mehlum L, Ramberg M, Tørmoen AJ, et al. Dialectical behavior therapy compared with enhanced usual care for adolescents with repeated suicidal and self-harming behavior: outcomes over a one-year follow-up. *J Am Acad Child Adolesc Psychiatry*. 2016; 55(4): 295–300. doi:10.1016/j.jaac.2016.01.005

52. Saito E, Tebbett-Mock AA, McGee M. Dialectical behavior therapy decreases depressive symptoms among adolescents in an acute-care inpatient unit. *J Child Adolesc Psychopharmacol*. 2020; 30(4):244–249. doi:10.1089/cap.2019.0149

53. Shelton D, Kesten K, Zhang W, Trestman R. Impact of a dialectic behavior therapy-corrections modified (DBT-CM) upon behaviorally challenged incarcerated male adolescents. *J Child Adolesc Psychiatr Nurs*. 2011; 24(2): 105–113. doi:10.1111/j.1744-6171.2011.00275.x

54. Tebbett-Mock AA, Saito E, McGee M, Woloszyn P, Venuti M. Efficacy of dialectical behavior therapy versus treatment as usual for acute-care inpatient adolescents. *J Am Acad Child Adolesc Psychiatry*. 2020; 59(1): 149–156. doi:10.1016/j.jaac.2019.01.020

55. Navarro-Haro MV, Botella C, Guillen V, et al. Dialectical behavior therapy in the treatment of borderline personality disorder and eating disorders comorbidity: a pilot study in a naturalistic setting. *Cognit Ther Res*. 2018; 42(5): 636–649. doi:10.1007/s10608-018-9906-9

56. Priebe S, Bhatti N, Barnicot K, et al. Effectiveness and cost-effectiveness of dialectical behaviour therapy for self-harming patients with personality disorder: a pragmatic randomised controlled trial. *Psychother Psychosom*. 2012; 81(6): 356–365. doi:10.1159/000338897

57. Verheul R, Van Den Bosch LM, Koeter MW, De Ridder MA, Stijnen T, Van Den Brink W. Dialectical behaviour therapy for women with borderline personality disorder: 12-month, randomised clinical trial in The Netherlands. *Br J Psychiatry*. 2003; 182: 135–140. doi:10.1192/bjp.182.2.135

58. Bianchini V, Cofini V, Curto M, et al. Dialectical behaviour therapy (DBT) for forensic psychiatric patients: an Italian pilot study. *Crim Behav Ment Health*. 2019; 29(2): 122–130. doi:10.1002/cbm.2102

59. Flynn D, Kells M, Joyce M, et al. Standard 12 month dialectical behaviour therapy for adults with borderline personality disorder in a public community mental health setting. *Borderline Personal Disord Emot Dysregul*. 2017; 4: 19. doi:10.1186/s40479-017-0070-8

60. Lin TJ, Ko HC, Wu JY, Oei TP, Lane HY, Chen CH. The effectiveness of dialectical behavior therapy skills training group vs. cognitive therapy group on reducing depression and suicide attempts for borderline personality disorder in Taiwan. *Arch Suicide Res*. 2019; 23(1): 82–99. doi:10.1080/13811118.2018.1436104

61. Probst T, O'Rourke T, Decker V, et al. Effectiveness of a 5-week inpatient dialectical behavior therapy for borderline personality disorder. *J Psychiatr Pract*. 2019; 25(3): 192–198. doi:10.1097/PRA.0000000000000383

62. Sinnaeve R, van den Bosch LMC, Hakkaart-van Roijen L, Vansteelandt K. Effectiveness of step-down versus outpatient dialectical behaviour therapy for patients with severe

levels of borderline personality disorder: a pragmatic randomized controlled trial. *Borderline Personal Disord Emot Dysregul.* 2018; 5:12. doi:10.1186/s40479-018-0089-5

63. Uliaszek AA, Rashid T, Williams GE, Gulamani T. Group therapy for university students: a randomized control trial of dialectical behavior therapy and positive psychotherapy. *Behav Res Ther.* 2016; 77: 78–85. doi:10.1016/j.brat.2015.12.003

64. McMain SF, Guimond T, Barnhart R, Habinski L, Streiner DL. A randomized trial of brief dialectical behaviour therapy skills training in suicidal patients suffering from borderline disorder. *Acta Psychiatr Scand.* 2017; 135(2): 138–148. doi:10.1111/acps.12664

65. Linehan MM, Layden MA, Newman CF, Freeman A, Norcross JC. Plunging in where angels fear to tread. *Contemp Psychol.* 1995; 40(5): 426–428. doi:10.1037/003631

12
Schema Therapy

Anja Schaich, Eva Fassbinder, and Arnoud Arntz

Key Points

- Schema therapy (ST) is an integrative therapy based on a cognitive model that integrates cognitive, behavioral, psychodynamic, and experiential therapies with insights, methods, and techniques from attachment and other developmental theories.
- ST has become one of the major evidence-based treatments for patients with personality disorders (PDs).
- Schemas are mental representations of oneself, one's relationships with others, and the world.
- ST assumes that aversive childhood experiences and the frustration of basic needs during childhood can lead to the development of early maladaptive schemas (EMS) and schema modes.
- Maladaptive schemas, schema modes and associated coping strategies lead to problems in adulthood.
- Assessment involves understanding the patient's current symptoms, important relationships, and early life history.
- Cases are conceptualized using the schema mode model and are explained to the patient using this model.
- The therapeutic relationship has an essential role in revealing and modifying dysfunctional interpersonal relationships and the patient's relationships in the outside world.
- The therapeutic relationship is built using empathic confrontation and limited reparenting.
- Therapists use an eclectic group of interventions to facilitate change, including: cognitive-behavioral interventions; behavioral techniques (e.g., role-play, behavioral experiments, skills training, problem-solving, behavioral activation, or relaxation techniques); and experiential techniques such as chair dialogues and imagery rescripting.
- ST is well accepted by both therapists and patients and has very low dropout rates.

Introduction

Schema therapy (ST; formerly also called schema-focused therapy [SFT]) has become one of the major evidence-based treatments for patients with personality disorders

(PDs).[1] ST assumes that aversive childhood experiences and the frustration of basic needs in early childhood, in interaction with biological and cultural factors, lead to the development of dysfunctional schemas, in ST usually called "early maladaptive schemas" (EMS). Schemas are mental representations of oneself, of one's relationships with others, and of the world, that strongly influence information processing and resulting emotions and cognitions. When an EMS gets activated, this leads to emotional distress. In order to prevent or deal with this emotional distress, the individual develops specific coping strategies (surrender, avoidance, overcompensation) that help to reduce emotional pain. However, these coping strategies also block access to primary feelings and needs, and result in unmet needs and problems that persist into adult life.

ST is an integrative therapy, based on a cognitive model that integrates cognitive, behavioral, psychodynamic, and experiential therapies with insights, methods, and techniques from attachment and other developmental theories. A special focus is placed on the therapeutic relationship as well as on the use of experiential techniques such as chair dialogues and imagery rescripting. ST can be seen as a transdiagnostic approach, but there are disorder-specific case conceptualizations for most of the PDs.[2] ST has proven effective in the treatment of PDs in multiple studies, with most studies conducted for patients with borderline personality disorder (BPD) and Cluster C PDs (avoidant, dependent, and obsessive-compulsive PD).[3-5] This chapter provides an overview of the outcome data of ST, the theoretical background and the development of ST, followed by a description of the treatment plan and the practical application of ST. The case formulation and the therapeutic techniques will be illustrated by case examples.

Effectiveness of Schema Therapy for Personality Disorders

ST has proven effective in the treatment of PDs in several studies. Most of the studies were conducted on patients with BPD. ST for BPD was investigated in two randomized controlled trials (RCTs),[6,7] one case study,[8] one observational study,[9] five pilot studies,[10-12] and two implementation studies.[13,14] ST was successful in reducing BPD symptom severity and general psychopathology as well improving the quality of life. A meta-analysis, including all studies published up to 2013, showed a very large pre–post effect size of d = 2.38 regarding the reduction of BPD symptomatology and a very low dropout rate of 10 percent.[3]

In one of the RCTs, ST was compared to transference-focused psychotherapy (TFP) (N = 86). In both conditions, patients received three years of treatment with two therapy sessions per week. Patients in both conditions showed a reduction in BPD symptom severity and a composite measure of general and personality psychopathology, as well as an improvement in the quality of life. ST outperformed TFP regarding all of these outcome variables and showed a lower dropout rate[15] and higher cost-efficiency than TPF.[16] An implementation study (N = 62) indicated that ST is effective, also with shorter treatment duration and a lower session frequency.[13]

In a second RCT (N = 32), patients with BPD received either treatment as usual (TAU), or an additional 30 sessions of ST in a group format (GST) over the course of eight months.[7] There were no dropouts in the GST conditions and higher remission rates of BPD diagnoses. The GST condition also outperformed the TAU condition demonstrating a reduction of general psychopathology and the improvement of psychosocial functioning. Two pilot studies (N = 18 and N = 10) on GST also indicated improvement of BPD symptoms, general psychopathology, schemas and schema modes, quality of life, and happiness.[10,12] In three studies, GST was also successful in treating inpatients with BPD (N = 92) by reducing BPD symptom severity and general psychopathology.[11]

In a recent not yet published multicenter RCT (N = 494), GST alone, as well as combined individual and group therapy for BPD patients, were compared to TAU for their effectiveness and cost-effectiveness.[17] The first results showed a greater reduction of BPD symptoms and general psychopathology as well as greater improvement of psychosocial functioning in the ST conditions compared to the TAU conditions. In the combined individual and group ST condition, the attrition rate was lower, and effects were generally better, than in the other conditions.[18] Another RCT using a combined individual and group format is currently being conducted, comparing ST to dialectical behavior therapy.[19]

In a first naturalistic observational study and qualitative study on a ST eHealth program (priovi®), patients with BPD (N = 14) received individual ST over the duration of one year in combination with the eHealth program.[20] The treatment proved effective in the reduction of BPD symptom severity and was well accepted by both patients and therapists.[9]

There are also studies on patients with other PDs than BPD. One RCT compared ST with clarification-oriented psychotherapy (COP) and TAU (N = 323) for patients with PDs (90 percent Cluster C).[21] ST outperformed both TAU and COP regarding the reduction of PD symptomatology and depressive disorders. The patients that received ST also showed a higher general and psychosocial functioning at follow-up, and the dropout rate was lower in the ST condition. Furthermore, ST proved more cost-effective than TAU and COP. A multiple-baseline study investigating older patients with Cluster C PDs (N = 8) showed a reduction regarding dysfunctional core beliefs and general psychopathology, as well as an improvement regarding quality of life, schemas, and PD diagnosis. A multicenter RCT among high-security forensic patients suffering from PDs (74 percent antisocial PD), compared ST to TAU.[22] Preliminary results indicate superiority of ST in reducing PD pathology, recidivism risk, and promoting reentry into the community.[22] An RCT on GST for avoidant PD and social phobia[23] and one on GST for older patients with Cluster B and Cluster C PDs are currently being conducted.[24] The results on ST for patients with BPD and other PDs until 2016 were summarized in three reviews.[3-5]

Qualitative studies demonstrate that ST is well accepted both by therapists and patients with PDs.[25,26] Patients experience ST as effective,[26] and experiential techniques (like chair dialogues and imagery rescripting) as intense but highly valuable.[26,27] Patients reported that imagery rescripting had led to a better understanding of their problems and schemas, as well as to an improvement in their emotional regulation skills and their interpersonal relationships.[28] See Box 12.1, p. 316 for a summary of the evidence for ST.

Origin and Theoretical Background of Schema Therapy

Jeffrey Young started developing ST in the early 1980s in order to meet the needs of patients with pervasive, complex, and rigid psychological problems regarding emotion regulation and interpersonal relationships, who did not sufficiently profit from standard cognitive-behavioral therapy (CBT).[1] Young observed that these patients exhibited dysfunctional behavior patterns that often had persisted since their childhood and which

---

Box 12.1   Levels of Evidence for Effectiveness of Schema Therapy for Personality Disorders

---

Published studies on ST until 07/2020

- Level I: 2 reviews,[4,5] 1 meta-analysis[3]
- Level II: 3 RCTs[6,7,21]
- Level III: 5 pilot studies,[10-12] 2 implementation studies[13,14]
- Level IV: 1 case study,[8] 1 observational study,[9] 1 multiple-baseline-study[22]
- Level V: 3 qualitative studies[25,26,28]

Key; Level of Evidence:
Level I: Systematic review or meta-analysis of randomized controlled trials
Level II: Randomized controlled trial
Level III: Non-randomized controlled, cohort/follow-up studies
Level IV: Case series or case control
Level V: Mechanism based reasoning
Center for Evidenced based Medicine
https://www.cebm.ox.ac.uk/resources/levels-of-evidence/ocebm-levels-of-evidence

---

also blocked the therapeutic process. A substantial number of these patients also met the diagnosis of a personality disorder.

As Young tried to understand why these patients did not profit from CBT, he discovered that they seemed to have developed coping strategies as a response to adverse experiences in their past. These led to difficulties in the therapeutic relationship and the therapeutic process for multiple reasons; some learned to suppress or avoid their emotions or thoughts and were therefore not able or willing to follow CBT protocol on observing, recording, and sharing their thoughts and feelings. Due to coping strategies developed as a response to adverse interpersonal experiences such as mistrust, dependency, hostility, or controlling behavior, patients had trouble engaging in a collaborative relationship with their therapists. Young encountered other difficulties: patients' complaints were vague and hard to capture, which made it difficult to fit them in traditional CBT treatment targets. A lack of psychological flexibility, inherent to PDs, also made them less responsive to CBT techniques and prevented changes in the short treatment period characteristic for CBT. In order to meet the needs of these patients, Young developed ST.

The Development of Schema Therapy

Young addressed the problems patients with PDs encountered with traditional CBT by extending CBT techniques with elements from other therapeutic theories such as attachment, interpersonal, and object-relation theory, and enriched the treatment by integrating experiential techniques from gestalt and emotion-focused therapy.

Maladaptive Schemas

ST assumes that the frustration of basic childhood needs interacts with biological and cultural influences, leading to the development of EMSs that promote persistent psychological problems in adulthood. Basic emotional needs[2] include: (1) secure attachment, stability, and care; (2) autonomy, competence, and identity; (3) realistic limits; (4) expression and validation of emotions, needs, and opinions; and (5) play and spontaneity.

EMSs are defined as dysfunctional knowledge structures, acquired early in life, that govern cognitive processes such as attention, interpretation, or memory consolidation. EMSs contain both explicit information such as dysfunctional beliefs as well as implicit knowledge, and behavioral-procedural and emotional information.[2] Schemas are developed during childhood or adolescence and are elaborated throughout the lifetime. Schemas tend to act as filters for information by processing information in a way that fits the schema, which make them self-sustaining and very resistant to change. Schemas can be triggered by internal or external stimuli, especially if they show similarities with past situations that led to the development of the schema.

Young[1] described 18 EMSs, organized into five domains that are related to the five core needs (see Table 12.1 for an overview; for a detailed description of EMSs see Young, Klosko and Weishaar[1] and Arntz and Jacob[2]).

Strategies for Coping with Schema Activation

The activation of an EMS is usually accompanied by psychological distress and unwanted emotions. In order to cope with psychological distress, an individual may react with one of three types of coping: (1) *schema surrender:* the individual yields to the schema; (2) *schema avoidance:* the individual avoids the full activation and awareness of the schema;

Table 12.1. Early Maladaptive Schemas and Schema Domains (from Arntz and Jacob[2])

Basic Emotional Needs	Schema Domain	Schemas
Secure attachment, stability, and care	*Disconnection and rejection*	Abandonment/instability Mistrust/abuse Emotional deprivation Defectiveness/shame Social isolation/alienation
Autonomy, competence, identity	*Impaired autonomy and achievement*	Dependency/incompetence Vulnerability to harm and illness Enmeshment/undeveloped self Failure
Realistic limits	*Impaired limits*	Entitlement/grandiosity Insufficient self-control/self-discipline
Expression and validation of emotions, needs and opinions	*Other-directedness*	Subjugation Self-sacrifice Approval-seeking
Play and spontaneity	*Hypervigilance and inhibition*	Negativity/pessimism Emotional inhibition Unrelenting standards Punitiveness

or (3) *schema overcompensation:* the individual fights the schema by thinking, feeling, behaving and relating as if the opposite of the schema were true.

These coping styles are typically developed during childhood as an adaptive way to help the child survive and endure distressing situations and emotions (e.g., dissociation during an abusive experience). In adulthood, however, these former "survival strategies" have become rigid, inflexible, and automatically activated behaviors that prevent healthy interpersonal relationships, functional emotion regulation, and satisfaction of emotional core needs.

Schema Modes

In patients with PDs, usually, multiple schemas and coping strategies are active at the same time, and patients tend to switch between schemas quickly. Therefore, Young added the schema mode model approach to schema theory.[1] A schema mode is the combination of an activated schema and a coping strategy, and describes the moment-to-moment emotional-cognitive-behavioral state of the patient. There are four categories of modes in the basic approach of the mode model:

1. Dysfunctional child modes
2. Dysfunctional parent modes
3. Dysfunctional coping modes
4. Healthy modes

Dysfunctional Child Modes
Dysfunctional child modes are developed when basic emotional needs were frustrated in childhood. These modes are accompanied by intense emotions like fear, loneliness, helplessness, sadness, or mistrust in the *vulnerable child modes.* Other child modes include the *angry child, enraged child, impulsive child,* and *undisciplined child modes.* Dysfunctional child modes result from surrendering to an EMS.

Dysfunctional Parent Modes
The dysfunctional parent modes include internalized negative beliefs about oneself that are developed during childhood due to behavior and reactions of significant others like parents, teachers, or peers. There are *punitive parent* and *demanding parent modes.* Dysfunctional parent modes are associated with high standards, self-devaluations, self-hatred, guilt, or shame. Dysfunctional parent modes result from surrendering to two specific EMSs: punitiveness and unrelenting standards.

Dysfunctional Coping Modes
The dysfunctional coping modes result when the coping strategy with the EMS activation is an avoidance or overcompensation type. These coping strategies, when strong enough, overshadow the EMS, and the experience and behavior of the person is dominated by the coping strategy rather than by the EMS. These coping strategies are usually developed during childhood and serve as "survival strategies." In adulthood, they

aim to prevent, numb, or invert the intense emotions activated by child modes and parent modes.

Healthy Modes

There are two modes that represent functional states: the *healthy adult mode* and the *happy child mode*. In the healthy adult mode, patients can deal with emotions and needs adequately and engage in healthy relationships. In the happy child mode, patients can enjoy fun, play, and spontaneity. All skills, resources, and healthy insights of patients are summarized in the healthy modes. The healthy modes are usually weak in the beginning of ST and grow stronger during the course of therapy.

Prototype schema mode models are available for a range of psychological disorders and are personalized for individual patients to serve as a case conceptualization at the beginning of ST. In clinical practice, the schema mode model is a helpful tool that is easily understood. It helps both patients and therapists to explain and sort the frequent and sudden shifts in cognition, emotion, and behavior (see Figure 12.1).

The most important modes are displayed in Table 12.2, p. 320. The names of the modes are typically tailored to fit the feelings and behaviors of individual patients and are detailed elsewhere.[1,2,29,30]

Aims of Schema Therapy

The main goals of ST are to help patients to satisfy their needs more functionally, to learn to cope with situations in which need fulfillment is not possible, and to change EMSs

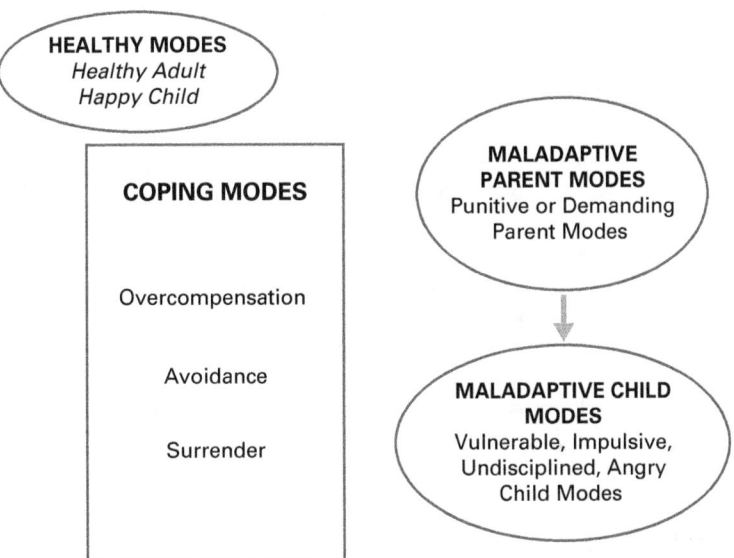

Figure 12.1. Schema Mode Model (Adapted from Arntz and Jacob[2])

Table 12.2. Schema Modes (Modified after Arntz and Jacob[2])

CHILD MODES

Vulnerability

Lonely child	Feels alone, socially unaccepted, unloved, and unlovable.
Abandoned, abused child	Feels abandoned, sad, anxious, helpless, hopeless, and threatened; fear to be left alone, to be mistreated, or to be neglected.
Dependent child	Feels incapable and overwhelmed by adult responsibilities.

Anger

Angry/enraged child	Feels angry, enraged, frustrated, and impatient because the core needs of the vulnerable child are not fulfilled. Loss of control over anger leading to inappropriate verbal or behavioral expressions of anger or aggression.

Lack Discipline

Impulsive child	Lacks the ability to delay gratification and engage in long-term goals, acts impulsively to get need fulfillment.
Undisciplined child	Feels frustrated quickly, has difficulties with rules, discipline, and finishing routine tasks, gives up easily.

Happiness

Happy child	Feels happy and content as core needs have been met. Feels loved, valued, understood, hopeful, optimistic, and spontaneous. Has a sense of belonging and connection to others.

DYSFUNCTIONAL PARENT MODES

Punishment

Punitive parent	Internalized punitive messages of significant others leading to self-devaluation, self-contempt, self-hatred, shame, and guilt. Feels like the expression of needs, emotions, or mistakes need to be punished.

Criticism

Demanding parent	Internalized extremely high standards of perfection and efficiency, modesty, or achievement. Criticizes or induces guilt when feelings, needs, or spontaneity are expressed.

MALADAPTIVE COPING MODES

Surrender

Compliant surrender	Is reassurance-seeking and acts passively and submissively in order to avoid conflicts or rejection.

Avoidance

Detached protector	Tries to achieve distance from emotions by withdrawing from relationships and dysfunctional emotion control strategies (e.g., substance use, dissociation, distraction).
Avoidant protector	Avoids social interaction, challenging situations, and conflicts, as well as intensive sensations or activities.
Angry protector	Tries to keep others at distance by angry and aggressive behavior.
Detached self-soother	Tries to avoid emotions by engaging in activities that soothe, stimulate, or distract (e.g., addictive or compulsive behaviors like gambling, sports, eating, TV, fantasies, sex).

Overcompensation

Self-aggrandizer	Behaves in a grandiose, arrogant, and self-confident manner. Acts competitive, highlights own strengths and achievements and others' mistakes and weaknesses. Lacks empathy for other peoples' needs and feelings. Expects and demands special treatment.

Table 12.2. Continued

Attention and approval Seeking mode	Acts extravagant, inappropriate, and exaggerated in order to get other peoples' attention and approval.
Perfectionistic over-controller	Tries to prevent misfortune, criticism, mistakes, or guilt by perfectionistic behavior, rumination, worrying, excessive planning, and control.
Suspicious over-controller	Tries to prevent threat by suspiciousness, vigilance, and looking for signs of malevolence in others.
Bully and attack	Tries to prevent loss of control and being harmed by being aggressive and intimidating toward others.

HEALTHY ADULT MODE

In this mode, patients are able to functionally perform tasks like working and parenting, take responsibility, and are able to commit. They pursue and enjoy adult activities like intellectual and cultural interests, sex, sports, and health maintenance.

and modes. For each mode, there are mode-specific goals and therapeutic tasks (see Figure 12.2).

Child Modes

In order to heal and correct EMSs, patients are instructed to emotionally process childhood maltreatment, frustrated needs, and allow emotions. Needs and emotions are then validated and fulfilled to enable corrective experiences. Patients with *angry, undisciplined,* and *impulsive child modes* are instructed to learn more adaptive ways to

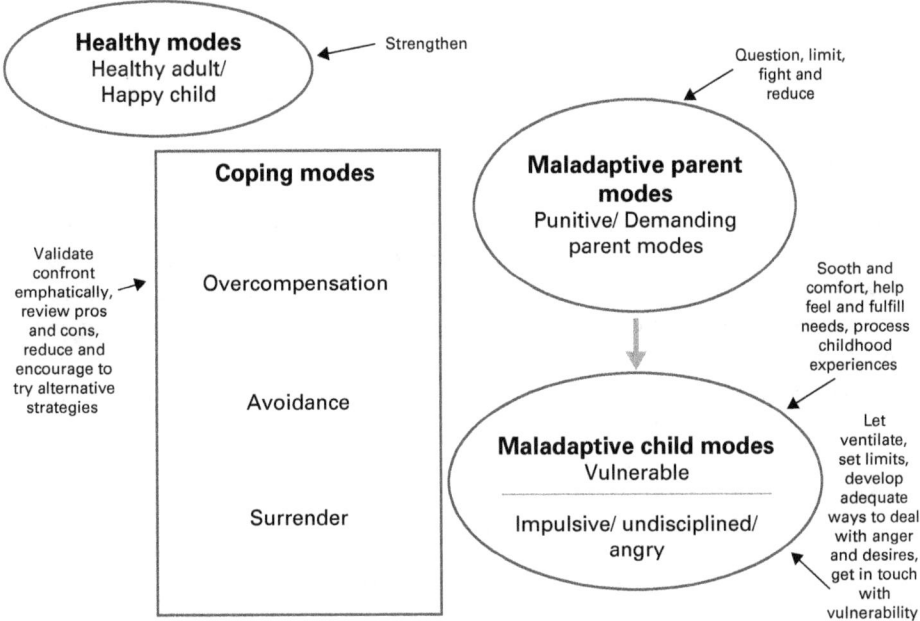

Figure 12.2. Schema Mode Model with Mode Specific Treatment Aims (Modified after Arntz and Jacob[2])

express and fulfill their needs. This may also include setting limits, but the primary therapeutic task is to reach and soothe the vulnerable child mode underneath these externalizing modes.

Parent Modes

Therapists help patients to fight, restrict, and contradict the *punitive* and *demanding parent modes* and to develop self-compassion and a more adequate and healthy self-concept to replace the dysfunctional parent mode.

Coping Modes

Therapists acknowledge these modes as previously adaptive and carefully weigh their pros and cons together with patients, and try to reach the parent and child modes that are warded off by these coping modes. The more child modes are processed, the less these coping modes are needed. Patients are assisted to replace dysfunctional coping modes with healthier, more flexible strategies.

Healthy Modes

The aim is to help the healthy adult mode to become the predominant mode. The aim is to strengthen the healthy adult mode in order to help patients engage in healthy relationships and enable them to deal with the child, parent, and coping modes on their own. As the healthy adult mode grows stronger, the therapist becomes less important toward the end of the treatment. In order to build resilience, the happy child mode is promoted and patients are guided to include joy and spontaneity in their lives.

Indications and Contraindications for Schema Therapy

ST is suitable for patients with long-enduring, pervasive, maladaptive emotional and interpersonal patterns, which are commonly seen in people with PDs or other complex and chronic psychological problems. ST was developed as a transdiagnostic approach to treat a variety of problem constellations. However, there are also prototype models for the conceptualization and treatment of most PDs.

Patients with acute, circumscribed problems that are not part of a persistent pattern can be treated with approaches that are less complex than ST. Also, limited efficacy is expected in states that prevent emotional learning such as pronounced substance abuse, low body-mass index (BMI), or severe medical or neurological diseases. It is important to consider psychosocial circumstances that may aggravate treatment including environmental stressors, such as ongoing contact with violent perpetrators, unstable living arrangements, housing insecurity, or difficult financial circumstances (see Box 12.2, p. 323 for a summary of indications and contraindications).

Techniques and Treatment Course of Schema Therapy

General Treatment Plan

During the first sessions, current symptoms, important relationships, and the life history are assessed. Using the schema mode model, an individual case conceptualization is developed, in which current problems and developmental information are incorporated.

Box 12.2 Indications and Contraindications for Schema Therapy

Indications

- Personality disorders
- Pervasive maladaptive emotional and interpersonal patterns
- Complex and chronic course of psychological problems (e.g., trauma)

Contraindications

- States that prevent emotional learning (e.g., severe substance abuse, low body-mass index (BMI), or severe medical or neurological diseases)
- Severe ongoing psychosocial stressors (e.g., contact with violent perpetrators, unstable living arrangements, housing insecurity)

When the individual's schema mode model is developed, all problems that patients report, as well as all distressing interpersonal situations that arise during the treatment, are explained using the mode model. Appropriate treatment interventions are chosen according to the mode-specific goals.

In most cases, the coping modes are addressed first, as they block the access to the vulnerable child mode. As these coping modes have been protecting patients for many years, they are often reluctant to lower their "shield." Therefore, it is important for therapists to proceed patiently and carefully. Therapists need to acknowledge the adaptive value of these modes and validate them in the context of the patients' life history, but they also need to emphasize the disadvantages these modes have for the patients' life today (e.g., using empathic confrontation, pros and cons). As soon as the patients reduce their coping modes, therapists can get access to the vulnerable child mode. Therapists can validate the emotions and needs of the child mode and help patients using experiential techniques. Through the therapeutic relationship, therapists can help patients heal the emotional wounds of the past, so that patients can experience a new way of relating to their current needs and emotions. By doing this, new adaptive schemas are learned and needs can be better fulfilled in patients' everyday lives. At the same time, dysfunctional parent modes are reduced and their influence is weakened. In the later phase of the treatment, behavior-based techniques are included that help patients to enter and stay in the healthy adult mode. The healthy adult mode is strengthened during the entire course of treatment, and patients are gradually encouraged to take over responsibility for their treatment and lives.

In the remainder of the chapter, case conceptualizations and therapeutic and relationship techniques will be presented. They will be illustrated by two patients diagnosed with BPD and Cluster C personality disorders, because these PDs have been studied in RCTs. The general ST approach to treatment is reviewed in Box 12.3 (see p. 324).

Case Conceptualization

For most PDs and forensic patients, prototype schema mode models are available[2] that have been researched empirically.[31,32] However, these rough frames for case conceptualizations have to be adapted to the individual patients with their specific symptoms and

> ## Box 12.3 Schema Therapy Treatment Approach
>
> - Development and socialization to individual mode model
> - Derive treatment aims from mode model
> - Validate, question, reduce coping modes
> - Soothe and comfort child modes
> - Reduce parent modes
> - Strengthen healthy modes

life histories. In order to capture all major problems, the prototype schema mode model can be extended by adding additional modes as appropriate. In doing this, therapists should focus on the most relevant modes that capture the patients' symptomatology, and try to keep the model as simple as possible (e.g., four to six problematic modes). For disorders with no disorder-specific mode model available (e.g., chronic axis-I disorders) therapists can use the general mode approach and choose the relevant modes for the individual patients.

Research on schema mode conceptualizations for specific PDs indicates that, for some, associations with self-reported vulnerable modes could not be found.[31] It has been hypothesized that patients with strong overcompensation modes may be unaware of, deny, or be unwilling to report vulnerable experiences.[31] Some typical modes for each personality disorder[1] are described and illustrated by case examples of one patient with BPD and one with combined obsessive-compulsive and avoidant PD.

Borderline Personality Disorder

A typical maladaptive schema mode in patients with BPD is the abandoned, abused child mode, which is accompanied by feelings of abandonment and threat. Other typical child modes include the angry child mode, representing the rage about the unjust treatment of these patients during their childhood, and the impulsive child mode, characterized by a tendency to pursue immediate need fulfillment. Typical parent modes include the punitive parent mode, incorporating extreme self-devaluation and self-hatred. As a coping mode, the detached protector mode has the function to protect patients from the emotions of the child and parent modes and includes behavior like social withdrawal, avoidance, self-injury, substance abuse, dissociation, or binge eating to numb emotions.

Case Example 1: Patient with BPD and Histrionic Traits

Clara, a 25-year-old physiotherapist, comes to treatment with a variety of problems, including anxiety and depression. She wears dark makeup, a short skirt, and her hair is dyed red. She reports being "devastated" because of the breakup with her boyfriend and being "bullied and excluded" at work. She complains about the lack of support she receives from her friends during her crises, and feeling "abandoned and alone." This causes frequent "breakdowns," during which she calls her friends and leaves desperate messages. If they don't calm her down "in time" she would "lose it": "I feel so lonely and desperate then, like, I can't breathe. I feel worthless; then I smoke, I drink, I binge, I burn my skin with cigarettes . . . anything that makes these feelings go away or makes me feel for a moment." She reports that she sometimes threatens her friends: "I can be really evil when I am desperate like that, just out of control. I yell, I leave messages telling them that I will hurt myself if they don't call back. Afterwards, I feel extremely sorry and beg them for forgiveness. I'm not worth their friendship; I'm such a bad person."

Clara grew up with her mother and her brother, who is ten years older. Clara was overweight as a child and was ridiculed and excluded by her classmates. In order to feel less alone, she tried to "dress up" with extravagant makeup and clothes, and told interesting or disturbing stories. Clara's mother suffered from depression and an alcohol dependency. She hit and punished her children harshly, sometimes for no reason. Clara's brother was very important to her, but he was much older and he "ignored" and "babied" her. In order to get her brother's attention, she dressed up "as an adult" and flirted with his friends. Clara experienced several stepfathers come and go during her childhood. Most of them were physically and some sexually abusive toward her; she liked only one of them. Clara tried to make him stay by charming him and begging him, but ultimately he left the family, too; that was when Clara first hurt herself and started stealing alcohol from her mother.

Clara's Mode Model

The therapist and Clara develop a mode model (see Figure 12.3). Clara picks individual names for each of her modes. Clara's anxiety to be abandoned and her loneliness are captured in the abandoned/abused child mode called "little lonely Clara." Clara's outbursts are conceptualized in the impulsive child mode, which Clara calls "Little out-of-control Clara." These modes had developed because major early childhood needs were frustrated. Clara experienced verbal and physical abuse from her mother, her stepfathers, and peers. These internalized self-devaluating messages, shame, and self-hatred form Clara's punitive parent mode, called "the Dragon." Her coping modes include an

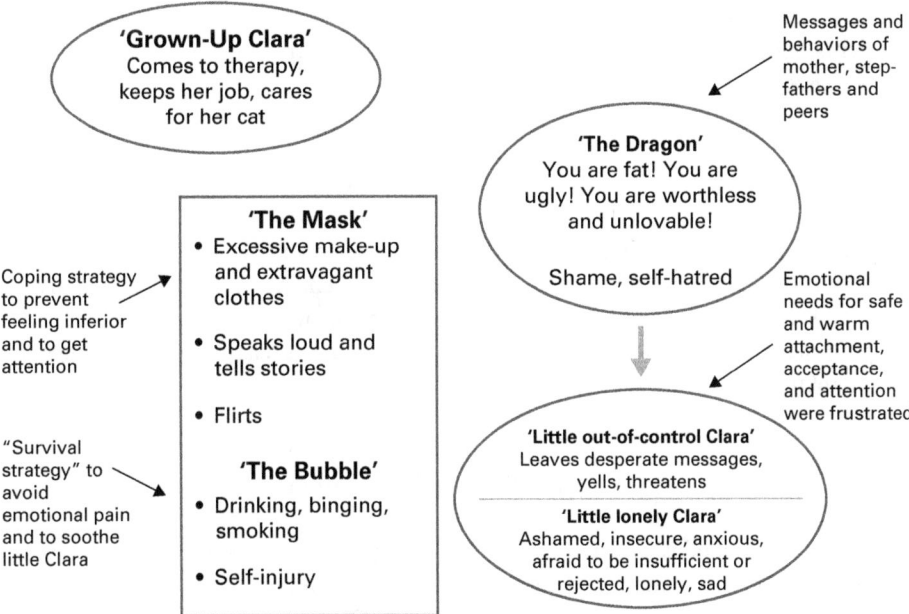

Figure 12.3. Clara's Schema Mode Model

over-compensator mode that Clara calls "the Mask." As Clara's drinking and bingeing both serve to detach and self-soothe, her detached protector and detached self-soothing modes are combined in what Clara calls "the Bubble," in order to simplify the model. She developed these coping modes early in her childhood to soothe her and protect her from emotional pain; review Figure 12.3.

Histrionic Personality Disorder

Typical schema modes in patients with histrionic personality disorder (HPD) are the abandoned/abused child mode, an impulsive/undisciplined child mode, and an attention and approval-seeking mode, representing behavior patterns like dramatic or sexualized behavior. Bamelis, Renner, Heidkamp, and Arntz[31] only found the approval-seeking mode being associated with HPD. The authors hypothesized that patients with strong overcompensation modes, like with HPD, may be unaware of, deny, or be unwilling to report vulnerable experiences.[31]

Narcissistic Personality Disorder

Typical schema modes in patients with narcissistic personality disorder (NPD) are the lonely child mode and a demanding parent mode. Coping modes include: a self-aggrandizer mode, reflecting the fantasies of grandiosity and devaluations of others that are characteristically seen in patients with NPD; and a detached self-soother mode in which patients with NPD stimulate themselves by gambling, substance use, sex/pornography, excessive playing of sports, or excessive work. An attention- and approval-seeking mode is also associated with NPD (described by Bamelis, Renner, Heidkamp, and Arntz[31]). Instead of the lonely child mode, Bamelis et al. found the undisciplined child mode to be associated with NPD. Similar to HPD, this could be because NPD patients, with strong overcompensation modes, may have trouble reporting vulnerable experiences.[31]

Dependent Personality Disorder

Typical schema modes in patients with dependent personality disorder (DPD) are an abandoned/abused or dependent child mode, and a demanding and punitive parent mode, which induces guilt whenever patients put their own needs first. The primary coping mode is the compliant surrender mode, but an association of DPD with the avoidant protector mode was also found.[31]

Avoidant Personality Disorder

Typical schema modes in patients with avoidant personality disorder (AVPD) are a lonely child or an abandoned/abused child mode and a punitive parent mode, which often induces guilt and shame in patients with AVPD. Coping modes are the avoidant protector mode, in which patients try to distance themselves from needs, feelings, and thoughts, and the compliant surrender mode, in which patients surrender and adapt to other people's ideas. Bamelis, Renner, Heidkamp, and Arntz[31] also found associations with the detached protector mode and the suspicious over-controller mode.

Obsessive-compulsive Personality Disorder

The typical modes in patients with obsessive-compulsive personality disorder (OCPD) are the lonely child mode and the demanding parent mode. The predominant coping mode is the perfectionistic over-controller mode with which patients try to prevent mistakes or misfortunes. Other common coping modes are the detached self-soother and the self-aggrandizer modes. In the self-aggrandizer mode, patients regard other people as less reliable and thorough than themselves. No association with vulnerable modes could be found, because patients with OCPD often have strong overcompensation modes and may be unaware, deny, or be unwilling to report vulnerable experiences.[31]

Case Example 2: Patient with Combined Avoidant and Obsessive-compulsive Personality Disorder

Paul, a 40-year-old bank accountant, comes to treatment because of his chronic back pain and because he has been feeling depressed "since childhood." He complains about his coworkers who "come in late and spend half of the day drinking coffee and chatting." He is annoyed that they get credit and approval when he is the one who is "the first in, and the last out every single day." He explains that he has "no time or energy for hobbies." He spends his evenings and weekends either cleaning his apartment or feeling too "knocked out" for anything other than watching TV or playing video games. He has some old friends, but often cancels his plans with them to avoid "spending a fortune in a pub."

Paul grew up with his parents and his little sister. He was a quiet child who preferred to spend his time reading fantasy books in his room. His father was the director of Paul's school and paid a lot of attention to Paul's grades in order to "keep up appearances." He was self-centered and got physically abusive when the children did not live up to his standards. He did not tolerate it when Paul read "nonsense books" or when the children played "childish games"; he always found "something more useful" for them to do. His father closely supervised tasks like cleaning, tidying, and doing homework, making Paul redo them until they were perfect. Paul's mother reacted passively to her husband's outbursts and always took her husband's side. She was a stay-at-home-mom, very engaged in her church, and spent her free time on charity work instead of on her children. Paul never felt loved or wanted and felt lonely through all of his childhood.

Paul's Mode Model

Paul and his therapist develop a schema mode model that captures both his OCPD and his APD (see Figure 12.4, p. 328). The therapist uses the disorder-specific mode model for OCPD with the internalized messages of his father forming the demanding parent mode, which Paul called "the Dictator," and the perfectionistic over-controller mode, which Paul called "Mister Perfect." The therapist also includes Paul's lonely/inferior child mode called "little Paul" and his avoidant protector mode that Paul calls the "Switch-Off." With this individualized mode model, all of Paul's problematic modes are captured and explained in one case conceptualization (Figure 12.4, p. 328).

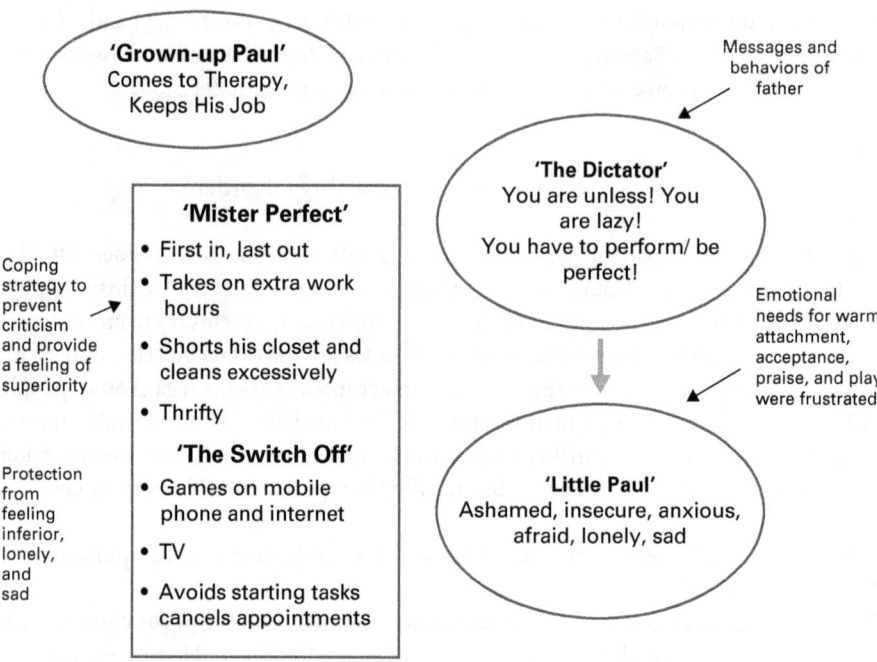

Figure 12.4. Paul's Schema Mode Model

Paranoid Personality Disorder

Typical schema modes in patients with paranoid personality disorder (PPD) are an abandoned/abused or an angry child mode, as well as a punitive parent mode. The predominant coping modes are the suspicious over-controller mode, which reflects the paranoid experiential and behavioral patterns, and the avoidant protector mode, which represents the social withdrawal characteristic seen in patients with PPD. Bamelis, Renner, Heidkamp, and Arntz[31] only found associations between PPD and the angry child mode and the suspicious over-controller mode. Patients with PPD have strong overcompensation modes that may explain the lack of an association with vulnerable modes.[31]

Therapeutic Relationship

EMSs typically develop because of deprivation or interpersonal trauma at the hands of significant others or early childhood caregivers. The therapeutic relationship has an essential role in revealing and modifying dysfunctional interpersonal relationships. In ST, the therapeutic relationship serves as a source of interpersonal information and corrective emotional and interpersonal experiences that help to change the EMSs. Therapists use validation, caring, and support, within the therapeutic relationship, to provide a safe environment, while also creating possibilities for patients to try and practice new interpersonal behaviors. Therapists also confront patients with objective reality and set limits, as is necessary. The most important techniques in achieving this balance are *limited reparenting* and *empathic confrontation*.[1]

Limited Reparenting

Limited reparenting refers to a therapeutic attitude of behaving as a good parental figure toward patients throughout the treatment, while at the same time respecting the limits of a professional therapist–patient relationship. By adopting this attitude, therapists model appropriate parental responses and behaviors. Therapists help patients become aware of and express their emotions and needs. Therapists validate the patients' emotions and adapt their behavior to the needs of the individual patient (e.g., attention, limits, and autonomy). This may include support, empathy, praise, and providing secure attachment, but also setting adequate limits and encouraging autonomy. In the course of the treatment, patients internalize therapists' reactions toward their emotions and needs. As their healthy adult mode grows stronger, they can take over the role of a good parent to themselves.

Case Example Clara: Limited Reparenting
During her childhood, Clara experienced unreliability, abuse, and abandonment. Her mother was physically and emotionally abusive. Her stepfathers were sexually abusive and abandoned her. Clara did not experience love or support and had to work hard to receive any kind of attention. For this reason, it is particularly important that the therapist offers a reliable, warm-hearted, and authentically caring relationship. The therapist shows real interest in Clara's feelings and opinions and praises her for progress. In her impulsive child mode, Clara needs a reliable structure and clear limits.

Empathic Confrontation

Empathic confrontation refers to the way in which therapists react to problematic behavior or views of the patients. Therapists show understanding and validate the patients' feelings and needs that led to the problematic behavior, linking them to their early life history and schema mode model. At the same time, therapists also confront patients with the consequences of their behavior in a friendly but explicit way; therapists reveal to patients their own reactions and feelings concerning the patients' behavior, after checking that their reactions are not connected with their own dysfunctional schemas (careful self-disclosure). By doing so, therapists emphasize that the patients' behavior, and not the patients themselves, is addressed, and they check the patients' emotional reactions every step of the way.

Case Example Paul: Empathic Confrontation
As a first homework exercise, Paul is asked to copy and personalize the mode model which was co-created by the therapist and Paul. For the second time, he reports not having started on the assignment.

The therapist points out that this might be Paul's avoidant protector mode.

Therapist: Paul, I think your coping mode, the "Switch-Off," prevents you from starting the homework assignment.

Pointing to the mode model, the therapist continues:

Therapist: We talked about how, in this mode, you tend to avoid getting started on tasks or cancel appointments with friends and instead default to watching TV or playing video games. In your past, the "Switch-Off" was really important to protect "Little Paul" from all the pressure your father put on you. I think that you currently still hear the messages of "the Dictator," even while in therapy. Am I right?

Paul: I guess so.

Therapist: I understand. At the same time, the "Switch-Off" prevents you from learning new things and meeting people. The feelings of inferiority, shame, and loneliness stay with you.

Paul: Yes, usually, "the Dictator" lashes out especially hard after the "Switch-Off" . . . and not meeting people does make me feel lonely.

Therapist: You know Paul, I really care for you and I want you to feel safe. The homework assignments help me to get to know you and to help you. There is no right or wrong when you are here with me in therapy; you can't fail any assignments and there is no need to be perfect. What do you think about that?

Treatment Techniques

Experiential Techniques

Experiential techniques, especially *chair dialogues* and *imagery exercises*, are a core feature of ST. They are used to understand and change the intense emotions that accompany schemas and modes as well as to process traumatic childhood memories. In a later phase of the treatment, chair dialogues and imagery work can also be used to clarify and work on present problems and to strengthen the healthy adult mode. Both chair dialogues and imagery work are powerful techniques that elicit intense emotions. Therefore, therapists need to plan enough time for these techniques, so that patients have the opportunity to process the material during the exercises and also for debriefing afterwards.

Chair Dialogues

The idea of chair dialogues originates from psychodrama,[33] and was utilized by Fritz Pearls[34] within gestalt therapy as a major intervention that he called "The Empty Chair." In ST, chair dialogues are most often used to explore the different modes of patients in order to sort the problematic situations they encountered, to fight the parent modes, to empathically confront the coping modes, to soothe child modes, and to strengthen the healthy adult mode. The chairs represent the different modes; by letting patients switch chairs, they can experience and express the modes that are relevant to a specific problem. While this helps patients and therapists to clarify what modes play a role in a problematic situation, the technique is also used to bring about change, for instance by breaking through coping modes, combating punitive and demanding parent modes, limiting externalizing child modes, validating vulnerable child modes, and strengthening the healthy adult mode.

Case Example Paul: Chair Dialogue
After the empathic confrontation, the therapist uses the situation for a chair dialogue.

Therapist: Let's have a closer look at what happens when you want to start a task like the homework assignment. What did you notice first?

Paul: I thought: "This is the first homework assignment, this really needs to be good," and also that I'm lazy because I hadn't started it earlier.

Therapist: Have a look at the schema mode model. Which mode do you think this was?

Paul: Um . . . "the Dictator"?

Therapist: I think you're right. (Stands up and gets an extra chair.) This is the chair of your demanding parent mode, "the Dictator." What did you notice then?

Paul: I felt bad, because I was already late with the assignment and there was no way that I could complete it before our session.

Therapist: I think that is the mode of "little Paul." (Gets another chair.) Paul, could you please take a seat here? (Paul switches chairs.) On this chair, you are "little Paul" and I will address you as such. "Little Paul," what do you hear "the Dictator" say?

Paul: He says: "You're useless and lazy! You have to perform and be perfect!"

Therapist: And how does it feel when you hear these nasty things, "little Paul"?

Paul: Bad, I feel bad . . . , overwhelmed and anxious . . . , and I am ashamed.

Therapist: I understand, these messages really hurt and put a lot of pressure on you. Because of the emotional pain inflicted by "the Dictator," your two survival strategies "Mister Perfect" and the "Switch-Off" came to help you, right? (Gets two more chairs.) Where do I put these chairs?

Paul: Right here, between me and "the Dictator."

Therapist (putting the chairs of the coping modes between the chair of "Little Paul" and "the Dictator"): Like that? How does that feel?

Paul: Well, I do feel protected a little, because I see and hear "the Dictator" a little less behind those two chairs. (Paul points to the chairs of the coping mode.) I feel kind of locked up back here and still feel the pressure; "Mister Perfect" is really exhausting and the "Switch-Off" causes "the Dictator" to yell harder. I feel sad and lonely.

Therapist: That must be hard! Back here, the coping modes make you feel a little safer, but you don't really get what you need. What do you need?

Paul: "The Dictator" to be gone!

Therapist: You are right. I'm going to send him away! (He addresses the chair of "the Dictator.") "Dictator," you are not helping "Little Paul," you have to shut up and leave! (The therapist carries the chair of "the Dictator" out of the therapy room and closes the door.) How does this feel, "little Paul"?

Paul: Better.

Therapist (kneels besides Paul): You know, "little Paul," I really care for you and I think you are amazing just the way you are. How does this feel?

Paul: Pretty OK. I feel warmer and calmer.

Therapist: What else do you need?

Paul: Um . . . I feel pretty cramped; maybe those two can back off just a little. (Paul gets up and pushes the chairs of the coping modes to the side a little.)

Therapist: How does this feel?

Paul: Better, I feel like I can breathe again.

After the chair dialogue, the therapist instructs Paul to take a seat in his regular chair and asks about his experiences. They decide that they will keep working on reducing "the Dictator's" influence, increase care for "Little Paul's" feelings and needs, and develop healthier strategies so that the "Switch-Off" and "Mister Perfect" can step aside more often.

Imagery Exercises

Imagery-related techniques were first introduced by Joseph Wolpe in the late 1960s in behavior-modification therapy.[35] In ST, imagery exercises include diagnostic imagery and imagery rescripting.

Diagnostic Imagery Exercises

Diagnostic imagery exercises are usually used at the beginning of the treatment in order to explore the origin of dysfunctional emotional-cognitive behavior patterns. Therapists can use a current or recent emotionally disturbing situation, reported by their patients, and ask the patients to imagine that situation with their eyes closed. The therapists encourage vividness and intensity of the imagery by asking patients to describe in detail their experiences, bodily sensations, emotions, and thoughts using first-person language and the present tense. When the emotion is elicited, the therapists ask the patients to let go of the current situation, stay with the feeling and to "float back" to their childhood to see if an image associated with this feeling emerges (affect bridge). With the emergence and exploration of this childhood image, the patients are encouraged to express their feelings and needs. Diagnostic imagery exercises can also be performed without an affect bridge (e.g., by asking a patient to image a disturbing situation with a parent). Diagnostic exercises (without rescripting) are not recommended at the beginning of the treatment (in some patient groups, e.g., BPD), because these exercises can leave patients overwhelmed by emotions that they cannot adequately regulate.

Imagery Rescripting

Imagery rescripting is used to reprocess aversive childhood memories in order to change maladaptive schemas. The term "rescripting" refers to the rewriting of the original memory. The aim of the rescripting is not to erase the original memory but to change the meaning associated with the aversive memory. The basic version of imagery rescripting has two phases: (1) recalling imagery of an unpleasant situation; and (2) rescripting the situation to a better ending.

During the first phase, the therapist may elicit through an affect bridge or the patient chooses to recall a disturbing childhood memory with a strong relation to the patient's maladaptive schemas. The therapist instructs the patient to describe this situation in detail, using first-person language and present tense. The patient is encouraged to express their sensory experiences, emotions, cognitions, and needs from the child's perspective. In ST, it is not necessary for patients to relive the whole trauma. As soon as the emotions and needs are sufficiently activated, the second phase, the rescripting, can begin.

During the second phase, the emotionally disturbing memory is changed to elicit a positive ending where the emotional needs of the child are met. During this phase, an auxiliary person is introduced to step into the image. The use of an auxiliary person originally comes from psychodrama.[36] The auxiliary person first creates safety for the child by stopping, confronting, and banishing the perpetrator. The auxiliary person then comforts and soothes the child. The child is encouraged to express all emotions and needs, and the auxiliary person takes care of any needs the child may have. Also, the child is provided with explanations and corrective information on the needs, emotions, and rights of children. In patients with PDs, at the beginning of the treatment, this auxiliary person is usually the therapist; in a later stage of therapy, it can be another real or fictive person, and ultimately, patients themselves, in their healthy adult modes, can take over.

When patients in their healthy adult modes do the rescripting, the imagery rescripting exercise is conducted in three phases: (1) recalling imagery of an unpleasant situation from the perspective of the child; (2) rescripting the situation to a better ending by the patients themselves in their healthy adult modes; and (3) rewinding the scene and experiencing the rescripting from the child's perspective. In this third phase, the patient switches back to the perspective of the child and experiences how the grown-up patient in healthy adult mode protects and takes care of the child. From the child's perspective, the patient might experience further needs that she or he wants to have met, and can ask the adult self to meet these needs.

Case Example Clara: Imagery Rescripting

Clara talks about an "emotional breakdown" at work. When she got out of her office, her colleagues already went off to lunch. Clara felt hurt and excluded and spent her lunchtime crying and bingeing in her office. When she heard her colleagues coming back, she refreshed her makeup, burst out of her office, and told everyone to listen to the "insane experiences" she had the other night. When her colleagues tried to cut her short in order to get back to work, she felt ashamed, left work early, called her friends, and left them desperate messages. Clara felt sad and unhappy with her behavior.

The therapist proposed to use this situation for an imagery rescripting exercise by performing an affect bridge to a childhood situation. She asks Clara to sit comfortably and imagine the situation in detail until the moment she notices that her colleagues left and she feels sad and lonely. When the emotion is activated adequately, the therapist asks Clara to stay with the emotion, to wipe out the present situation, and to recall or fall back to a similar situation of her childhood. Clara reports that she can picture herself when she was eight years old. The therapist lets Clara describe in detail what she sees, hears, smells, tastes, feels, thinks, and needs. Clara tells about how she came home from school crying after she had been excluded and bullied during a lunch break. Instead of comforting Clara, her mother yelled at her, called her "fat and ugly," and told her that "no one in their right mind" would want to be friends with her. The therapist enters the picture, stands next to Clara, and asks her if it is OK to put her hand on her shoulder. The therapist addresses the mother: "Stop right now! You are not allowed to treat little Clara like this and say those ugly things! This makes her feel ashamed and sad!" As the mother keeps saying mean things and tries to hit Clara, the therapist steps between her and Clara, pulls out her magic wand, and transforms Clara's mother into a tiny version of herself. She asks Clara if she can see the miniature version of her mother jumping up and down, complaining inaudibly in a squeaky voice. Clara giggles a little and confirms seeing the transformation. The therapist picks up the miniature version of the mother and sends her off to "parenting camp" where she has to learn how to be a good parent to little Clara.

The therapist turns to Clara and asks her how this feels and what she needs. Clara answers that she already feels safer, but that she wants to leave the house and go to the playground. The therapist takes Clara by the hand and goes with her to her favorite playground. They sit on the swings and the therapist tells Clara that it is not her fault, but her mother's problem, and that Clara is an adorable little girl and that her feelings are important. The therapist continues to ask about Clara's feelings and needs and fulfills them until Clara feels calm and at peace.

Cognitive Techniques

Cognitive techniques are used to educate patients on schemas, coping styles, modes, needs, and emotions. All CBT techniques may be used as long as they are adapted to the mode model and ST goals. Examples of cognitive techniques are identification and re-appraisal of schemas and mode-related distortions, pros and cons list of coping modes, diaries and flashcards.

Case Example Paul: Pro and Cons of Paul's Avoidant Protector Mode

The therapist and Paul write down advantages and disadvantages of Paul's avoidant pro-tector mode called the "Switch-Off" (see Table 12.3).

Case Example Clara: Audio Flashcard

After the imagery rescripting exercise, the therapist takes time to debrief Clara's experi-ences. The therapist validates her feelings and praises her for her courage to feel and show her emotions and needs. She asks what she takes from the exercise and Clara answers: "That I AM okay and I AM important and it's okay that I wish that someone takes care of me. Unfortunately, I tend to forget this. And then 'the Mask' automatically steps in and others are annoyed in the long run." The therapist proposes to prepare an audio flash-card, in which "Grown-Up Clara" records a message for "little Clara," so that she will be prepared for such difficult situations. Clara uses her mobile phone to record the message: "Dear 'little Clara,' I know that you feel sad and lonely right now. Please know that all of your feelings are OK, and that you are important and OK just the way you are. It is OK that you want someone to be there for you and give you some attention. 'The Mask' does not help you to get 'true contact,' so let us try something else: I know that it comforts you to cuddle your cat. You can cuddle her now and play with her, feel her warm and fluffy fur. If you want to, you can call your best friend Nina and set up a date to do something nice. Remember that you are not alone anymore."

Behavioral Techniques

Behavioral techniques include all techniques of behavior therapy that aim at learning new behavior, including role-play, behavioral experiments, skills training, problem-solving, behavioral activation, or relaxation techniques.[2] In ST, these behavioral tech-niques are adjusted to the mode model. Behavioral techniques can be used to break

Table 12.3. Paul's "Switch-off" Mode: Pros and Cons List

Pros	Cons
Unpleasant feelings are numbed.	I feel depressed and lonely because I avoid people and activities.
I don't hear the "Dictator" as loud.	The "Dictator" lashes out twice as hard later.
Stress is reduced.	I am bored and lonely because watching TV and video games are my only hobbies.
Prevents me from being disappointed or from failing.	I can't learn new things.

behavioral patterns that patients display when they are in coping modes. Also, behavioral techniques can help patients to spend more time in the healthy adult mode. Behavioral patterns that patients display when they are in coping modes are usually very rigid; these patients don't yet have healthy alternatives to deal with (potential) EMS activation because the healthy adult mode is usually weak at the beginning of treatment. Therefore, behavioral techniques are typically used in later stages of the treatment. Often dysfunctional behavioral patterns reduce in intensity after successfully addressing the child and parental modes. Nevertheless, some behavioral patterns have become so habitual that they don't disappear spontaneously, even after the underlying problems have been addressed. Therefore, behavioral patterns often need explicit attention at the final stage of treatment.

Case Example Clara: Role-play

Clara likes to ask her colleagues, in her healthy adult mode, to wait for her because she would like to accompany them to lunch. In a role-play with video feedback, the therapist and Clara experiment with different ways Clara can approach her colleagues. Clara tries different ways of using her voice and gestures until she feels confident and authentic. As homework, Clara decides to try these new behaviors at work the next day.

Case Example Paul: Behavioral Experiment

Paul would like to invite a friend to his apartment but feels that he has to perfectly clean it before the friend's visit. The therapist and Paul set up a behavioral experiment. They develop a cleaning schedule in which Paul only spends one hour tidying up before his friend arrives. They also set up an observational task to determine if his friend behaves any differently compared with earlier visits. Paul performs the experiment as a homework assignment and they review the results in the next session. Paul reports having had a nice evening and not having noticed any signs that indicated that his friend acted differently or even noticed that he only spent one hour tidying up, instead of all day.

Conclusion

ST is an evidence-based psychotherapy for patients with PDs. These patients show persistent dysfunctional schemas that often lead to problems in interpersonal relationships as well as in the therapist–patient relationship (e.g. poor cooperation, overcompensation, avoidance, overdependence). A strength of ST is the ability to understand these problem behaviors occurring both within and outside therapy sessions, by seeing them in the light of the developmental history of the patients and by using the schema mode model. The mode model gives a clear structure for the development of an individual case conceptualization and guides the treatment; each mode has mode-specific tasks therapists should follow. In addition to cognitive and behavioral techniques, experiential techniques are frequently used, especially chair dialogues and imagery rescripting. ST has a special focus on the therapeutic relationship ("limited reparenting"). By using these techniques, the learning process can be intensified to promote behavioral, cognitive, and emotional change. ST's need-oriented approach is well accepted by therapists and patients. Review Box 12.4, p. 336 for resources related to ST.

Conflict of Interest/Disclosure: The authors of this chapter have no financial conflicts and nothing to disclose.

Box 12.4 Resources for Clinicians, Patients, and Families

- Arntz A, Jacob G. *Schema Therapy in Practice: An Introductory Guide to the Schema Mode Approach*. Hoboken, New Jersey: Wiley; 2017.
- Arntz A, Van Genderen H. *Schema Therapy for Borderline Personality Disorder*. 2nd ed. Chichester, West Sussex: Wiley; 2020.
- International Society of Schema Therapy e.V. https://schematherapysociety. org/.
- Jacob G, Van Genderen H, Seebauer L. *Breaking Negative Thinking Patterns: A Schema Therapy Self-help and Support Book*. Chichester, West Sussex: John Wiley & Sons; 2014.
- Schema Therapy Step by Step. https://www.schematherapy.nl/shop/schema-therapy-step-by-step/.
- Young JE, Klosko JS, Weishaar ME. *Schema Therapy: A Practitioner's Guide*. New York, NY: Guilford Press; 2003.

References

1. Young JE, Klosko JS, Weishaar ME. *Schema Therapy: A Practitioner's Guide*. New York, NY: Guilford Press; 2003.

2. Arntz A, Jacob G. *Schema Therapy in Practice: An Introductory Guide to the Schema Mode Approach*. Hoboken, New Jersey: John Wiley & Sons; 2017.

3. Jacob GA, Arntz A. Schema therapy for personality disorders—a review. *Int J Cogn Ther*. 2013;(2):171–185.

4. Sempertegui GA, Karreman A, Arntz A, Bekker MH. Schema therapy for borderline personality disorder: a comprehensive review of its empirical foundations, effectiveness and implementation possibilities. *Clin Psychol Rev*. 2013;(3):426–447.

5. Taylor CD, Bee P, Haddock G. Does schema therapy change schemas and symptoms? A systematic review across mental health disorders. *Psychol Psychother*. 2017;(3):456–479.

6. Giesen-Bloo J, Van Dyck R, Spinhoven P, et al. Outpatient psychotherapy for borderline personality disorder: randomized trial of schema-focused therapy vs transference-focused psychotherapy. *Arch Gen Psychiatry*. 2006;(6):649–658.

7. Farrell JM, Shaw IA, Webber MA. A schema-focused approach to group psychotherapy for outpatients with borderline personality disorder: a randomized controlled trial. *J Behav Ther Exp Psychiatry*. 2009;(2):317–328.

8. Nordahl HM, Nysæter TE. Schema therapy for patients with borderline personality disorder: a single case series. *J Behav Ther Exp Psychiatry*. 2005;(3):254–264.

9. Jacob GA, Hauer A, Köhne S, et al. A schema therapy–based eHealth program for patients with borderline personality disorder (priovi): naturalistic single-arm observational study. *JMIR Ment Health*. 2018;(4):e10983.

10. Dickhaut V, Arntz A. Combined group and individual schema therapy for borderline personality disorder: a pilot study. *J Behav Ther Exp Psychiatry*. 2014;(2):242–251.

11. Reiss N, Lieb K, Arntz A, Shaw IA, Farrell J. Responding to the treatment challenge of patients with severe BPD: results of three pilot studies of inpatient schema therapy. *Behav Cogn Psychother*. 2014;(3):355–367.

12. Fassbinder E, Schuetze M, Kranich A, et al. Feasibility of group schema therapy for outpatients with severe borderline personality disorder in Germany: a pilot study with three year follow-up. *Front Psychol.* 2016;(7):1851.

13. Nadort M, Arntz A, Smit JH, et al. Implementation of outpatient schema therapy for borderline personality disorder with versus without crisis support by the therapist outside office hours: a randomized trial. *Behav Res Ther.* 2009;(11):961–973.

14. Nenadić I, Lamberth S, Reiss N. Group schema therapy for personality disorders: a pilot study for implementation in acute psychiatric in-patient settings. *Psychiatry Res.* 2017 Jul;253:9–12. doi:10.1016/j.psychres.2017.01.093.

15. Giesen-Bloo J, Arntz A, Schouten E. The borderline personality disorder checklist: psychometric evaluation and factorial structure in clinical and nonclinical samples. In: Giesen-Bloo J, eds. *Crossing Borders: Theory, Assessment and Treatment in Borderline Personality Disorder.* Maastricht, Limburg: Datawyse/Universitaire Pers Maastricht; 2006:85–102.

16. Van Asselt AD, Dirksen CD, Arntz A, et al. Out-patient psychotherapy for borderline personality disorder: cost-effectiveness of schema-focused therapy v. transference-focused psychotherapy. *Br J Psychiatry.* 2008;(6):450–457.

17. Wetzelaer P, Farrell J, Evers SM, et al. Design of an international multicentre RCT on group schema therapy for borderline personality disorder. *BMC Psychiatry.* 2014;(1):319.

18. Arntz A. Schema therapy: latest research findings and clinical applications. Presented at: *WCBCT*; July 18, 2019; Berlin.

19. Fassbinder E, Assmann N, Schaich A, et al. PRO*BPD: effectiveness of outpatient treatment programs for borderline personality disorder: a comparison of Schema therapy and dialectical behavior therapy: study protocol for a randomized trial. *BMC Psychiatry.* 2018;(1):341.

20. Fassbinder E, Hauer A, Schaich A, Schweiger U, Jacob GA, Arntz A. Integration of e-health tools into face-to-face psychotherapy for borderline personality disorder: a chance to close the gap between demand and supply? *J Clin Psychol.* 2015;(8):764–777.

21. Bamelis LL, Evers SM, Spinhoven P, Arntz A. Results of a multicenter randomized controlled trial of the clinical effectiveness of schema therapy for personality disorders. *Am J Psychiatry.* 2014;(3):305–322.

22. Bernstein, D. P., Keulen-de Vos, M., Clercx, M., de Vogel, V., Kersten, G. C., Lancel, M., Jonkers, P.P., Bogaerts, S., Slaats, M., Broers, N.J., Deenen, T.A.M. & Arntz, A. (2021). Schema therapy for violent PD offenders: a randomized clinical trial. Psychological medicine, 1–15.

23. Baljé A, Greeven A, van Giezen A, Korrelboom K, Arntz A, Spinhoven P. Group schema therapy versus group cognitive behavioral therapy for social anxiety disorder with comorbid avoidant personality disorder: study protocol for a randomized controlled trial. *Trials.* 2016;(1):487.

24. Van Dijk S, Veenstra M, Bouman R, et al. Group schema-focused therapy enriched with psychomotor therapy versus treatment as usual for older adults with cluster B and/or C personality disorders: a randomized trial. *BMC Psychiatry.* 2019;(1):1–14.

25. De Klerk N, Abma TA, Bamelis LL, Arntz A. Schema therapy for personality disorders: a qualitative study of patients' and therapists' perspectives. *Behav Cogn Psychother.* 2017;(1):31–45.

26. Tan YM, Lee CW, Averbeck LE, et al. Schema therapy for borderline personality disorder: A qualitative study of patients' perceptions. *PloS one.* 2018;(11):e0206039.

27. Ten Napel-Schutz M, C, Abma TA, Bamelis L, Arntz A. Personality disorder patients' perspectives on the introduction of imagery within schema therapy: a qualitative study of patients' experiences. *Cogn Behav Pract.* 2011;(4):482–490.

28. Schaich A, Braakmann D, Richter A, et al. Experiences of patients with borderline personality disorder with imagery rescripting in the context of schema therapy: a qualitative study. Accepted for publication in *Front Psychiatry.* 2020; 11:1358. doi:10.3389/fpsyt.2020.550833

29. Arntz A, Van Genderen H. *Schema Therapy for Borderline Personality Disorder.* 2nd ed. Chichester, West Sussex: John Wiley & Sons; 2020.

30. Bernstein DP, Arntz A, de Vos M. Schema focused therapy in forensic settings: Theoretical model and recommendations for best clinical practice. *Int J Forensic Ment Health.* 2007;(2):169–183.

31. Bamelis LL, Renner F, Heidkamp D, Arntz A. Extended schema mode conceptualizations for specific personality disorders: an empirical study. *J Pers Disord.* 2011;(1):41–58.

32. Lobbestael J, Van Vreeswijk MF, Arntz A. An empirical test of schema mode conceptualizations in personality disorders. *Behav Res Ther.* 2008;(7):854–860.

33. Moreno J. *Psychodrama.* Vol 1. Rev. ed. Beacon, NY: Beacon House; 1964.

34. Fagan J, Shepherd IL. *Gestalt Therapy Now: Theory, Techniques, Applications.* New York, NY: Harper & Row; 1970.

35. Wolpe J. *Psychotherapy by Reciprocal Inhibition*: Stanford, CA: Stanford University Press; 1958:130–135.

36. Moreno JL, Moreno ZT. *Psychodrama.* Vol. 3. Beacon, NY: Beacon House; 1969.

13

Good Psychiatric Management (GPM) for Borderline Personality Disorder

Richard G. Hersh, Benjamin McCommon, Emma Golkin, and Jennifer Sotsky

> **Key Points**
>
> - Good psychiatric management (GPM) is an empirically validated treatment for patients with borderline personality disorder (BPD).
> - GPM was developed as a study control intervention informed by the 2001 American Psychiatric Association Guideline for the Treatment of Patients with Borderline Personality Disorder, inspired by the work of BPD researcher John Gunderson.
> - The wide gap between the need for competent clinicians able to treat patients with BPD, and the current undersupply of those sufficiently trained to do so, strengthens GPM's public health mission.
> - GPM can be taught as focused didactics and training in most mental health training programs. It is more accessible, requires less time devoted to training, and costs less to implement compared to other evidence-based trainings for the treatment of BPD.
> - GPM is designed with essential elements that can be learned relatively easily, quickly, and for a limited cost. Often, one day of training is all that is needed.
> - A central tenet of GPM is the use of multiple strategies to avoid common iatrogenic complications in the treatment of patients with BPD. Things to be avoided include: destabilizing unfocused treatments; derailing psychiatric hospitalizations; problematic polypharmacy; patient's relative passivity; and an insufficient focus on meaningful work or studies.
> - GPM promotes clinician flexibility, in contrast to the other relatively prescriptive evidence-based treatments for BPD.
> - The GPM approach includes: diagnosis sharing and psychoeducation; the establishment of treatment goals; the adjustment of the intensity and duration of the treatment; the management of self-harm and suicidality; the integration of psychotherapy elements; case-management techniques; and guidance for pharmacotherapy and management of co-occurring conditions.
> - GPM has an evidence base for use with patients with BPD, however its essential principles have been used to treat patients with other primary or co-occurring disorders.

Overview of Good Psychiatric Management for Borderline Personality Disorder

Good psychiatric management (GPM) for borderline personality disorder (BPD) evolved from its original iteration, first titled *general psychiatric management*. The 2001 Practice Guideline for the Treatment of Patients with Borderline Personality Disorder[1] and Gunderson's *Borderline Personality Disorder: A Clinical Guide*[2] together were the foundation of GPM. GPM was compared to dialectical behavior therapy (DBT) in a one-year randomized controlled study of patients with BPD and recent suicidal activity.[3] The results of this study, published in 2009, revealed that a well-considered, straightforward treatment intervention conceptualized as a study control, could demonstrate an efficacy comparable to a specialized, state-of-the-art intervention performed by highly skilled clinicians. A follow-up study confirmed that the benefits observed for patients in both arms of the study persisted over two years following completion of the treatment.[4] Since publication of the study in 2009, "general psychiatric management" was redubbed "good psychiatric management," suggesting an allusion to Winnicott's hypothesis about the "good enough" mothering.[5] The basic idea is that a treatment designed for the generalist clinician has a utility of its own and a relevant place in the offerings for patients with BPD that is not necessarily an intervention for specialists or self-designated experts in this field: GPM should be "good enough" for most patients.

Much of GPM's overarching perspective and many of its essential principles reflect the attitude and work of the late John Gunderson, a leading figure over decades in the advance of BPD nosology and treatment.[6] Gunderson's approach was marked by an attitude of proactively addressing common iatrogenic complications in the treatment of patients with BPD, and a simultaneous broad embrace of different treatment philosophies and modalities. GPM stresses the centrality of a general psychiatric management approach to the treatment of a specific psychiatric disorder (e.g., BPD). Of note, GPM's approach to the pharmacotherapy of patients with BPD deviates significantly from the Practice Guideline's more ambitious expectations for the utility of medications. The revised edition of Gunderson's *Borderline Personality Disorder: A Clinical Guide,* coauthored with Paul Links, harnessed the research and clinical wisdom emerging in that period, as traditional psychoanalytic theory and practice, which once dominated the field of personality disorders, faded in relevance.[7] The *Handbook of Good Psychiatric Management for Borderline Personality Disorder,* by Gunderson with Links, published in 2014, offered an updated overview of the treatment that included extensive case illustrations.[8]

GPM's central tenets implicitly address the commonly observed iatrogenic complications of treatment of patients with BPD. These complications can include: destabilizing treatments using more orthodox psychoanalytic practices; frequent and derailing psychiatric hospitalizations; highly problematic polypharmacy; and the risks of a patient's relative passivity, including an insufficient focus on meaningful work or studies. GPM's appreciation of these concerning complications followed organically from the accumulating research evidence of this period. Attempts to use more traditional psychoanalytic methods yielded concerning outcomes in well-regarded research.[9] The changing patterns of psychiatric hospitalization related to larger currents in healthcare economics led to the gradual demise of most long-term psychiatric hospitalization options for patients with BPD. Currently, hospitalizations for BPD are more likely to last days rather than months, and repeated hospitalizations are associated with concerning interruptions for patients in their social and vocational lives. Hospitalizations often create more problems than they solve.

The explosion in psychiatric prescribing practices over the past generation contributed to the frequently observed pattern of questionable, and often counterproductive, polypharmacy in patients with BPD. This phenomenon was marked by side effects including medication abuse or dependence, obesity, hypersomnolence, or diminished libido. Also, concerning data emerged from large prospective studies of patients with BPD,[10,11] which underscored that while core symptoms of the disorder might remit in time, these patients continued to have significant challenges in key areas of functioning. In particular, marked difficulties were observed in the ability of many patients with BPD to identify and keep meaningful work, with an associated loss of life structure, self-esteem, and income.

Choi-Kain, Albert, and Gunderson[12] examined the requirements for learning and practicing the evidence-based treatments for BPD. The specialized training for these interventions can be costly and time-consuming; moreover, the designs of these treatments are also relatively expensive and customarily require more than one clinical encounter per week. Iliakis et al.[13] put into context the high demand for treatment and the low availability of practitioners trained to treat BPD patients, even in the most well-resourced Western countries. These observations about the barriers to learning and offering evidence-based interventions, and the associated imbalance between patients in need and clinicians available to provide treatment, have been reflected in epidemiologic studies.[14] With rare exceptions, useful training for work with patients with personality-disorder pathology is limited in mental health training programs.[15]

GPM's mission has a central public health focus informed by ample data about the significant representation of BPD patients in most mental health settings. It is fair to observe that BPD is common, with estimations of prevalence rates in the psychiatric outpatient setting of 10–12 percent and in the psychiatric inpatient setting of 20–22 percent, often undiagnosed, and routinely untreated.[16,17] This pattern has created a chronic public health crisis: a group of patients with a disorder with high morbidity and mortality, who are frequently seen in psychiatric emergency departments, inpatient units and outpatient psychiatric settings, and in the general medical setting. BPD is often not diagnosed, and even when diagnosed, patients are frequently unaware of their condition because of clinicians' reluctance to share their diagnostic impression, even when reliably made.

This chapter will offer: (1) a summary of the level of evidence for the effectiveness of GPM; (2) an overview of the central tenets of GPM and its core theoretical underpinnings; (3) the indications for treatment with GPM; (4) an outline of the basics of the GPM treatment approach with a focus on diagnosis sharing and psychoeducation, the establishment of treatment goals, the adjustment of the intensity and duration of the treatment, the management of self-harm and suicidality, the integration of psychotherapy elements from the other empirically validated treatments for BPD, case-management techniques, and GPM's guide for pharmacotherapy and management of co-occurring conditions; and (5) relevant resources for clinicians, patients, and their families.

Level of Evidence for Effectiveness

The evidence for GPM's efficacy is based on a single but rigorous randomized trial that compared a year of treatment with GPM to a year of DBT.[3] This trial, conducted by

Shelley McMain and collaborators in 2009, was then followed up by continued assessments of the participants over two years (after study completion) to evaluate for lasting change.[4] The authors posited that DBT would be more effective than GPM, but they expected GPM to perform well. Interestingly, they found GPM and DBT to be equally effective across all patient outcomes including the primary metrics of frequency and severity of suicidal and non-suicidal self-injurious episodes.[3] Critically, these improvements were shown to persist for patients in both treatment modalities over the two-year follow-up period with no significant differences.[4] Based on the Strength of Recommendation Taxonomy (SORT) approach published by the *Journal of the American Board of Family Practice*, we assign GPM an A-level recommendation for its consistent and patient-centric evidence.[18]

McMain and her collaborators randomized 180 patients diagnosed with BPD who had at least two suicidal or non-suicidal self-injurious episodes in the past five years to receive one year of DBT or GPM. Both treatments included once weekly individual therapy as well as weekly supervision for clinicians. In order to see differences in the treatments, components specific to each treatment were reserved for that condition, and adherence scales were used to evaluate treatment fidelity. DBT was administered with its standard elements such as a skills-training group, use of dialectical strategies, prioritization of focus on self-harm and suicidality, and explicit behavioral strategies such as diary cards and behavioral analyses. Similarly, GPM utilized psychodynamic attentiveness to anger and countertransference reactions, as well as APA guidelines for prescribing. However, both treatments readily employed their overlapping elements, including psychoeducation and diagnostic disclosure, a helpful clinical approach, here-and-now focus, collaborative crisis-management protocols, validation, emotion focus, and patient and clinician accountability to roles.[3] As already noted, at the end of a year, no significant differences in clinical outcomes were found between the patients receiving DBT and those receiving GPM. Patients with BPD in both treatment arms showed significant reductions in the frequency and severity of suicidal (OR 0.23, P = 0.01) and non-suicidal self-injurious episodes (OR 0.52, p = 0.03), as well as significant improvements in secondary outcomes including BPD symptoms, the experience of symptom distress, depression, anger, and interpersonal functioning. There was also a reduction in general healthcare utilization including general emergency department (ED) visits and ED visits for suicidal behavior (OR = 0.43, P<0.0001). The authors used an intent-to-treat analysis but also analyzed the outcomes per protocol to see if there were any significant differences for those who actually received treatment. Still, no differences in the treatment arms were found.[3]

In McMain et al.'s follow-up study, patients were assessed at 6, 12, 18, and 24 months after treatment completion using multiple structured interviews and instruments. The authors found that the effects of treatment persisted for patients on all assessed outcomes through the two-year follow-up period.[4] Participants also continued to improve on measures of interpersonal functioning, anger, depression, and quality of life. This longitudinal assessment lends even more credibility to the original finding that GPM and DBT are equally effective. It is important to note that although quality of life ratings improved after both treatments, participants still exhibited considerable functional impairment, as indicated by low rates of full-time employment and continuing reliance on disability benefits. This continues to be an area of focus for all BPD treatments.

Although the McMain et al. study is only a single positive trial, the strength of GPM is also bolstered by the well-documented efficacy of DBT, to which it was compared.

High-fidelity DBT has been rigorously studied, with more than 18 controlled trials since its introduction in 1993. A recent meta-analysis of these trials affirmed DBT's efficacy at reducing suicidal behavior and the frequency of psychiatric crisis visits.[19] As GPM and DBT have many core elements in common, it is logical that their overlapping components could explain the positive and persistent change seen in patients in the McMain trial. Although DBT prioritizes a focus on self-harm and suicidality and GPM on interpersonal problems, outcome measures related to self-destructive behavior and interpersonal functioning did not differ between the treatment groups. Thus, it is plausible that it was the common core features of these two treatments that drove lasting change for patients.

A major limitation of the 2009 trial is that both treatment groups had experienced therapists (average of 14–15 years) who had worked with BPD patients in the past and who were recruited for their "expertise, aptitude, and interest" in treating BPD. GPM is designed as a generalist treatment that can be quickly learned and is suitable for any provider in the community. Thus, the question remains whether GPM will remain as effective if administered by less-experienced therapists. Other limitations include that the sample was mostly female and that suicidal/non-suicidal self-injury measures were self-reported, which could be subject to responder bias.

Unlike the more specialized psychotherapies for BPD, GPM can be learned from a single-day training course or a slim handbook. This accessibility seems to have a positive impact on clinicians and their ability to work with BPD patients. Keuroghlian et al.[20] conducted a study of 297 providers learning GPM and found that after a single-day training, clinicians had increased confidence in their ability to treat BPD, had corrected negative misconceptions about borderline pathology, and decreased their dislike of and motivation to avoid people with BPD. These attitudinal changes were shown to persist for at least six months following the one-day GPM training.[21] These data are encouraging, as the current need for providers who are able to treat BPD far exceeds the clinicians trained in the specialized psychotherapies.

GPM is rooted in the theory that a streamlined, generalist approach that conserves core principles of the more specialized psychotherapies can benefit the majority of patients with BPD. This theory proved true in the McMain trial when GPM performed on par with DBT. It is further supported by a similar study by Bateman and Fonagy designed to evaluate mentalization-based treatment (MBT) in comparison with another generalist treatment called structural case management (SCM). SCM has some overlap with GPM in its focus on case management and supportive psychotherapy techniques. The authors compared SCM to MBT and found that SCM performed well across all patient outcomes, although there were steeper improvements for MBT.[22] Although this is not evidence specific to GPM, it lends further support to the theoretical underpinnings of GPM and buttresses the strong results of the McMain et al. trial on which we have based our recommendation. Review Box 13.1, p. 344 for a summary of the level of evidence for GPM.

GPM's Central Theory and Orientation

In recent years, the development of a number of empirically validated treatments for patients with BPD has understandably been a source of optimism for patients, families, and clinicians.[23] In addition, important prospective studies have shown that patients

---

Box 13.1 Level of Evidence

- GPM has a small but strong evidence base centered around a rigorous, single-blind trial showing that GPM was equally effective in the treatment of BPD compared to DBT (Level A).
- A two-year follow-up study revealed GPM and DBT were equally effective across a range of primary outcomes (reduction in frequency and severity of suicidal and non-suicidal self-injurious episodes) and secondary outcomes (general healthcare utilization, improvements in BPD symptoms, distress from symptoms, depression, anger, and interpersonal functioning; Level A).
- The strength of GPM is also bolstered by the well-documented efficacy of DBT, to which it was compared. DBT has been rigorously studied, with more than 18 controlled trials (Level B).
- There is evidence that learning GPM positively impacts clinicians' attitudes and beliefs about BPD. Keuroghlian et al.[20] found that after a one-day GPM training for which clinicians could volunteer, clinicians reported a decreased inclination to avoid patients with BPD, a reduced belief that the BPD prognosis is hopeless, and increased feelings of competence and ability to make a positive difference with BPD patients. These benefits persisted at six-month follow-up (Level C).

Key: Levels of Evidence; Strength of recommendation taxonomy (SORT)*
Level of Evidence A: Good quality patient-oriented evidence.
Level of Evidence B: Limited quality patient-oriented evidence.
Level of Evidence C: Based on consensus, usual practice, opinion, disease-oriented evidence, or case series for studies of diagnosis.
*Ebell MH, Siwek J, Weiss BD, Woolf SH, Susman J, Ewigman B, Bowman M. Simplifying the language of evidence to improve patient care. *J Fam Pract.* 2004 Feb 1;53(2):111–120.

---

with BPD (whether or not they are engaged in various treatments) will have significant reduction of symptoms over time at rates not expected for a condition labeled in the DSM-5 as a "relatively stable" pattern of behaviors.[10,11] These observations together have directly confronted the long-standing conventional wisdom that BPD is an untreatable condition and one that is highly likely to persist in patients over time. Unfortunately, many clinicians will conclude that BPD is, by definition, both persistent and untreatable because of their exposure primarily to only those individuals with the more intractable presentations of the disorder. Data from prospective GPM studies supports the hypothesis that most clinicians should be able to treat most patients with BPD traits or BPD, and that only a smaller subset of BPD patients will require treatment by experts with more labor-intensive or extended interventions.

GPM's flexibility rests in its eclectic embrace of elements of other well-described treatment interventions. GPM borrows from traditional case management, specifically the employment of active, practical help conducted during a treatment session. Elements of cognitive-behavioral therapy (CBT) and DBT are also used extensively, including chain analyses, diary cards, and coaching. Concepts and interventions derived from the psychoanalytically informed MBT and transference-focused psychotherapy (TFP) are also used in GPM: from MBT, a focus on attachment as a key understanding and exploration of attributions patients may make about themselves and others; and from TFP, an appreciation of defense mechanisms, including splitting, projection, and projective identification, and a close monitoring of countertransference currents.

GPM has a central theory about the factors contributing to BPD symptoms and to impairment in functioning, which stresses the contribution of interpersonal hypersensitivity. This theory posits that the patient with BPD will alternate between four states: (1) feeling connected, (2) feeling threatened, (3) feeling alone, and (4) feeling despair. These four states are associated with specific reactions, and a patient's pattern of traversing between these states will correlate with specific stimuli from others, including the therapist. Providing psychoeducation to patients and families about interpersonal hypersensitivity and exploring with patients specific material related to BPD symptoms is an anchoring set of interventions in GPM. This includes discussing affective instability, unstable interpersonal relationships, perceived abandonment, and intense anger as understood through the prism of interpersonal hypersensitivity.

GPM is offered as an initial intervention that should suffice for most patients. Because GPM includes frequent assessments of treatment progress, there will be situations when the GPM clinician recommends referral to another treatment. In many treatment settings, it is not practical to offer extended, expensive, labor-intensive treatments to all patients with BPD pathology; the specialized interventions including DBT, TFP, MBT, and schema therapy (ST) would therefore be reserved for a subset of patients who do not progress with GPM.

GPM's public health mission includes an openness to adjunctive treatments of different kinds, allowing administrators and clinicians to build on mental health or substance-abuse infrastructure already in place. GPM would not hew to a model of an inviolate patient–therapist dyad, but would rather work to integrate adjunctive treatments like 12-step programs, skills groups, behavior-modification programs like Weight Watchers, or family psychoeducation programs. GPM clinicians will be also open to practical, cautious pharmacotherapy.

It is possible to understand GPM's overarching approach by appreciating its emergence from an extended period of widespread iatrogenically-induced complications. The treatment of patients with BPD was marked by extended, not always fruitful, hospitalizations, concerning polypharmacy often conducted with little or no empirical support, and aimless, unstructured psychotherapies. Many of GPM's central tenets directly address these iatrogenic complications; accumulated wisdom had suggested that while the empirically validated interventions had begun to emerge in the past three decades, a convincing literature had also emerged that underscored what *not* to do in the clinical management of patients with BPD. Review Box 13.2, p. 346 for a summary of the theory behind GPM.

Indications for Treatment with GPM

GPM was developed as an introductory, and often sufficient, treatment of patients with BPD. GPM can be conceptualized as a reasonable "first-pass" treatment intervention for a wide swath of patients with BPD traits or meeting criteria for the DSM-5 BPD disorder. GPM's limited core principles and the premium placed on flexibility together can allow clinicians to offer this as a reasonable intervention for many, maybe most patients, while

Box 13.2 Summary of the Theoretical Orientation

- GPM embraces an eclectic approach to treatment, encouraging use of CBT, DBT, case management, and psychodynamic elements, when indicated.
- GPMs overarching hypothesis and organizing interventions are based on the centrality of interpersonal hypersensitivity. GPM posits that BPD symptoms, associated iatrogenic complications, and effective treatments are all tied directly to management of interpersonal hypersensitivity.
- Most clinicians should be able to competently treat patients with BPD without extensive and expensive training. One day of training is typically all that is needed.
- The appreciation of the natural course of BPD, informed by data from prospective studies, supports a hypothesis that most BPD patients will not need intensive treatment and can be successfully treated with limited, but informed, interventions.
- GPM can be the initial intervention for most patients with BPD. Intensive treatments such as DBT, MBT, TFP or ST can be reserved for those patients who do not respond to GPM.
- Patient's engagement in adjunctive treatments (pharmacotherapy, group therapy, self-help groups, family treatment) is advantageous and highly likely to benefit the effectiveness of a primary GPM approach.
- GPM actively reduces the risk of iatrogenic complications of treatment for BPD, with a proactive approach to reducing polypharmacy, unhelpful psychiatric hospitalization, or aimless, unfocused individual psychotherapy.

remaining sensitive to the heterogeneity of presentations and range of severity of illness among patients with BPD pathology.

That said, there are some patients with primary or co-occurring BPD who would not be considered appropriate candidates for the treatment. Broadly speaking, the patient with BPD and a co-occurring condition that would preclude the patient's ability to use GPM as designed would likely be referred to an intervention for the co-occurring condition at the outset. There are clearly patients with BPD who require a higher level of care than GPM can accommodate; these might be patients referred to day programs, intensive outpatient programs, or residential facilities. Also, some co-occurring conditions would likely require a sequenced treatment, with a specialized intervention first, and then possibly GPM might be employed once a particular set of symptoms has been adequately addressed. For example, certain patients with active substance-use disorders, likely in the moderate to severe categories, should probably access substance-use disorder specialty services before their BPD symptoms are addressed with a GPM model. Similarly, those patients with co-occurring eating disorders with prominent medical complications, including seriously underweight or medically unstable patients with anorexia nervosa, or patients with bulimia nervosa causing metabolic instability, would be referred to eating-disorder treatments at the outset.

Because the best-known empirically validated treatments for BPD, including DBT, MBT, TFP and ST, all require multiple meetings per week for the patient, GPM in some situations may be more convenient, affordable, or both. Because of GPM's inherent adaptability, a clinician could transition from one of these treatments to a less-intensive GPM format, while still including certain essential elements of the other treatments as part of a more eclectic approach. In some systems, a treatment for BPD requiring more than one encounter per week is simply not available; GPM could serve as a reasonable option when constraints would not allow alternative approaches.

Choi-Kain, Albert, and Gunderson[12] wrote about the benefits of a sequenced approach to patients with BPD. In their proposal, GPM can be used as an introductory treatment and also as an alternative for those patients with the most intractable presentations who do not respond to higher levels of care or more intensive treatment choices. While perhaps counterintuitive, they propose that there are some patients who would benefit from use of fewer resources, with more modest treatment goals understood as essentially custodial care. In this case, if the patient were to become better able to use a more intensively resourced treatment, then that could be a possibility after careful deliberation.

The 2019 volume *Applications of Good Psychiatric Management for Borderline Personality Disorder: A Practical Guide*[24] extended the scope of GPM principles to settings beyond the familiar outpatient, individual psychotherapy modality. While there has not yet been research that explicitly examines the use of GPM in inpatient units, ED, and consultation-liaison services, among other examples offered, the contributing authors describe their efforts to employ GPM elements in working in these settings. In addition, this volume explores the utility of GPM principles in the treatment of patients with primary or co-occurring narcissistic disorders. The integration of GPM and other empirically validated treatments for BPD, as described in this chapter, underscores the potential benefits of eclectic treatment approaches, including sequenced treatments. To this end, those practicing GPM resist the oft-criticized "silo" approach to the treatment of patients with BPD. Review Box 13.3 for a summary of the indications for GPM.

Box 13.3 Indications for Treatment

- GPM can usually be the initial treatment approach when treating BPD or mild co-occurring disorders with a BPD diagnosis.
- GPM is a second-line treatment for BPD when a co-occurring condition is severe or has prominent symptoms (e.g., eating disorder, active psychosis, untreated mania, or moderate to severe substance-use disorders).
- GPM is a reasonable alternative when logistical concerns, such as finances, travel, or an inability to meet more than once weekly, preclude a recommendation for other evidence-based treatments.
- GPM is a viable alternative when a patient with BPD has had extensive, intensive treatment(s) that have not helped, or when a less expensive treatment is needed.
- The scope of GPM's utility has moved beyond an individual treatment for patients with BPD; it can be used in other settings, with a wider range of patients, and in concert with other treatment interventions.

Basics of the GPM Treatment Approach

The GPM clinician's interventions are organized by eight basic components of the treatment approach: (1) forthright sharing of the BPD diagnosis; (2) psychoeducation for the patient (and, when indicated, with family members) including a focus on an interpersonal hypersensitivity hypothesis about BPD symptoms; (3) the establishment of personal and treatment goals; (4) flexible duration and intensity; (5) a consistent, measured management of self-harm or suicidal threats or behaviors; (6) psychotherapy integrating elements from the other evidence-based interventions for BPD; (7) case management; and (8) conservative pharmacotherapy and a deliberate management of co-occurring conditions.

Diagnostic Sharing and Psychoeducation

GPM, like other evidence-supported treatments for BPD, requires sharing of the diagnosis of BPD as part of the initial consultation. Clinicians are encouraged to be direct about their consideration of BPD as a relevant possible diagnosis for their patients, and can offer to review diagnostic criteria together with patients to decide which are applicable. If other psychiatric disorders are also diagnosed, these are also shared with patients, including the possible difficulty of treating comorbid disorders if BPD is not also addressed; the limited effectiveness of medications for BPD; and the possibly reduced effectiveness of medications for comorbid disorders when BPD is present. If a patient does not meet full diagnostic criteria for BPD, GPM advises that treatment for BPD nonetheless is likely to be useful if a patient endorses some combination of prominent rejection sensitivity, self-destructive behavior, or intense anger. A patient is not required to accept the diagnosis of BPD in order for GPM treatment to be considered, as long as the patient is interested in working on problems related to BPD for which a GPM approach is likely to be helpful.

GPM also explicitly incorporates psychoeducation about BPD and available treatments, which is seen as part of an informed-consent process that encourages patients to collaborate in decision-making about treatment planning. Psychoeducation also is viewed as crucial to engendering hope, reducing stigma, and fostering the start of a therapeutic alliance. Although GPM has been studied as an outpatient treatment, diagnostic sharing and psychoeducation about BPD is appropriate and feasible in other settings, including inpatient psychiatric units, EDs, and consultation-liaison services.[25-27]

Psychoeducation should include the genetic heritability of BPD and the limited available neurobiological findings, including increased amygdala activation in response to facial expression and decreased ventromedial frontal cortex activity during a self-control task when feeling sad (overactive "emotional brain" vs. underactive "thinking brain").[28-30] BPD can be described as a "good prognosis" disorder, for which multiple effective treatments are available. Even without specific treatment, symptoms of BPD resolve over time and functioning may improve: after six years, nearly 70 percent of patients with BPD no longer meet diagnostic criteria, but after 16 years, only 40 percent of patients with BPD will have good functioning in work and relationships.[31,32] Treatments for BPD can be thought of as ways to speed up resolution of symptoms and increase the odds of attaining a better life. Also, as part of instilling hope, patients can be told that if they do not receive full benefit from one treatment for BPD, it will be reasonable to consider trying another evidence-supported approach. Review Box 13.4 as a brief summary of the basics of the GPM treatment approach.

Andrew: Discussing the Diagnosis of BPD

Andrew is a college freshman who was accompanied to the campus mental health center by his resident advisor for increasing suicidal feelings. In his initial session with the social worker there, he said he thought he had "depression" but described mood instability, episodes of superficial cutting, and occasional bulimia symptoms. Recently, he was also experiencing turmoil in a long-distance relationship with his girlfriend from high school. After careful assessment, the social worker explained to Andrew GPM's model of interpersonal hypersensitivity and rejection sensitivity. Andrew felt this was relevant to him, and he met most criteria of BPD when they reviewed them together. Andrew met some but not all criteria for major depressive disorder (MDD). The social worker explained how MDD and BPD can occur together, but that they have different treatment and that BPD is unlikely to improve with treatments for MDD alone, such as medication. He described the significant heritability of BPD and the evidence-supported treatments available to address Andrew's BPD.

Box 13.4 Basics of the Treatment Approach

- GPM emphasizes diagnostic sharing and psychoeducation to help the patient, and possibly the family, to become an active partner in treatment. Psychoeducation is about BPD and its treatment but also about practical aspects of life.
- The GPM approach to the working alliance is to promote a climate of collaboration, conveying an attitude that change is expected, which also fosters patient responsibility and accountability.
- GPM focuses on interpersonal hypersensitivity to link interpersonal interactions to problematic thoughts, feelings, and behaviors. This provides an easily understandable guide to treatment for patients with BPD and clinicians.
- Decreased symptoms and improved self-control facilitate treatment goals focused on the patient's life outside of therapy, especially initially functioning at work or school, and subsequently on interpersonal relationships.
- Case-management approaches ensure that practical problems in the patient's life, often caused or exacerbated by BPD and interpersonal hypersensitivity, are adequately addressed.
- GPM supports a multimodal treatment incorporating supportive and behavioral approaches, case management, and limited psychopharmacology.
- GPM clinicians are encouraged to be flexible, pragmatic, and eclectic, and open to family interventions and group psychotherapy.
- The duration and intensity of GPM treatment are flexibly adjusted based on the patient's progress. If little or no improvement is observed, reconsideration of the treatment approach is advised.

Psychoeducation about Interpersonal Hypersensitivity and Rejection Sensitivity

GPM uses the model of interpersonal hypersensitivity to provide guidance for clinicians and patients to understand the symptoms and problems of functioning in patients with BPD and find effective interventions for them.[33] Patients are seen as shifting among four self-states caused by interpersonal stressors to which patient responses are informed by the chronic presence of rejection sensitivity: (1) connectedness, (2) feeling threatened, (3) aloneness, and (4) despair. The initial self-state of *connectedness* is characterized by feelings of being cared for by others, but this is fragile due to dependence on idealized views of others and hypervigilance to perceived rejection. If the patient experiences actual or perceived separation, criticism, hostility, or anger from others, this can quickly cause a shift to *feeling threatened*, leading to anxiety, help-seeking, devaluation, and self-injury as a form of communication. If support from others is obtained, the patient can return to the state of connectedness, but this will always remain fragile due to ongoing rejection sensitivity. If support is lacking, which can occur because the manifestations of feeling threatened may lead to the withdrawal of others who might have been potential sources of support, aloneness emerges. In *aloneness,* the patient experiences a loss of containment from supportive others, resulting in dissociation, paranoia, impulsive behaviors to avoid annihilating feelings of abandonment, and help rejection linked to aggressive negative self-assessments. This can proceed to *despair,* including anhedonia, hopelessness, and suicidality, which may require rescue by others or containment by emergency services. At any point, including sometimes remarkably quickly in emergency rooms, if the patient experiences support and an alleviation of rejection, a return to fragile connectedness is possible, subject to the inevitable return of interpersonal stressors that fuel this repeated cycle.

The model of interpersonal hypersensitivity is used to understand and guide interventions throughout GPM treatment. In the initial evaluation, psychoeducation to describe this cycle provides to patients with BPD a coherent explanation for their chaotic symptoms and life experiences, of which they are well aware but usually feel at a loss to understand. During treatment, for patients with limited sources of support to rely on when they feel threatened, identification of new sources of support can be a relevant approach. Alternatively, ways to reduce withdrawal from existing sources of support are likely to be important. This includes helping the patient notice reactions in the cycle that may be alienating or ineffective and substitute more effective actions to gain support or an improved self-concept. Increased self-reliance is encouraged by achieving better functioning in work or schooling, leading to less susceptibility to the problems of interpersonal hypersensitivity. For this reason, GPM advises patients to focus on work improvements before addressing problems in interpersonal relationships, which are seen as more triggering of rejection sensitivity. Although GPM provides a framework for managing acute suicidality and self-harm, which are core symptoms of BPD, improvement in how the patient handles interpersonal hypersensitivity is viewed as the most important approach to reliably reduce recurrences of suicidality and self-harm.

GPM encourages certain clinician attitudes informed by an expectation of rejection sensitivity and interpersonal hypersensitivity in patients with BPD: (1) being active while avoiding extremes of withdrawal or overreaction; (2) being thoughtful, both as a form of containment and a model of "thinking first" to the patient; and (3) considering the therapy relationship as both a real relationship and a professional relationship and imparting this understanding to the patient, allowing exploration of the patient's experience of the therapeutic relationship as another application of the model of interpersonal hypersensitivity.

Dora: Interpersonal Hypersensitivity and Self-Destructive Behavior

Dora is a lesbian woman in her late 20s who, for several years, has been seeing a social worker for treatment of BPD. Early in treatment, she had several episodes of hyperglycemia requiring emergency room visits, after stormy break-ups, when she stopped taking her medications for diabetes mellitus. The social worker emphasized the importance of the model of interpersonal hypersensitivity to understand this self-destructive behavior. Gradually, Dora recognized her pattern of becoming quickly dependent on a new girlfriend. Her fragile state of connectedness was often disrupted by her rejection sensitivity to a new girlfriend not being perfectly responsive to texts or phone calls. She would shift to feeling threatened, and she would desperately reach out to friends for reassurance. If support was not immediately forthcoming or if a break-up actually happened, she experienced aloneness and might no longer answer her phone. In the context of despair and suicidal thoughts, she felt worthless and would stop administering her diabetes medication. Dora usually came to sessions explaining that she had been too upset to complete diary cards; she and the social worker would discuss a recent upsetting event and perform a chain analysis to better understand her impulsive behavior.

Establishing Treatment Goals

GPM's focus on life outside of therapy leads to encouragement of treatment goals beyond intrapsychic exploration, self-understanding, or symptom reduction. After chronic experiences of cycles of interpersonal hypersensitivity, patients with BPD may perceive themselves as weak and excessively dependent on the support of others. Conveying an expectation of change introduces the need for collaborative development of realistic, incremental goals as an important strategy to counter negative self-perceptions of being unable to function effectively in life. Also, movement toward having a more satisfying life is seen as the most likely way to promote persistent symptom reduction and improved self-control with diminished impulsivity.

For some patients, due to their fragmented identities and chaotic lives, setting goals itself can be the initial treatment goal. In this case, the clinician may need to be a consistent source of motivation for considering what first steps may be reasonable to consider. Initial goals may focus on basic self-care using case-management approaches, bolstering the patient's self-esteem and engendering hope. This may be especially important for patients whose response to interpersonal hypersensitivity has included chronic withdrawal from work and relationships. GPM encourages goals of improvement in work functioning prior to goals in relationships, consistent with vocational functioning as a positive prognostic factor in BPD.[34] At first, patients are expected to be able to more easily address their difficulties with interpersonal hypersensitivity in work settings, developing skills and a sense of efficacy that then can be used in more charged intimate relationships.

Bettina: Setting Goals

Bettina is a young woman living at home after dropping out of college. She was previously diagnosed with BPD by a therapist at her college mental health center. She was referred to a psychologist at her local clinic. She is interested in gaining "self-knowledge" about her episodes of rage and impulsivity, which she considers as resulting from the trauma of having parents who are not adequately supportive. Currently, Bettina is mostly smoking marijuana and writing songs, having made no efforts to perform or sell them. After assessment, the psychologist agrees with the BPD diagnosis and explains that treatment goals need to extend beyond symptom reduction or gaining insight. He encourages Bettina to think about possible goals related to returning to school, working, or developing relationships. She is surprised about the focus on life outside of treatment, and grudgingly agrees to work with the psychologist on forming treatment goals. In the first few sessions, in an effort to foster accountability and greater responsibility, he continues to focus discussion on Bettina's life outside of treatment, including her thoughts and efforts related to productive activity and improved relationships.

Duration and Intensity of Treatment

GPM is meant to be a flexible treatment that can be adapted in practical ways to the treatment goals of patients and their ability to participate in treatment. Treatment is usually expected to begin on a weekly basis, but this can be flexibly adjusted based on the patient's level of severity, motivation, and circumstances. For example, a motivated patient with more acuity might be seen twice per week, although GPM advises against ongoing treatments at more than twice per week as being too likely to foster an excessive focus on therapy itself over improvements in the patient's life outside of therapy. Alternatively, a patient who is more stable might be able to continue less-frequent treatment, or patients in school or traveling for work might need periods of less-intensive treatment or breaks in treatment.

In GPM, the duration of treatment will depend crucially on whether progress is being made. At the beginning of treatment, the clinician will have conveyed an expectation of change and the need for collaborative monitoring of progress toward treatment goals. In general, improvements are expected to follow a trajectory of: reduced subjective distress in the first few weeks; reduced problematic behavior in the first few months; reduced devaluation, withdrawal, and dependency in interpersonal relationships in the first six months to a year; and improved functioning in school or work beginning after six to 18 months. If progress is completely lacking during these timeframes, this should lead to a collaborative discussion with the patient, including a reconsideration of the treatment approach and possible referral to a different treatment modality. If progress has occurred, patients may wish to continue GPM at a reduced frequency, or referral to more intensive treatments for specific problems that have not yet been addressed can be considered.

Yolanda: Flexible Duration and Intensity of Treatment

When Yolanda was a nursing student, she saw a psychologist at her school's counseling service for her BPD. Yolanda had previously investigated DBT treatment at a local clinic, but felt that the commitment to two sessions per week for many months would not be realistic for her. Yolanda wanted to be able to travel for electives at other institutions, and she did not feel that she could make a commitment to attend the DBT treatment as recommended. Yolanda and her psychologist at the school counseling center agreed to a weekly GPM treatment as long as Yolanda was available locally for sessions, with the understanding that they would review this plan periodically. During the next several months, they focused on how binge eating and hopelessness were influenced by her rejection sensitivity. When Yolanda was away for her electives, she made a point of returning to see her psychologist monthly. After graduating nursing school, she took a job that allowed her the flexibility to begin a weekly DBT skills group. She found both receiving and giving peer support to be helpful, and she continued seeing the psychologist for individual sessions about once per month.

Management of Self-Harm or Threats of Suicide or Suicidal Behavior

GPM emphasizes that suicidal thinking, self-harm, and suicide gestures and attempts are to be expected in patients with BPD pathology. This is supported by data underscoring that patients with BPD have both high rates of suicidal behavior and of completed suicide. As mentioned, one of GPM's central tenets is the avoidance of problematic iatrogenic complications. These complications can often involve management of suicidal behaviors. One familiar concerning pattern is repeated, counterproductive psychiatric hospitalizations in the context of a patient's self-injury or suicidal thinking. The clinician's over-involvement and risk of boundary violations can also occur in work with the suicidal BPD patient; alternatively, there can be risk when a clinician is moved to ignore the suicidal BPD patient, thereby becoming vulnerable to accusations of dereliction of duty or abandonment.

GPM outlines a simple and helpful calculus of chronic and acute risks of suicide in BPD. This theory describes the expectable chronic suicidal thinking experienced by many patients with BPD, the distinction between suicidality and non-suicidal self-injurious behaviors, and those acute risks that, when added to the BPD patient's chronic suicidal thinking, should be the target of specific interventions. The acute risks described in this model can include the worsening of a BPD patient's mood disorder, the addition of active, concerning substance use, or the emergence of persistent psychotic thinking beyond the well-described transient psychosis or paranoid thinking under stress experienced by many BPD patients. This "acute-on-chronic" model is designed to help the clinician calculate increased risks and to intervene with either additional outpatient or, when indicated, inpatient treatment.

GPM stresses that self-injury or suicide gestures or attempts should be explored as communications of the patient's internal distress. GPM advises against a ritualized, formulaic discussion of the patient's suicidality as in a "safety check" model. Instead, the emergence of material related to suicidality is seen as an opportunity to revisit the interpersonal hypersensitivity construct and the practical interventions informed by that theory.

The GPM clinician will be clear at the outset when working with the patient with BPD about limitations in between session contact and support. This discussion would be coupled with practical advice about safety planning and alternative sources of support (friends, hotlines, 12-step meetings). When the patient does engage in self-injury or suicidal behavior, following an assessment of safety, the GPM clinician will work with the patient using chain analysis to identify contributing factors leading to this behavior, integrating the central hypothesis about interpersonal hypersensitivity in this intervention. In addition, in these situations the therapist will revisit the safety plan in place and work collaboratively with the patient to identify additional coping mechanisms, sources of support, or emergency services, when indicated.

Jose: Managing Self-Harm and Suicidal Behaviors

Jose is a medical resident in his late 20s who was given a diagnosis of BPD and alcohol use disorder while in college. During his college years, Jose had repeated episodes of self-injury, mostly superficial cutting, that led to repeated psychiatric hospitalizations, which were often disruptive. Jose's first therapist became visibly alarmed any time Jose shared with her his chronic suicidal thoughts, leading to a number of ED visits. Jose had another therapist at his medical school's counseling center whom Jose experienced as dismissive and hostile whenever the topic of suicidality came up in their sessions. Jose's new psychiatrist uses GPM principles in her approach to suicidality and self-harm. She explains to Jose that she takes seriously the risk of suicidality in patients with BPD, and she underscores the particular risks associated with interpersonal stress, substance misuse, or depression. The psychiatrist outlines what she calls an "acute-on-chronic" way of assessing suicidality. She enlists Jose to look together at variables that could either increase or decrease his suicide risk level. When Jose does have an episode of increased suicidal thinking and self-injury, his psychiatrist engages him in a detailed exploration of the chain of events that precipitated the events. They revisit the interpersonal hypersensitivity theory and attempt to identify how Jose's suicidality might be linked to an experience of perceived hostility or criticism at work. Jose's psychiatrist stresses the importance of their exploration of Jose's suicidal thoughts and behaviors, at the same time being clear about her limitations. She encourages Jose to develop ways to manage his suicidality including identification of close friends and local 12-step meetings as alternative ways to manage escalating distress.

Eclectic Psychotherapy Integrating Elements of Other Evidence-based Interventions

GPM encourages an eclectic approach to treatment that allows for flexibly combining distinct treatment components that each can play a pragmatic role in addressing a patient's multiple difficulties. The core elements of GPM already establish multimodality: psychotherapy that is psychodynamically informed but includes supportive techniques and CBT approaches such as behavioral chain analyses; case management that addresses practical problems of patients in their lives outside of therapy; and judicious psychopharmacology that recognizes the limits of medications for patients with BPD.

GPM's recommended psychotherapeutic interventions borrow liberally from the other empirically validated treatments for BPD. GPM has elements of psychodynamic treatments, including MBT and TFP, and of cognitive-behavioral therapies. GPM advocates for use of DBT's concept of the BPD patient's deficits in skills, encouraging active coaching at times and homework between sessions emphasizing self-monitoring and use of practical, readily teachable tools. GPM also integrates MBT's focus on attachment, as evidenced by the centrality of the interpersonal hypersensitivity model proposed. The MBT process of exploration of the patient's attributions about self and others, asking the patient to consider internal states, is part of GPM's principle of enlisting the patient to "think first" before acting. From TFP, GPM integrates a psychotherapeutic focus on establishing an expectation for engagement and activity as a challenge to avoidance and chronic acting out through passivity. The TFP prioritization of monitoring and maintaining boundaries and the active exploration of countertransference currents can inform the GPM therapist's priorities.

Beyond these core elements, GPM encourages family involvement and patient participation in group psychotherapy. GPM's approach to family involvement emphasizes psychoeducation more than formal family therapy and may include coaching on practical interventions addressing interpersonal hypersensitivity to reduce stress and improve support. GPM is open to the possible benefits of participation in a wide range of psychotherapy groups including general supportive groups, 12-step groups, or skills-focused groups such as DBT. From a GPM perspective, the specific content of a group or immediate support may be less crucial than the opportunity for a patient to listen to and learn from other people. This may also give the patient a valuable chance to work on communication skills and interpersonal hypersensitivity.

Daisy: Eclectic Use of Psychotherapy Skills

Daisy is a married homemaker in her early 30s with two young children. She was diagnosed with MDD after the birth of her second child; at this time the treating psychiatrist shared with Daisy and her husband his impression that Daisy had both a mood disorder and borderline and narcissistic personality disorder traits. Daisy responded well to treatment with antidepressant medication, but she continued to have ongoing symptoms of unstable relationships, reckless driving, and periodic non-suicidal, self-injurious behavior, specifically cutting herself to relieve acute distress.

One year of pastoral counseling was helpful to Daisy in only a limited way. She appreciated the counselor's advice and praise for her parenting skills, but she continued to have unstable moods and her self-injury was a source of great distress for Daisy's husband. Daisy's psychiatrist recommend that Daisy transfer her care to a social worker trained in GPM so that she could receive treatment specifically targeting her personality disorder symptoms.

Daisy's new treater outlines a number of recommendations for their work together that mark a change from the model offered by her pastoral counselor. Daisy's new therapist asks her to keep a daily log of her mood; they use this log at their weekly meeting to examine the events that precede Daisy's episodes of self-injury. While Daisy in the past had texted her pastoral counselor on weekends for support when she was feeling impulsive, Daisy's new therapist describes the limitations on contact between sessions. Daisy's therapist introduces the idea that Daisy should identify ways to manage her intermittent feelings of distress, suggesting possible distractions or alternative coping mechanisms so that Daisy can avoid the self-injurious behavior that so distresses her husband. Daisy and her therapist explore Daisy's understanding of the effect of her behavior on others. This is a process that feels new to Daisy as she considers how her self-injury impacts her husband.

Every three months, Daisy and her husband meet together with Daisy's therapist. This meeting is framed as an opportunity for education for Daisy's husband about her personality disorder symptoms. There is also meeting time set aside for coaching for Daisy and her husband as they examine how Daisy's sensitivity to perceived criticism and feelings of isolation contribute to her risk for impulsive or self-injurious acts.

Applying Case-management Strategies

GPM emphasizes a focus on the patient's life outside of therapy. Psychosocial stressors are a common feature of BPD, resulting from the destructive symptoms generated by interpersonal hypersensitivity. Interpersonal hypersensitivity often leads to serious impairments in basic functioning beyond what might be expected from the patient's intellectual, educational, or socioeconomic background. In line with GPM's emphasis on practical help and eclecticism, the clinician is encouraged to apply case-management strategies when needed. The case-management approach might include assistance with activities of daily living, work, family, intimate relationships and friendships, health maintenance, financial management, and leisure-time activities. Patients may need help with social skills, making family connections, seeking education or employment, obtaining medical care, help with budgeting, or problem-solving about grooming, cleaning, cooking, shopping, and transportation.

Patients may be caught up in chaotic relationships in a desperate attempt to stave off their dysphoric states resulting from rejection sensitivity; they may resist addressing practical matters needed to provide the necessary basic foundations of life to be able to improve their interpersonal hypersensitivity. The clinician can take active steps with the patient during sessions in the patient's problem areas, working on practical tasks not usually considered part of traditional psychotherapy or medication management. Examples might include helping fill out a health insurance form, reviewing a resume, investigating online health options or calling a medical clinic, or making a budget. In general, patients are advised that it is important to focus on basic areas first, laying a groundwork for efforts in work or schooling and, eventually, in intimate relationships.

Christine: Use of Case Management

Christine is a woman in her 30s with BPD who had found her two years of exploratory psychodynamic psychotherapy to be superficially of interest, but of little help in managing the challenges of her day-to-day life. Christine's BPD was marked by significant elements of rejection sensitivity and avoidance. She worked only part-time and relied on financial support from her church for much of her monthly expenses.

Christine's new therapist described his different approach to treating patients with BPD. While Christine anticipated continued exploration of her background and motivation as central to her therapy for her BPD, her new therapist focused on the many concrete issues, starting with Christine's budget and bill-paying. Christine's therapist began by looking together at Christine's overdue bills, a source of great to distress to her, and together they contacted her creditors and arranged repayment plans. They together called the local Medicaid office to clarify how much income Christine could earn without compromising her healthcare benefits. Given Christine's clear need for increased income, her therapist then asked her to bring in her college transcript, so that they could look at what kinds of work Christine might pursue. In this process, Christine felt an increased sense of accountability. At times she felt overwhelmed when faced with the ways her BPD had contributed to her impaired functioning. Nevertheless, she grudgingly agreed to continue to work with her therapist to address the many practical difficulties she faced. Over time, Christine's therapist devoted less time to his case-management role; when they shifted to a more exploratory orientation, her therapist nevertheless continued to engage with Christine in solving specific tasks.

Pharmacotherapy and Management of Co-occurring Conditions

GPM offers clear and practical guidance for clinicians prescribing medications to patients with BPD. GPM's approach is informed by the well-documented pattern of polypharmacy in this population. This pattern is notable, given the very limited data supporting the use of medications to address core BPD symptoms. The risks associated with polypharmacy for patients with BPD is considerable, including risks of obesity, metabolic syndrome, benzodiazepine or sedative-hypnotic abuse or dependence, and diminished libido, among others. GPM's prescribing algorithm stresses a careful and conservative approach. This algorithm stresses the need to avoid prescribing in crisis, which is a common pattern. In addition, a gentle pressure to stop those medications that are identified as ineffective would be a priority. GPM's conservative approach is consistent with the emerging movement of "collaborative de-prescribing," originally developed for geriatric patients but since recommended for those many patients with BPD who take multiple medications, often without significant benefit.[35]

GPM endorses a measured attitude for the prescriber. There is an expectation that patients with BPD will have strong feelings about medications, medication seeking as well as medication refusing. From the start, key recommendations include providing ample psychoeducation about medications, including their limitations. Another goal would be active prescribing collaboration that can limit polypharmacy or excessive doses when prescribing. Patients are asked to monitor the impact of medication on particular target symptoms and are aware that medications will be stopped if it appears they are not useful.

Because BPD is often co-occurring with other psychiatric disorders, GPM offers guidance about how best to prioritize treatment. In general, the treatment of a co-occurring condition such as a mood, anxiety, eating disorder, or substance-use disorder would be the priority if it is determined that the presence of the co-occurring condition would somehow prevent the clinician from conducting an effective GPM treatment. Treating acute mania, severe substance abuse, or an eating disorder associated with medical instability are examples of co-occurring conditions that would require a sustained treatment first; recommendations for a GPM intervention would follow for co-occurring BPD symptoms. There are many cases when the co-occurring condition is significant but does not preclude GPM. In these situations, the provider would actively enlist the involvement of other clinicians or treatment programs to address the comorbidity. Consistent collaboration between clinicians in these situations would be expected for exchange of information, coordination of care, and minimization of potential splitting.

Lance: Conservative Pharmacotherapy and Management
of Co-occurring Conditions

Lance is a gay man with BPD working as pharmaceutical salesman. Now in his mid-30s, Lance was diagnosed with BPD and an alcohol use disorder as a late adolescent. He has been taking medication for many years. Lance has been prescribed medications from many different drug categories; he now takes an antidepressant, a stimulant, a sedative-hypnotic for sleep, and an atypical antipsychotic used as an adjunctive agent for his antidepressant. While his most alarming symptoms, including impulsive overdoses and unprotected sex, have resolved in recent years, he continues to seek treatment because of recurrent volatile romantic attachments and long-standing feelings of emptiness. Lance's alcohol use has been effectively reduced over time using a motivational interviewing (MI) coach.

When Lance is transferred to a new city, he begins treatment with a prescriber who shares with Lance her thinking about a conservative approach to medications informed by GPM principles. She stresses the very limited data supporting the effectiveness of medication for the BPD symptoms Lance endorses, including distress related to dating and feelings of emptiness. She reviews with Lance her plan to avoid impulsive prescribing, encouraging Lance to investigate other strategies for managing romantic turmoil. She explicitly outlines her desire to work with Lance to begin to taper some of the medications. Lance speaks freely about his anxiety about tapering any of his medications; at the same time, he feels burdened by the sexual side effects of his antidepressant and the persistent weight gain he attributes to the atypical antipsychotic agent.

Over a few months, Lance is able to slowly stop two of his four medications: the stimulant and sedative-hypnotic. After a difficult dating experience, Lance asks to restart his nightly "sleeping pill." His prescriber works with him to identify behavioral techniques to avoid restarting this medication. Lance also discloses that he has been using alcohol nightly. He and his psychiatrist explore whether Lance can manage this on own, possibly restarting a treatment focused on MI, or whether he requires a higher level of care. Lance is able to access adjunctive MI treatment and returns to rare use of alcohol, while using new techniques to manage his distress.

Conclusion

GPM is a an empirically validated treatment for patients with BPD, conceptualized as an intervention that can be mastered by clinicians of varying levels of training, to be delivered with maximum flexibility. GPM borrows from other evidence-based treatments for BPD and encourages integration of other treatment modalities in the patient's care. GPM's overarching approach aims to address the well-described pitfalls in the treatment of patients with BPD. Over decades, experts in the field have identified a number of treatment interventions routinely used with patients with BPD that appeared either to be of little benefit or, in some cases, added concerning complications. These pitfalls can include: failing to make a BPD diagnosis or share the BPD diagnosis with patient or family, even when reliably made; reflexive polypharmacy, often associated with burdensome medication side effects; recurrent, disruptive psychiatric hospitalizations; and aimless, unfocused psychotherapies. GPM is designed to proactively address these common pitfalls, with a deliberate, common-sense approach. GPM embraces a public health mission, aiming to extend informed, practical treatment to a growing group of clinicians with a goal of improving care for a broad group of patients. Review Box 13.5 for GPM resources.

Conflict of Interest/Disclosure: The authors of this chapter have no financial conflicts and nothing to disclose.

Box 13.5 Relevant Resources and Web Links for Clinicians, Patients and Their Families

---

- The Gunderson Personality Disorder Institute at McLean Hospital in Belmont, MA. https://www.mcleanhospital.org/training/gunderson-institute. Founded in 2013 with the goal of elevating awareness and training of the evidence-based treatments for BPD. They offer conferences and workshops for clinicians interested in learning GPM, among other treatment interventions.
- The National Education Alliance for Borderline Personality Disorder (NEABPD). https://www.borderlinepersonalitydisorder.org/professionals/6-module-online-course-for-professionals/. NEABPD offers an extensive archive of materials related to the assessment and treatment of BPD including information about training in GPM, including a six-module online course for professionals.
- Gunderson J, Links, P. *Handbook of Good Psychiatric Management for Borderline Personality Disorder*. Washington, DC: American Psychiatric Association; 2014, and Choi-Kain L, Gunderson J, eds. *Applications of Good Psychiatric Management for Borderline Personality Disorder*. Washington, DC: American Psychiatric Association; 2019, are essential texts on this subject.

References

1. American Psychiatric Association Practice Guidelines. Practice guideline for the treatment of patients with borderline personality disorder. American Psychiatric Association. *Am J Psychiatry*. 2001;158(10 Suppl):1–52.

2. Gunderson JG, Links PS. *Borderline Personality Disorder: A Clinical Guide*. Arlington, VA: American Psychiatric Association; 2001

3. McMain SF, Links PS, Gnam WH, et al. A randomized trial of dialectical behavior therapy versus general psychiatric management for borderline personality disorder. *Am J Psychiatry*. 2009;166(12):1365–1374.

4. McMain SF, Guimond T, Streiner DL, Cardish RJ, Links PS. Dialectical behavior therapy compared with general psychiatric management for borderline personality disorder: clinical outcomes and functioning over a 2-year follow-up. *Am J Psychiatry*. 2012;169(6):650–661.

5. Winnicott DW. Transitional objects and transitional phenomena: a study of the first not-me possession. *Int J Psychoanal*. 1953;34(2):89–97.

6. Gunderson JG. The emergence of a generalist model to meet public health needs for patients with borderline personality disorder. *Am J Psychiatry*. 2016;173(5):452–458.

7. Gunderson JG, Links P. *Borderline Personality Disorder: A Clinical Guide*. 2nd ed. Arlington, VA: American Psychiatric Association; 2008.

8. Gunderson JG, Links P. *Handbook of Good Psychiatric Management for Borderline Personality Disorder*. Washington, DC.: American Psychiatric Association; 2014.

9. Kernberg OF. Psychotherapy and psychoanalysis: final report of the Menninger Foundation's psychotherapy research project. *Bull Menninger Clin*. 1972;36(1-2):275–275.

10. Zanarini MC, Frankenburg FR, Hennen J, Reich DB, Silk KR. The McLean Study of Adult Development (MSAD): overview and implications of the first six years of prospective follow-up. *J Personal Disord*. 2005;19(5):505–523.

11. Skodol AE, Gunderson JG, Shea MT, et al. The Collaborative Longitudinal Personality Disorders Study (CLPS): overview and implications. *J Personal Disord*. 2005;19(5):487–504.

12. Choi-Kain LW, Albert EB, Gunderson JG. Evidence-based treatments for borderline personality disorder: implementation, integration, and stepped care. *Harv Rev Psychiatry*. 2016;24(5):342–356.

13. Iliakis EA, Sonley AKI, Ilagan GS, Choi-Kain LW. Treatment of borderline personality disorder: is supply adequate to meet public health needs? *Psychiatric Services*. 2019;70(9):772–781.

14. Grant BF, Chou SP, Goldstein RB, et al. Prevalence, correlates, disability, and comorbidity of DSM-IV borderline personality disorder: results from the Wave 2 National Epidemiologic Survey on Alcohol and Related Conditions. *J Clin Psychiatry*. 2008;69(4):533–545.

15. Sansone RA, Kay J, Anderson JL. Resident didactic education in borderline personality disorder: is it sufficient? *Academic Psychiatry*. 2013;37(4):287–288.

16. Zimmerman M, Rothschild L, Chelminski I. The prevalence of DSM-IV personality disorders in psychiatric outpatients. *Am J Psychiatry*. 2005;162(10):1911–1918.

17. Ellison WD, Rosenstein LK, Morgan TA, Zimmerman M. Community and clinical epidemiology of borderline personality disorder. *Psychiatr Clin North Am*. 2018;41(4):561–573.

18. Ebell MH, Siwek J, Weiss BD, et al. Strength of recommendation taxonomy (SORT): a patient-centered approach to grading evidence in the medical literature. *J Am Board Fam Pract*. 2004;17(1):59–67.

19. DeCou CR, Comtois KA, Landes SJ. Dialectical behavior therapy is effective for the treatment of suicidal behavior: a meta-analysis. *Behav Ther*. 2019;50(1):60–72.

20. Keuroghlian AS, Palmer BA, Choi-Kain LW, Borba CP, Links PS, Gunderson JG. The effect of attending good psychiatric management (GPM) workshops on attitudes toward patients with borderline personality disorder. *J Pers Disord*. 2016;30(4):567–576.

21. Masland SR, Price D, MacDonald J, Finch E, Gunderson J, Choi-Kain L. Enduring effects of one-day training in good psychiatric management on clinician attitudes about borderline personality disorder. *J Nerv Ment Dis*. 2018;206(11):865–869.

22. Bateman A, Fonagy P. Randomized controlled trial of outpatient mentalization-based treatment versus structured clinical management for borderline personality disorder. *Am J Psychiatry*. 2009;166(12):1355–1364.

23. Choi-Kain LW, Finch EF, Masland SR, Jenkins JA, Unruh BT. What works in the treatment of borderline personality disorder. *Curr Behav Neurosci Rep*. 2017;4(1):21–30.

24. Choi-Kain, L, Gunderson JG, eds. *Applications of Good Psychiatric Management for Borderline Personality Disorder: A Practical Guide*. Washington, DC.: American Psychiatric Association; 2019.

25. Gunderson JG, Palmer BA. Inpatient psychiatric units. In: Choi-Kain, LW, Gunderson, JG, eds. *Applications of Good Psychiatric Management for Borderline Personality Disorder: A Practical Guide*. Washington, DC: American Psychiatric Association; 2019:11–36.

26. Hong, V. Emergency departments. In: Choi-Kain, LW, Gunderson, JG, eds. *Applications of Good Psychiatric Management for Borderline Personality Disorder: A Practical Guide*. Washington, DC: American Psychiatric Association; 2019:37–56.

27. Jenkins JA, Iliakis EA, Choi-Kain LW. Consultation-liaison service. In: Choi-Kain LW, Gunderson JG, eds. *Applications of Good Psychiatric Management for Borderline Personality Disorder: A Practical Guide.* Washington, DC: American Psychiatric Association; 2019:57–83.

28. Distel MA, Rebollo-Mesa I, Willemsen G, Derom CA, Trull TJ, Martin NG, et al. Familial resemblance of borderline personality disorder features: genetic or cultural transmission? *PLoS One. 2009;4*(4):e5334.

29. Donegan NH, Sanislow CA, Blumberg HP, et al. Amygdala hyperreactivity in borderline personality disorder: implications for emotional dysregulation. *Bio Psychiatry.* 2003;54(11):1284–1293.

30. Silbersweig D, Clarkin JF, Goldstein M, et al. Failure of frontolimbic inhibitory function in the context of negative emotion in borderline personality disorder. *Am J Psychiatry.* 2007;164(12):1832–1841.

31. Zanarini MC, Frankenburg FR, Hennen J, Silk KR. The longitudinal course of borderline psychopathology: 6-year prospective follow-up of the phenomenology of borderline personality disorder. *Am J Psychiatry.* 2003;160(2):274–283.

32. Zanarini MC, Frankenburg FR, Reich DB, Fitzmaurice G. Attainment and stability of sustained symptomatic remission and recovery among patients with borderline personality disorder and axis II comparison subjects: a 16-year prospective follow up study. *Am J Psychiatry.* 2012;169(5):476–483.

33. Gunderson JG, Lyons-Ruth K. BPD's interpersonal hypersensitivity phenotype: a gene-environment-developmental model. *J Pers Disord.* 2008;22(1):22–41.

34. Ng FYY, Townsend ML, Miller, CE, et al. The lived experience of recovery in borderline personality disorder: a qualitative study. *Bord Personal Disord Emot Dysregul.* 2019;6:10.

35. Fineberg SK, Gupta S, Leavitt J. Collaborative deprescribing in borderline personality disorder: a narrative review. *Harv Rev Psychiatry.* 2019;27(2):75–86.

14

Employing Psychodynamic Process-oriented Group Psychotherapy with Personality Disorders

Kenneth M. Pollock and Robert E. Feinstein

Key Points

- All individuals possess and/or manifest personality disorder–like traits that can be treated in groups irrespective of whether or not members have a diagnosable PD and/or are participating for various other distressing problems in their lives.
- Psychodynamic-oriented groups for patients with personality traits or disorders that focus on here-and-now processes possess unique properties that provide multiple opportunities for therapist interventions, exceeding those available in individual psychotherapy.
- Unique properties can maximally be utilized when the therapist actively promotes interactions between group members; review Table 14.1, p. 367.
- Process-oriented groups allow therapists with different orientations to utilize the unique properties of groups to see and therapeutically intervene in multiple and varied problematic interpersonal relationships. Case vignettes demonstrate the unique properties that are offered.
- All forms of group therapy share four core psychotherapeutic functions helpful to patients with PDs. Groups can (1) offer support, (2) reduce dysfunctional life-long patterns, (3) strengthen and encourage growing of the self, and (4) be used to repair and improve interpersonal relationships.
- There are three overarching transtheoretical strategies that guide therapist interventions: (1) awareness and consciousness raising; (2) promoting interactions between members; and (3) facilitating members' authentic expressions. These can be applied in all groups with patients who have PDs.
- Countertransference phenomena in groups are more complex than in individual therapy, offering both increased potential therapeutic opportunities and/or increased pitfalls.
- Totalistic countertransference can be experienced with an individual group member, subgroups, and the group-as-a-whole. It can be employed as an aid to diagnosis and, with the unique properties of group, to make *the implicit, explicit*

(i.e., to make the pre-conscious, conscious) and foster treatment of emotional, behavioral, and interpersonal issues. A countertransference self-assessment tool is presented in Table 14.2, p. 383.
- A Toolbox is presented in Box 14.1, p. 384. It contains specific statements and interventions that can be used as an aid to group interventions: (1) making the implicit, explicit; (2) promoting group interactions; and (3) encouraging self-reflection.
- Fifteen key conceptual and operational guidelines, both summarizing and reflecting the essential elements of the model as outline in the chapter are presented. They constitute a mini "How-To" handbook for conducting a group.

Introduction

Personality disorders (PDs) are a constellation of problematic character traits that endure in a pattern over time, existing in sufficient quantity and magnitude so as to impair and/or create significant dysfunction in one or more facets of an individual's life. Patients with dysfunctional personality traits or a PD typically suffer with dysregulated emotions, distorted thinking, maladaptive behaviors, and problematic interpersonal relationships. PD traits and the distress that accompanies them, as well as the maladaptive functioning that often motivates patients with PDs to enter group treatment. Ultimately, the diagnosis of a PD is a function of the number of traits, their degree or intensity, and the breadth of psychosocial impairment. Many people with PD traits who access psychotherapy are not formally diagnosed as having a PD. Kernberg suggested that "even mature, relatively healthy, and successfully analyzed individuals, without a PD, may present with regressive reactions in group. . . . [T]hese phenomena (traits) point to patients uniquely regressing in groups in contrast to what takes place in ordinary dyadic and triadic interactions"[1]

Most patients entering treatment have a "mixed personality disorder" or a combination of PD traits. The mixed diagnosis is given when a patient has the characteristic traits of several personality disorders but does not fully meet the criteria for any specific one.[2]

A Brief History of Personality Theory and Treatment

To understand group therapy in the treatment of personality traits and the PDs, it's useful to consider some of the theory and history of individual psychotherapy for the PDs. For more than a century, people have been treated in individual psychotherapy for psychological distress and for every mental-health diagnostic label that has existed. Regardless of the primary complaint, some patients have been given a formal PD diagnosis, while others have not. More often than not, the inclusion or exclusion of a diagnosis of PD versus trait descriptions has been based upon differences between clinicians working in different settings. Medical or psychiatric clinicians working in institutional settings will often diagnose a PD. Other clinicians, with a more psychosocial orientation, will refrain from giving a PD diagnosis in order to protect a patient from the stigma of this diagnosis, preferring to think about these patients as having particular character problems or personality traits.

Aside from the psychoses and bipolar disorders, many problems treated in psychotherapy were historically referred to as neuroses. By current perspectives, a large proportion of these neurotic individuals would now be considered as having PDs or a subset of traits comorbid with their primary problem. This nomenclature was due to the predominance of psychoanalytic thinking and the use of the term "neurosis." Historically therapists would employ the term "personality disorder" interchangeably with "neurosis," and/or discuss the existence of PDs as being a facet of neurosis or vice versa.[3–5] Writing in 1992, Tyrer summed up the ever-changing and complex world of the inextricable relationships between these terms when he entitled a journal article, "The Core Elements of Neurosis: Mixed Anxiety-depression (Cotheymia) and Personality Disorder."[4] Both behavioral and psychodynamic theoreticians did *not* focus heavily on the PDs as diagnoses warranting specialized treatment in diagnostically homogenous settings, until after the emergence of the *Diagnostic and Statistical Manual of Mental Disorders (DSM) III*,[6] and the behavioral work of Wolpe,[7–9] Beck,[10] Ellis,[11] and Linehan.[12]

Based on these authors, and an increasing demand for scientific evidence, several structured, manualized, evidence-based, individual psychotherapy approaches emerged. One of the earliest individual psychodynamic treatments for PDs was developed by Kernberg, which came to be known as transference-focused psychotherapy (TFP).[13] Some treatments for the PDs were behaviorally oriented, such as cognitive therapy (CT)[10] and dialectical behavior therapy (DBT).[12] Young,[14] and Fonagy and Bateman[15] attempted to eclectically integrate behavioral and psychodynamic thinking. All of these formalized treatment approaches were systematically studied for their efficacy in comparison to what critics conceived of as essentially non-evidence-based, "unscientific" psychoanalysis. See Chapters 5 and 6 for overviews of these primarily individual evidence-based therapies.

These therapies were originally focused on treating borderline personality disorders (BPDs). They have more recently been broadened and modified to treat patients with PDs as well as other diagnoses. Most have employed group therapy as adjunctive to individual treatment, with the exception of TFP that remains solely an individual treatment. Practitioners treating patient with PDs have seen the economic and clinical benefits of group therapy, during which patients could benefit from sharing, support, observation of others, and the recognition that others shared their plights. Review Yalom and Lescz for a discussion of the essentially supportive therapeutic factors associated with all groups.[16]

Overview of Group Therapy for Treating Personality Disorder

PDs have been treated in group therapy since early in the 20th century. Group therapists were not employing diagnoses in any specific way other than as character formulations congruent with various psychoanalytic schools.[16] Non-psychotic outpatients were almost always treated in groups heterogeneous as to diagnosis. There was initially no meaningful structured or programmatic focus on treatment of the PDs. Many patients were referred to groups using psychodynamic or existential-humanistic approaches associated with the work of Rogers[17] and Perls et al.[18] This remained the case until the emergence and dissemination of the specific individual evidence-based therapies for the PDs in the 1980s and 1990s.

Other group-therapist theoreticians were influenced by self-psychology[19] and the role of the leader as a model.[20,21] Additionally, there were two other significant theoretical and technical developments that had major effects on group therapy. In Great Britain, the post-Freudians conceptualized a group as a single organism and developed theories and interventions centering around the group unconscious, labeling their approach as "group analysis."[22,23] Kurt Lewin, a social psychologist at the Massachusetts Institute of

Technology, with his students, examined group processes and dynamics, emphasizing a focus upon the relationship between group members, the existence of subgroups, and the creation of a group culture.[24] Out of the collective work of these authors emerged a host of different process-oriented offerings, including sensitivity training, T-group, personal growth groups, and encounter groups.[25,26] Their proponents argued that these approaches were not psychotherapy; nevertheless they all did involve experiences that most observers would conclude are therapeutic. This is especially the case when one defines growth as a core element of group treatment.

In sum, the various early streams of group therapy were heterogenous to diagnosis, but treated patients seeking help for distress associated with either personality traits and/or the PDs. Some groups were member-centered, while others remained leader-centered, and employed group processes as useful in the treatment to various extents. All of the later structured, programmatic groups for PDs, such as DBT, were leader-centered, and originally diagnostically homogeneous, focusing on patients with BPD. Each member received specific attention in every group, and the therapist functioned as something like a "master of ceremonies."

A Model for Intervention in Groups with Patients Who Have a PD

The premise of this proposed intervention model is: "Groups that focus on here-and-now processes possess unique properties, which provide multiple opportunities for therapist interventions, exceeding those available in individual psychotherapy." Unique properties can be utilized maximally when the therapist actively promotes interactions between group members. This model has a psychodynamic orientation but also, in terms of interventions, fits with a wide range of theoretical and other technical approaches including those that are more cognitive or behavioral. It is broad-based and has an eclectic set of assumptions and premises about personality and group therapy. These unique properties distinguish group from individual therapy and offer new and different views of the patient, as well as a wide array of interventional opportunities not possible in individual treatment.

Unique Therapeutic Opportunities Offered by Group Therapy as Compared to Individual Treatment

Premises of the current model include:

1. *Psychotherapy groups have many unique properties which both encourage and allow for a limitless range and depth of therapeutic interventions that do not exist in individual therapy.* This is especially true for treatment of patients with PDs, as their deficits are pervasive and powerfully manifested in many interpersonal contexts. The impact of patients with PDs, on a group and on the therapist, will often be so great and challenging that many therapists suggest that having more than one patient with BPD or narcissistic personality disorder (NPD) in a group is a "bad idea." In a wry, humorous vein, it is not unusual to hear group therapists comment, "It takes a whole group to treat a patient with BPD." In this vein, the reader is urged to carefully review the section on countertransference. Table 14.1, p. 367 describes the unique properties of a group, the therapeutic opportunities it can provide, and some observations about group patients who have a PD.

Table 14.1. Unique Properties of Groups That Permit Interventions Unavailable in Individual Therapy

Unique Group Interventions	Typical Maladaptive Responses To Interventions*
1. Encourage Receiving Feedback Therapist can facilitate patients asking for and receiving candid feedback from multiple others.	Patients with NPD, ASPD, BPD, and AVPD might feel criticized or are rejection-sensitive; a patient with BPD or HPD might feel abandoned; a patient with PPD might feel suspicious of positive feedback.
2. Giving Feedback Guide/teach members how to give authentic, interpersonal, constructive feedback, not advice or intellectual opinions. Learning that giving useful feedback, even when difficult for others to absorb can be growth enhancing for the receiver, the giver, and the members who are watching.	Patients with PPD, NPD, and BPD will have difficulty offering genuine feedback and may be overly devaluing or critical; NPD and ASPD patients may give feedback so as to be admired or to exploit others.
3. Risk-taking Facilitate intra- and interpersonal risk-taking by helping members face and express feelings, thoughts, or behaviors that may be difficult to own, or to express to others-trying out new behaviors and ways of being a person. The aim is learning to *tolerate* the anxiety of risk taking, not to eliminate it.	All patient with PDs will need to take risks to get out of their comfort zones and learn how others actually see them. Those PD's with higher anxiety may experience emotional paralysis inhibiting therapeutic risk-taking.
4. Recognition of Repetitive Dysfunctional Patterns Help members reflect on how they unwittingly "author" their own dissatisfying outcomes. Assist them in becoming aware how maladaptive scripts, themes, beliefs, or life patterns are repetitive or disabling and how these enduring patterns are reenacted in the group in ways that closely replicate their real lives.	All patients with PD have masochistic or self-destructive traits and have repetitive styles and maladaptive behaviors that are largely responsible for their dysfunction.
5. Struggle to Make Real Connections with Others Support members in recognizing and experiencing the centrality and power of being able to establish an open and present connection with others, including caring and love-helping them to drop walls between self and the other.	Interpersonal relations are impaired in all patients with a PD. Patients with DPD, AVPD, and HPD rely too much on others for help; NPD and ASPD exploit or may devalue others and find it difficult to authentically connect; BPD, ASPD, and NPD have stormy interpersonal relations and struggle to make long-lasting connections.
6. Reducing the Need for "Other-Validation" Assist members in explicitly examining their fear of being judged negatively (as inadequate); to acknowledge how lifelong opinions of themselves have been determined by how others view them; stop allowing others to determine how one feels about oneself.	ASPD, NPD, BPD, and HPD require excessive validation and admiration to maintain self-esteem. AVPD, DPD, HPD, and OCPD look to others for validation to feel safe. PPD, SCPD, and AVPD are wary of accepting validation out of fear of criticism.
7. Decrease Interpersonal Distortions Help members examine and re-evaluate their emotional reactions to other group members, by considering who they represent in their past and outside lives.	*All* PDs have interpersonal distortions of self and others. SPD, SAD, and PPD may be paralyzed in expressing thoughts and feelings.

(continued)

Table 14.1. Continued

Unique Group Interventions	Typical Maladaptive Responses To Interventions*
8. Normalization Helping all members realize that many others experience similar problems, distress, needs, thoughts, feelings, and behaviors, and that they are not alone. Also, normalization can reduce a sense of shame.	"No man is an island"; health dependency is normal while denying this is problematic. Normalize that others are needed for love, play, and work.
9. Staying in Difficult Conversations Through support of the group therapist and group members, learning to tolerate, not eliminate, anxiety and fear of anger from and toward others; how to in present in the room while maintaining a clear sense of self during difficult or painful discussions including how to negotiate and resolve conflict.	Patients with a PD avoid or cannot authentically stay in difficult, especially painful or angry conversations. This issue is commonly with patients who have AVPD, DPD, and OCPD. Those with NPD and ASPD struggle with anger from others; those with PPD, SCPD, SPD, and AVPD tend to withdraw.
10. Become a Witness With help of therapist and group, increases one's ability to listen, share and empathize, to witness and feel pain and powerlessness of others without being able to alleviate the person's suffering. This includes being able to learn how to accept, rather than anxiously brush off the the witnessing by others of oneself.	The psychological presence required for witnessing and empathy are particularly impaired for NPD, ASPD, and PPD. This is not as big a problem for those with HPD and BPD, OCPD, DPD, and AVPD.

*In the broadest sense, maladaptive reactions to appropriate interventions, require especially thoughtful therapist follow-through, in essence, the therapist may choose to persevere to obtain an adapative reaction rather than accept "defeat". This can range from noting and postponing a push at the moment, through to soliciting and involving other members reactions to the maladaptive reaction.

PD = personality disorder; SPD = schizotypal PD; SCPD = schizoid PD; PPD = paranoid PD; NPD = narcissistic PD; HPD = histrionic PD; ASPD = antisocial PD; DPD = dependent PD; OCPD = obsessive compulsive PD; AVPD = avoidant PD.

2. *Group therapy is a microcosm of life outside of the group.* Patients in a group will think, behave, and feel similarly to how they interact in "real life" (e.g., in the kitchen, at play, in the living room, in the bedroom, the office, or in an athletic setting). This also happens in individual therapy, but it may take more time for patients to reveal the wide range of their real selves interacting with others. At the same time, the individual therapist, by definition (being just one person), is precluded from providing the evocative stimuli to many group members who are of different ages, genders, cultures, and personalities.

3. *Groups that focus on here-and-now processes are analogous to current dysfunctional "real life" group experiences.* How patients act in group therapy is often an in vivo recapitulation of problematic relationships and interactions that exist in the multitudes of groups settings within patients' lives, (e.g., replicating their interactions in families, friendships, work, and leisure groups). In group therapy, with the support of members and therapist, patients can struggle to heal their dysfunctional interpersonal relationships. Groups also bring to the fore the norms, prohibitions, rivalries, implicit contracts, and mythologies from the outside world that can simultaneously be encountered therapeutically in the circle.

4. *There are four parallel and potentially psychotherapeutic processes available to members of groups. These are:* (1) support; (2) strengthening and growing of the self; (3) reducing dysfunctional patterns; and (4) repairing and improving interpersonal relationships.

5. *Groups provide a supportive arena for patients with a PD to engage in self-understanding and exploration of how they can become emotionally dysregulated and fall prey to maladaptive coping styles and behaviors.* Groups engender regression in individual members by stimulating powerful emotional reactions, thoughts, and behaviors, triggering each individual's historic intra- and interpersonal problems.

6. *Emotionally healthy people (not just those with PDs) will inevitably manifest maladaptive personality traits and behaviors that are often revealed and can be modified in group.*

7. *Groups that are member-centered (as contrasted with therapist-centered) can be facilitated to function in an increasingly autonomous way that promotes a therapeutic focus on relationships, especially around problems such as dependency, attachment, and differentiation.* There is a dramatic difference between "individual psychotherapy in a circle" in which the therapist functions as a master of ceremonies (working with each patient individually), as contrasted with group therapy where the leader and group members respond to interpersonal processes as they occur. In such a process-oriented group, members (with the facilitative assistance of the therapist) contribute significantly to much of the direction, structure, and learning that can occur.[22,23]

8. *Groups function at both an implicit and explicit level.* Thoughts, feelings, and thematic content range along a continuum from the conscious, to slightly beneath the surface, (preconscious), to the more deeply unconscious, including the "unthought known."[27] These phenomena can occur at all different levels and may be experienced by an individual, by one or more subgroups, or by the group-as-a-whole.

9. *Groups allow therapists with different orientations to utilize their unique properties to see and then therapeutically intervene in multiple and varied problematic, interpersonal relationships.* For example, a behaviorist might focus on an aggressive behavior exhibited in an interpersonal relationship with a specific group member, and ask the aggressor member if he/she wants feedback. Alternatively, the members might provide unsolicited feedback (depending upon the specific therapist intervention). A psychodynamic therapist, in response to the same aggression, might ask a group patient to describe what they imagine another group member is feeling or experiencing, and follow this up by asking that group member what they are actually experiencing. In either case, something psychotherapeutic can occur. Similarly, all of the four core psychotherapeutic functions can be applied in groups, each being compatible with diverse theoretical approaches (see Common Group Psychotherapy Goals for Patients with PDs).

Common Group Psychotherapy Goals for Patients with PDs

All forms of group therapy share four core psychotherapeutic functions helpful to patients with PDs. Groups can (1) offer support, (2) help reduce dysfunctional patterns, (3) strengthen and encourage growing of the self, and (4) repair and improve interpersonal relationships.

Support

Groups with patients who have PDs offer multiple opportunities for sharing, comforting, witnessing, and reducing the isolation of being alone with one's problems. They offer opportunities for a patient to obtain support from others while modeling new, adaptive behaviors observed in other members (and in the therapist). There are dimensions of support that groups can offer that individual treatment cannot, including member-to-member support, leader-to-member support, and group-to-member support. The member-to-group support experiences are particularly important for patients with PDs who have experienced exclusion from multiple groups all their lives and who need to learn how to join and function in groups for work and other important life activities.

Reducing Dysfunctional Patterns

Dysfunctional, unregulated emotions, negative thoughts, maladaptive behaviors, and disturbing interpersonal relations experienced toward the self and others are endemic to patients who have PDs. Patients with BPD experience emotional dysregulation and hypersensitivity to rejection. Those with narcissistic personality disorders (NPDs) may reveal their entitlement and feel wounded even when constructive criticism is offered. Patients with schizoid personality disorder (SPD) and paranoid personality disorder (PPD) may display maladaptive responses of vigilance and anxious withdrawal. Patients with dependent personality disorder (DPD) may reveal their excessive dependence on group members, constant nonverbal requests for being taken care of, and a long-standing fear of making independent decisions. Those with antisocial personality disorder (ASPD) may reveal their dishonesty and be confronted with honestly facing themselves, including their disregard and inability to empathize with others. In these ways, here-and-now groups, by their very essence, make dysfunctional patterns of life palpable and open to examination. With recognition and confrontations of these difficulties in a group setting, opportunities for support, learning, and modeling from other group members, many patterns associated with the PDs can be modified toward healthier and more adaptive responses.

Strengthen and Grow the Self

A stronger sense of self or agency rests upon increased differentiation from others. This is the experience of being able to "own" oneself, to act with purpose and to be effective in life, while permitting oneself to "march to one's own drummer." Being oneself is frequently a challenge for those with PDs; they typically have deficits in over- or under-reliance on themselves and others. They transcendently feel that they are just "not OK," and attribute the experiences of being different as a general explanation of their emotional dysregulation and failures in building happier lives. The aim of all PD groups, whether explicit or not, is to strengthen each member's sense of a healthy self, with agency and efficacy, to be able to experience an increase in personal causation.[28]

Ultimately, a highly differentiated self reflects the ability to be more self-validating rather than needing to be other-validated. A mature and optimally functioning individual who has reached a higher level of differentiation manifests, internally and externally, the capacity to both see and balance two major wishes: (1) the wish for closeness, intimacy, healthy dependency; and (2) the wish to be one's own person, live as one wants, while not being overly influenced by the views of others.[29] Paradoxically, the capacity to be differentiated is a necessary condition for closeness and intimacy. Without it, the intricate and sometimes entangled connection between two people become either parasitically symbiotic or estranged and difficult. This idea is expressed by David Schnarch when he writes "differentiation manifests as an individual characteristic in four distinct ways: 1) being able to maintain a clear sense of self while being close (physically and emotionally), to significant others; 2) regulating one's own anxieties; 3) not being overly reactive to other's anxieties; and 4), a willingness to tolerate discomfort which enables growth."[29] Learning to tolerate rather than unrealistically try to eliminate anxiety is among the unique properties listed in Table 14.1, p. 367.

Group therapy processes reveal that most patients with PDs have some impairment related to differentiating themselves from others. These issues can be addressed in the open and explicit forum of the group circle, engaging the work of understanding while simultaneously taking incremental risks, in the here-and-now, in order to be more self-validating and accepting of healthy dependency on others. The multi-transferential nature of group therapy renders this a major advantage of group in comparison to individual psychotherapy.

Repair and Improve Interpersonal Relations

For a personality-disordered individual, groups that focus on here-and-now processes provide an arena in which, under the skillful eye of the therapist and with the help of other group members, the patient can openly struggle to repair damaged interpersonal relationships and/or develop their capacity for new and healthier relationships. The group itself is a safe emotional container that "holds"[30] the person while they are struggling to express painful, difficult, frequently anxiety-laden experiences and conflicts.

Repairing relationships may simultaneously involve difficult but valuable intra- and interpersonal explorations of disturbing communication, feelings, or behaviors. This fosters the patient's ability to deal effectively and respond helpfully to anger from others, developing the capacity and ability to offer a genuine apology, and a willingness to risk a confrontation while offering the ongoing potential for a future relationship.

Learning how to develop new and better interpersonal relationships involves paying attention to another, being empathic, and generally being both self-validating and non-judgmentally available to others. It means clearly communicating wishes, requests, hopes, and expectations, and having the capacity to negotiate differences, manage conflicts, and to express gratitude.[31] *Groups for PDs are an ideal forum for practicing repair of problematic relationships and for developing new meaningful ones. In effect, groups are a safe laboratory for experimenting with new ways of being, making mistakes, learning, and trying again.* In large measure, this is because the emotional stakes in the group are lower than in real life

Basic Interventional Strategies for Group Therapists

There are three overarching transtheoretical strategies that guide therapist interventions: (1) awareness and consciousness raising; (2) promoting interactions between members;

and (3) facilitating members' authentic expressions. These can be applied in all groups with patients who have PDs.

Awareness and Consciousness Raising

Intervening to increase awareness of self and others is part of consciousness raising. Awareness begins with the attempt to make honest observations of one's own emotions, thoughts, and behaviors that are dysfunctional or unhealthy, as well as being able to accurately see these aspects in others. This is, of course, the challenge both for the patient and the therapist who is assisting in facilitating the struggle. Awareness can be explicit (that which is readily observable by all) or be implicit (that which is dimly perceived, preconscious, under the surface, or unconscious). Change requires making explicit much of that which is implicit!

Consciousness raising[32] in group therapy mostly occurs through the therapist's facilitating personal, face-to-face interactions that can engender increased appreciation, awareness, and understanding of other people's emotions and experiences. Additionally, it is frequently accomplished through interpretative comments offered by the therapist that make the implicit, explicit. Group participants can and do begin to develop an awareness of psychological processes that will be observed and experienced by individuals and the entire group, as well as the therapist (see Table 14.1, p. 367). Group members may also become aware of subgroups based on sociocultural divisions, sex, age, gender, sexual preference, or education.

It is awareness, along all of these dimensions, that ultimately sets the agenda for what groups discuss and constructively struggle with in the service of attaining support, repair, and growth.

Promote Interaction Between Members

Groups for patients with PDs are particularly useful for promoting interactions between members, especially those focused on here-and-now reactions to one another. These interpersonal interactions reflect upon, and bring to the fore, a broad range of dysfunctional and unhealthy interpersonal interactions that are also operative in the outside world. In this way, groups recapitulate psychopathological dysfunctions in interpersonal relatedness. These are both observable and amenable to change in the safety of the circle. They can provide new targets and models for interpersonal relationships, which the patient can then translate into their life outside the circle.

Facilitate Members' Authentic Expressions

For groups to work and have maximal impact, it is important that patients strive and struggle to be authentic. Inauthenticity is often the handmaiden of other-validation, essentially reflecting low levels of differentiation from others and usually low core self-esteem. Hence, trying hard to be authentic in the circle is both the work of the group member and, at the same time, a mark of therapeutic gain. The will to struggle is itself a victory.

A differentiated position requires being minimally reactive to the other's anxiety, emotional self-regulation, and a willingness to be vulnerable; to take constructive risks; and to receive feedback (see Table 14.1, p. 367). This clearly implies that one of the primary functions of the therapist is to encourage patients with PDs to authentically express feelings, thoughts, and behaviors about themselves and others in the group. This needs to be the case especially when there is fear of judgment and rejection by others. Risk-taking means that the member needs to struggle to find his/her courage: to risk negative reactions from others. Facing and challenging the fear of being genuine fosters healing and authentic relationships. Countless patients report that being able to take interpersonal risks followed by a dialogue with group members left them feeling exhilarated, as though they had reached the summit of a steep mountain. The feedback and learning in the group that occurs in this emotional crucible is central to increased adaptation and higher levels of functioning in one's daily life.[33,34] In general, patients in the group are frequently willing to be open that they are afraid of "people's" reactions (other-validation at work)! It is often useful for the therapist to ask patients, along with others who might identify with them, to try to verbalize what effect the fear, if it comes true, will have upon them. This exploration, because of group supportiveness, can be freeing to the patient.

Therapist Boundaries of Expression: The Impact upon Who Can Say What to Whom

It is likely that the majority of experienced and well-trained psychotherapists, regardless of professional discipline and theoretical orientation, would strongly concur that there are constraints and limitations on what therapists can say, what is said unfiltered or spoken bluntly and directly to patients. While there are specific and explicit professional prohibitions on use of some language and behaviors for therapists, there is significantly greater latitude for group members to be openly emotional and to directly express their unfiltered wishes and feelings that therapists are constrained from expressing. In fact, group members can and should be proactively encouraged by the therapist to say whatever is on their mind. Specifically, and at the very center of the current approach, it is proposed that the therapist should employ the opportunities delineated and implied in Table 14.1, p. 367. These provide an agenda for genuine therapeutic interactions. What emerges as a result of employing the unique properties of a group are a host of thoughts, feelings, wishes, and maladaptive attitudes generally not acceptable for therapists to express (and unequivocally acceptable for other group members to express) and in themselves, are useful for patients to hear. They constitute much of the essential grist of the therapeutic interactions between group members.

For example, two group members may have open, angry conflicts with name-calling, and reflecting both patient's real experiences, actual behaviors, and problems in the outside world. If managed thoughtfully (though clarification, interpretation, mentalization, etc., by the therapist), these kinds of experiences can break through patients' resistance to seeing the maladaptive aspects of themselves and may serve to highlight specific triggers that characteristically lead to interpersonal dysfunction. Group analysis and feedback on these kinds of enactments can enable patients to see part of themselves (previously avoided) more clearly and reveal—in the power of the moment—the distorted, maladaptive ways that they relate to others. These situations also offer real *in vivo* opportunities to practice (remember, groups are analogous laboratories paralleling real life), repairing a relationship in group, as a model for repairing a conflicted, difficult relationship outside the group.

The Challenges and Therapeutic Opportunities of Employing Unique Properties of Groups

A group therapist needs to be able to recognize personality-disordered emotional dysregulation, distorted thoughts, destructive behavior, and maladaptive personal styles brought into the group, as well as be able to recognize the patients' reports about these problems in their lives outside the group. Therapists need to recognize and learn how to utilize the unique properties of groups to help them manage and treat specific maladaptive traits and/or specific PDs. A few clinical examples are provided to help clarify how these unique properties may be employed. The unique properties utilized in these vignettes are from Table 14.1, p. 367 and indicated in the text by quotation marks.

Case I. Avoidant Traits with Severe Social Anxiety

A stay-at-home father and sculptor is afraid to approach art galleries to sell his work. In group therapy, he is very quiet. When pursued by the group members to talk about himself, he will say that he is afraid of rejection and being judged critically (his fear of "risk-taking"). He also describes himself as a major procrastinator. These are patterns in his life that are repeated in group therapy. He is described by others as a "quiet" member. In considering the therapeutic opportunities, the therapist may encourage the patient to take risks and go outside his comfort zone by taking incrementally small steps that involve expression of his feelings toward others in the group. He may also need to identify his negative beliefs about himself and the origins of these feelings.

The therapist might consider asking the patient to try expressing or doing something at home or in the group that involves "risk-taking" but is only a "little scary." The patient might, openly in the group, accept the therapist's suggestions (when he actually agrees it would be a good idea) to take a small risk. When asked, "Can you take a small risk to see if you will be rejected or criticized in group or take a similar risk at home?" he says yes. In the next group session, when asked if he has taken any small risks, the patient reports "no," he has avoided this. His answer to "why not?" (by a member) is that he could not find an "opening."

At this point, the therapist might ask other members in the group circle if they have had fears similar to the patient, including similar fears "in this group." This is an attempt to employ "normalization." Almost always, one or more members will talk about similar fears and what has happened to them. At the same time, one or more members will talk to the patient in an empathic, supportive way, identifying how they feel badly for him (e.g., that they understand how he feels ("witnessing"). The therapist can then ask the avoidant patient his reaction to the other group member who "witnessed" him. This patient then took the risk of showing himself as he became emotional, tearful, and expressed gratitude for the support. The therapist asks him if he felt shame or worried that group members were judging him. The patient responded, "yes." The therapist suggested to the patient that he might say "out loud" who in the group he felt was the least judgmental toward him (using "risk-taking," "making connections," and "accepting being witnessed"). The therapist also asked him to "give feedback" to another member by openly acknowledging who he felt safe with. To go further, the therapist asked the member who had just been named as "safest" to share how she felt about being identified in this way (practicing "making connections and risk-taking"). Finally, the therapist asked the entire group if "anyone felt jealous" when the "safe" member was picked by the socially anxious member (struggling to "make connections" and hopefully "decrease interpersonal distortions").

Case II. Narcissistic Traits: Considering Narcissistic Personality Disorder

Phil is an attorney in private practice whose wife left him for another woman. A middle-aged male, he frequently expresses a brief identification with another member's travails in her marriage or in her life, in general. On many occasions, he appears for a moment to express empathy, then it is quickly followed by a segue into a lengthy soliloquy about his own troubled marriage and his non-responsive, angry wife. He frequently proceeds to repetitively describe how she treats him, with little change in the story each time he retells it. He also complains endlessly, saying at the beginning of many group sessions that he has felt consistently "dropped" by the group. After weeks of repeating the same pattern of professing concern for another, then changing the topic to himself (e.g., what the authors call "narcissistic oxygen robbery"), a number of members appeared to be annoyed, disengaged, or not listening. This was often expressed by group members via nonverbal facial cues and restless movements indicating boredom.

Seeking to help Phil "receive feedback," the therapist says, "A number of people look distracted or annoyed while Phil is speaking. Phil, would you like to know how people are feeling about you: the way you are being perceived by the group?" He says, "Yes." The therapist asks him to choose a member he wants to obtain feedback from. The therapist is asking him if he wants to "receive feedback," while also promoting his "struggling to make real connections with others." Phil is also being offering an additional choice; giving him the power to select who he wants to hear from. His choice opens an opportunity for another member to "give him feedback." The therapist is hoping/expecting Phil will get honest feedback. This situation will also likely provide the therapist an opportunity to intervene by helping him to "recognize his repetitive patterns." Phil is also asked if he will "receive [in this case] negative feedback." The therapist may also ask Phil to ask the other group members if they also feel emotional pain when receiving negative feedback. The therapist is "normalizing" Phil's fear. This also involves the person he asked to "give feedback" and to "take a risk," and practice "giving negative constructive feedback."

Subsequently, the rest of the group can be asked to share what they felt about him, again, asking group members to "give feedback" to Phil. Other group members (not the therapist) ask Phil if he wants to "receive [their] feedback" in addition to the first person who gave him feedback. He again says, "Yes." Other members then collectively "take a risk" and "give feedback" to Phil; to wit, that they had trouble listening to him but had been afraid to tell him; Phil additionally is seeking honest feedback from others. Some group members then tell Phil that they had been experiencing him as behaving both narcissistically and manipulative in order to get attention. One other member wondered aloud if he had a "repetitive pattern" of manipulatively attention-seeking with his wife, speculating that this could have been a real "turn-off" to her (as it was to most group members).

Other patients with NPDs might have reacted differently than Phil with a range of different coping styles or defenses. They might withdraw, become angry, wounded, or project their anger onto others. A patient with NPD may feel angry and cheated by the group no matter how hard he tries to feel differently, with little ability to sensitively recognize how he is affecting others and the group processes. Someone with a severe NPD may be furious, hostile, and savagely attacking of others. This response would be on the severe end of the NPD continuum. On the healthier side (of the NPD continuum), Phil thoughtfully "received feedback," albeit with some embarrassment, shame, and pain. He attempted to understand what he was doing, its origins, and the place seeking-attention has had in his life. He responded in a useful way, acknowledging his need to be center stage. Within a matter of weeks, he demonstrated significant growth and a wish to repair any damage he had done to his relationships in the group.

Case III. Paranoid Personality Disorder, Mixed with Schizoid Traits and Post-traumatic

Stress Disorder (PTSD-Paranoid PD)

John, a 64-year-old carpenter, had a history of military combat trauma. He was married for 40 years and came to group following his wife's demands for a separation and his fear of losing her. He is unequivocal about how he sees life saying, "Trust No One." He also says, "If I lose my vigilance and caution with other people, I will lose my life." He is neither delusional nor psychotic. He asked the therapist to help him be with others, and learn how to treat them in new and healthier ways. His style is polite. He is well spoken and communicates in a totally functional and logical manner, avoiding expressing or showing his emotions as he refuses or is unable to appear vulnerable. By John's report, the only exception, when he does trust people, is small children who are "innocent" and do not have "questionable motivations." "Once kids get older," he says, "they lose their innocence and are no longer trustworthy." He currently mistrusts his own adult children.

John joined the group because it was recommended by a psychiatrist at the VA as a way to help him learn to trust others. He grudgingly recognizes he must do this in order to win back and pacify his wife, whom he also does not trust emotionally. During his first few group sessions, John remained silent. Finally, after several meetings, and in response to member inquiries, he said he joined because his wife gave him an ultimatum. He reported that she wanted a separation unless he changed and got help. He told the group that he trusts "no one." The therapist suggested to the group that they would need to understand that John was "reluctant to be vulnerable." The therapist asked the entire group, "Could you accept John's wariness and cautious nature and his initial mistrust of all of us here while he is working on things?" Note that this intervention was an attempt by the therapist to ask other group members to both "witness" his difficulty and "connect to the patient." This was also an effort to reduce John's sense of being abnormal ("normalization" and "struggling to connect," and simultaneously lowering his need for "other-validation"). This indirect and carefully considered intervention represents the therapist's effort to employ group processes rather than directly focusing on this patient with a PPD. This involves the entire group becoming part of his treatment by talking about themselves in a way that might ultimately make group a safe place for John to struggle constructively with his goals. This approach also opens up a path to all group members to work on differentiation and reduce their needs for "other-validation," while helping John "decrease his interpersonal distortions," and all group members practice "staying in a difficult conversation."

In response to this intervention, several group members spontaneously said they had felt similarly in the past ("normalization") and sometimes still felt that way; others expressed empathy for John; while still others said that they still experienced being mistrustful. Many agreed ("normalization") that mistrust was related to fears of being judged by others. Several emphasized that the judgments of others (seeking "other-validation") was extremely important to them. The therapist asked, "Do people in here feel they put too much importance on what other members feel about them?" Everyone in the circle raised their hands and laughed. The therapist interventions were aimed at having group members talk openly and be vulnerable ("risk-taking"). The group was also being encouraged to work indirectly with John by becoming a "witness" to his mistrust, as other members shared ("normalize") their similar mistrust issues and their need for "other-validation" versus self-validation. This intervention helped John listen to others, who were clearly respecting his vigilance, while avoiding, at this early stage in group, making him feel vulnerable by pushing him to talk. Because John was not being challenged to be open, he was able to "witness" discussions about trust and open expressions of vulnerability in a supportive environment. These interactions, during which John observes (perhaps even empathetically witnesses other members struggling with his problem) likely constitutes "therapy by proxy."

At the conclusion of this particular interaction, the therapist commented that the need for "other-validation" was a "repetitive pattern" in many people's lives, often interfering with their ability to be authentic and just say what they feel or want. The therapist added that a "repetition of dysfunctional patterns" such as powerful dependence on being "other-validated" unwittingly prevents the "other from knowing you" well enough to meet "your" needs. Indirectly, the entire interventional pattern employed by the therapist was aimed at helping John eventually trust the group. Ultimately, the intent of these interventions were to help John trust *himself* enough to "struggle to connect" to the group. In a subsequent private individual session, John reported that he "really enjoyed" the group and that he found it "interesting." He also began to gradually open up about his feelings and personal history. He and other group members became explicitly clear that their safety with others was a function of each person's differentiation and its inextricable linkage to core self-esteem.

Case IV: Borderline PD and PTSD

Following six months of incremental progress in group, Kate, a nurse whose mother had physically abused her, was increasingly able to connect to others, engage in dialogue, and express empathy. However, for unclear reasons, Kate went through a period of quiet withdrawal, regressing to what had been her original way-of-being in group and in her life. She began missing groups, ostensibly because she had to work evenings. Notably, two other members had recently left group and two new members joined. After a few weeks, when she returned, the therapist commented, "I wonder what is going on in the group that has led Kate to withdraw and stay quiet." The therapist's intervention was not just made to her individually but was offered to her and the rest of the group, as though they were two interacting subgroups. The intervention could have been made solely to Kate, asking about her withdrawal. Instead, the therapist chose to treat it as a group issue, with the idea that her withdrawal reflected both an individual as well as group problem. A few members spoke up, "struggling to make a connection" and "taking a risk" by expressing their concern, and the effects on them personally, of her withdrawal and silence. If the therapist had simply asked the patient why she had withdrawn, it is likely that she would have become the "patient" of the therapist and the rest of the group. Kate said that she had "trouble" with the loss of the old members, and also accepting the new members; she was "uncomfortable" and did not know if she wanted to attend anymore. The conversation, although started by the therapist, was carried by the members who "struggled to make a connections" with her. The therapist was fostering "giving and receiving feedback" as a way to "make connections." Rather than speaking up weeks ago, Kate had simply gone mute and absent. The members said they wished she had spoken sooner. Some identified with her; others said they were hurt by her, saying "we are not good enough for you ourselves . . . so you want to leave?" Kate went quiet, left group early and did not return for weeks.

When she finally returned, she said she was "angry" and that she walked out because the group was "punishing" her for open expression of her not wanting new members. A long dialogue followed during which people told Kate that she was cared about and that they wanted her to stay. They also said Kate "missed" and had difficulty recognizing and accepting how much others genuinely cared about her. She struggled to listen to this ("making connections," "risk-taking," "giving feedback"). The following week, she said that she had "reconsidered everything" and realized that she doesn't see love when it is coming in her direction. She reported that she felt rejected after a member she liked had left the group, and felt guarded with the new members. She said it had been difficult for her to speak up a few weeks past, and then "the group became angry with me. It was the same thing that happened when I told my mother how I felt. She beat me. I was punished by the group for saying what I felt. That's why I walked out and didn't come back until now. I could not tolerate the anger" ("staying in difficult conversations" and "recognizing [her] repetitive patterns").

Case V: Antisocial Personality Disorder (ASPD) with Narcissistic Features

Zack, a stockbroker, came into group feeling that others, especially at work and in the world in general, were mistreating him. Under a thinly veiled disguise of raising legitimate issues, he frequently complained about the behavior of other group members; "You talk too much, are boring, and should stop complaining." Often highly articulate and with anger just below the surface, he would raise one problem after another, often about the group or with its leader. It was evident that he was camouflaging his own internal difficulties. He frequently attacked and undermined the therapist while narcissistically "robbing the group of its oxygen." He would persistently take over the group conversation and process. He never revealed or expressed his own vulnerability, although he frequently complained of being mistreated by group members and others in his life. He was intellectually facile.

On the first occasion when he "highjacked" the group, he raised the question about "unreasonable boundary setting by the therapist." On the face of it, this was an appropriate expression. However, over the course of months, he increasingly brought up other controversial topics about the therapist and/or two other group members. He suggested that they were homophobic, that they were in a subgroup who did not "like him." Additionally, he offered a host of other seemingly legitimate complaints. When members asked him about whether he felt hurt or angry, or raised a question about what he "really" needed from others and from the group, he conveyed negligible feelings without showing any hint of vulnerability. When others told him they were hurt by his behaviors and attitude, he would attack them and turn things around. He felt the group was emotionally unavailable and acting unreasonably. At the same time, he was unavailable and apparently unreachable, while clearly desperate for the attentions of the therapist and other members. He was ultimately unable to experience anyone's attempt at "making a real connection" despite many members' sincere attempt to be a "witness" to his obvious but camouflaged pain.

Zack was clearly displaying an ASPD that the therapist and group experienced as a mix of cruelty, sadism, playing the victim, little caring, and exploitation of others, while all the time superficially demonstrating a polite manner. The therapist had strong negative countertransference reactions for many weeks, including internal anger, helplessness, and self-doubt. On multiple occasions, the therapist and group members tried to respond by "giving feedback" and by "reinforcing a desire to be connected," in the hope this would decrease his "interpersonal distortions." This was rarely, if ever, effective. Feeling and showing significant emotional openness and empathy, the therapist attempted, without success, to acknowledge this patient's emptiness and suffering. He suggested that the patient must have suffered unbearable torment and pain when he was a child. These attempts did not appear to scratch the surface of this deeply impaired man. Patients with this antisocial style repeatedly demonstrate that they do not do well in groups, can prevent the work of others, and may not be treatable in any setting. Patients with ASPD probably need to be excluded from entering a group. If they manage to join because they are able to literally con others, and are later discovered to have ASPD, they may need to leave the group.

Recognizing and Addressing Countertransference in Groups: Opportunities and Pitfalls

Group therapy, especially groups that deal with the here-and-now processes, by their very nature present a number of countertransference-inducing stimuli that differ from and are more complex than those that occur in individual therapy. They also offer a multiplicity of additional therapeutic opportunities.

Freud described countertransference as the analyst's own reactions to the patient, based on the therapist's problematic life. He considered countertransference a weakness in the therapist, to be eliminated by self-analysis or mental-health treatment.[35] This has been described as "classic countertransference." Winnicott[36] took this concept a step further when he described "objective countertransference," the therapist's real (appropriate), non-neurotic reactions to a patient. In 1965, Kernberg summarized and extended these definitions of countertransference.[37] He described Freud's "classic countertransference" as the therapist's unhelpful, unconscious reaction to the patient, based on the therapist's transference to the patient, which becomes an impediment to the treatment. He then also coined the term "totalistic countertransference" to include Winnicott's "objective" emotional reactions experienced by the analyst and other unconsciously experienced countertransference transmitted by the patient.[37] Kernberg also described how countertransference reactions, felt by a therapist, can be generated by the patient and transmitted to the therapist via the patient's use of projection and projective identification.

Classic Countertransference in Group Therapy

In a group setting, "classic countertransference" can also be seen as interfering with a therapist's ability to be an effective group therapist. For example, a therapist may react to his therapy group with distorted and similar reactions coming from past experience with the therapist's own family group or based on early life traumatic experiences with other groups (e.g., in school or on a team). Recall one of the current intervention model's premises: "People, including both patients and therapists, are the same in every room." Therapists always need to be mindful and attend to how their past group (e.g., family of origin) experiences can interfere with their functioning effectively in a current group. For example, a group therapist observed an intense interpersonal struggle between two angry and defensive women members. They were arguing about who was guilty of the first insult. The therapist noted his uncharacteristic difficulty in finding a useful way to intervene, ostensibly because of the intensity and rapidity of their escalating fight. He felt a sense of powerlessness and anxiety about his ability to therapeutically intervene in this conflict. He was, at that moment, able to recall his past unsuccessful attempts to mediate arguments between his mother and older sister. He remembered feeling that mediation was his family "job." He recalled feeling helpless and anxious about not resolving their conflicts. The results of his sacrificing himself by trying to intervene were that he was "always a failure," because both his mother and sister became angry and blamed him whenever he tried to help. In this current group situation, his fears of intervening, emanating from his past, were a "classic countertransference" that could easily lead him to fail at successfully helping these two angry women group members.

In addition, group therapists may sometime experience classic countertransference (impatient annoyance toward the entire group) when the group is (in the therapist's mind, based on the therapist's past experiences) avoiding talking about something the therapist thinks is important. Conversely, group therapists may feel prideful or even grandiose about their ability to induce their groups to engage in intense, meaningful, and interconnected interaction as a result of their "brilliant" interventions. As with individual therapists, group therapists need to recognize, reflect, and resolve any classic group countertransference, seek group supervision, or seek their own psychotherapy to get help.

Totalistic Group Countertransference

A group therapist may also have "totalistic countertransference reactions," both positive and negative, to multiple members of the group, often at times to a subgroup, and frequently to the entire group. This can be even more complex, as a therapist will frequently need to deal simultaneously with totalistic countertransference feelings coming from an individual group member, a subgroup, and/or from the group-as-a-whole. Group members can also induce *countertransference-by-proxy,* during which the therapist experiences the reaction(s) (through observation and identification) with others in the group who are interacting. For example, one group member might be harshly criticizing another group member, while the observing therapist might identify with one side/one member or identify with the other side/other member—or with both—during their interactions. The group therapist may feel angry at the member doing the criticizing, who is also acting sadistically, while simultaneously experiencing a wish to take care of the other member(s) who is being attacked. The therapist's challenge is, at one and the same time, to be useful to each person in the transaction, to help them understand their conflict, while simultaneously being aware of the way the rest of the group experiences the conflict and its meaning and to be able to intervene therapeutically on all of these levels! The challenge to the therapist is to avoid countertransference-determined interventions and be able to make explicit the implicit, at the individual, dyad, and group levels. A tall task, but circumstances such as these often offer the richest therapeutic opportunities. One therapist, in sharing her reaction to such a circumstance, intervened by saying, "How are we all going to handle what is happening right now between Jane and Andrew? My question, includes Jane and Andrew?" (making the implicit explicit by asking members to figure it out).

Complex Countertransference

Consider another common circumstance, in which a subgroup is interacting with another subgroup, while one member, Jennifer, is sitting quietly, eyes glazed, looking out the window. When Jennifer is asked by a group member what she is feeling, she says, "I feel excluded and invisible." Jennifer may be experiencing feelings from her own past that are consistent with her long-standing core belief that she is always excluded. The therapist may be identifying with Jennifer's feeling excluded while also considering her reaction (positive, negative, or mixed) to each of the subgroups. The therapist may additionally have a third countertransference reaction to other members of the subgroups, who also feel excluded. The therapist will have to decide where to intervene (Jennifer, versus the subgroup, versus other group members) and then follow up with the others.

Therapist have affective responses to maladaptive reactions from members which were described previously in column II of Table 14.1, p. 367. The therapist needs to pay particular attention to his/her own reactions as many of these counter-transference reactions may include therapist anger, feelings of helplessness, and/or inadequacy. It is these very phenomena which can result in the therapist reacting therapeutically or counter-therapeutically. An example of "acting-in" would be for the therapist to push harder, possibly with a covert micro-agression. On the other hand, the therapist, might then respond by asking other members how they felt about the reaction which just occurred, often eliciting comments that may prove helpful to the patient who just responded maladaptively.

Countertransference to Patients with a Personality Disorder in Group

Betan and his associates focused on totalistic countertransference in individual psychotherapy and conducted research that sought to measure countertransference psychometrically.[38] They discovered that there is a high degree of common, specific, therapist totalistic countertransference reactions that are transmitted to the therapist by each patient who is diagnosed as belonging to one of the three personality disorder clusters[38] as described in the DSM. They identified eight "clinically and conceptually coherent reactions" or countertransference reactions induced by the patients that were commonly experienced by many therapists, regardless of theoretical orientation. In other words, certain types of patients, within specific personality disorder clusters, engender commonly expectable totalistic countertransference reactions in their therapists. Given this commonality of therapist reactions to different PD clusters, the researchers concluded that totalistic countertransference reactions could be used therapeutically as an aid to both diagnosis and treatment. Their research findings indicated several major countertransference factors evoked by patients with a PD, included therapists feeling "overwhelmed and disorganized," "helpless and inadequate," "positive," "sexualized," "disengaged," "mistreated," "special/overinvolved " and "parental/protective" [38] Cluster A (odd/eccentric) personalities showed a significant association with the criticized/mistreated factor. Cluster B (dramatic/erratic) PDs are associated with the overwhelmed/disorganized, helpless/inadequate, special/overinvolved, disengaged, and negatively correlated with positive countertransference. Cluster C (anxious/fearful) PDs are associated with the parental/protective factor.

These findings suggest a special value that countertransference has in group therapy. The common reactions experienced by the group to a member with a PD can serve as a useful, consensually based reason for encouraging group members to ask for and/or offer similar feedback to other members of the group. Betan and his colleagues' research offers an evidence-based finding for the value of interpersonal feedback, demonstrating that PD patients in the group are likely experiencing many similar reactions from others in their lives outside the group. This clearly opens the clinical reality that feedback from the group, in which the patient can constructively struggle with reactions from others (assisted by therapeutic interventions), can facilitate support, growth, and repair (see Table 14.1, p. 367). Constructive struggle within the group can help members emerge with a healthier template for real-world functioning outside the group.

All these illustrations reveal that classic countertransference can interfere with the therapist's ability to be an effective group therapist. Totalistic countertransference reactions can be both informative and useful when they are clearly recognized as coming from the patient. The challenge is to be aware and effectively manage or utilize both of these reactions for the benefit of the individuals and the group. A useful, brief countertransference self-assessment instrument is presented in Table 14.2, p. 383.[39]

There are a few different ways the clinician can utilize this instrument. These include:

1. Read and reflect on the table's contents.
2. Ask yourself about how prone you might be to common fears and needs listed.
3. Rank your "Therapist Needs" elements from highest to lowest and ask yourself (being as honest you can) the extent to which the highest-ranked need is operative in your behavior in groups (either as a member or a leader).
4. Read the "problematic intervention" column. Based on knowing yourself, choose which one of those listed is your most likely problematic intervention. Write it down on a card and bring it to your next group. Look at the card before the group starts, and reflect after the group ends, on your ability to avoid using this problematic intervention. The authors have employed this self-assessment instrument in classrooms, asking residents or graduate students to rate themselves and then share and discuss relevant data in clusters of two or three people for ten minutes.

A Mini-Handbook: Tips, Considerations, Interventions and Cautions

The essential theoretical and interventional themes and elements of this chapter are presented below. They are intended as core guidelines for use by the group therapist.

1. *There are many common, specific interventions that can be employed by group therapists. Most are aimed at one or more of these three goals: (1) making the implicit, explicit; (2) promoting interactions; and (3) encouraging self-reflection.* Box 14.1 (see pg. 384) offers a compendium of actual verbatim interventions based upon the

Table 14.2. Assessing My Own Counter Transference: Personal Challenges Confronted by Therapists in Groups: A Worksheet*

Need(s) of the Leader/ therapist	Fears	Problematic Intervention	Therapeutic Intervention
To be liked	Members will not like the leader	Acting "chummy" or as a good mother	Leader strives for neutrality, freeing members from manipulative niceness
To prevent regressive behavior and acting out	Members will act crazy or be disruptive or act out	Leader becomes over-controlling in order to stop the behavior	Leader helps members examine and react to the meaning of regressive behaviors
Prevent expression of hostility	Anger will get out of control leading to violence	Leader actively suppresses or ignores the anger or hostility	The leader aggressively and gently pushes for members to contend with and explore anger and hostility
To prevent resistance	Members will be silent, avoidant, quit the group, complain about the leader, miss sessions	Leader controls the group interaction too quickly, responds to meet dependency needs, or encourages inappropriate dependency	The leader helps members explore both individual and group level resistance and allows people to struggle with their discomfort rather than gratifying it
To impress the group with authority and knowledge	Members will view the leader as incompetent	The leader tries to act like a "doctor" or a "supervisor"	The leader acts as a resource person: resist doing anything for the group which the group can do for itself
To resist processes that do not go through the leader	That the group can function without the leader and doesn't really need the leader	The leader acts as a "master of ceremonies"	The leader stays out of the interaction except to say things other members don't see, or say things to promote interactions
To prevent the discussion of taboo topics, e.g., sexual attraction between people, etc.	Talk will either get out of hand or go nowhere or make the leader very uncomfortable personally	The leader controls content (consciously or unconsciously); suppressing the expressions of members	The leader helps members explore and discuss topics no matter how embarrassing
To avoid being seen as human or having problems	Members will see the leader's problems and feelings, and the leader will experience shame	Leader becomes defensive, puts up a wall, pretends that he/she is not feeling and human	The leader shows their humanity is not phony or overly self-disclosing

* To use this table circle the problematic interventions you are prone to make. Read all items left to right.

Kenneth M Pollock, PhD, CGP and John Koenig, NP, CGP, developed at New York Medical College, 2009.

Ideas in this Exercise are based on a personal communication with Suzi Lego, RN, PhD, 1980.

Box 14.1   Tool Box-A Partial list of Group Interventions

1. What does it feel like to be here?
2. Sometimes a question is really a statement. What is the statement behind your question?
3. Is there some chance that you were just wrapping a feeling inside a question?
4. Is there a possibility that Martha may be speaking for others? She could very possibly be a spokesperson for feelings that exist in many people here.
5. What do you need from Tom, right now?
6. How are you feeling about me (or him or her or the group) right now? Or, would you like to know how X (or others) are feeling about you right now?
7. Where did you get that idea? (referring to a feeling or opinion one has about oneself).
8. Would you be willing to tell Donna what your reactions are to her right now?
9. How many people in here give too much power to other people's judgments and reactions to you? Raise hands.
10. Discussing the topic of difficult authorities outside the group may be a safer, more comfortable way to discuss it inside the group.
11. What is the group silence saying?
12. How emotionally safe is it in here right now? How safe is it for people to say exactly what they are feeling?
13. You are being experienced by others in a way which is different than how you want to be experienced (directed at an individual). Shall we try to figure that out?
14. You are getting a very different reaction from others than you want. What do we do with this?
15. If your father (mother, wife, etc.) could see your face right now, what would they see?
16. The group is making Sally into a patient now, and Sally is going along with that. I wonder if this isn't really a comfortable way for the group to manage its anxiety about other issues that are present here?
17. Who, specifically, in this room are you most emotionally safe with? Unsafe?
18. Are there "insiders" and "outsiders" in this circle? Who are they?
19. Do you want to take a risk now? (directed at an individual). Try saying something about yourself or to another which is difficult to say.
20. If you had to choose, Rhonda, who in this group would you feel safest with even though they might be angry with you?
21. You seemed to have been tuning out when Rob was speaking (directed an individual or several group members). It looks like the group is making Sarah tune out.
22. Mia appears to be carrying all of the group's angry feelings.
23. What is it *not* safe to talk about in here?
24. How would people describe the weather or climate in the group right now?
25. Is this group being helpful to you (to people) so far? How useful is it? (directed to an individual or total group).

26. Some group members (or the group-as-a-whole) appear to be dissatisfied or disconnected.
27. It looks like we have some informal subgroups in here. Can people name them?
28. Are you feeling understood by other(s) in the group? (directed to an individual).
29. The group and Michael have an unwritten agreement that he will not speak. Am I correct?
30. Two of the subgroups we have here are the "talkers," who speak, and "the quiet people," who don't speak. Hmmm. How is this working for each of you two groups?
31. There is an unspoken agreement between group members to be nice and polite . . .
32. How do the members and Patty feel about her, having come late?
33. What just happened? I sense that there is an elephant in the room that we're all quietly agreeing not to talk about it (in response to a palpable, but nevertheless implicit event that has just taken place, which no one is mentioning).
34. You look tuned out. What does this mean? Mary looks tuned out. What's the meaning of this?
35. The group is interviewing John in order to find out how "it" feels.
36. Your facial expression changed when David said he felt bored (directed to an individual).
37. How is the group (how do people) feeling about being here today?
38. What's your reaction to Edward? (directed to an individual).
39. Would you like some feedback from someone? Who? Tell him/her why you picked them? Are you going to trust what they say if it is *positive*?
40. The discussion of this topic (e.g., politics, or almost any other content area other than the here-and-now of the group) has something to do with what is going on in here right now.
41. Who is the angriest person here?
42. Would you like some of that? Do you want to own some of that action? (The therapist is asking if a person who is not in a discussion wants to join it because they probably have relevant treatment issues.)
43. Talking about stuff outside the group is a safe way of avoiding what's going on inside.

Note: This list of interventions was compiled by Tom Brandt, CSW, Michael Arena, DO, Ken Pollock, Ph.D., and Joan Koenig, NP, during the years 1991–1994 at New York Medical College.

observations of several experienced group therapists. Many of these statements or interventions are essentially those that follow from these therapists' attempts to utilize the various unique properties of groups. Using the specific language in Box 14.1 (see pg. 384) may foster one, two or, all three of these goals in the same statement. See if you can identify which statements facilitate reaching one or more of these goals.

2. *The degree to which therapists are psychologically present, connected, and authentic— not hidden behind a "professional shield"—will maximize their effectiveness as group*

therapists. The position of being genuine and revealing oneself openly is riskier, although often necessary when conducting a group.

3. *Even the most experienced therapists need to remind themselves to pay attention to and utilize the multiple levels of countertransference experienced in group.*

4. *The therapist should present a policy of "no socializing outside the group."* This is always useful, especially when working with patients who have PDs, because many of them are inclined toward boundary crossing and/or violations. Sometimes a boundary is broken in subtle ways by members, including communicating by e-mail, phone, chatting in the parking lot, having coffee together, and so forth. Patients with PDs may entice other group members into sexual relationships or business deals. When boundary "rules" are broken, many useful issues are brought to the fore, including those of trust and attachment. Almost all boundary violations, when they become known, typically offer important therapeutic opportunities to address interpersonal difficulties.

5. *Therapeutic efficacy is improved if a group stays predominantly in the here-and-now rather than the there-and-then.* This can be a major challenge, because there is often a tendency for groups to stick with outside events to avoid interacting with one another. They may also collude in staying out of the here-and-now when each group member, one member after another, sequentially bring up outside psychological events.

   It is often more comfortable and safer for the group to treat one member as a "patient" and to counsel him or her (or one another), rather than dealing with their identification or feelings toward her/him, and how her/his problem plays out within the group. In other words, talking to and about the patient as a topic itself is often a defense against talking to one another about how members are feeling and thinking about themselves and the other(s). Clearly, these phenomena call for interventions aimed at bringing the discussion into the here-and-now!

   Sometimes, there are important outside experiences that impact the country (an election) or the world (Covid-19) that need to be brought into group. In such cases, therapists should attend to ways these events impact group functioning. In addition, therapist interventions can center around encouraging members to share their own current feelings and reactions to what other members say and feel, and how they express them.

6. *The best opportunities for growth, repair, and support occur when something goes "wrong" in the group.* This can happen in hundreds of different ways, ranging from lateness, to difficult behavior by someone, two members becoming friends outside the group, or if there is an affair between two group members. Something going wrong may also involve a therapist's behavior (e.g., the therapists arrives late, is overly defensive, has aggressive outbursts, or calls someone by the wrong name). Sometimes, regardless of the actor(s), acting out can be so problematic that it threatens to rupture the group itself. Therapists need not always be the enforcer of group rules. Instead, they can be a resource to help members explore the meanings of what has happened. This does *not* mean therapists should stand by when egregious behaviors occur. The challenge is to walk the line between boundary-setter and facilitator of good therapeutic work.

7. *Constantly promote member interaction with one another.* Clearly, there are occasions when doing individual therapy in the circle is needed. However, so-called "star-formation" treatment in groups, when the leader and the group move from one person to another, with the leader at the center, does not take advantage of the unique properties of groups. It does not promote the powerful and therapeutically rich phenomena that occur when members are connecting and encountering one another. The leader-centered method can deprive group members of the opportunity to work on many of their own goals, especially those having to do with improving and/or practicing the development of meaningful interpersonal relationships with others who are not the therapist. Utilize the unique properties list in Table 14.1 to foster member-centered groups, through promotion of interaction.

8. *Therapist interventions should be directed toward talking about personal and interpersonal feelings toward each other or issues within the group.* Focusing on a topic, especially a psychologically important one, or issues of the day can be an unwitting, albeit subtle defense against encountering more central issues occurring in the group. Frequently, the content of the topic may be a clue to what is being avoided. For example, a discussion may emerge about how some people have felt invisible to their bosses at work. The therapist might say: "Perhaps the group is indirectly discussing feeling invisible or not being seen in here. Does anyone in this group feel or experience this?"

9. *Pay attention to the challenge of therapist over-responsivity to dependency needs and anxiety.* This often plays out in the form of members asking one question after another that appear information-seeking but are actually associated with dependency concerns and autonomy difficulties implicitly beneath the surface. It is tempting for the therapist to try to reduce dependency by providing either structure or answers, often in the form of "psycho-education." When the therapist plays into this, it can be understood as a "conscious collusion" with the group generated by the therapist's own issues (e.g., classic countertransference). A suggested intervention might be: "I'm wondering if these questions may be a way of expressing some anxiety over what might be seen as my failure to provide sufficient structure or directions in here. . . . Perhaps I am being experienced as abdicating my responsibility to direct things. . . . Anyone feeling like that?"

10. *It is almost always useful to assume that when a patient is expressing some strong feeling or opinion about the group and/or the therapist, that they are a spokesperson for others in the group who think or feel the same way.* This typically calls for an intervention such as: "I wonder if Peter is voicing feelings other people are having as well?"

11. *Therapist anxiety regarding silences can often lead to interventions explicitly aimed at inducing members to talk, but whose real purpose is to reduce the therapist's anxiety.* Silences are reflective of something that has potential psychotherapeutic value, but only if addressed out loud. Therapists should be cautious if they break silence, and almost always, when they do, it should be with a statement or question about the silence and its meanings. For example, "What does this silence say?" or "How are people feeling right now in here?"

12. *Therapist negative feelings toward a patient, including the therapist believing the patient is taking up too much time, can manifest in covert attempts to "direct" the group.* This is typically a form of therapist defensive avoidance of the issues at hand

in the circle. It is both a countertransference "moment" but also a therapeutic opportunity. Therapist "stage-managing" can subvert autonomous development of members as well suppress important potential feedback to that member (e.g., the therapist, in response to his or her own anxiety or anger, directs the conversation away from an annoying, domineering, or a monopolizing patient). A useful intervention involves identification of at least one other member who appears to be distracted or bored, and then saying, "Paul, I notice that whenever Susan is talking you seem distracted." Most of the time, Paul will respond by indicating his problematic reactions to Susan. This can begin a useful discussion involving feedback to Susan or Paul from other members as well.

13. *Speak the unspeakable; this is the leader's job. If there is an "elephant" in the room, it must be addressed.* Therapists often fear that if they make something explicit that is implicit, it will be too uncomfortable for the person(s) involved. The challenge is to find a way to encourage the group to bring out the "elephant." For example, consider the case of Phil's "narcissistic robbery of group oxygen." Group members were having difficulty with Phil's disingenuous empathy followed with his efforts to control the group by being the center of attention. Other members would consistently have looks of displeasure or boredom on their faces, but no one said anything. The therapist could say, "There is an elephant in the room right now. . . . Does anyone care to identify what it is?" If a member speaks up, others also might also say they agree, and dialogue about the phenomenon, as well as difficult but useful feedback, might follow.

14. *The leader needs to fight any tendency to be defensive in the face of personal attacks.* Typically, therapist defensiveness is manifested by "professional-sounding" comments, self-justification, or "interviewing" the attacker. Ostensibly, this is done to help the patient, but actually is a way of detoxifying the therapist's feeling hurt. Resist being defensive by trying to understand your countertransference. Why it is affecting me that way? Does it relate to my own history?

15. *Wait a few minutes until after group starts to bring up group business or therapy issues that are on your agenda.* Something more important to the group could be pre-empted if you do not wait.

16. *Theory is your friend and guide.* It is like a map, template, or compass. It can assist you to both understand and help your patients.

Conclusion

Ultimately, group therapy can be a powerful tool for the treatment of personality traits and many PDs. It requires additional knowledge and skills that go beyond those needed to conduct effective individual therapy. This chapter is not an argument that group psychotherapy is more efficacious than individual treatment for the PDs. However, it is proposed that there are things that the clinician can accomplish in group that are not available in individual therapy. Groups are especially useful to patients with PDs who need a lot of help knowing themselves, empathizing and being with others, repairing damaged relationships, staying in difficult conversations, and finding new, safe opportunities (with guidance from others) to practice developing meaningful and rewarding interpersonal relationships. The unique properties of group and specific group therapeutic strategies can

---

Box 14.2 Resources for Patients, Families and Clinicians

American Group Psychotherapy Association. https://www.AGPA.org. This organization offers limitless opportunities for professional development.

American Group Psychotherapy Association. Group Treatment of Personality Disorder. https://www.agpa.org/home/practice-resources/evidence-based-practice-in-group-psychotherapy/personality-disorders.

Mclean Hospital: Group therapy for borderline personality disorder. Mclean Hospital website. https://www.mcleanhospital.org/video/group-therapy-borderline-personality-disorder.

Rutan JS, Stone WN, Shay JJ. *Psychodynamic Group Psychotherapy*. New York, NY: Guilford; 2014.

---

be employed by group leaders to provide many opportunities for patients with PDs to change and grow personally.

It is common when treating a patient with a PD for a patient to benefit from being in both individual and group therapy. Many of the programmatic treatments for PDs recommend both individual and group therapy. Therapists who do both group and individual therapy commonly acknowledge a synergy between the two. It is also important to recognize that groups may not be an appropriate choice for some patients with a PD. For example, patients with ASPD are generally not good candidates for group, and the same may be true for patients who have complex, difficult, mixed PDs.

Readers who have not yet been in a group as a member are encouraged to participate in one, whether it be therapy, an experiential workshop, or a T-group. Groups can be both personally and professionally helpful in facilitating group therapy skill development and personal growth of the therapist. Review Box 14.2 for additional resources related to group therapy for the PDs.

Conflict of Interest/Disclosure: The authors of this chapter have no financial conflicts and nothing to disclose.

References

1. Kernberg OF. Aggression, trauma, and hatred in the treatment of borderline patients. *Psychiatr Clin North Am*. 1994;17(4):701–714. PMID: 7877899 Review.

2. Clark L, Vanderbleek E, Shapiro J, et al. The brave new world of personality disorder-trait specified: effects of additional definitions on coverage prevalence and co-morbidity. *Psychopathol Rev*. 2015; 2(1); 52–82. doi:10.5127/pr.036314

3. Mielimąka M, Rutkowski K, Cyranka K, et al. Effectiveness of intensive group psychotherapy in treatment of neurotic and personality disorders. *Psychiatr Pol*. 2015;49(1):29–48. doi: 10.12740/PP/26093. PMID: 25844408

4. Tyrer P, Seivewright N, Ferguson B, Tyrer J. The general neurotic syndrome: a coaxial diagnosis of anxiety, depression and personality disorder. *Acta Psychiatr Scand*. 1992;85(3):201–206. doi:10.1111/j.1600-0447.1992.tb08595.x

5. Tyrer P, Casey P, Gall J. Relationship between neurosis and personality disorder. *Br J Psychiatry*. 1983;142(4):404–408. doi:10.1192/bjp.142.4.404

6. Janet BW, Spitzer RL, Gibbon M, Skodal A, Williams JB. *Diagnostic and Statistical Manual of Mental Disorders*. 3rd ed. DSM III. Washington, DC: American Psychiatric Association; 1980.

7. Wolpe J. *The Practice of Behavior Therapy*. 1st ed. Oxford, UK: Pergamon Press; 1969.

8. Wolpe J, Lazarus A. *Behavior Therapy Techniques*. 1st ed. Oxford, UK: Pergamon Press; 1966.

9. Wolpe J. Reciprocal inhibition as the main basis of psychotherapeutic effects. *AMA Arch Neurol Psychiatry*. 1954;72(2):205–226. doi:10.1001/archneurpsyc.1954.02330020073007

10. Beck AT. *Cognitive Therapy and the Emotional Disorders*. New York, NY: Meridian; 1976.

11. Ellis A. *Overcoming Resistance: A Rational Emotive Behavior Therapy Integrated Approach*. 2nd ed. New York, NY: Springer; 2002.

12. Linehan MM, Armstrong HE, Suarez A, Allmon D, Heard HL. Cognitive behavioral treatment of chronically parasuicidal borderline patients. *Arch Gen Psychiatry*. 1991:Dec 1;48(12):1060–1064.

13. Kernberg OF, Selzer MA, Koenigsberg HW, Carr AC, Appelbaum AH. *Psychodynamic Psychotherapy of Borderline Patients*. New York, NY: Basic Books; 1989.

14. Young JE, Klosko JS, Weishaar ME. *Schema Therapy: A Practitioners Guide*. New York, NY: Guilford Press; 2003.

15. Fonagy P, Bateman AW. Mechanisms of change in mentalization-based treatment of BPD. *J Clin Psychol*. 2006;62(4):411–430. doi: 10.1002/jclp.20241

16. Yalom ID, Leszcz M. *The Theory and Practice of Group Psychotherapy*. New York, NY: Basic Books; 2005.

17. Rogers C. Psychology: A study of a science. In: Koch S., ed. *A Theory of Therapy, Personality Relationships as Developed in the Client-centered Framework*. Vol. 3. New York, NY: McGraw Hill; 1959:184–256.

18. Perls F, Hefferline R, Goodman P. *Gestalt Therapy: Excitement and Growth in the Human Personality*. Gouldsborom, ME: The Gestalt Journal Press; 1951.

19. Kohut H, Seitz PFD. Concepts and theories of psychoanalysis. In: Wepman JM, Heine RW, eds. *Concepts of Personality*. Chicago, IL: Aldine; 1963:113–141.

20. Spotnitz H. *The Couch and the Circle: A Story of Group Psychotherapy*. New York, NY: Knopf; 1961.

21. Ormont LR. *The Technique of Group Treatment*. Madison, CT: Psychosocial Press; 2001.

22. Foulkes SH. *Selected Papers of S.H. Foulkes: Psychoanalysis and Group Analysis*. Foulkes E, ed. London, UK: Karnac; 1990.

23. Bion WR. *Experiences in Groups, Human Relations*. Vols. I–IV, 1948–1951. Reprinted in *Experiences in Groups and Other Papers*. New York, NY: Basic Books; 1961.

24. Lewin K. *Resolving Social Conflicts: Selected Papers on Group Dynamics*. Lewin GW, ed. New York, NY: Harper & Row; 1948.

25. Bradford LP, Gibb JR, Benne KD. *T-Group Theory and Laboratory Method: Innovations in Re-education*. 1st ed. Hoboken, NJ: Wiley; 1964.

26. Lieberman MA, Yalom ID, Miles MB. *Encounter Groups: First Facts*. New York, NY: Basic Books; 1973.

27. Bollas C. The unthought known. In: Bollas C, ed. *The Shadow of the Object: Psychoanalysis of the Unthought Known*. New York, NY: Columbia University Press; 1987:277.

28. De Charms R. *Personal Causation: The Internal Affective Determinants of Behavior.* Milton Park, Abingdon, UK: Routledge; 2013.

29. Schnarch D. Desire problems: a systemic perspective. In: Leiblum SR, Rosen RC, eds. *Principles and Practices of Sex Therapy.* 3rd ed. New York, NY: Guilford Press; 2000:17–56.

30. Winnicott DW. *Holding and Interpretation: Fragment of an Analysis.* New York, NY: Grove Press; 1989.

31. Linehan MM. *DBT Skills Training Manual.* 2nd ed. New York, NY: Guilford Press; 2015.

32. Prochaska JO, DiClemente CC. Transtheoretical therapy: toward a more integrative model of change. *Psychol Psychother.* 1982;19(3):276.

33. Guignon C. Authenticity, moral values, and psychotherapy. In: Guignon, CB, ed. *The Cambridge Companion to Heidegger.* New York, NY: Cambridge University Press; 1993:215–239.

34. Sapriel L. Creating an embodied, authentic self: integrating mindfulness with psychotherapy when working with trauma. In: Levine, TB-Y, ed. *Gestalt Therapy: Advances in Theory and Practice.* New York, NY: Routledge; 2012:107–122.

35. Freud S. The dynamics of the transference. In: Strachey J, ed. The Standard Edition of the Complete Psychological Works of Sigmund Freud, Volume XII (1911-1913): The Case of Schreber, Papers on Technique and Other Works. London, UK: Hogarth Press; 1958:97–108.

36. Winnicott DW. *Hate in the Countertransference.* London, UK: Tavistock; 1947.

37. Kernberg O. (1965). Notes on countertransference. *J Am Psychoanal Assoc.* 1965;13(1):38–56.

38. Betan E, Kegley AM, Conklin CZ, Weste D. Countertransference phenomena and personality in clinical practice: an empirical investigation. *Amer J. Psychiatry.* 2005;162:890–898.

39. Pollock K, Koenig J. How not to do individual psychotherapy in a circle. Paper presented at: the Annual Meeting of The American Group Psychotherapy Association; 2004.

15

Psychopharmacology of Personality Disorders

Tawny L. Smith and Samantha M. Catanzano

Key Points

General Principles

- Psychotherapy is the mainstay of treatment for personality disorders (PDs).
- When a pharmacologic agent(s) is used, it should be adjunctive to psychotherapeutic interventions.
- The choice of medication management should be determined by the presence of psychiatric comorbidities and the dominant symptom domain(s).
- It is important to reassess the ongoing need for pharmacologic agents, especially in the absence of a psychiatric comorbidity.

Cluster A: Paranoid, Schizoid, Schizotypal Personality Disorder

- In general, individuals with a Cluster A personality disorder are less likely than other PDs to seek psychiatric treatment.
- Antipsychotic medications may have a role in improving the positive and negative symptoms associated with schizoid personality disorder, but data are limited to open-label and small randomized controlled trials.
- Due to a lack of information, the role of medications to treat schizotypal or paranoid PDs is largely unknown.

Cluster B: Antisocial, Histrionic, and Narcissistic (except Borderline) Personality Disorder

- There is limited data supporting the use of medications in antisocial personality disorder, with most focusing on the management of aggression.
- Divalproex, oxcarbazepine, carbamazepine, levetiracetam, phenytoin, and lithium may be beneficial in reducing aggression, but studies are limited in number and scope.
- Pharmacologic management of histrionic and narcissistic personality disorders is unsupported.

Cluster B: Borderline Personality Disorder (BPD)

- The use of medication(s) as a first-line or solo interventions for BPD is not supported and should only be used adjunctive to psychotherapy.
- Use of antidepressants in BPD has fallen out of favor and should be reserved for individuals with an antidepressant responsive psychiatric comorbidity, such as depression or anxiety.
- Some antiepileptic mood stabilizers (e.g., divalproex and topiramate) may reduce irritability and/or aggression in individuals with BPD.
- Second generation antipsychotics may have a role in reducing impulsivity, as well as cognitive distortions in BPD.

Cluster C: Avoidant, Dependent, Obsessive-Compulsive Personality Disorder

- Unlike other PDs, Cluster C PDs have higher rates of treatment-seeking behavior.
- There is a significant overlap in avoidant personality disorder (AVPD) and social anxiety disorder symptoms. While there are no pharmacologic studies specific to AVPD, there is a general consensus to approach pharmacologic management similar to social anxiety disorder (e.g., antidepressants).
- There is a significant overlap in obsessive-compulsive personality disorder (OCPD) and obsessive-compulsive disorder (OCD). The use of antidepressants to treat OCPD is largely extrapolated from OCD data.
- Studies regarding pharmacological treatment of DPD are nonexistent.

Introduction

Historically, the *Diagnostic and Statistical Manual of Mental Disorders-IV* (DSM-IV) "Axis I" diagnoses were thought of as disorders that might be responsive to pharmacologic interventions, whereas "Axis II" or personality disorders (PDs) were considered psychological disorders requiring psychotherapeutic interventions.[1,2] However, PDs consist of symptom clusters that are often similar or identical to symptoms seen in pharmacologically responsive mental health disorders. While some aspects of PDs may differ in their pathophysiologic etiology from mental health disorders, there have been neurobiologic similarities for some traits (e.g., impulsivity, aggression, schizotypy) that suggest pharmacologic interventions may have a role in PDs.

Currently, there are no FDA approved medications for PDs; however, individuals with PDs, especially Borderline Personality Disorder (BPD), are frequently prescribed psychotropic medications off-label. More recent guidelines recommend cautious use of medications, with the primary goal of providing symptom stabilization to allow the patient to better engage in psychotherapeutic interventions.[3] Despite recommendation for judicious use of medications, polypharmacy can be common, especially in BPD.[4]

Recommendations for adjunctive pharmacotherapy tend to target specific symptom domains—affective dysregulation, cognitive-perceptual, and impulsive aggression—which are more likely to respond to pharmacologic interventions. Effects tend to be modest, making it essential to weigh risks and benefits and reserve pharmacologic management for those with more severe or impairing symptoms.

In this chapter we will review the available evidence for the use of pharmacologic agents for DSM-5 Clusters A, B, and C personality disorders.[5]

Cluster A: Paranoid, Schizoid, Schizotypal PDs

Cluster A PDs are comprised of paranoid, schizoid, and schizotypal personality types. Individuals with Cluster A disorders can be characterized by social antipathy, a failure to form close relationships, and a general lack of empathy, with little awareness of these deficits.[6] As a result, individuals with Cluster A disorders are less likely to seek treatment compared to other PDs and hence are a challenging population to study. Overall, research regarding pharmacologic management of Cluster A disorders is sparse, with schizotypal personality disorder (SPD) having been studied the most.

Schizotypal Personality Disorder

Because of the genetic, neurobiologic, and symptom overlap between SPD and schizophrenia, as well as a >20 percent conversion rate from SPD to schizophrenia-related illnesses, one might assume that antipsychotics would be effective for SPD. In fact, several open-label trials with both first and second generation antipsychotics have supported this assumption.[6–8] Haloperidol and thiothixene have been the most studied first generation antipsychotics (FGAs) for SPD. Unfortunately, >70 percent of the individuals in these trials had a comorbid BPD or other comorbid psychiatric disorders that greatly confounds these positive study findings.[8] These studies are also older and plagued with high dropout rates.

The use of second generation antipsychotics (SGAs) for SPD has also been studied. Keshevan conducted a 26-week open-label study using olanzapine with 11 patients diagnosed with SPD.[9] Eight of the 11 completed the trial and demonstrated significant improvements in both positive and negative symptoms, and depressive symptoms, as well as an improvement in overall functioning. As one might expect, weight gain was significant with an average increase of 7.33 ± 9.6 kg on an average olanzapine dose of 9.32 ± 2.75 mg/day. Other metabolic parameters were not reported. There are no randomized control trials (RCTs) for olanzapine use in SPD.

The potential benefit of low-dose risperidone in SPD has been explored in two different RCTs. In a 9-week trial conducted by Koenigsburg and colleagues,[10] risperidone (up to 2 mg/day) led to a greater decrease in positive and negative symptoms versus placebo. In a 10-week RCT conducted by McClure et al.,[11] risperidone failed to demonstrate a cognitive benefit over placebo. Note that 23 of the 31 subjects in this trial had also been enrolled in Koenigsburg's risperidone RCT. Lastly, in a RCT of a single, low-dose risperidone, amilsupride, or placebo, only the amilsupride group demonstrated improvement in cognitive measures; however, this study was not designed to assess the potential impact of antipsychotics on cognition and should therefore be considered preliminary and requiring further study.[12]

A more recently published RCT demonstrated improvement in cognitive and functional skills with guanfacine augmentation in individuals with SPD.[13] Specifically, the 15 subjects who received guanfacine in combination with cognitive remediation and social-skills training experienced greater improvement in reasoning, problem-solving, and functional skills versus those who received placebo (n = 13). Because cognitive deficits are a marker for functional outcomes, these findings are promising, but warrant further study.

Paranoid and Schizoid Personality Disorders

Unfortunately, there are no published pharmacologic trials for paranoid and schizoid PD. There is only one retrospective case series of 15 individuals with paranoid PD reported in the literature.[14] In this small case series, seven patients received an antipsychotic during their hospital stay. Four patients had an available six-week Clinical Global Impression Improvement (CGI-I) scale assessment and all demonstrated improvement. Three of the four patients continued to show benefit at the last follow-up visit (up to 15 weeks). There are no published case series for pharmacologic interventions for schizoid PD.

In summary, there is a dearth of pharmacologic studies for Cluster A PDs. With the general lack of information regarding pharmacologic management of paranoid and schizoid PD, it is unclear if medications would be helpful; this question requires further study. SPD is the best studied of the three, with open-label data and a few small RCTs supporting the use of low-dose antipsychotics to address positive and negative symptoms. Similar to what we see in schizophrenia, antipsychotics do not impact cognitive symptoms of SPD as robustly, if at all. Guanfacine or another alpha-2 agonist may be helpful in this regard but warrant further study. Should our understanding of SPD continue to be linked with schizophrenia-spectrum disorder, we suspect that pharmacologic management of SPD will continue to advance.

Cluster B: Antisocial, Borderline, Histrionic, and Narcissistic Personality Disorders

The four PDs comprising Cluster B include antisocial, borderline, histrionic, and narcissistic. PDs categorized within Cluster B possess key emotional and behavioral dysregulation that separate them from other clusters.[15] Borderline personality disorder is most studied related to pharmacologic treatment interventions and is discussed in the section on BPD. Defining features and potential therapeutic modalities of the remaining Cluster B disorders are discussed.

Antisocial Personality Disorder

Antisocial personality disorder (ASPD) is broadly defined as "a pervasive pattern of disregard and violation of the rights of others."[5] Individuals with ASPD can be characterized by traits of impulsivity, high negative emotionality, and low conscientiousness.[16] Variable interpersonal and social disturbances are also present. Patients with ASPD are less likely to present in healthcare settings and seek treatment, resulting in a paucity of data.[17] Because of the historical correlation with criminality and ASPD, the majority of studies have focused on treatment of incarcerated patients, which is difficult to generalize to the community setting.[15] Medication management of ASPD is challenging due to the heterogeneous nature of the disorder and uncertainty surrounding the potential underlying neurobiochemical processes. Therefore, current evidence examines pharmacological treatment of antisocial personality disorder in the context of symptom clusters (e.g., aggression, impulsivity).

Most studies have examined the pharmacological impact of reducing aggressive behavior. Impulsivity has been less studied and is often combined within measurements of aggression. Furthermore, evidence specifically in ASPD patient subtypes is limited due to the challenging nature of diagnosis. Most studies evaluate the effects of anticonvulsants, known for their GABA-modulating activity that may positively impact aggression.[18] Fewer studies exist for antidepressants or serotonin modulators. Anticonvulsants, including divalproex, levetiracetam, and oxcarbazepine, and the antidepressant fluoxetine demonstrated improvement in aggression.[19] Carbamazepine, phenytoin, and valproate were also compared in a small parallel design study and demonstrated a reduction in average aggression score over a six-week treatment course.[20] Lithium has also demonstrated reduction in aggressive behavior over the course of three months, however evidence is limited to patients in an institutionalized setting.[1,21]

Evidence surrounding antipsychotic use in ASPD is minimal. One retrospective study in the UK identified that low doses of clozapine significantly reduced violence toward others in a small group of patients with ASPD without concurrent schizophrenia or those at a forensic hospital.[22] Despite positive results, this study is limited by a small sample size, lack of generalizability, and potential confounding effects with concurrent treatment modalities.

Variable evidence exists regarding treatment of comorbidities specifically in the context of ASPD, with the most common co-occurring conditions including substance use, anxiety, and depressive disorders.[16] Particular attention is required to ensure that patients with ASPD are offered guideline-directed treatment for anxiety and depressive disorders, as the chronicity of these disorders often exacerbates problems associated with ASPD.[16] One study examining the use of tiagabine in individuals on parole or probation with antisocial behavior and co-occurring substance use disorder showed a decrease in aggression over a five-week period.[18] Various studies have also examined amantadine, bromocriptine, desipramine, naltrexone, and nortriptyline in the context of co-occurring alcohol or cocaine dependence.[23] Limitations of all studies include small sample sizes, lack of generalizability, uncertainty of ASPD diagnosis, and short study durations in the context of a chronic, often fluctuating disorder.

In general, limited evidence exists to support pharmacological treatment for ASPD or associated symptom clusters. Instead, treatment should focus on guideline recommendations for co-occurring disorders. Whether treating ASPD psychologically or pharmacologically, particular attention must be paid to the possible influence of treatment compliance and dropout, misuse of prescribed medication, and drug interactions related to alcohol and illicit substances.

Histrionic and Narcissistic Personality Disorders

Histrionic personality disorder (HPD) is characterized by a pattern of "excessive emotionality and attention-seeking behavior."[5] Patients with HPD demonstrate rapidly changing and shallow emotions and inappropriate sexual or provocative behavior, as well as high rates of suggestibility, impulsivity, and reward dependence.[24,25] Despite the presence of attention-seeking behavior, similar to other PDs categorized in Cluster B, patients with HPDs are more likely to be resistant to seeking medical treatment.[1] Narcissistic personality disorder (NPD) is defined by a pattern of grandiosity, extreme entitlement, and lack of empathy.[5] Patients may hold a sense of self-importance, believe that he or she is special, and often require excessive admiration. Patients with NPD are at greater risk for suicide and follow the trend of "treatment rejecting" behaviors associated with other Cluster B PDs.[26]

First-line treatment for HPD and NPD includes psychotherapy focused on interpersonal processes.[25,27] For patients with co-occurring BPD, dialectical behavioral therapy is the preferred modality.[28] Pharmacological treatment is generally considered unsupported for HPD and NPD, with no randomized controlled trials currently existing. Due to lack of evidence supporting pharmacotherapy in the treatment of HPD, medication use is primarily focused around treatment of somatic symptoms and co-occurring somatization disorder, as well as treatment of affective conditions such as anxiety and depression.[5,29] Similarly, patients with NPD also demonstrate high levels of comorbid anxiety and depressive symptoms as well as bipolar disorder, substance use disorder, and other PDs.[28] When symptoms of anxiety and depression are present, treatment with selective serotonin reuptake inhibitors (SSRIs) or tricyclic antidepressants (TCAs) may be beneficial, although SSRIs may be preferable due to improved tolerability profiles.[1,3] No evidence exists for the role of mood stabilizers and antipsychotics for patients with HPD or NPD outside of co-occurring mood disorders.[25]

In summary, psychotherapeutic approaches are the recommend treatment approach for patients with HPD and NPD. Appropriate boundary setting and validating patient concerns is key to maintaining a therapeutic relationship. When pharmacotherapeutic options are employed, use should focus around evidence-based treatment approaches for co-occurring mental health disorders.[30]

Borderline Personality Disorder

BPD is characterized by a persistent pattern of affect instability, impulsivity, tumultuous interpersonal relationships, poor self-esteem, and self-harming or suicidal behaviors.[31] The rate of psychiatric comorbidities in BPD is high, especially substance use and affective disorders, which can elevate the risk of suicide attempts and completed suicides.[32,33] Other PDs, eating disorders, and anxiety disorders are also frequently seen comorbidities with BPD.

There are more data evaluating the use of pharmacologic interventions for BPD than any other PD. However, psychotherapy is still the mainstay intervention for BPD. Older guidelines were more permissive of psychotropic use in BPD,[3,34] with more recent guidelines recommending minimal use of adjunctive medications (see Table 15.1, p. 399 for guideline summaries).[35,36]

Small sample sizes and short duration of treatment for BPD pharmacologic studies, as well as their inconsistent findings, are the basis for limiting the use of these medications. Despite this, pharmacologic interventions are common in BPD, with reports of 90–99 percent of patients being prescribed at least one psychotropic medication, and polypharmacy being a frequent occurrence.[37]

Antidepressants, mood stabilizers, and antipsychotics are frequently prescribed for BPD, often targeting hallmark symptoms such as affective instability, impulsivity, or

Table 15.1. Pharmacotherapeutic Recommendations for Borderline Personality Disorder

Guideline (year)	Target Symptom Cluster	Medication Class Recommended	Level of Evidence	Specific Agents
American Psychiatric Association (2001)[34]	Affective Instability	AD MS	Level C originally Now insufficient evidence: Clinician should use clinical judgment	1st line: SSRIs (fluoxetine, sertraline) venlafaxine 2nd line: MAOIs (phenelzine, tranylcypromine) 2nd line or adjunctive: lithium, carbamazepine, divalproex
	Aggression Impulsivity	AD AP MS	Level C originally Now insufficient evidence: Clinician should use clinical judgment	1st line: SSRIs (fluoxetine, sertraline) After 2 SSRI failure: augment with AP, lithium or other MS
	Cognitive-Perceptual Disturbances	AP (low dose)	Level C originally Now Insufficient evidence: Clinician should use clinical judgment	FGA (haloperidol, perphenazine, thiothixene, flupentoxol, loxapine, chlorpromazine, trifluoperazine) SGA (clozapine, olanzapine, risperidone)
World Federation of Societies of Biologic Psychiatry (2007)[3]	Affective Instability	AD MS	Level C originally Now Insufficient evidence: Clinician should use clinical judgment	SSRI (not enough evidence to recommend a specific drug) Topiramate, lamotrigine, divalproex
	Aggression Impulsivity	MS AP	Level C originally Now Insufficient evidence: Clinician should use clinical judgment	Topiramate, lamotrigine, divalproex AP (doses lower than in schizophrenia; olanzapine studied the most, but insufficient data to differentiate). SGA>FGA
	Cognitive-Perceptual Disturbances	AP	Level C originally Insufficient evidence: Clinician should use clinical judgment	AP (doses lower than in schizophrenia; olanzapine studied the most, but insufficient data to differentiate). SGA>FGA
National Institute for Health and Clinical Excellence (2009)[36]			Level B	Avoid pharmacotherapy, except in acute crisis (< 1 week) Stop or reduce pharmacotherapy if no comorbid disorder
National Health and Medical Research Council (2012)[35]			Level B	Do not use pharmacotherapy 1st line or as sole treatment

AD = antidepressant; AP = antipsychotic; FGA = first generation antipsychotic; MAOI = monoamine oxidase inhibitor; SGA = second generation antipsychotic; SSRI = selective serotonin reuptake inhibitor
Key: Levels of Evidence; Strength of recommendation taxonomy (SORT)*

Level of Evidence A: Good quality patient-oriented evidence.

Level of Evidence B: Limited quality patient-oriented evidence.

Level of Evidence C: Based on consensus, usual practice, opinion, disease-oriented evidence, or case series for studies of diagnosis.

*Ebell MH, Siwek J, Weiss BD, Woolf SH, Susman J, Ewigman B, Bowman M. Simplifying the language of evidence to improve patient care. *J Fam Pract.* 2004 Feb 1;53(2):111–120.)

cognitive distortions.[38] In this section, we will explore the evidence behind the use of antidepressants, mood stabilizers/antiepileptics, and antipsychotics, because these are commonly used medications in the management of BPD symptoms. We will also briefly discuss emerging data on other possible pharmacologic interventions. Finally, because of the elevated polypharmacy risk, we will provide general approaches to prescribing, as well as deprescribing, recommendations for patients with BPD.

Antidepressants

Considering the core symptoms of BPD, such as affective dysregulation, it's not surprising that the use antidepressants (ADs) in BPD has been investigated and that they are frequently prescribed for patients with BPD. Despite SSRIs and venlafaxine being a treatment of choice for affect dysregulation and impulsive-behavior symptoms of BPD, in an older guideline,[34] literature supporting the use of antidepressants to treat the core BPD symptoms has been underwhelming.[39] In fact the most recent Cochrane Review[31] suggests that fluoxetine, fluvoxamine, mianserin, or phenelzine were not beneficial in BPD. The TCA amitriptyline was the only antidepressant in the Cochrane Review with data showing a reduction in depressive pathology. TCAs are, however, not recommended for use in BPD due to their toxicity and the risk of suicide when taken in an overdose. Published later that same year, a small open-label pilot of 18 subjects supported the use of duloxetine for BPD for "affective instability," "impulsivity," and "outbursts of anger." Because this was a small pilot, these efficacy findings would need to be replicated in a RCT to be a recommended intervention. Subsequent meta-analyses and systematic reviews have also failed to demonstrate the value of ADs to treat overall BPD pathology or symptom clusters.[40,41] These data likely explain the shift away from guidelines recommending ADs as first-line pharmacologic interventions to treat different BPD symptom domains.[38] That being said, a co-occurring depressive disorder is common in BPD, with some estimates as high as 77 percent.[42] Depressive symptoms tend to be more severe, with higher rates of anger/hostility and lower self-esteem when compared to those without BPD.[42] As previously noted, anxiety disorders are also highly comorbid with BPD. The use of antidepressants would be appropriate to address these AD-responsive comorbidities, with the caveat that AD efficacy may be more modest than reported in a non-BPD population.

Anticonvulsants and Mood Stabilizers

Affective instability (i.e., depression and anxiety) and impulsive aggression (i.e., suicide attempts, self-injurious behavior) in patients with BPD are often symptoms that bring individuals to seek care from healthcare providers. Mood stabilizers are frequently used to address these symptoms across various psychiatric diagnoses. Meta-analyses have found that, as a drug class, open-label trials and RCTs support anticonvulsants/mood stabilizers to address these symptom clusters, with larger effects seen for female patients.[31,41,43] However, when agents are examined individually, there are differences seen among them both in terms of efficacy for target symptoms and safety concerns. For instance, lithium, a gold standard for the treatment of bipolar disorder, did not show benefit for BPD in the only available placebo-controlled trial.[44] There are also great concerns about the lethality of lithium in overdose. Carbamazepine has shown benefit for impulsive aggression in one small RCT, but also carries concerns regarding overdose risk, is notorious for drug–drug interactions, and is considered a major teratogen. Divalproex (DVP), lamotrigine (LTG), and topiramate (TOP) have the most available data for use in

BPD. Unfortunately, like the AD trials, these studies tend to be small, short in duration, use varying rating scales, and have produced conflicting findings.

Divalproex

Divalproex (DVP) is an antiepileptic medication with mood-stabilizing properties. Its benefits as a mood stabilizer and effect on aggressive behaviors led to it being investigated for use in BPD.[45] Hollander and colleagues[45] evaluated the use of DVP versus placebo to reduce impulsive aggression across a variety psychiatric diagnoses, specifically Cluster B PDs, intermittent explosive disorder, and post-traumatic stress disorder. Unfortunately, when all diagnoses were examined together, DVP did not demonstrate a statistically significant improvement in symptoms. However, when patients with a Cluster B diagnosis were evaluated separately, improvements in irritability and aggression were seen in the DVP group, with an average dose of 1404 mg/day and 65.5 mg/ml serum concentration at final evaluation. Similarly, in a double-blind, placebo-controlled RCT of 30 subjects with BPD and bipolar II disorder, DVP improved irritability/agitation and aggressiveness, as well as interpersonal sensitivity, on an average dose of 850 mg ± 249 mg/day.[46] This trial was included as one of the two trials in the 2010 Cochrane Review[31] that concluded that subjects on DVP demonstrated a reduction in interpersonal problems (one RCT, n = 30) and anger (one RCT, n = 16). Of note, the results for these two symptom clusters could not be pooled due to significant heterogeneity in the data. Depressive symptoms also improved in the DVP group (n = 32) versus placebo (n = 14), but not anxiety symptoms. It is interesting to note that, in one small study published after the Cochrane review was conducted, DVP extended release (ER) failed to show benefit over placebo in any symptom domain for individuals with BPD with insufficient symptom reduction after a 4-week DBT program, which adds some concerns about its utility in this patient population.[47] There have been no additional studies evaluating DVP use published since 2012.

Treatment emergent adverse effects reported in the BPD trials were similar to what is seen in non-BPD DVP studies. Somnolence, headache, and nausea were commonly reported, and increases in liver enzymes, asthenia, depression, increased appetite, nausea, nervousness, and tremor were statistically more prevalent in the DVP group versus placebo.[46]

While intuitively, DVP would seem like a possible pharmacologic intervention for BPD, the studies supporting its use in BPD are older, small, and less-robust than more recent studies. DVP has a possible role in reducing impulsive aggression but has not definitely demonstrated benefit for affective instability. Weighing questionable benefits against possible adverse effects (i.e., teratogenicity), the use of DVP in a population of patients, most of whom are women of childbearing age, would need to be done cautiously, even in individuals with a comorbid bipolar diagnosis.[48]

Lamotrigine

Lamotrigine (LTG) is also an anticonvulsant that is approved for maintenance treatment of bipolar disorder. Its efficacy as a mood stabilizer, relative safety in pregnancy, and low risk of toxicity in overdose make it an appealing option for use in BPD. Early RCTs were small and short term, but promising, demonstrating benefit specifically for the core BPD symptoms, affect instability and impulsivity/aggression. However, individuals with psychiatric comorbidities were excluded, which makes the generalizability of their findings questionable.[49] In a larger, more recent RCT of subjects with BPD (n = 276) and more inclusive comorbidities, LTG failed to separate from placebo on any primary or secondary outcome measures at 12 and 52 weeks.[49] A recent meta-analysis, which includes three RCTs, concluded that LTG was well tolerated but did not differ in overall symptom improvement from placebo at 12 weeks or study end.[49] LTG also failed to separate from placebo in the secondary analysis measuring impulsivity/aggression. The findings from the more recent study as well as this meta-analysis calls into question the utility of LTG for BPD in the absence of other psychiatric comorbidities, such as bipolar disorder.

Topiramate

Despite the lack of RCT data supporting topiramate (TOP) as a mood stabilizer in bipolar disorder, there have been five trials supporting its use in BPD, three short-term,[50-52] and two 18-month follow-up studies.[53,54] With TOP doses ranging from 200–250 mg/day, reductions in irritability and anger have been reported. Both male and female samples showed a statistically significant improvement in anger in the eight-week trials; however, a larger effect was seen in female patients.[50,52] In both of these trials, anger scores decreased dramatically at the sixth week and continued to improve throughout of the duration of the trial, suggesting that a dose of at least 200 mg is likely needed for appreciable impact on anger. In the 18-month observational study of male patients, anger symptoms continued to improve over time.[53] An eight-week trial in a female-only, placebo-controlled RCT, as well the open-label, 18-month follow-up of the same cohort, also reported improvement in global functioning, hostility, interpersonal sensitivity, and somatization symptoms in patients with concurrent BPD and comorbid mood disorders.[51,54]

Overall, TOP was well tolerated and bothersome side effects were generally reported as mild in severity. TOP is notorious for appetite reduction and weight loss, both of which were appreciated in the short- and long-term BPD trials.[50-54] Parasthesia, dizziness, and headache were also reported. Surprisingly, cognitive complaints were not frequent and did not lead to treatment discontinuation, but this may be due to the use of doses below 300 mg/day in the trials.[55]

It is important to highlight that while the five trials appear very promising regarding the potential role of TOP for BPD, they were all conducted by the same research group. That being said, TOP has shown promise for off-label use in binge eating disorder and alcohol use disorder, which may make it a more desirable treatment option in patients with BPD who have one or both of these common comorbidities. Caution is warranted regarding the use of TOP in women of childbearing age, as it can lower the effectiveness of estrogen-containing oral contraceptives and has also been associated with cleft lip and/or palate with use during the first trimester.[48,56]

Antipsychotics

Antipsychotics may be beneficial when targeting impulsivity dysregulation in patients with BPD, such as aggression and self-damaging behaviors. Antipsychotics have also demonstrated efficacy in the treatment of psychotic symptoms associated with BPD, including cognitive and perceptual disturbances. These symptoms may include paranoid, referential, or suspicious thinking. In addition to target symptom clusters, antipsychotics have also been studied in addressing overall BPD severity, symptoms of depression, mania and psychosis, and improvement in psychosocial functioning.[57] National guidelines recommend use of antipsychotics as first-line when cognitive-perceptual disturbances are present, while they are typically reserved as third-line therapy for the management of impulsivity control.[19]

The evidence surrounding the use of antipsychotics in BPD is limited to a few randomized controlled and open-label trials, and even fewer comparative studies. Additionally, many of the studies have several limitations, including lack of assurance in the diagnostic criteria for BPD and potential confounding comorbid psychotic disorders. Furthermore, the body of literature exploring antipsychotic treatment in BPD is restricted by duration of treatment and sample size, with few studies assessing long-term outcomes post-treatment.[19]

FGAs have fallen largely out of favor due to lack of efficacy beyond acute periods of symptoms exacerbation, in addition to greater risk of extrapyramidal side effects and possible worsening of depressive symptoms. Outside of improvement in impulsivity and acute aggression, haloperidol has limited efficacy in the treatment of overall symptom severity in BPD. Lack of recent studies and high dropout rates limit its applicability among newer data with SGAs. Other FGAs that have been studied for BPD include chlorpromazine, thiothixene, and thioridazine, which have demonstrated similar improvement in hostility and are again limited by older trial data and lack of significant impact on overall BPD symptoms.[19] Loxapine has recently emerged as a potential treatment of interest given its recent reformulation as an inhalant. However, trials in BPD have only examined its use for the treatment of acute aggression in the emergency setting.[19]

SGAs have been the primary target of recent studies and overall seem to have more favorable data and side-effect profiles.[19] The largest body of evidence among SGAs exists for olanzapine; it has repeatedly demonstrated improvements in global functioning, affective instability, anxiety and anger, interpersonal sensitivity, and impulsive-aggressive behaviors. Four comparator drug studies exist comparing olanzapine to aripiprazole, asenapine, haloperidol, and sertraline. Olanzapine has demonstrated superiority to asenapine for paranoid ideation and dissociation and greater efficacy against aripiprazole related to cooperativeness and excitement.[57] No differences were found when compared to haloperidol, and both olanzapine and sertraline demonstrated improvements in multiple symptoms domains. Placebo-controlled trials of olanzapine have demonstrated improvements in anger, impulsivity, and global symptoms; however, adverse effects, including dry mouth, sedation, and weight gain, are notably more common with olanzapine.[19] Additionally, a Cochrane Review in 2010 noted an increase in self-harming behavior when olanzapine was used in the treatment of BPD.[31] While self-harming behavior may be an inherent symptom of BPD, other SGAs have demonstrated a reduction in these behaviors with treatment.[19]

Quetiapine and aripiprazole are other common SGAs studied for BPD. Quetiapine has been studied in both open-label and placebo-controlled trials. Studies for quetiapine have generally demonstrated overall tolerability and efficacy across a wide dose range for multiple symptoms including impulsivity, aggression, affective instability, and overall BPD severity.[19,58] No comparator trials exist for quetiapine, but a recent retrospective analysis identified quetiapine as one of the most common psychotropics prescribed for patients with BPD.[38] Aripiprazole has been studied in several RCTs and is one of the few SGAs with evidence expanding beyond 12 weeks. Three placebo-controlled trials demonstrated improvement in BPD psychopathology, social and global functioning, mood symptoms, and aggressiveness. When compared to olanzapine, both drugs demonstrated improvement in overall severity, and aripiprazole was superior for cognitive-perceptual symptoms including paranoid ideation.[19] Unlike olanzapine, which has shown an increase in self-harming behavior, aripiprazole has demonstrated reduction in self-injurious behaviors.[19]

Risperidone and its metabolite 9OH-risperidone (paliperidone) have limited evidence in the treatment of BPD. Risperidone has been examined in several open-label trials where improvements were noted primarily for impulsivity, aggression, and affective instability.[19] Only one RCT has been performed that includes risperidone, which only showed improvement in cognitive-perceptual disturbances.

Paliperidone extended release oral formulation and the long-acting intramuscular formulation paliperidone palmitate have both been examined in open-label studies. Both formulations showed reduction in global BPD symptoms, impulsivity, and cognitive-perceptual disturbances.[59,60]

Asenapine has been studied in one open-label trial and one comparator trial versus olanzapine.[61] In the open-label study of eight patients, asenapine reduced the overall symptomatology over the course of eight weeks. No effect was noted for depressive symptoms; however, no serious adverse events were reported, and patients also experienced weight reduction during treatment.[57] When compared to olanzapine, asenapine was superior on measures of affective instability.

Despite the potential efficacy of other SGAs, ziprasidone has failed to demonstrate efficacy in two studies. One RCT found no difference compared to placebo in overall BPD severity during a 12-week treatment period.[62] An open-label study in a psychiatric emergency setting showed reduction in acute exacerbations related to mood cognitive-perceptual symptoms, but did not measure any effect on overall BPD symptomatology. [19]

While clozapine has demonstrated improvements for BPD symptoms, potential safety risks within the BPD population must be addressed. Open-label studies have shown clozapine to be an effective agent in improving impulsivity, affective instability, self-injurious behaviors, and cognitive-perceptual disturbances.[19] Additionally, a recent naturalistic study explored the effects of clozapine over two years of treatment and found that psychiatric hospital admissions and psychiatric bed days were significantly reduced.[19] However, given the likelihood of low adherence to pharmacotherapeutic treatment and required monitoring, use of clozapine is particularly risky in patients with BPD. Currently, no studies exist for the newer SGAs lurasidone, cariprazine, or lumateperone. Only a single case report has indicated a potential role for cariprazine in reducing anxiety, affective instability, and anger in BPD.[63] Ongoing studies examining brexpiprazole in BPD have not yet been published.[57]

In summary, antipsychotics may be particularly helpful in addressing symptoms of impulsivity and aggressiveness as well as cognitive-perceptual disturbances. While FGAs may be beneficial for the reduction of acute aggression and hostility, preference remains for use of SGAs in the treatment of overall BPD symptomology given the larger body of literature and improved tolerability compared to FGAs. The role of SGAs on affective instability varies between agents, and aripiprazole may have the strongest evidence on improvement of depressive and anxiety symptoms. To date, olanzapine and aripiprazole have the highest evidence for their use in BPD, particularly for psychotic symptoms and aggression. Quetiapine and clozapine have also demonstrated efficacy; however, safety concerns and treatment adherence demand important attention when considering clozapine. Side-effect profile and required monitoring must be considered when choosing an agent.

Benzodiazepines

Several guidelines recommend against the routine use of benzodiazepines in the treatment of BPD due to greater risk of misuse and dependence, as well as the presence of other psychiatric comorbidities that may be negatively impacted by benzodiazepine use.[30] Additionally, benzodiazepines have the ability to reduce inhibitions and worsen symptoms of impulsivity and suicidality.[1] Outside of inpatient crisis situations, the use of benzodiazepines to manage anxiety or insomnia symptoms is highly discouraged for patients with BPD.

Miscellaneous Pharmacologic Agents

Other psychotropic agents including naltrexone, omega-3 fatty acids, oxytocin, and memantine have been studied in recent years in the treatment of BPD. The opioid antagonist's naloxone and naltrexone have been evaluated for their effects on dissociative symptoms in BPD. Both medications have demonstrated positive results compared to placebo, although improvements were not deemed statistically significant. Despite potential benefits, data are limited to a few small studies.[19]

Omega-3 fatty acids, including eicosapentaenoic acid (EPA) and docosahexaenoic acid (DHA), have demonstrated efficacy in the treatment of depression, and recently have received attention for their potential role in the treatment of BPD. EHA and DHA have been studied as monotherapy and in conjunction with DVP. In patients with BPD, omega-3 fatty acids have demonstrated improvements in depressive symptoms, aggressive behaviors, impulsivity, anger, and self-injury. It is interesting to note that one study evaluating the long-term efficacy of these agents in combination with DVP suggests a lasting effect of omega-3 supplementation on anger symptoms in BPD after treatment discontinuation.[19]

Oxytocin is a neuropeptide that modulates activity in areas of the brain associated with social cognition, such as the amygdala and inula.[64] Low oxytocin levels have been associated with poor social relationships in individuals with schizophrenia and autism.[65] While somewhat different deficits, interpersonal problems are also a core symptom seen in BPD. Oxytocin has also been implicated in emotional dysregulation, another prominent BPD symptom. With this in mind, Carrasco and colleagues measured oxytocin levels and expression of oxytocin receptors in individuals with moderate to severe BPD and found reductions in both of these measures compared to healthy controls.[66] Similar findings in other studies have led to an increase interest in exploring the use of intranasal (IN) oxytocin in patients with BPD. A systematic review conducted by Peled-Avron et al.[65] reported oxytocin IN improved social skills in five of eight small trials reviewed. In a more recent placebo-controlled, single-dose IN oxytocin RCT, Domes and colleagues[67] reported improvements in affective empathy and approach behavior motivation, but not cognitive empathy. While the use of IN oxytocin has some promising findings, Peled-Avron et al.'s systematic review also suggested that IN oxytocin resulted in reduced emotional response to threat cues and lower trust levels, and led to more antisocial than prosocial behaviors for those with lower self-esteem and a history of childhood trauma, which is cause for concern regarding its use in this population. It is also important to note that although there are nine oxytocin studies, they are all small studies, done predominately with female patients, often with only a single IN oxytocin dose given, and not done in conjunction with other first-line interventions (e.g., psychotherapy). Needless to say, the exact role of oxytocin in BPD is likely complex and remains largely uncertain at this point in time.

Glutamatergic overactivity has been linked with impulsivity across a variety of psychiatric disorders, including BPD, and presents a potentially novel treatment target.[68] Memantine is an N-methyl-D-aspartate (NMDA) receptor blocker that selectively blocks glutamate overactivity while maintaining normal synaptic function.[69] To date, there has only been one double-blind, placebo-controlled RCT investigating the effect of memantine as an adjunct to treatment as usual (consisting of antidepressants, mood stabilizers, and/or antipsychotics, as well as psychotherapy).[69] In this eight-week trial, memantine augmentation significantly reduced BPD symptoms. Its low abuse potential and tolerability profile make it an appealing novel treatment option for use in BPD; however, findings should be considered preliminary and warrant further study.

Ketamine, another glutamatergic modulator, has demonstrated efficacy for rapid reduction of suicidal ideation and depressive symptoms. Its misuse potential and short-lived effects are two significant downsides to its use. The potential anti-suicide benefits of ketamine in BPD are currently being explored in one ongoing clinical trial.[70] Should ketamine prove to be an effective anti-suicide intervention in BPD, it could potentially serve as a useful tool especially in acute suicidality in response to a stressor or crisis. This would be a niche specific to ketamine, as no other medication has demonstrated efficacy for suicidality and self-harm in BPD.[35]

Prescribing Approaches for BPD

Despite most pharmacotherapy trials being low quality, and reviews reporting inconsistent findings, the off-label use of psychotropic medications is commonplace in BPD. In fact, despite guidelines recommending evidence-based psychotherapies as a first line, pharmacotherapy is often the primary intervention used by clinicians.[71] Riffer and colleagues[38] reported that 96.4 percent of their study population were prescribed at least one psychotropic medication, with an average of 2.8 medications per patient.[38] Similar findings have been reported by others.[4] One could postulate that medication-responsive, psychiatric comorbidities seen with BPD could drive the use of medications; however, Riffer et al. also reported that use of psychotropics in patients with BPD was not related to comorbidities.[38] In fact, there was no difference in the types of or the total number of psychotropics prescribed in those with or without a psychiatric comorbidity. One possible explanation for this is that it may be derived from clinicians feeling the need to quickly address symptoms with a pharmacologic intervention each time a patient is in crisis. For instance, clinicians may feel the need to intervene quickly in patients with an elevated risk of self-harm or suicidal ideation. Unfortunately, crises can be frequent with BPD, and patients may be better served by learning techniques to manage crises; this a skill learned with BPD-focused psychotherapy. Medication changes or additions during a crisis should only be used as adjunctive treatment (see Box 15.1, p. 407 for general prescribing principles in BPD).

Polypharmacy

Polypharmacy in individuals with BPD may occur when clinicians mistake persistent symptoms of emptiness, loneliness, and chronic dysphoria as treatment refractory depression; this may lead to the prescriber to using combinations of medications in an attempt to address these symptoms.[3] Another possible explanation for polypharmacy may be a result of a symptom-based approach to prescribing medications, a practice supported in guidelines.[37] No single agent addresses all BPD symptom domains, so it is easy

---

Box 15.1   Key Points for Prescribing Medications in BPD

- Psychotherapy is the mainstay of treatment for BPD.
- When medications are used to address BPD symptom clusters, it should be adjunctive and for a defined period of time.
- The choice of medication management should be driven by the presence of psychiatric comorbidities and dominant symptom domain.
- It is important to recognize the pattern of polypharmacy that often results during the treatment of patients with BPD.
- Establish clear goals and expectations about the use of medications.
- Avoid "as needed" use of medications, especially benzodiazepines.
- Make one medication change or adjustment at a time when possible, and allow time for response.
- Resist the urge to make medication adjustments with every crisis.
- Reassess the ongoing need for psychotropic agents, especially in the absence of a psychiatric comorbidity.

---

to pick a mood stabilizer for aggressive behaviors, an antipsychotic for cognitive distortions, and a benzodiazepine for anxious distress. Caution is warranted regarding this approach, as it can easily lead to unwarranted polypharmacy. In the Riffer and colleague's study, 62.8 percent of the patients were prescribed three or more medications, with some on as many as nine medications, which is not supported by evidence.[38]

To avoid the "medication pile up," prescribers are encouraged to provide a clear explanation of the disorder and set realistic expectations about the use of medications, emphasizing that psychotherapy is the mainstay of treatment, and medications are adjunctive. Like prescribing medications for other psychiatric disorders, it's important to provide education about what symptom(s) is being targeted, expected onset of action, potential side effects, and general limitations to using medications. Providers should consider making one medication change at a time and waiting enough time to appreciate the impact an intervention may have on symptoms. It is likely that symptom improvement is subtle and occurs over time.[72] Also, if symptoms are not adequately addressed, switching medications is preferred rather than adding more medications; this is a conservative approach, especially in light of little available data regarding combination treatment. Similarly, if a medication is not well tolerated, switching medications versus adding an antidote is recommended. It is also important to educate patients that more medication is not always better and can lead to an increase in drug interactions and adverse events.

While the goal is to maintain patients on as few medications as possible, inevitably providers we will care for patients with BPD who are receiving polypharmacy. When a provider is first meeting a patient, unless there are safety concerns, it may be best to resist the urge to make medication changes at the first appointment. The provider should take time to obtain a thorough medication history including information on which medications have worked well and which haven't proven effective, as well as the side effects the patient has experienced. When streamlining medications, it's important to involve the patient in treatment-plan decisions using shared decision making techniques.[4] This means the provider should take time to assess the patient's knowledge and beliefs about medications, his or her understanding of their risks and benefits, and her or his perceptions of each medication. Ideally, the provider and patient should collaboratively weigh the pros and cons of each medication and develop an agreed-upon deprescribing plan.

As Needed Medication

Patients with BPD are also more likely to receive "as needed" (PRN) medications, despite a lack of evidence supporting this practice.[4] In general, patients with BPD are more likely to receive PRN medications, compared to other PDs, and are also more likely to continue to use these medications over extended periods of time. While one might assume this could be an indication of their effectiveness, BPD recovery is actually associated with less PRN medication use. This implies that the need for ongoing PRNs may instead be an indication of continued active symptoms.[4] If PRN medications for specific target symptoms are prescribed, it is important to provide clear instructions while setting an expectation for very short-term or limited use.[4]

Whether prescribing PRN or scheduled medications, providers are encouraged to limit pill counts for patients. Having large quantities of medications may elevate the risk of overuse or overdose. This is especially important for medications like TCAs or lithium that can be fatal in overdose.

Short-term Use

With the limited data surrounding long-term use in BPD and potential for long-term adverse effects of agents, providers should also determine if an ongoing or maintenance medication is needed. If a medication was added during a crisis, and the crisis has subsided, it behooves the provider to evaluate the continued need for medication. The National Institute for Clinical Excellence guidelines actually recommend that medications for patients with BPD not be given for periods greater than one week.[36] This is especially important when the patient is engaged in BPD-focused psychotherapy, which may reduce or eliminate the need for ongoing medications.

Tapering of medications should be gradual to avoid discontinuation symptoms, but also to monitor for symptom exacerbation. Patients with BPD may also feel reliant on the medications; a slow taper gives the patient to time to process their fears of being on less medication with the provider or therapist.[4]

Cluster C: Avoidant, Dependent, Obsessive-Compulsive Personality Disorders

The three Cluster C PDs include avoidant, dependent, and obsessive-compulsive personality disorder (OCPD). Cluster C PDs share in common anxious or fearful features.[30] Unlike PDs previously described, patients with Cluster C PDs tend to have higher rates of treatment-seeking behavior.[17] While avoidant personality disorder (AVPD) is the most prevalent disorder within Cluster C, there is significant overlap with social anxiety symptoms. Likewise, OCPD shares similar features with obsessive-compulsive disorder (OCD), and most data is derived by studying patients with both OCPD and OCD.[73]

Avoidant Personality Disorder

Avoidant Personality Disorder (AVPD) is described by a pattern of social inhibition, social phobia, feelings of inadequacy, and hypersensitivity to criticism. There is a significant relationship between AVPD and social anxiety disorder, and controversy exists regarding the degree of separation between them.[73,74] No randomized controlled trials exist examining pharmacological treatment modalities in patients with AVPD. Due to the overlap with AVPD and social anxiety disorders, there is reasonable consensus defending the application of treatments that are largely related to social anxiety disorders. Thus, the current evidence below is extrapolated from that population.

Utilization of antidepressants in the treatment of social phobia is well established. International guidelines and published reviews have identified numerous studies comparing various SSRIs, serotonin-norepinephrine reuptake inhibitors (SNRIs), and monoamine oxidase inhibitors (MAOIs) on reduction of social anxiety symptoms. The majority of evidence supports SSRIs and the SNRI venlafaxine for reduction of a variety of social anxiety–related symptoms, with or without concurrent improvement in social functioning. Paroxetine has the most available studies, followed by sertraline, fluvoxamine, venlafaxine, escitalopram, and fluoxetine.[1,3] Only paroxetine has been studied in comparator trials versus escitalopram and venlafaxine; however, these comparisons have not resulted in significant differences between treatment arms. MOAIs, including brofaromine, moclobemide, and phenelzine, have also been studied and demonstrated benefit.[1,3] However, only phenelzine is available in the United States, and risk of drug interactions and increased side effects have limited its applicability in treating social phobias.[1,3]

In addition to the effectiveness of SSRIs and venlafaxine, the gabapentinoids, including gabapentin and pregabalin, have also demonstrated efficacy in the reduction of social anxiety symptoms. While pharmacological agents such as buspirone, drug classes such as beta-blockers, and benzodiazepines have benefit in other anxiety disorders (e.g., generalized anxiety disorder, performance anxiety, and panic disorder), there is a lack of efficacy in social anxiety disorder. These agents are unlikely to elicit a response in those with AVPD and are not recommended in the absence of co-occurring conditions.[1]

Few studies have examined benefits of combined psychotherapy and pharmacological treatment for social anxiety. The earliest study compared phenelzine plus CBT versus placebo groups. The combination of phenelzine plus CBT was better versus either placebo condition, with similar dropout rates.[3] Two studies have compared SSRIs (fluoxetine and sertraline) plus CBT versus placebo groups with mixed results on improved efficacy for combination threatment.[3] Only one study specifically included subjects with AVPD.[75] This 2016 study compared paroxetine, cognitive therapy, combined paroxetine and cognitive therapy, or placebo in patients with social anxiety disorder with and without AVPD. The study, which was conducted in outpatients over 16 weeks, found that cognitive therapy was superior to paroxetine or placebo, but not combination treatment. Presence of AVPD did not reduce the outcome measures.[75]

Dependent Personality Disorder

Dependent Personality Disorder (DPD) is the least common of Cluster C disorders.[5,30] Patients with DPD often exhibit submissive and clinging behavior, extreme fears of separation, and an inability to assume responsibility for everyday decisions and major areas of life. Evidence for both behavioral and pharmacological interventions in DPD is scarce. Studies regarding pharmacological treatment of DPD is nonexistent.

Pharmacotherapeutic approaches should focus on management of comorbid diagnoses. Patients with DPD are more likely to be diagnosed with depression, panic disorder, somatization, substance use disorders, and other PDs.[76] However, studies are lacking examining the optimal medication treatment of comorbid mental health conditions in those with DPD. In the absence of supportive literature, it is reasonable to approach pharmacological treatment by following vetted guideline-directed treatment for concurrent psychiatric diagnoses.[30,76]

Obsessive-compulsive Personality Disorder

Obsessive-compulsive Personality Disorder (OCPD) is characterized by a preoccupation with order, perfectionism, and interpersonal control causing a moderate level of impairment.[5,30] Higher rates have been reported in those with a comorbid diagnosis of OCD and those in an inpatient psychiatric setting.[77,78] Despite a relatively high prevalence rate, overall data on behavioral and pharmacological treatment for OCPD is limited, with most investigations exploring the role of psychotherapy. There has also been demonstration of improvement in OCPD anxiety symptoms when group CBT therapy is employed with SSRI treatment.[77] Pharmacological treatment is limited by lack of RCTs.

Current treatment has primarily focused on SSRIs and mood stabilizers. An early study examined the effects of fluvoxamine on depressive symptoms in outpatients with major depressive disorder (MDD) in which greater than 50 percent of subjects had comorbid OCPD. The OCPD group demonstrated significant reductions in depressive symptoms after eight weeks of treatment.[79] Another early study compared 24 weeks of sertraline versus citalopram in outpatients with OCPD, OCD, and MDD. In both groups, OCPD traits reduced over the duration of the study, with citalopram appearing to be most effective.[80] In 2002, a case report described the positive effects of carbamazepine in reducing OCPD symptoms after several months of treatment.[81] Use of antidepressants is largely extrapolated from existing data among patients with OCD and other anxiety disorders. In particular, SSRIs may be helpful, particularly when comorbid anxiety or depressive disorders are present.[3,15]

Similar to Cluster B PDs, psychotherapy approaches should be a key component of the treatment approach in patients with Cluster C PDs. In patients with OCPD or AVPD, use of SSRIs is reasonable given the overlap of symptomology and associated comorbidities with OCD and social anxiety disorders. Other pharmacotherapeutic options must focus on evidence-based treatment approaches for co-occurring mental health disorders, specifically anxiety and depressive disorders. Assessment and treatment of co-occurring substance use disorders is also pertinent, particularly in those with DPD.[30]

Addressing Comorbidities

An important consideration in treating PDs includes attention to the management of comorbid conditions, particularly concurrent psychiatric diagnoses. Comorbid mood, anxiety, and substance use disorders can impact the severity of global symptoms of BPD as well as the degree of somatization and interpersonal sensitivity.[19] It is important to note that many studies examining pharmacotherapeutic interventions in PDs are often limited by exclusion criteria that prevent analysis of these treatments on those with comorbid diagnoses.[57,58] When possible, the choice of medication management should be driven by the presence of psychiatric comorbidities, including other PDs, and dominant symptom domain. Pharmacologic suggestions for BPD with comorbid psychiatric conditions are provided in Table 15.2 (see pg. 411).

Table 15.2. Pharmacotherapeutic Recommendations for Comorbidities with BPD

Comorbid Diagnosis	Medication Class(es)	Considerations
Anxiety/Depression	SSRIs SNRIs	Possibly higher consideration to duloxetine given potential benefit for core BPD symptoms in a pilot study Fluoxetine, fluvoxamine, and sertraline most studied in BPD
Bipolar Disorder	Mood stabilizers	Lamotrigine→not effective in treating mania Divalproex→concerns for use in women of childbearing age Lithium → concerns for toxicity & routine blood levels
Psychotic Disorder	Antipsychotics	SGA > FGA Lower doses likely needed if psychotic features d/t BPD
Substance Use Disorder	Anticonvulsants Naltrexone	Topiramate for AUD (off-label)
Binge Eating Disorder	SSRIs Topiramate	Off-label use

SSRIs = Selective serotonin reuptake inhibitors; SNRIs = serotonin and norepinephrine reuptake inhibitors; BPD = Borderline Personality Disorder; SGA = Second Generation Antipsychotics; FGA = Firest Generation Antipsychotics; AUD = Alcohol Use Disorder

Conclusion

Psychotherapy should be the primary therapeutic intervention for all PDs; the role of medication, if used, is adjunctive and judicious. There are no data supporting the use of medications in Cluster A PD, with the exception of SPD. Antipsychotics may be beneficial in SPD largely due to the neurobiologic and symptom overlap with schizophrenia. Similar to Cluster A PD, there is little to no data supporting the use of pharmacologic agents in the management of Cluster B PD, with the exception of BPD. For Cluster C PD, use of medications in DPD is also not supported; however, antidepressants may have a role in managing AVPD and OCPD.

Evidence-based literature supporting pharmacologic management of PDs has largely focused on BPD. While BPD has the most available data involving the use of psychotropics in this patient population, many studies are small and short in duration. Studies are also older and utilize a variety of rating scales, making it difficult to compare outcomes.

Guidelines recommend judicious use of medications but acknowledge that medications may be useful to target BPD specific symptoms. Recommendations have shifted away from the use of antidepressants across symptom domains, and more inclusive of mood stabilizers and antipsychotics. However, widespread use of all of these classes of medications continues. More recent data challenges the utility of mood stabilizers, specifically lamotrigine. While TOP and DVP may be beneficial for use, especially in the presence of certain psychiatric comorbidities, there are concerns about use of these drugs in women of childbearing age. Antipsychotics may play a role in the treatment of BPD, but concerns about side effects such as metabolic disturbances or movement disorders needs to be taken into consideration, especially with longer term use.

While there are controversies about which medications are best, there is a general consensus that polypharmacy does not have clear evidence in BPD and is likely more harmful than beneficial. Polypharmacy in BPD is the norm in clinical practice, with some reporting continued polypharmacy even over extended periods of time.

Guidelines recommend that prescribers assess the continued need for medication(s) over time. Using shared decision making with the patient for treatment planning can assist in avoiding polypharmacy or aid in simplifying medication regimens.

As our knowledge about the psychopathology of BPD and other PDs grows, it may lead us to new drug targets and the possibility of a more clearly defined role for pharmacologic interventions. Review Box 15.2 for resources for patient. families, and clinicians.

Conflict of Interest/Disclosure: The authors of this chapter have no financial conflicts and nothing to disclose.

Box 15.2 Resource Box for Patients, Families, and Clinicians

Patient and Family Resources

- National Institute of Mental Health. Borderline Personality Disorder.
  https://www.nimh.n0ih.gov/health/publications/borderline-personality-
     disorder/index.shtml#pub.
- NewYork-Presbyterian. Diagnosis and Treatment.
  https://www.nyp.org/bpdresourcecenter/treatment.
- Mayo Clinic: Borderline Personality Disorder.
  https://www.mayoclinic.org/diseases-conditions/borderline-personality-
     disorder/diagnosis-treatment/drc-20370242.
- National Alliance on Mental Illness. Types of Medication. 2020.
  https://www.nami.org/About-Mental-Illness/Treatments/Mental-Health-
     Medications/Types-of-Medication.

Clinician Resources

- European Guidelines for Personality Disorders: Past, Present, and Future. Posted 2019.
  https://bpded.biomedcentral.com/articles/10.1186/s40479-019-0106-3.
- Canadian Agency for Drugs and Technologies in Health. Treatment of Personality Disorders in Adults. Posted 2018.
  https://cadth.ca/sites/default/files/pdf/htis/2018/RB1199%20
     Personality%20Disorders%20Final.pdf
- Australian Government National Health and Medical Research Council. Caring for People with Borderline Personality Disorder. Posted 2013.
  https://bpdfoundation.org.au/images/mh25b_bpd_reference_guide_
     130530.pdf.
- National Institute for Health and Clinical Excellence Guidelines. Borderline Personality Disorder. Posted 2009.
  https://www.nice.org.uk/guidance/cg78/resources/borderline-personality-
     disorder-recognition-and-management-pdf-975635141317.
- World Federation of Societies of Biological Psychiatry. Guidelines for Biological Treatment of Personality Disorders. Posted 2007.
  https://www.wfsbp.org/fileadmin/user_upload/Treatment_Guidelines/
     Guidelines_Personality_Disorders.pdf.

References

1. Ripoll LH, Triebwasser J, Siever LJ. Evidence-based pharmacotherapy for personality disorders. *Int J Neuropsychopharmacol.* 2011;14(09):1257–1288. doi:10.1017/S1461145711000071

2. *Diagnostic and Statistical Manual of Mental Disorders: DSM-IV-TR.* Washington, DC: American Psychiatric Association; 2000.

3. Herpertz SC, Zanarini M, Schulz CS, et al. World Federation of Societies of Biological Psychiatry (WFSBP) guidelines for biological treatment of personality disorders. *World J Biol Psychiatry.* 2007;8(4):212–244. doi:10.1080/15622970701685224

4. Fineberg SK, Gupta S, Leavitt J. Collaborative deprescribing in borderline personality disorder: a narrative review. *Harv Rev Psychiatry.* 2019;27(2):75–86. doi:10.1097/HRP.0000000000000200

5. *Diagnostic and Statistical Manual of Mental Disorders: DSM-5.* Washington, DC: American Psychiatric Publishing; 2013. http://ebookcentral.proquest.com/lib/utxa/detail.action?docID=1811753.

6. Koch J, Modesitt T, Palmer M, et al. Review of pharmacologic treatment in cluster A personality disorders. *Ment Health Clin.* 2016;6(2):75–81. doi:10.9740/mhc.2016.03.75

7. Kirchner SK, Roeh A, Nolden J, Hasan A. Diagnosis and treatment of schizotypal personality disorder: evidence from a systematic review. *Npj Schizophr.* 2018;4(1):20. doi:10.1038/s41537-018-0062-8

8. Jakobsen KD, Skyum E, Hashemi N, Schjerning O, Fink-Jensen A, Nielsen J. Antipsychotic treatment of schizotypy and schizotypal personality disorder: a systematic review. *J Psychopharmacol (Oxf).* 2017;31(4):397–405. doi:10.1177/0269881117695879

9. Keshavan M. Efficacy and tolerability of olanzapine in the treatment of schizotypal personality disorder. *Schizophr Res.* 2004;71(1):97–101. doi:10.1016/j.schres.2003.12.008

10. Koenigsberg HW, Goodman M, Trestman RL. Risperidone in the treatment of schizotypal personality disorder. *J Clin Psychiatry.* 2003 June;64(6):628. doi:10.4088/jcp.v64n0602

11. McClure MM, Koenigsberg HW, Reynolds D, et al. The effects of risperidone on the cognitive performance of individuals with schizotypal personality disorder. *J Clin Psychopharmacol.* 2009;29(4):396–398. doi:10.1097/JCP.0b013e3181accfd9

12. Koychev I, McMullen K, Lees J, et al. A validation of cognitive biomarkers for the early identification of cognitive enhancing agents in schizotypy: a three-center double-blind placebo-controlled study. *Eur Neuropsychopharmacol.* 2012;22(7):469–481. doi:10.1016/j.euroneuro.2011.10.005

13. McClure MM, Graff F, Triebwasser J, et al. Guanfacine augmentation of a combined intervention of computerized cognitive remediation therapy and social skills training for schizotypal personality disorder. *Am J Psychiatry.* 2019;176(4):307–314. doi:10.1176/appi.ajp.2018.18030349

14. Birkeland SF. Psychopharmacological treatment and course in paranoid personality disorder: a case series. *Int Clin Psychopharmacol.* 2013;28(5):283–285. doi:10.1097/YIC.0b013e328363f676

15. Bateman AW, Gunderson J, Mulder R. Treatment of personality disorder. *The Lancet.* 2015;385(9969):735–743. doi:10.1016/S0140-6736(14)61394-5

16. National Collaborating Centre for Mental Health (Great Britain), National Institute for Health and Clinical Excellence (Great Britain), eds. *Antisocial Personality Disorder: Treatment, Management and Prevention.* Leicester, UK: British Psychological Society; 2010.

17. Tyrer P, Mitchard S, Methuen C, Ranger M. Treatment rejecting and treatment seeking personality disorders: type R and type S. *J Personal Disord*. 2003;17(3):263–268. doi:10.1521/pedi.17.3.263.22152

18. Gowin JL, Green CE, Alcorn JL, Swann AC, Moeller FG, Lane SD. Chronic tiagabine administration and aggressive responding in individuals with a history of substance abuse and antisocial behavior. *J Psychopharmacol (Oxf)*. 2012;26(7):982–993. doi:10.1177/0269881111408962

19. Bozzatello P, Rocca P, De Rosa ML, Bellino S. Current and emerging medications for borderline personality disorder: is pharmacotherapy alone enough? *Expert Opin Pharmacother*. 2020;21(1):47–61. doi:10.1080/14656566.2019.1686482

20. Stanford MS, Helfritz LE, Conklin SM, et al. A comparison of anticonvulsants in the treatment of impulsive aggression. *Exp Clin Psychopharmacol*. 2005;13(1):72–77. doi:10.1037/1064-1297.13.1.72

21. Sheard MH, Marini JL, Bridges CI, Wagner E. The effect of lithium on impulsive aggressive behavior in man. *Am J Psychiatry*. 1976;133(12):1409–1413. doi:10.1176/ajp.133.12.1409

22. Brown D, Larkin F, Sengupta S, et al. Clozapine: an effective treatment for seriously violent and psychopathic men with antisocial personality disorder in a UK high-security hospital. *CNS Spectr*. 2014;19(5):391–402. doi:10.1017/S1092852914000157

23. Khalifa N, Duggan C, Stoffers J, et al. Pharmacological interventions for antisocial personality disorder. *Cochrane Database Syst Rev*. 2010;(8). doi:10.1002/14651858.CD007667.pub2

24. Department of Psychiatry, Washington University in St. Louis School of Medicine, St. Louis, USA, Svrakic D, Veterans Affairs Medical Center, Saint Louis, Missouri, USA, et al. An integrative model of personality disorder: Part 3: mechanism-based approach to the pharmacotherapy of personality disorder: an emerging concept. *Psychiatr Danub*. 2019;3(31):290–307. doi:10.24869/psyd.2019.290

25. French JH, Shrestha S. *Histrionic Personality Disorder*. In *StatPearls [Internet]*. StatPearls Publishing; 2019. http://www.ncbi.nlm.nih.gov/books/NBK542325/.

26. Dhawan N, Kunik ME, Oldham J, Coverdale J. Prevalence and treatment of narcissistic personality disorder in the community: a systematic review. *Compr Psychiatry*. 2010;51(4):333–339. doi:10.1016/j.comppsych.2009.09.003

27. Sulz S. Hysterie I: histrionische persönlichkeitsstörung. Der *Nervenarzt*. 2010;81(7):879–888. doi:10.1007/s00115-010-3016-6

28. Caligor E, Levy KN, Yeomans FE. Narcissistic personality disorder: diagnostic and clinical challenges. *Am J Psychiatry*. 2015;172(5):415–422. doi:10.1176/appi.ajp.2014.14060723

29. Morrison J. Histrionic personality disorder in women with somatization disorder. *Psychosomatics*. 1989;30(4):433–437. doi:10.1016/S0033-3182(89)72250-7

30. Angstman KB, Rasmussen NH. Personality disorders: review and clinical application in daily practice. **Am Fam Physician**. 2011;84(11):8.

31. Lieb K, Völlm B, Rücker G, Timmer A, Stoffers JM. Pharmacotherapy for borderline personality disorder: Cochrane systematic review of randomised trials. *Br J Psychiatry*. 2010;196(1):4–12. doi:10.1192/bjp.bp.108.062984

32. Leichsenring F, Leibing E, Kruse J, New AS, Leweke F. Borderline personality disorder. *The Lancet*. 2011;377(9759):74–84. doi:10.1016/S0140-6736(10)61422-5

33. Sher L, Fisher AM, Kelliher CH, et al. Clinical features and psychiatric comorbidities of borderline personality disorder patients with versus without a history of suicide attempt. *Psychiatry Res*. 2016;246:261–266.

34. Oldham JM, Gabbard GO, Goin MK, et al. practice guideline for treatment of patients with borderline personality disorder. *Am J Psychiatry*. 2001;158(10).

35. National Health and Medical Research Council. *Clinical Practice Guideline for the Management of Borderline Personality Disorder*. Melbourne: National Health and Medical Research Council; 2012. https://bpdfoundation.org.au/images/mh25_borderline_personality_guideline.pdf.

36. National Collaborating Centre for Mental Health (UK). *Borderline Personality Disorder: Treatment and Management*. British Psychological Society; 2009. http://www.ncbi.nlm.nih.gov/books/NBK55403/.

37. Starcevic V, Janca A. Pharmacotherapy of borderline personality disorder: replacing confusion with prudent pragmatism. *Curr Opin Psychiatry*. 2018;31(1):69–73. doi:10.1097/YCO.0000000000000373

38. Riffer F, Farkas M, Streibl L, Kaiser E, Sprung M. Psychopharmacological treatment of patients with borderline personality disorder: comparing data from routine clinical care with recommended guidelines. *Int J Psychiatry Clin Pract*. 2019;23(3):178–188. doi:10.1080/13651501.2019.1576904

39. Tyrer P, Silk KR. A comparison of UK and US guidelines for drug treatment in borderline personality disorder. *Int Rev Psychiatry Abingdon Engl*. 2011;23(4):388–394. doi:10.3109/09540261.2011.606540

40. Hancock-Johnson E, Griffiths C, Picchioni M. A focused systematic review of pharmacological treatment for borderline personality disorder. *CNS Drugs*. 2017;31(5):345–356. doi:10.1007/s40263-017-0425-0

41. Vita A, De Peri L, Sacchetti E. Antipsychotics, antidepressants, anticonvulsants, and placebo on the symptom dimensions of borderline personality disorder: a meta-analysis of randomized controlled and open-label trials. *J Clin Psychopharmacol*. 2011;31(5):613–624. doi:10.1097/JCP.0b013e31822c1636

42. Rao S, Broadbear J. Borderline personality disorder and depressive disorder. *Australas Psychiatry*. 2019 Dec;27(6):573–577. doi:10.1177/1039856219878643

43. Ingenhoven T, Lafay P, Rinne T, Passchier J, Duivenvoorden H. Effectiveness of pharmacotherapy for severe personality disorders: meta-analyses of randomized controlled trials. *J Clin Psychiatry*. 2010;71(01):14–25. doi:10.4088/JCP.08r04526gre

44. Paris J. Clinical trials of treatment for personality disorders. *Psychiatr Clin North Am*. 2008;31(3):517–526. doi:10.1016/j.psc.2008.03.013

45. Hollander E, Tracy KA, Swann AC, et al. Divalproex in the treatment of impulsive aggression: efficacy in Cluster B personality disorders. *Neuropsychopharmacology*. 2003;28(0):1186–1197. doi:10.1038/sj.npp.1300153

46. Frankenburg Z. Divalproex sodium treatment of women with borderline personality disorder and bipolar II disorder: a double-blind placebo-controlled pilot study. *J Clin Psychiatry*. 2002:63(5) 442–446.

47. Moen R, Freitag M, Miller M, et al. Efficacy of extended-release divalproex combined with "condensed" dialectical behavior therapy for individuals with borderline personality disorder. *Ann Clin Psychiatry Off J Am Acad Clin Psychiatr*. 2012;24(4):255–260.

48. Tomson T, Battino D, Bonizzoni E, et al. Comparative risk of major congenital malformations with eight different antiepileptic drugs: a prospective cohort study of the EURAP registry. *Lancet Neurol*. 2018;17(6):530–538. doi:10.1016/S1474-4422(18)30107-8

49. Pahwa M, Nuñez NA, Joseph B, et al. Efficacy and tolerability of lamotrigine in borderline personality disorder: a systematic review and meta-analysis. *Psychopharmacol Bull*. 2020;50(4):118–136.

50. Nickel M. Topiramate reduced aggression in female patients with borderline personality disorder. *Eur Arch Psychiatry Clin Neurosci*. 2007;257(17):432. doi:10.1007/s00406-007-0735-1

51. Loew TH, Nickel MK, Muehlbacher M, et al. Topiramate treatment for women with borderline personality disorder: a double-blind, placebo-controlled study. *J Clin Psychopharmacol*. 2006;26(1):61–66. doi:10.1097/01.jcp.0000195113.61291.48

52. Nickel MK, Nickel C, Kaplan P, et al. Treatment of aggression with topiramate in male borderline patients: A double-blind, placebo-controlled study. *Biol Psychiatry*. 2005;57(5):495–499. doi:10.1016/j.biopsych.2004.11.044

53. Nickel MK, Loew TH. Treatment of aggression with topiramate in male borderline patients, part II: 18-month follow-up. *Eur Psychiatry*. 2008;23(2):115–117. doi:10.1016/j.eurpsy.2007.09.004

54. Loew TH, Nickel MK. Topiramate treatment of women with borderline personality disorder, part II: an open 18-month follow-up. *J Clin Psychopharmacol*. 2008;28(3):355–357. doi:10.1097/JCP.0b013e318173a8fb

55. Thompson PJ. Effects of topiramate on cognitive function. *J Neurol Neurosurg Psychiatry*. 2000;69(5):636–641. doi:10.1136/jnnp.69.5.636

56. Bhakta J, Bainbridge J, Borgelt L. Teratogenic medications and concurrent contraceptive use in women of childbearing ability with epilepsy. *Epilepsy Behav*. 2015;52:212–217. doi:10.1016/j.yebeh.2015.08.004

57. Stoffers-Winterling J, Storebø OJ, Lieb K. Pharmacotherapy for borderline personality disorder: an update of published, unpublished and ongoing studies. *Curr Psychiatry Rep*. 2020;22(8). doi:10.1007/s11920-020-01164-1

58. Bellino S, Paradiso E, Bogetto F. Efficacy and tolerability of quetiapine in the treatment of borderline personality disorder: a pilot study. J Clin Psychiatry. 2006;67(7):1042–1046.

59. Bellino S, Bozzatello P, Rinaldi C, Bogetto F. Paliperidone ER in the treatment of borderline personality disorder: a pilot study of efficacy and tolerability. *Depress Res Treat*. 2011;2011. doi:10.1155/2011/680194

60. Palomares N, Montes A, Díaz-Marsá M, Carrasco JL. Effectiveness of long-acting paliperidone palmitate in borderline personality disorder. *Int Clin Psychopharmacol*. 2015;30(6):338–341. doi:10.1097/YIC.0000000000000095

61. Bozzatello P, Rocca P, Uscinska M, Bellino S. Efficacy and tolerability of asenapine compared with olanzapine in borderline personality disorder: an open-label randomized controlled trial. *CNS Drugs*. 2017;31(9):809–819. doi:10.1007/s40263-017-0458-4

62. Pascual JC, Soler J, Puigdemont D, et al. Ziprasidone in the treatment of borderline personality disorder: a double-blind, placebo-controlled, randomized study. *J Clin Psychiatry*. 2008;69(4):603–608. doi:10.4088/jcp.v69n0412

63. Grant JE, Chamberlain SR. Cariprazine treatment of borderline personality disorder: a case report. *Psychiatry Clin Neurosci*. n/a(n/a). doi:10.1111/pcn.13094

64. Brüne M. On the role of oxytocin in borderline personality disorder. *Br J Clin Psychol*. 2016;55(3):287–304. doi:10.1111/bjc.12100

65. Peled-Avron L, Abu-Akel A, Shamay-Tsoory S. Exogenous effects of oxytocin in five psychiatric disorders: a systematic review, meta-analyses and a personalized approach through the lens of the social salience hypothesis. *Neurosci Biobehav Rev*. 2020;114:70–95. doi:10.1016/j.neubiorev.2020.04.023

66. Carrasco JL, Buenache E, MacDowell KS, et al. Decreased oxytocin plasma levels and oxytocin receptor expression in borderline personality disorder. *Acta Psychiatr Scand*. 2020;142(4):319–325. doi:10.1111/acps.13222

67. Domes G, Ower N, von Dawans B, et al. Effects of intranasal oxytocin administration on empathy and approach motivation in women with borderline personality disorder: a randomized controlled trial. *Transl Psychiatry*. 2019;9(1):328. doi:10.1038/s41398-019-0658-4

68. Krause-Utz A, Winter D, Niedtfeld I, Schmahl C. The latest neuroimaging findings in borderline personality disorder. *Curr Psychiatry Rep*. 2014;16(3):438. doi:10.1007/s11920-014-0438-z

69. Kulkarni J, Thomas N, Hudaib A-R, et al. Effect of the glutamate NMDA receptor antagonist memantine as adjunctive treatment in borderline personality disorder: an exploratory, randomised, double-blind, placebo-controlled trial. *CNS Drugs*. 2018;32(2):179–187. doi:10.1007/s40263-018-0506-8

70. Ketamine in borderline personality disorder. Posted January 10, 2018. ClinicalTrials.gov. NCT03395314. https://clinicaltrials.gov/ct2/show/NCT03395314.

71. Rogers B, Acton T. "I think we're all guinea pigs really": a qualitative study of medication and borderline personality disorder. *J Psychiatr Ment Health Nurs*. 2012;19(4):341–347. doi:10.1111/j.1365-2850.2011.01800.x

72. Silk KR. The process of managing medications in patients with borderline personality disorder. *J Psychiatr Pract*. 2011;17(5):311–319. doi:10.1097/01.pra.0000405361.88257.4a

73. Widiger, TA, ed. *The Oxford Handbook of Personality Disorders*. Oxford University Press; 2012. doi:10.1093/oxfordhb/9780199735013.001.0001

74. Lampe L. Avoidant personality disorder as a social anxiety phenotype: risk factors, associations and treatment. *Curr Opin Psychiatry*. 2016;29(1):64–69. doi:10.1097/YCO.0000000000000211

75. Nordahl HM, Vogel PA, Morken G, Stiles TC, Sandvik P, Wells A. Paroxetine, cognitive therapy or their combination in the treatment of social anxiety disorder with and without avoidant personality disorder: a randomized clinical trial. *Psychother Psychosom*. 2016;85(6):346–356. doi:10.1159/000447013

76. Maccaferri GE, Dunker-Scheuner D, De Roten Y, Despland J-N, Sachse R, Kramer U. Psychotherapy of dependent personality disorder: the relationship of patient–therapist interactions to outcome. *Psychiatry*. Published online October 15, 2019:1–16. doi:10.1080/00332747.2019.1675376

77. Diedrich A, Voderholzer U. Obsessive-compulsive personality disorder: a current review. *Curr Psychiatry Rep*. 2015;17(2):2. doi:10.1007/s11920-014-0547-8

78. Bulli F, Melli G, Cavalletti V, Stopani E, Carraresi C. Comorbid personality disorders in obsessive-compulsive disorder and its symptom dimensions. *Psychiatr Q*. 2016;87(2):365–376. doi:10.1007/s11126-015-9393-z

79. Ansseau M, Troisfontaines B, Papart P, von Frenckell R. Compulsive personality as predictor of response to serotoninergic antidepressants. *BMJ*. 1991;303(6805):760–761.

80. Ekselius L, von Knorring L. Personality disorder comorbidity with major depression and response to treatment with sertraline or citalopram. *Int Clin Psychopharmacol*. 1998;13(5):205–212.

81. Greve KW, Adams D. Treatment of features of obsessive-compulsive personality disorder using carbamazepine. *Psychiatry Clin Neurosci*. 2002;56(2):207–208. doi:10.1046/j.1440-1819.2002.00946.x

III

PERSONALITY DISORDERS

16

Paranoid Personalities (Vigilant Style)

Royce Lee and Edwin Santos

Key Points

- Suspiciousness and hostility are key symptoms in PPD.
- Clinicians should consider PPD as a Cluster B disorder is miscategorized in the DSM-5 Cluster A section. By this simple thought experiment, we think that the thoughtful clinician can more fully anticipate the clinical problems and opportunities that treatment of PPD entails.
- PPD is common in clinics, inpatient hospitals, and forensic settings, but is often missed.
- The neurobiology of PPD is shared with PTSD.
- Sensitivity to shame in interpersonal contexts drives many of the problematic behaviors associated with PPD.
- Psychological trauma, structural violence, and social stress are risk factors for PPD.

Introduction and Historical Context

This chapter is intended as a concise reference for clinicians, trainees, and experts with an interest in paranoid personality disorder (PPD). We will explore what is too often the long-neglected elephant in the room: PPD is often misdiagnosed in the clinic, even when mistrust and suspiciousness are the pervasive dynamic in the treatment relationship. PPD's belated recognition is often associated with a pained sigh by the clinician who has finally seen the obvious. Like many of the personality disorders, the PPD construct is, in its most lucid and useful form, a dimensional construct. This has led to proposals to remove its categorical representation from the *Diagnostic and Statistical Manual of Mental Disorders* (DSM-5).[1] Nonetheless, PPD tells an important story involving social cognition, social dynamics, and trauma exposure. Its ubiquity in the clinic means that any expert in personality disorders should be able to grapple with PPD.

One reason to suspect that PPD will remain in the lexicon in the future comes from its origins in the past. Paranoia stems from the Greek *para* or "deranged" and *noeo* or "thinking," encompassing a wide range of maladies from delirium to monomania.[2] However, the ancients also described individuals with paranoid beliefs with otherwise preserved reasoning and intellect. While Hippocrates conceptualized melancholy as near wholly affective in nature, Galen observed many melancholics with paranoid thoughts.[3] Unlike more severe conditions like schizophrenia, delusional melancholics' psychological disturbances are separate from global cognitive and sensory capacities. In a subtle distinction, the 9th-century Persian physician Al-Razi distinguished melancholia from madness (*junun*) based on the former's retention of reason, carving out a space for paranoia in those who might superficially be considered sane.[4]

Karl Jaspers's "delusional atmosphere"[5] and Kraepelin's "strife with the world"[2] bring into focus a group of individuals captured by the PPD construct. From these historical descriptions, a portrait of the disorder emerges that is characterized by suspiciousness, mostly preserved mental and neurological function, and a hostile engagement with, rather than indifference to, other humans and society in general.

Clinical Illustrations

Case 1: Mr. A

A 50-year-old Caucasian research scientist, Mr. A, appears for an evaluation of his treatment-resistant depression. He is dressed impressively at the first appointment and comes prepared with extensive documentation of his clinical history. He is an incisive thinker, and his work productivity reveals his ambitions to excel in his work. His personal and professional life are marked by a consistent pattern of escalating conflict, fed by mostly private ruminations about the ill intentions of others, and an accumulating history of slights, ill intentions, and subtle sabotage of his success and happiness. A history of repeated work problems seems at odds with the promise of his intellect and strong work ethic. Themes in treatment that emerge quickly are feelings of entitlement and betrayal. He is initially diagnosed with narcissistic personality disorder (NPD), recurrent major depression, and post-traumatic stress disorder (PTSD). In the first few months of treatment, outbursts of hostility, such as secretive but unrealistic homicidal fantasies, and problematic verbal outbursts at work are identified. These symptoms respond to treatment with selective serotonin reuptake inhibitors (SSRIs) and supportive psychotherapy.

Over the next year, the patient's recurring tendency to fear retribution and abandonment, in even the smallest of transgressions (e.g., a missed refill authorization or irritating letter from the billing office) reveals a mistrust of the clinician. His suspicious motives endure, despite repeated protests to the opposite, and even factual demonstrations of it. His therapist decides to try schema therapy as a treatment method. Collaborative work between the two quickly identifies an underlying schema of defectiveness and an intense avoidance of feelings of shame.

Repeated breaks and repairs in the therapeutic alliance over the next two years make the pattern explicit; Mr. A can begrudgingly acknowledge this. With increased trust, it becomes possible to address his PTSD for the first time in therapy, although he refuses to engage in prolonged exposure therapy. Over time, his mediations have been simplified, and dramatic swings in moods are reduced in frequency and amplitude.

Case 2: Mr. B

A 35-year-old African American plumber, Mr. B, has recently been discharged from the hospital after a traumatic gunshot injury. He is given a diagnosis of PTSD based on prominent symptoms of hyperarousal and avoidance and starts a treatment course of prolonged exposure therapy. However, the therapist notices that sessions are quickly derailed despite an initial acknowledgment of the need to address his hyperarousal symptoms; this is despite a demonstrated ability to talk about traumatic events without excessive distress or arousal. Further exploration reveals a history of severe psychological and physical abuse as a child, and a heavy dose of exposure to community and structural violence. His relationships are transactional. Due to a pervasive mistrust, he is unable to name any associate he can count on as a friend, nor a family member with benign intentions. He makes a convincing case for the validity of his convictions based on past experience. During sessions Mr. B is not consistently aloof, but rather tries to test his clinician for trustworthiness, and at times disengages or seems unreachable. Mr. B requests a letter to excuse a missed court appearance due to the side effects of medications. This is difficult to verify. Writing the letter provides the opportunity to discuss trust in the relationship. The gambit seems to have the desired effect. Mr. B becomes more comfortable in sessions talking about the great difficulty he has trusting and confiding in his clinician and resisting his intuitive response to flee or abandon the treatment. After six months, he is finally comfortable enough to start taking sertraline, 50 mg per day, for symptoms of PTSD. The medications improved his mood and reduced the severity of his PTSD symptoms.

Case Analyses

These two prototypical cases illustrate how context modifies the presentation of PPD. Commonalities between the two cases include a history of childhood trauma and the importance of comorbid PTSD. In both cases, recognition of PPD allows for an important shift in the treatment after a period of slow engagement. For the patient, this is a move away from defensive reactions. For the clinician, this is an alert to see the hypersensitivity of the patient and to perceived ruptures of trust. In neither case did the recognition of PPD lead to psychopharmacological intervention, other than treatment of comorbid conditions. In both cases the question of comorbid personality disorders is important. In the case of Mr. A, NPD is a relevant piece of the diagnostic puzzle. In the case of Mr. B, the question of antisocial personality disorder (ASPD) is raised, but must be contextualized in the context of community and structural violence. A trauma-informed approach is appropriate for both cases, but must take into account the unique interpersonal dynamic of PPD.

Epidemiology

The prevalence of PPD ranges from 1.21 to 4.4 percent in the community, between 2–10 percent of outpatients and 10–30 percent of psychiatric inpatients.[6] Even higher rates (23 percent) are found in prisoners.[7] As with other personality disorders, PPD's prevalence increases with higher levels of psychiatric acuity. It is more commonly diagnosed in black individuals (odds ratio relative to white = 2.5), Native American (OR = 3.12), and in those with low income (OR = 3.55).[8] The pattern of differences suggests that socioeconomic stress is an important risk factor, a hypothesis that is confirmed by empirical studies reviewed in later sections of this chapter.[6]

The dimensional view of PPD[9] posits that clinical PPD represents the severe end of a continuum of PPD-related traits in the population, such as suspicion. Epidemiological studies of suspiciousness find that it is generally higher in males and divorced individuals, and decreases with age and level of education.[10] Paranoid ideation is found in between 10–30 percent of the population in studies worldwide, with more severe paranoia found in about 2 percent.[6,11,12] In the community, PPD is associated with committing acts of physical[13,14] and sexual[13] violence. PPD is also associated with elevated risk for completed suicide,[15] although the risk associated with PPD may not be as great as borderline personality disorder (BPD).[6]

Diagnostic Considerations

Some aspects of the descriptive psychopathology of PPD have shifted over time, while others have remained unchanged. In the first edition of the DSM (1952),[16] PPD was described tersely as traits of "suspiciousness, envy, extreme jealousy, and stubbornness." At the time, these characteristics were explained in terms of the psychoanalytic defense mechanism of projection.[17] DSM-II carried PPD forward, emphasizing "hypersensitivity, rigidity, unwarranted suspicion, jealousy, envy, excessive self-importance."[18] The DSM-III added rigidity, social domineering, and interpersonal suspicion in interpersonal situations and introduced explicit diagnostic criteria.[19] DSM-IV and DSM-5 narrowed the focus somewhat to core traits of distrust and hypervigilance, de-emphasizing affective aspects of the disorder.[20,21] Indeed, examination of the progression of diagnostic criteria reveals that the PPD construct has become more and more monothetic, to a degree perhaps unmatched by other personality disorder constructs. All seven criteria in the DSM-5 describe suspiciousness in different domains, and only indirectly refer to associated traits of cognitive rigidity (unforgiving of slights) and hostility.

This analysis of the DSM diagnostic criteria for PPD offers an important insight for clinicians on the lookout for the disorder. Although the cognitive traits of PPD align it with schizophrenia-spectrum disorders, its affective and interpersonal facets make it a closer relative to Cluster B personality disorders. Indeed, we previously used factor analysis on a sample of 1,675 male and female adults, enriched for personality disorder.[22] Examination of the cognitive, affective, and interpersonal criteria surprisingly recapitulated the structure of DSM-IV, with each factor respectively conforming largely to Cluster A, B, and C personality disorders. However, PPD symptoms loaded most strongly with other symptoms in the Cluster B group (antisocial, narcissistic, borderline) and only weakly with other Cluster A personality disorders (schizoid, schizotypal). Thus, in the clinic, individuals with PPD may look and feel more like patients with borderline, narcissistic, or antisocial personality disorders. This may explain why clinicians frequently miss or do not even consider the diagnosis, perhaps priming themselves to recognize a bizarre, thought-disordered individual rather than a hostile, embittered one.

Subtyping of PPD has not yet been formalized. A study using finite mixture modeling in a sample of personality-disordered individuals has provided some evidence for two subtypes: one with high levels of paranoia but not aggression or antisocial features, and another with high levels of paranoia along with aggression and antisocial features.[23] These provocative findings echo the high rates of PPD found in aggressive individuals and point to the utility of accounting for impulsive aggression in treatment planning.

The interrater reliability of the diagnosis ranges from a low of 0.35 to a high of 0.57, making it one of the less-reliable personality disorder diagnoses.[6] However, the reliability of assessments of PPD traits is higher, between 0.75 and 0.85. Given the higher reliability of dimensional-trait assessments, could a dimensional approach to PPD be more useful? Serious proposals have been made to reconsider PPD as a trait characterized by dimensionality in the population, with those at the extreme high end meeting clinical criteria for a disorder.[9,24]

Studies examining the question of dimensionality in PPD have found somewhat mixed results and will not be reviewed in detail here. In summary, the taxonometric structure supports a dimensional structure in a well-conducted community study in the United States. However, evidence has also been found for a cubic-frequency distribution of traits in a Korean sample; a cubic distribution would suggest a construct that may intermediate between these two types.[6] The idea of PPD as exhibiting both dimensional and categorical properties could be explained if PPD in fact combined lower-order traits, whose interaction would lead to nonlinear expression of symptoms. Supporting this idea is the preponderance of evidence that paranoid thoughts are best characterized as a dimensional trait in the population. Paranoid traits themselves may include separable traits of suspiciousness and hostility.[25] If so, it would seem that dimensional assessments of PPD-related symptoms should measure hostility and suspiciousness separately, not suspicious thoughts, in order to capture the same set of behaviors as contained in the PPD construct.

In summary, the diagnostician faces a challenge in the assessment of PPD. On the one hand, PPD common enough in the clinic to warrant staying alert to its presence. On the other hand, a categorical diagnosis of PPD may be unreliable from clinician to clinician. The fact that many cases are missed, even by experts, indicates that diagnosticians should be alert to the possibility that false negatives warrant reassessment as more data becomes available in the course of treatment. A way of grappling with this problem may be to assess PPD-related traits in tandem with the disorder, and when doing so, to bear in mind the importance of assessing both suspiciousness and hostility. Tracking where the patient lies on the continuum of these traits will position the clinician to recognize the disorder when it presents, as well as to track its severity over the course of treatment.

Common Comorbidities

Considering PPD in its dimensional form is most important when considering the comorbidities that define the negative space surrounding the disorder. In these cases, we have found that PPD provides the missing piece of the picture crucial for treatment planning. The four comorbidities that warrant specific attention are PTSD, BPD, ASPD, and intermittent explosive disorder (IED).

The close relationship between PTSD and PPD makes PTSD arguably the most important comorbidity. In a study of U.S. veterans diagnosed with PTSD, PPD was the most common personality-disorder diagnosis, with 17 percent of cases with PTSD meeting diagnostic criteria for PPD.[26] These data are supported by analysis of data from the National Epidemiologic Survey on Alcohol and Related Conditions, which found that 13 percent of adults with PTSD in the United States belonged to a latent class characterized by PPD and symptoms of cognitive rigidity.[27] Viewing the comorbidity relationship from the perspective of PPD, 29 percent of PPD patients have comorbid

PTSD.[28] Although most clinicians associate PTSD with BPD, in fact more individuals with PPD have PTSD than those with BPD. High rates of PPD in this population reveal that disrupted trust in traumatized individuals and groups is a significant problem. Providing further evidence of the need to think carefully about the interaction between the two disorders, it appears that treatment of PTSD can strongly impact PPD. In a longitudinal study that followed a cohort of patients with PTSD and comorbid personality disorders, of the 19 patients with PPD at baseline, 9 (53%) of the patients no longer met criteria for PPD after 14 weeks of evidence based psychotherapy.[29] This is a startling finding, given other evidence of the chronic and treatment refractory nature of PPD. This close relationship, whereby treatment for one disorder has powerful effects on another, points to the need for further research into alternative diagnostic systems, such as the proposed category of developmental trauma disorder, or complex PTSD. Supportive evidence for this comes from data from both clinical and epidemiological samples finding that individuals with PPD and PTSD have an earlier onset of trauma and trauma-related symptoms.[27,30]

Most patients with PPD will have a comorbid personality disorder. Of the 75 percent that do, avoidant (48 percent), borderline (48 percent), and narcissistic (35.9 percent) disorders are the most common.[31] The constancy between this data and our own data regarding the factor structure of personality-disorder symptoms[22] is striking, supporting both categorical and dimensional models. We previously have found that the elevated suicide risk that comes from comorbid BPD and PPD is due to the fact that BPD[6] is associated with higher suicide risk than PPD. This would suggest that interventions targeted for suicidal behavior, such as dialectical behavioral therapy (DBT), would be helpful in cases with comorbid PPD and BPD. Because PPD is associated with elevated risk for all other personality disorders,[32] one would expect to encounter such combinations frequently. The psychodynamic field has provided a rich descriptive, psychopathological model for PPD in the theory of borderline personality organization, (see Chapter 2), which stresses innately high levels of aggression and reactivity to shame.[33,34] Not surprisingly then, the personality disorder most associated with aggression is PPD, even more closely than ASPD.[35] In short, we would invite clinicians to consider PPD as a Cluster B personality disorder miscategorized in Cluster A. By this simple thought experiment, we think that the thoughtful clinician can more fully anticipate the clinical problems and opportunities that PPD entails.

Genetic, Biologic, and Neuropsychiatric Contributions

PPD is 66 percent heritable.[36] Self-reported suspiciousness, a dimensional facet of PPD, has an estimated heritability of 41 percent.[10] Thus, both the categorical and dimensional forms of PPD have a genetic component. Although genetic risk factors have not yet been established, clues about the neurobiology of PPD have emerged. Given the overlap between the suspiciousness of PPD symptoms and the paranoid delusions encountered in psychotic disorders, the question of PPD's relationship to schizophrenia has been a topic of interest. The biological links between PPD and schizophrenia as gleaned from family association studies are not very consistent; some studies find an increase in rates of PPD in probands of persons with schizophrenia,[37] but others repudiate this association.[38,39]

Unlike schizotypal personality disorder, PPD does not seem to have a strong genetic relationship with schizophrenia,[40] but may have a closer relationship with delusional disorder.[41] Thus, PPD, despite its superficial similarity to schizophrenia, likely has a different underlying mechanism.

Neurophysiological studies have found evidence for diminished amplitude of the visual and auditory P300 in patients with PPD, along with reduced working memory.[42] Amplitude of the P300 event-related potential (ERP) is an index of neurophysiological working memory resources from largely cortical, midline structures of the brain. Diminished P300 and reduced working memory are also found in schizophrenia. However, PPD is associated with normal mismatch negativity to auditory stimuli, which is reduced in schizophrenia.[43] Mismatch negativity is an increase in the amplitude of the N100 ERP to a second tone that does not match the preceding tone, and thus indexes salience in the environment. PPD subjects in this study did have faster latency of the N100 ERP. These two findings are consistent with increased arousal, or hypervigilance, in PPD.

Other data support the idea of a hypervigilant phenotype in PPD. Paranoid personality traits have been found to be associated with a tendency to perceive neutral faces as harshly negative,[44] a finding generally associated with psychopathologies characterized by anxiety and interpersonal hypersensitivity. We have previously found that PPD, but not other personality disorders, are associated with elevated central concentration of corticotropin-releasing hormone (CRH).[45] CRH is the master stress hormone, acting on both hypothalamic and cortical CRH receptors. Elevated central CRH drive has long been implicated in PTSD, and variation of the CRH R1 receptor has been linked to re-experiencing symptoms of PTSD in a large, genome-wide association study.[46] Elevated CRH drive is seen in adults with personality disorder who have reported high levels of childhood maltreatment, but without comorbid PTSD; this is associated with reduced peripheral responsiveness to adrenocorticotropic hormone (ACTH) challenge and decreased AM cortisol;[47] this neuroendocrine profile has also been found in PTSD. Thus, PPD and PTSD share neurobiological similarities and suggest a common underlying endophenotype, upregulated central CRH drive, but chronically downregulated peripheral hypothalamic-pituitary-adrenal axis reactivity. Hypervigilance to threat in PPD does not necessarily manifest as fear: quickness to anger in social interactions is more likely. A functional neuroimaging study has recently found that left-lateralized, ventrolateral, prefrontal cortex activity was decreased in PPD during cognitive reappraisal of anger-eliciting visual stimuli.[48] This decrease in a frontal "brake" mediated the relationship between PPD and runaway paranoid social cognition. This finding is of particular interest as it links suspiciousness with emotion regulation to potentially explain the hostility associated with PPD.

Such emotional reactivity likely carries a metabolic cost. One such cost is oxidative stress, the process by which the body attempts to neutralize potentially harmful, chemically reactive oxidative species created through the catabolism of monoamine neurotransmitters and other molecules. Recent research from our laboratory has implicated oxidative stress in Cluster B personality disorders,[49] including BPD and NPD. Reductions in the enzyme superoxide dismutate (SOD), an important antioxidant, have been reported in PPD,[42] along with altered gene expression of mitochondrial enzymes. Genetic polymorphisms of nitric oxide synthase 1 adaptor protein (NOS1AP), have been linked to PPD.[50] Brain NOS1AP is involved in the regulation of nitric oxide releasing following N-methyl-D-aspartate (NMDA) receptor activation, which has downstream effects on neural signaling and oxidative processes. The pathophysiological significance of altered oxidative stress pathways in PPD is not clear. It seems likely that it represents increased oxidative stress burden caused by PPD-related interpersonal hypersensitivity. However, the reverse is possible that oxidative stress affects brain development: childhood exposure to air pollution is associated with adult personality disorder symptoms.[51]

Computational models of psychopathology have been proposed to incorporate biological findings into systems that can be described in terms of system dynamics. As it turns out, the first computational model of psychopathology described in the literature was a model of a paranoia. This was simultaneously the first simulation of human conversation with a computer program, or what we today call a chatbot: PARRY, created by the psychiatrist Kenneth Colby in 1972.[52] The model contained two main components: a supersensitivity to shame that leads PARRY to enter a cognitive state characterized by suspiciousness of the user; and a heightened emotional state that drives suspiciousness but decays eventually. Thus, PARRY's suspicious nature was activated by a critical comment from a human user, leading to paranoid, hostile responses as long as its anger remained activated. This emotional state dissipated over time, so long as no more interactions triggered PARRY's suspicion. After dissipating, PARRY's hostility also became quiescent. Thus, PARRY incorporated a psychological model of shame avoidance and projection of hostility. While its programming was limited in comparison with contemporary computer models, PARRY was able to pass a Turing test, insofar as blinded psychiatrists were not able to distinguish scripts of PARRY's interaction with a human from those of a paranoid patient.[53]

PARRY provides clues to psychotherapeutic approaches to PPD. Computational models of BPD have been proposed, based on embodied cognition and its importance in predictive models during online social interactions.[54] Predictive coding models posit that mental activity serves to create a model of the environment based on prior experience; it is the experience of this model that defines and determines human experience. This activity includes perception of the environment through the sensory organs and by the sensory cortex, whose limited informational bandwidth is overcome through bottom-up and top-down predictive modeling, or simulation. Computational models of predictive encoding in psychosis have focused on aberrant prediction error,[55] the difference between observed outcomes of action (such as sampling the sensory environment) and expected, or predicted outcome (what one may expect to perceive in the environment based on past experience). Prediction error is minimized in a well-functioning neural network, based on updating of beliefs based on prior experience. However, prediction error is large in a delusional mind, as reflected in the discrepancy between the erroneous contents of a delusion and the actual state of the world.

A predictive model relevant to PPD would need to be based on social threat, based on a predictive model of intention understanding. One component of the model that has been discussed is hyperarousal (decreased N100 latency and elevated central CRH concentration). It is likely that serotonin signaling has a role in these processes, as evidenced by effects of SSRI medications on the processing of social cues.[56] To account for increased noise, as evidenced by decreased P300 amplitude and impaired working memory, altered striatal dopamine signaling and cortical NMDA receptor function would be included. Such a model would need to account for some of the behavioral responses first put forward by Kenneth Colby's PARRY. Fortunately, psychological models have been developed (see the next section on psychosocial factors).

Psychosocial and Cultural Factors

Psychological models of PPD and paranoia fit nicely into the computational and neurobiological model that we have sketched out. Salmon Akhtar has provided a lucid review of the psychodynamic, meta-psychological literature stressing the difference between the hostile, assertive outward posture of PPD and the internal experience of vulnerability and feared dependency.[57] Freud's conceptualization of paranoia that focused on repressed homosexual impulses has been rejected. However, the theme of suppressed shame in paranoia was carried forward in the object-relations model of a class of disorders characterized by borderline personality organization (BPO).[58] BPO's dimensional system of psychopathology included PPD features along with NPD and BPD features. From the field of cognitive psychology, Aaron Beck described PPD's foundational structure to be a dysfunctional core belief of incompetence, with attendant fears of vulnerability.[59] Jeffrey Young proposed a schema therapy model of PPD. Schemas are patterns of repeated thoughts, behaviors, emotions, and body states that emerge in development in response to environmental demands. In PPD they include schemas of defectiveness/shame, abuse/mistrust, and vulnerability to harm. In response to these, a person responds to the world with an understandable but dysfunctional defensive hostility. In summary, psychological theories of PPD show a high degree of consilience.

Empirical data also support a shame- and avoidance-based theoretical model. Social cognition researchers have found that experimental manipulations of social rank and physical vulnerability increase paranoid ideation.[6] Social vulnerability can cause paranoia. Epidemiological studies have repeatedly reported higher rates of PPD in African American and Native American groups.[60] These higher numbers are entirely accounted for by differences in socioeconomic status and exposure to childhood trauma.[61] Importantly, the elevated paranoia found in African Americans is reflected in the lived experience of black individuals in society, in which experienced racism is correlated with levels of paranoia.[62] It is entirely possible that social and cultural contexts could justify a "healthy paranoia."[63] One such context is income inequality, defined as the relative distribution of resources in a society. The degree of income inequality is correlated with levels of trust of others in society: the states with highest levels of income inequality endorsed the lowest mean levels of trust.[64]

Exposure to childhood trauma has been consistently linked to PPD. Longitudinal studies have linked PPD to parental maltreatment[65] as well as childhood malnutrition.[66] Consistent with the known comorbidity of PPD and PTSD, severe adult traumas are also associated with PPD.[67] These findings strongly suggest that social learning has an important role in the development of PPD, and that this learning may occur both early in life and in adulthood. Given that not all maltreated children and traumatized adults develop PPD, other risk factors are clearly required. These include the cognitive traits found to be associated with PPD, such as neuroticism;[10] impaired working memory;[42] impaired cognitive empathy, or perspective taking;[6] or facets of pathological narcissism.[68] This latter trait deserves special mention. A study using the Pathological Narcissism Inventory found that the severity of delusional ideation was correlated with the Hiding Self subscale. Hiding Self is a component of so-called vulnerable narcissism, which includes endorsements of hiding needs from others, not showing weakness, not relying on other people, and fearing being perceived as weak. Thus, we have returned to the initial psychodynamic models of PPD from contemporary cognitive psychological research, based on an underlying framework of shame, aversion, and interpersonal hypersensitivity.

Transference and Typical Reactions/Countertransference

The interpersonal aspects of PPD, outward hostility and avoidance of closeness, raises challenges to relationships, including treatment relationships. The rigid, habitual cycle of projection and withdrawal is chronic, having been reinforced by psychological traumas, and thus does not disappear with mere reassurance. Clinical encounters are thus expected to be characterized by low levels of trust and, at times, high levels of hostility.

Clinicians find themselves to be swiftly recruited into a supporting role in the internal drama of the PPD patient. This difficulty is described by projective identification, a meta-psychological theory accounting for predetermined countertransference reactions. In PPD, the projected identification on the therapist would be the hostile, persecutory other. According to this theory, the therapist may find him- or herself enacting alien, aggressive, or rejecting impulses. Some support for the aversive nature of countertransference in PPD has been demonstrated empirically in a study using the Therapist Response Questionnaire. In this study of 148 clinicians, they tended to characterize their reaction to PPD cases with a feeling of helplessness.[69] One must wonder if the helplessness that these clinicians noticed arises from frustration with being forced to identify with the projected hostile introjects, or something simpler: feeling left out of a closed system.

An alternative perspective on PPD's interpersonal dynamics comes from behavioral/reinforcement-learning theory. The conditioned avoidance response (CAR) is a rewarded escape response, conditioned by the escape, or avoidance, of an aversive unconditioned stimulus. Two properties of the CAR make it intriguing in the context of PPD: Escape conditioning relies on dopamine signaling, and it is highly resistant to extinction. The close comorbidity relationship between PPD and PTSD, as well as the developmental history of PPD, supports the validity of the CAR as a model of PPD.[6] In this framework, the individual with PPD, conditioned to expect punishment in relationships and rewarded to escape even the possibility of it, would be expected to automatically avoid the formation of a therapeutic relationship. This framework may help to explain why a long and/or intensive treatment course is likely necessary to treat PPD. It would also stress the importance of exposure-based learning in the therapeutic process.

Case Formulation and Diagnosis

Case formulation of PPD is best done in the framework of trauma-informed care (TIC). The biological findings, empirical data, and models of psychopathology reinforce the need to view PPD symptoms in the context of social learning. The clinician should take a long view of how a patient's once-adaptive response to social interaction is now incompatible with relationships and living. Cases of PPD in the TIC framework should be considered in the light of structural violence, the need to avoid retraumatizing clients who are alert to potential threats, the necessity to provide effective treatment of PTSD when needed, and, finally, as we have made a case for in this chapter, a sufficiently rich description of PPD to allow for treatment planning.

In our experience as clinicians and consultants on cases of PPD, the challenge of identification and diagnosis is real. However, when the diagnosis is missed, it is not due to ignorance. Rather, clinicians and teams can be so persuasively and quickly committed to reacting to the tough exterior of the PPD case that, in a state of distraction, they may fail to screen for it. Unfortunately, expertise is not sufficient to escape this process, as evidenced by the authors' own experience and analysis of post-hoc diagnoses of PPD made in even rigorous treatment and evaluation programs.[70] Fortunately, after screening, diagnosis is fairly straightforward, because the DSM-5 diagnostic criteria are monothetic.

Treatment

Synthesis of the available data leads to these recommendations regarding the overall approach to patients with PPD. Assessment is extremely important, particularly identification of comorbid treatable conditions such as PTSD, BPD, and IED. Proper screening, leading to early diagnosis, is the best hope to delay or prevent dropout from treatment. Medications, when provided, are off label for PPD, or prescribed for comorbid conditions. When off label, specific consent should be documented. Informed consent must disclose potential side effects, such as metabolic syndrome in the case of antipsychotic medications. Low-dose antipsychotic medications or SSRIs would be justifiable for severe cases, but the treatment course need not be long, especially if the patient sees little or no benefit from it. Beneficial effects are likely to be seen if there is prominent anger or aggression. However, psychotherapy is likely to be the approach that makes the largest impact. Trauma-focused, cognitive-behavioral therapy (CBT) for PTSD is likely to have the largest impact in cases with comorbid PTSD and PPD. Thoughtful adaptation of DBT, mentalization-based treatment (MBT), transference-focused psychotherapy, or schema therapy to the treatment of PPD is likely to be of some benefit, but requires considerable expertise. Next, we will explore some of these recommendations in greater detail.

Treatment planning using the TIC framework should take into account what is known about the patterns of treatment response observed in PPD patients. PPD sufferers are more likely than other personality-disorder cases, such as BPD, to drop out from intensive outpatient treatments.[71] Based on these experiences, clinicians may assume that patients with PPD are untreatable. However, such a pessimistic view should be tempered by data showing change in PPD symptoms over time. It is known that PPD traits decline substantially (46 percent) from adolescence to early adulthood.[72] As reviewed in this chapter, "remission" from PPD is reported even when treatment is targeting comorbid conditions such as PTSD.[29] Because PPD can adversely affect the treatment outcome of comorbid conditions such as eating disorder,[73] consideration of how PPD fits into the constellation of comorbid disorders is warranted.

Psychotherapy

Definitive randomized controlled trials targeting PPD are lacking. However, data from studies of existing evidence-based treatments of personality disorder are relevant to PPD.

Dialectical Behavioral Therapy

DBT is effective at reducing impulsive suicidality in BPD. However, individuals with PPD have lower levels of suicidality and impulsivity[6] and are cognitively rigid. Lynch and Cheavens have proposed an adaptation of DBT, radically open (RO) DBT, to address cognitive rigidity that characterizes non-BPD conditions such as PPD.[74] Their study includes description of a successful course of treatment in an individual with PPD and obsessive-compulsive personality disorder. DBT was modified to target the conditioned avoidance response. This included additional modules involving brief, in vivo exposure to criticism and feedback with the therapist, combined with skills training in opposition to an emotional action urge. Instead of escape and avoidance, "talking it out" with the therapist is practiced, thus countering the natural inclination of the patient to maintain maximal distance from the therapist. Exposures were brief (1–5 minutes) and relied on overt praise and encouragement of the client to reward participation. In vivo exposures included: confiding in others; increasing prosocial behaviors; noticing others' judgments and letting them go; and participating in activities that could evoke judgment. This treatment course was successful, with the client in remission from both PPD and obsessive-compulsive personality disorder at the end of treatment. RO DBT has been found to effective for personality disorder in a comparative trial.[75] At post-treatment and six-month measures, improvements were seen in interpersonal sensitivity and interpersonal aggression, as well as PPD-relevant traits such as decreased openness, cognitive rigidity, inhibited emotional expression, and aloof/distant relationships.

Schema Therapy

Cognitive-behavioral therapy-based approaches to PPD have been proposed,[59] but empirical data is lacking. Schema therapy is an adaptation of CBT for personality disorder. A comparative trial of schema therapy versus treatment as usual and clarification-oriented psychotherapy for personality disorder found that schema therapy was superior to these two alternatives with respect to recovery rate, and social and occupational functioning.[76] Although data specifically regarding PPD were not described, a comparison of schema therapy versus transference-focused psychotherapy found that schema therapy was more effective at reducing paranoid ideation.[77] One particularly appealing aspect of schema therapy for personality disorder is the degree to which the client is an informed, active participant in treatment and treatment formulation. These attributes are consistent with the growing emphasis on person-centered care. Although no reports regarding transference-focused psychotherapy (TFP) and PPD are yet available, a case description of a TFP treatment of a client with comorbid NPD and BPD, with some paranoid features, found that the approach increased reflective function, or mentalizing,[33] with emerging reflective concern about aggressive or negative feelings rather than habitual projections of them.

Mentalization-based Treatment

Many of the features of PPD are consistent with a hypermentalizing profile as described in MBT. Indeed, MBT has been applied to the treatment of psychotic delusions, targeting epistemic mistrust.[78] A blinded randomized control trial (RCT) of non-affective psychosis found equivocal results, although some improvement with MBT relative to control was seen at six months post-treatment.[79]

Pharmacotherapy

No double-blind, randomized controlled trials of any medications have been reported for PPD. No medications have regulatory approval. Given the confirmed relevance of the dopamine D2 receptor in schizophrenia,[80] antipsychotic medications could be a plausible approach. Risperidone has been found to have some beneficial effects in schizotypal personality disorder in a small, pilot RCT.[81] In a retrospective review of 15 consecutive cases of PPD, Clinical Global Impression (CGI) score was used to evaluate the effects of antipsychotic treatment in four patients who received flupentixol, bromperidol, or promazine compared with six patients who did not.[82] The mean treatment was for 15 weeks. At six weeks, the mean CGI of the four patients on antipsychotic medications decreased from 5.5 to 1.8, while the mean CGI of the six patients not on antipsychotic medications increased from 4.0 to 4.8. At 15-week follow-up, one of the four patients on antipsychotic medications worsened, while the other three remained improved. These results suggest that antipsychotic medications may be of some benefit for severe cases in the short term, though it is not clear how long such benefits last.

Serotonergic neuromodulation plays an important role in social cognition,[83] and thus it is biologically plausible that serotonin modulators could be beneficial in PPD. No rigorous RCTs of SSRIs in PPD have been conducted. Secondary analysis of studies of SSRIs have found some positive effects. In patients with depression and comorbid personality disorder, sertraline and citalopram treatment were found to be associated with both remission from PPD and significant decrease in the severity of PPD symptoms.[84] This evidence is consistent with the positive effects of SSRI treatment with fluoxetine on irritability and verbal aggression in adults with personality disorder, many of whom had comorbid PPD.[85] Benzodiazepines have not been studied in PPD. It is difficult to make predictions about their efficacy or toxicity. Given their propensity to worsen PTSD[86] and BPD,[87] two of the most common comorbidities of PPD, it seems unlikely that they would be of benefit. Benzodiazepines may be expected to aggravate the conditioned avoidant response in PPD.[88] Thus, it seems unlikely that benzodiazepines would be helpful in the treatment of PPD. A summary of the evidence for effective diagnosis and treatment is given in Box 16.1.

Box 16.1 Effectiveness of Treatment

- Antipsychotic medications have been proposed based on their efficacy for psychotic delusions and disease-level inference. A single open-label case series shows short term improvement in PPD patients; no blinded RCT data is available. Level of evidence C.
- SSRI medications are of interest based on disease-level inference and positive data for SSRIs in aggression and comorbid condition. Meta-analytic data reveals positive effects of SSRI medications on PPD-related symptoms. Level of evidence B.
- DBT is effective at treating BPD symptoms of anger and suicidality and is considered the gold standard treatment of personality disorder. Adaptation of DBT (Radically Open DBT) has been reported for PPD and related traits, but not yet studied in a rigorous RCT. Level of evidence B.
- MBT, ST, and TFP: The rationale for these treatments in PPD is quite strong, as both treatments are based on dimensional views of personality disorder that include components of PPD. Analysis of secondary data and from case reports provide indirect evidence of the efficacy of these psychotherapies for PPD. Level of evidence C.

Key: Levels of Evidence; Strength of recommendation taxonomy (SORT)*
Level of Evidence A: Good quality patient-oriented evidence.
Level of Evidence B: Limited quality patient-oriented evidence.
Level of Evidence C: Based on consensus, usual practice, opinion, disease-oriented evidence, or case series for studies of diagnosis.
*Ebell MH, Siwek J, Weiss BD, Woolf SH, Susman J, Ewigman B, Bowman M. Simplifying the language of evidence to improve patient care. *J Fam Pract*. 2004 Feb 1;53(2):111–120.

Box 16.2 Resources for Patients, Families, and Clinicians

Paranoid Personality Disorder Diagnosis

- Made of Millions website: https://www.madeofmillions.com/conditions/ paranoid-personality-disorder.
- Psychology Today website: https://www.psychologytoday.com/us/conditions/paranoid-personality-disorder.

Getting Help for Paranoid Personality

- Goodtherapy website: https://www.goodtherapy.org/learn-about-therapy/ issues/paranoid-personality/get-help.

Conclusion

PPD remains a compelling construct to understand. A review of the still-gathering evidence provides a portrait of a disorder that seems obscure, but in fact is more familiar than expected. Its superficial similarity to schizophrenia belies its true relationships with trauma and stress-related problems. Viewing PPD in this way brings into focus a coherent epidemiological, neurobiological, and psychological literature. The dimensional nature of PPD, and limitations of its categorical description, have limited opportunities to study it in rigorous clinical trials. However, PPD is positioned well in the pivot toward a dimensional diagnostic system. Coherence between theoretical models of PPD provide a plausible starting point for adaptation of personality disorder–specific psychotherapies that have shown to be effective for other disorders. Review Box 16.2 for resources for patients, families, and clinicians about PPD.

Conflict of Interest/Disclosure: The authors of this chapter have no financial conflicts and nothing to disclose.

References

1. Zimmerman M, Chelminski I, Young D, Dalrymple K, Martinez J. Impact of deleting 5 DSM-IV personality disorders on prevalence, comorbidity, and the association between personality disorder pathology and psychosocial morbidity. *J Clin Psychiatry*. 2012;73(2):202–207. doi:10.4088/jcp.11m07140

2. Akhtar S. Paranoid personality disorder: a synthesis of developmental, dynamic, and descriptive features. *Am J Psychother*. 1990;44(1):5–25. doi:10.1176/appi.psychotherapy.1990.44.1.5

3. Telles-Correia D, Marques JG. Melancholia before the twentieth century: fear and sorrow or partial insanity? *Front Psychol*. 03 February 2015;6:81. doi:10.3389/fpsyg.2015.00081

4. Abbasi Y, Omrani A. Mental health problems: journey from Baghdad to Europe. *Int Psychiatry*. 2013;10(04):100–101. doi:10.1192/s1749367600004094

5. Maj M. Karl Jaspers and the genesis of delusions in schizophrenia. *Schizophr Bull*. 2013 Mar;39(2):242–243. doi:10.1093/schbul/sbs190

6. Lee R. Mistrustful and misunderstood: a review of paranoid personality disorder. *Curr Behav Neurosci Reports*. 2017;4:151–165. doi:10.1007/s40473-017-0116-7

7. Esbec E, Echeburúa E. Violence and personality disorders: clinical and forensic implications. *Actas Esp Psiquiatr*. 2010;38(5):249–261.

8. Grant B, Hasin D, Stinson F, et al. Prevalence, correlates, and disability of personality disorders in the United States: results from the National Epidemiologic Survey on Alcohol and Related Conditions. *J Clin Psychiatry*. 2004;65(7):948–958. doi:10.4088/jcp.v65n0711

9. Lee RJ. Mistrustful and misunderstood: A review of paranoid personality disorder. *Curr Behav Neurosci Reports* 2017 Jun;4(2):151–165. doi:10.1007/s40473-017-0116-7

10. Bernstein D, Useda J. Paranoid personality disorder. In W O'Donohue, KA Fowler, SO Libenfeld, eds., *Personality Disorders: Toward the DSM–V*. New York: Sage; 2007.

11. Kendler K, Heath A, Martin N. A genetic epidemiologic study of self-report suspiciousness. *Compr Psychiatry*. 1987;28(3):187–196. doi:10.1016/0010-440x(87)90026-5.

12. Carroll A. Are you looking at me? Understanding and managing paranoid personality disorder. *Adv Psychiatr Treat*. 2009;15(1):40–48. doi:10.1192/apt.bp.107.005421

13. Coid JW, Ullrich S, Bebbington P, Fazel S, Keers R. Paranoid ideation and violence: meta-analysis of individual subject data of 7 population surveys. *Schizophr Bull*. 2016;42(4):907–915. doi:10.1093/schbul/sbw006

14. Bouthier M, Mahé V. [Paranoid personality disorder and criminal offense]. *Encephale*. 2019;45(2):162–168. doi:10.1016/j.encep.2018.07.005

15. Ghahramanlou-Holloway M, Lee-Tauler SY, LaCroix JM, et al. Dysfunctional personality disorder beliefs and lifetime suicide attempts among psychiatrically hospitalized military personnel. *Compr Psychiatry*. 2018;82:108–114. doi:10.1016/j.comppsych.2018.01.010

16. American Psychiatric Association. *Diagnostic and Statistical Manual of Mental Disorders*. Washington, DC: American Psychiatric Association; 1952.

17. O'Donohue W, Fowler KA, Lilienfeld SO. *Personality Disorders: Toward the DSM-V.*; New York: Sage; 2007. doi:10.4135/9781483328980

18. American Psychiatric Association. *Diagnostic and Statistical Manual of Mental Disorders*. 2nd ed., text rev. Washington, DC: American Psychiatric Association; 1968.

19. American Psychiatric Association. *Diagnostic and Statistical Manual of Mental Disorders*. 3rd ed., text rev. Washington, DC: American Psychiatric Association; 1980.

20. American Psychiatric Association. *Diagnostic and Statistical Manual of Mental Disorders (DSM-IV)*. Washington, DC: American Psychiatric Association; 2000.

21. American Psychiatric Association. *Diagnostic and Statistical Manual of Mental Disorders (DSM 5)*. Washington, DC: American Psychiatric Association; 2013. doi:10.1176/appi.books.9780890425596.744053

22. Perry C, Lee R. Childhood trauma in personality disorders. In: Spalletta G, Janiri D, F P, Sani G, eds. *Childhood Trauma in Mental Disorders*. Switzerland AG: Springer Nature; 2020.

23. Yun RJ, Stern BL, Lenzenweger MF, Tiersky LA. Refining personality disorder subtypes and classification using finite mixture modeling. *Personal Disord Theory, Res Treat*. 2013;4(2):121–128. doi:10.1037/a0029944

24. Triebwasser J, Chemerinski E, Roussos P, Siever LJ. Paranoid personality disorder. *J Pers Disord*. 2013;27(6):795–805. doi:10.1521/pedi_2012_26_055

25. Falkum E, Pedersen G, Karterud S. Diagnostic and Statistical Manual of Mental Disorders, Fourth Edition, paranoid personality disorder diagnosis: a unitary or a two-dimensional construct? *Compr Psychiatry*. 2009;50(6):533–541. doi:10.1016/j.comppsych.2009.01.003

26. Dunn NJ, Yanasak E, Schillaci J, et al. Personality disorders in veterans with post-traumatic stress disorder and depression. *J Trauma Stress*. 2004;17(1):75–82. doi:10.1023/B:JOTS.0000014680.54051.50

27. Tsai J, Harpaz-Rotem I, Pilver CE, et al. Latent class analysis of personality disorders in adults with posttraumatic stress disorder: results from the National Epidemiologic Survey on Alcohol and Related Conditions. *J Clin Psychiatry*. 2014;75(3):276–284. doi:10.4088/JCP.13m08466

28. Golier JA, Yehuda R, Bierer LM, et al. The relationship of borderline personality disorder to posttraumatic stress disorder and traumatic events. *Am J Psychiatry*. 2013;160(11):2018–2024. doi:10.1176/appi.ajp.160.11.2018

29. Markowitz JC, Petkova E, Biyanova T, Ding K, Suh EJ, Neria Y. Exploring personality diagnosis stability following acute psychotherapy for chronic posttraumatic stress disorder. *Depress Anxiety*. 2015;32(12):919–926. doi:10.1002/da.22436

30. Gómez-Beneyto M, Salazar-Fraile J, Martí-Sanjuan V, Gonzalez-Luján L. Posttraumatic stress disorder in primary care with special reference to personality disorder comorbidity. *Br J Gen Pract*. 2006;56(526):349–354.

31. Morey LC. Personality disorders in DSM-III and DSM-III-R: convergence, coverage, and internal consistency. *Am J Psychiatry*. 1988;145(5):573–577.

32. Muñoz-Negro JE, Prudent C, Gutiérrez B, Cervilla JA. Paranoia and risk of personality disorder in the general population. *Personal Ment Health*. 2019;13(2):107–116. doi:10.1002/pmh.1443

33. Diamond D, Yeomans FE, Stern B, et al. Transference focused psychotherapy for patients with comorbid narcissistic and borderline personality disorder. *Psychoanal Inq*. 2013;33(6):527–551. doi:10.1080/07351690.2013.815087

34. Kernberg OF. Factors in the psychoanalytic treatment of narcissistic personalities. *J Am Psychoanal Assoc*. 1970;18(1):51–85. doi:10.1177/000306517001800103

35. Berman ME, Fallon AE, Coccaro EF. The relationship between personality psychopathology and aggressive behavior in research volunteers. *J Abnorm Psychol*. 1998;107(4):651–658. doi:10.1037/0021-843X.107.4.651

36. Czajkowski N, Aggen SH, Krueger RF, et al. A twin study of normative personality and DSM-IV personality disorder criterion counts: evidence for separate genetic influences. *Am J Psychiatry*. 2018;175(7):649–656. doi:10.1176/appi.ajp.2017.17050493

37. Webb CT, Levinson DF. Schizotypal and paranoid personality disorder in the relatives of patients with schizophrenia and affective disorders: a review. *Schizophr Res*. 1993;11(1):81–92. doi:10.1016/0920-9964(93)90041-g

38. Tienari P, Wynne LC, Läksy K, et al. Genetic boundaries of the schizophrenia spectrum: evidence from the Finnish adoptive family study of schizophrenia. *Am J Psychiatry*. 2003;160(9):1587–1594. doi:10.1176/appi.ajp.160.9.1587

39. Hans SL, Auerbach JG, Styr B, et al. Offspring of parents with schizophrenia: mental disorders during childhood and adolescence. *Schizophr Bull*. 2004;30(2):303–315. doi:10.1093/oxfordjournals.schbul.a007080

30. Kendler KS, McGuire M, Gruenberg AM, O'Hare A, Spellman M, Walsh D. The Roscommon family study. III. Schizophrenia-related personality disorders in relatives. *Arch Gen Psychiatry*. 1993;50(10):781–788. doi:10.1001/archpsyc.1993.01820220033004

41. Winokur G. Familial psychopathology in delusional disorder. *Compr Psychiatry*. 1985;26(3):241–248. doi:10.1016/0010-440X(85)90069-0

42. Haghighatfard A, Andalib S, Amini Faskhodi M, et al. Gene expression study of mitochondrial complex I in schizophrenia and paranoid personality disorder. *World J Biol Psychiatry*. 2018;19(sup3):S133–S146. doi:10.1080/15622975.2017.1282171

43. Liu Y, Shen X, Zhu Y, et al. Mismatch negativity in paranoid, schizotypal, and antisocial personality disorders. *Neurophysiol Clin*. 2007;37(2):89–96. doi:10.1016/j.neucli.2007.03.001

44. Doustkam M, Pourheidari S, Mansouri A. Interpretation bias towards vague faces in individuals with paranoid personality disorder traits. *J Fundam Ment Heal*. 2017;19(6):437–442. doi:10.22038/jfmh.2017.9550

45. Lee RJ, Gollan J, Kasckow J, Geracioti T, Coccaro EF. CSF corticotropin-releasing factor in personality disorder: relationship with self-reported parental care. *Neuropsychopharmacology*. 2006;31(10):2289–2295. doi:10.1038/sj.npp.1301104

46. Gelernter J, Sun N, Polimanti R, et al. Genome-wide association study of post-traumatic stress disorder reexperiencing symptoms in >165,000 US veterans. *Nat Neurosci*. 2019;22(9):1394–1401. doi:10.1038/s41593-019-0447-7

47. Lee RJ, Hempel J, TenHarmsel A, Liu T, Mathé AA, Klock A. The neuroendocrinology of childhood trauma in personality disorder. *Psychoneuroendocrinology*. 2012;37(1):78–86. doi:10.1016/j.psyneuen.2011.05.006

48. Perchtold CM, Weiss EM, Rominger C, Fink A, Weber H, Papousek I. Cognitive reappraisal capacity mediates the relationship between prefrontal recruitment during reappraisal of anger-eliciting events and paranoia-proneness. *Brain Cogn*. 2019;132:108–117. doi:https://doi.org/10.1016/j.bandc.2019.04.001

49. Lee RJ, Gozal D, Coccaro EF, Fanning J. Narcissistic and borderline personality disorders: relationship with oxidative stress. *J Pers Disord*. 2020;34(Supplement):6–24. doi:10.1521/pedi.2020.34.supp.6

50. Wang Q, Liu G, Li J, et al. Effects of interaction of NOS1AP gene polymorphisms and childhood abuse on paranoid personality disorder features among male violent offenders in China. *J Psychiatr Res*. 2020;130:180–186. doi:10.1016/j.jpsychires.2020.07.026

51. Khan A, Plana-Ripoll O, Antonsen S, et al. Environmental pollution is associated with increased risk of psychiatric disorders in the US and Denmark. *PLOS Biol*. 2019;17(8):e3000353.

52. Colby KM. Modeling a paranoid mind. *Behav Brain Sci*. 1981;4(4):515–560. doi:10.1017/S0140525X00000169

53. Colby KM, Hilf FD, Weber S, Kraemer HC. Turing-like indistinguishability tests for the validation of a computer simulation of paranoid processes. *Artif Intell*. 1972;3:199–221. doi:10.1016/0004-3702(72)90049-5

54. Fineberg SK, Stahl D, Corlett P. Computational psychiatry in borderline personality disorder. *Curr Behav Neurosci reports*. 2017;4(1):31–40. doi:10.1007/s40473-017-0104-y

55. Sterzer P, Adams RA, Fletcher P, et al. The predictive coding account of psychosis. *Biological Psychiatry*. 2018 Nov 1;84(9):634–643. doi:10.1016/j.biopsych.2018.05.015

56. Harmer CJ, Bhagwagar Z, Perrett DI, Völlm BA, Cowen PJ, Goodwin GM. Acute SSRI administration affects the rrocessing of social cues in healthy volunteers. *Neuropsychopharmacology*. 2003;28(1):148–152. doi:10.1038/sj.npp.1300004

57. Akhtar S. Paranoid personality disorder: a synthesis of developmental, dynamic, and descriptive features. *Am J Psychother*. 1990;XLIV(1):5–25.

58. Kernberg O. Borderline personality organization. *J Am Psychoanal Assoc*. 1967;15(3):641–685. doi:10.1177/000306516701500309

59. Beck AT, Butler AC, Brown GK, Dahlsgaard KK, Newman CF, Beck JS. Dysfunctional beliefs discriminate personality disorders. *Behav Res Ther.* 2001;39(10):1213–1225. doi:10.1016/S0005-7967(00)00099-1

60. Grant BF, Hasin DS, Stinson FS, et al. Prevalence, correlates, and disability of personality disorders in the United States: results from the National Epidemiologic Survey on Alcohol and Related Conditions. *J Clin Psychiatry.* 2004;65(7):948–958. doi:10.4088/JCP.v65n0711

61. Iacovino JM, Jackson JJ, Oltmanns TF. The relative impact of socioeconomic status and childhood trauma on black-white differences in paranoid personality disorder symptoms. *J Abnorm Psychol.* 2014;123(1):225–230. doi:10.1037/a0035258

62. Combs DR. Perceived racism as a predictor of paranoia among African Americans. *J Black Psychol.* 2006;32(1):87–104. doi:10.1177/0095798405283175

63. Mosley DV, Owen KH, Rostosky SS, Reese RJ. Contextualizing behaviors associated with paranoia: perspectives of Black men. *Psychol Men Masc.* 2017;18(2):165–175. doi:10.1037/men0000052

64. NORC. *General Social Survey.* Chicago. https://gss.norc.org/

65. Johnson JG, Cohen P, Brown J, Smailes E, Bernstein DP. Childhood maltreatment increases risk for personality disorders during early adulthood. *Arch Gen Psychiatry.* 1999;56(7):600–606. doi:10.1001/archpsyc.56.7.600

66. Hock RS, Bryce CP, Fischer L, et al. Childhood malnutrition and maltreatment are linked with personality disorder symptoms in adulthood: results from a Barbados lifespan cohort. *Psychiatry Res.* 2018;269:301–308. doi:10.1016/j.psychres.2018.05.085

67. Munjiza J, Britvic D, Crawford MJ. Lasting personality pathology following exposure to severe trauma in adulthood: retrospective cohort study. *BMC Psychiatry.* 2019;19(1):3. doi:10.1186/s12888-018-1975-5

68. Tonna M, Paglia F, Ottoni R, Ossola P, De Panfilis C, Marchesi C. Delusional disorder: the role of personality and emotions on delusional ideation. *Compr Psychiatry.* 2018;85:78–83. doi:10.1016/j.comppsych.2018.07.002

69. Gazzillo F, Lingiardi V, Del Corno F, et al. Clinicians' emotional responses and Psychodynamic Diagnostic Manual adult personality disorders: a clinically relevant empirical investigation. *Psychotherapy.* 2015;52(2):238–246. doi:10.1037/a0038799

70. Oldham JM, Skodol A. Do patients with paranoid personality disorder seek psychoanalysis? In: Oldham, JM, Bone, S, eds. *Paranoia: New Psychoanalytic Perspectives.* Madison and Connecticut: International Universities Press; 1994:151–166.

71. Karterud S, Pedersen G, Bjordal E, et al. Day treatment of patients with personality disorders: experiences from a Norwegian treatment research network. *J Pers Disord.* 2003;17(3):243–262. doi:10.1521/pedi.17.3.243.22151

72. Johnson JG, Cohen P, Kasen S, Skodol AE, Hamagami F, Brook JS. Age-related change in personality disorder trait levels between early adolescence and adulthood: a community-based longitudinal investigation. *Acta Psychiatr Scand.* 2000;102(35):265–275. doi:10.1034/j.1600-0447.2000.102004265.x

73. Muzi L, Tieghi L, Rugo MA, Lingiardi V. Personality as a predictor of symptomatic change in a residential treatment setting for anorexia nervosa and bulimia nervosa. *Eat Weight Disord.* 2021;26:1195–1209. doi:10.1007/s40519-020-01023-1

74. Lynch TR, Cheavens JS. Dialectical behavior therapy for comorbid personality disorders. *J Clin Psychol.* 2008;64(2):154–167. doi:10.1002/jclp.20449

75. Lynch TR, Cheavens JS, Cukrowicz KC, Thorp SR, Bronner L, Beyer J. Treatment of older adults with co-morbid personality disorder and depression: a dialectical behavior therapy approach. *Int J Geriatr Psychiatry.* 2007;22(2):131–143. doi:10.1002/gps.1703

76. Bamelis LLM, Evers SMAA, Spinhoven P, Arntz A. Results of a multicenter randomized controlled trial of the clinical effectiveness of schema therapy for personality disorders. *Am J Psychiatry.* 2014;171(3):305–322. doi:10.1176/appi.ajp.2013.12040518

77. Giesen-Bloo J, Van Dyck R, Spinhoven P, et al. Outpatient psychotherapy for borderline personality disorder: randomized trial of schema-focused therapy vs. transference-focused psychotherapy. *Arch Gen Psychiatry.* 2006;63(6):649–658. doi:10.1001/archpsyc.63.6.649

78. Weijers JG, ten Kate C, Debbané M, et al. Mentalization and psychosis: a rationale for the use of mentalization theory to understand and treat non-affective psychotic disorder. *J Contemp Psychother.* 2020;50(3):223–232. doi:10.1007/s10879-019-09449-0

79. Weijers J, Ten Kate C, Viechtbauer W, Rampaart LJA, Eurelings EHM, Selten JP. Mentalization-based treatment for psychotic disorder: a rater-blinded, multi-center, randomized controlled trial. *Psychol Med.* 29 May 2020:1–10. doi: 10.1017/S0033291720001506

80. Ripke S, Neale BM, Corvin A, et al. Biological insights from 108 schizophrenia-associated genetic loci. *Nature.* 2014;511(7510):421–427. doi:10.1038/nature13595

81. Koenigsberg HW, Reynolds D, Goodman M, et al. Risperidone in the treatment of schizotypal personality disorder. *J Clin Psychiatry.* 2003;64(6):628–634. doi:10.4088/jcp.v64n0602

82. Birkeland SF. Psychopharmacological treatment and course in paranoid personality disorder: a case series. *Int Clin Psychopharmacol.* 2013;28(5):283–285. doi:10.1097/YIC.0b013e328363f676

83. Coccaro EF, Lee RJ. 5-HT2c agonist, lorcaserin, reduces aggressive responding in intermittent explosive disorder: A pilot study. *Hum Psychopharmacol Clin Exp.* 2019;34(6):e2714. doi:10.1002/hup.2714

84. Ekselius L, von Knorring L. Personality disorder comorbidity with major depression and response to treatment with sertraline or citalopram. *Int Clin Psychopharmacol.* 1998;13(5):205–211. doi:10.1097/00004850-199809000-00003

85. Coccaro EF, Lee RJ, Kavoussi RJ. A double-blind, randomized, placebo-controlled trial of fluoxetine in patients with intermittent explosive disorder. *J Clin Psychiatry.* 2009 Apr 21;70(5):653–662. doi:10.4088/JCP.08m04150

86. Guina J, Rossetter SR, Derhodes BJ, Nahhas RW, Welton RS. Benzodiazepines for PTSD: a systematic review and meta-analysis. *J Psychiatr Pract.* 2015;21:281–303. doi:10.1097/PRA.0000000000000091

87. Cowdry RW, Gardner DL. Pharmacotherapy of borderline personality disorder. Alprazolam, carbamazepine, trifluoperazine, and tranylcypromine. *Arch Gen Psychiatry.* 1988;45(2):111–119. doi:10.1001/archpsyc.1988.01800260015002

88. Li M, He W, Mead A. An investigation of the behavioral mechanisms of antipsychotic action using a drug-drug conditioning paradigm. *Behav Pharmacol.* 2009;20(2):184–194. doi:10.1097/FBP.0b013e32832a8f66

17

Some Thoughts about Schizoid Dynamics

Nancy McWilliams

Key Points

- This chapter discusses inferential, phenomenologically oriented psychoanalytic understanding of schizoid issues. It is not on schizoid personality disorder.
- People with significant schizoid tendencies are more common than is typically thought and run the gamut from psychotically disturbed to enviably robust.
- Mental health professionals have had a tendency to equate the schizoid with the mentally primitive, and the primitive with the insane, which is often not the case.
- The term "schizoid" refers to the complex intrapsychic life of the introverted individual, rather than to a preference for introspection and solitary pursuits, which are more or less surface phenomena.
- Highest-functioning "schizoid" people are often found in the arts, the theoretical sciences, psychoanalysis, and the philosophical and spiritual disciplines. They can often times be much healthier in every meaningful respect (life satisfaction, sense of agency, affect regulation, self and object constancy, personal relationships, and creativity) than those with neurotic psychologies.
- The psychoanalytic use of the term "schizoid" derives from the observations of "schisms" between the internal life (a deep longing for closeness and compelling fantasies of intimate involvement) and the externally observable life (overtly detached and self-sufficient).
- Schizoid versions of personality structure are characterized by a constitutionally sensitive temperament, and feelings of hyperpermeability, both noticeable from birth and influenced by a genetic disposition.
- The painful experiences of patients with a schizoid personality structure may have been repeatedly disconfirmed by caregivers who, if their temperament differs from that of their children, cannot identify with their acute sensitivities and consequently treat them with impatience, exasperation, and even scorn.
- Because schizoid individuals tend to feel safe with comparatively few others, any threat to or loss of their connection with the people with whom they do feel comfortable can be devastating.
- A common precipitant of a schizoid person's seeking treatment is loss.
- Schizoid individuals can be remarkably attuned to unconscious primal thoughts, feelings, impulses, and nonverbal processes in others.
- Schizoid people tend to feel connected with their surroundings, or a oneness with the universe, in a profound and interpenetrating way.

- The schizoid–hysterical romance is based on admiration and idealization of traits in each other.
- A hysterically organized woman idealizes the capacity of the schizoid man to stand alone, to "speak truth to power," contain affect, and tap into levels of creative imagination that she can only dream of. The schizoid man admires her warmth, comfort with others, empathy, grace in expressing emotion without awkwardness or shame, and capacity to experience her own creativity in a relationship.
- See Box 17.1, p. 454 for the therapeutic implications for the treatment of schizoid individuals.

Reprinted with permission (with minor formatting revisions): McWilliams, N. (2006). Some thoughts about schizoid dynamics. *The Psychoanalytic Review*. 93(1): 1–24.

Introduction

For many years, I have been trying to develop a fuller understanding of the subjectivities of individuals with schizoid psychologies. I am not referring to the type of schizoid personality disorder that appears in descriptive psychiatric taxonomies like the *Diagnostic and Statistical Manual of Mental Disorders*,[1] but to the more inferential, phenomenologically oriented, psychoanalytic understanding of schizoid issues. I have always been more interested in exploring individual differences than in arguing about what is and is not pathology. I have found that when individuals with schizoid dynamics—whether patients, colleagues, or personal friends—sense that their disclosures will not be disdained or "criminalized" (Barbara Nicholls, personal communication, Jun 16, 2004), they are willing to share with me a lot about their inner world. As is true in many other realms, when one becomes open to seeing something, one sees it everywhere.

I have come to believe that people with significant schizoid tendencies are more common than is typically thought, and that there is a range of mental and emotional health in such people that runs from psychotically disturbed to enviably robust. Although I have become persuaded that schizoid individuals do not have "neurotic-level" conflicts,[2] the highest-functioning schizoid people, of whom there are many, seem much healthier in every meaningful respect (life satisfaction, sense of agency, affect regulation, self and object constancy, personal relationships, and creativity) than many people with certifiably neurotic psychologies. Although the Jungian concept of "introversion" is perhaps a less stigmatizing term, I prefer "schizoid" because it implicitly refers to the complex intrapsychic life of the introverted individual, rather than to a preference for introspection and solitary pursuits, which are more or less surface phenomena.

One of the reasons that mental health professionals often don't notice the existence of high-level schizoid psychology is that many people with schizoid dynamics hide, or "pass," among nonschizoid others. Not only does their psychology involve a kind of allergy to being the object of someone else's intrusive gaze, they have learned to fear that they will be exposed as "weird" or "crazy." Given that nonschizoid observers tend to attribute pathology to people who are more reclusive and eccentric than they are, the schizoid person's fears of being scrutinized and found abnormal or less-than-sane are realistic. In addition, some schizoid people worry about their own sanity, whether or not they have ever lost it. Their fears of being categorized as "psychotic" may constitute the projection of a conviction that their inner experience is so private, unrecognized, unmirrored, and intolerable to others that their isolation equates with madness.

Many nonprofessionals regard schizoid people as peculiar and incomprehensible. But to add insult to injury, mental health professionals have had a tendency to equate the schizoid with the mentally primitive, and the primitive with the insane. Melanie Klein's[3] brilliant understanding of the "paranoid-schizoid position" as the precursor of the capacity to comprehend the separateness of others (the "depressive position") has contributed to this belief, as has the general tendency in the field to see developmentally earlier phenomena as inherently "immature" or "archaic."[4] In addition, we have tended to suspect schizoid personality manifestations as being possible precursors of a schizophrenic psychosis. Behaviors common in schizoid personality can certainly mimic the early stages of schizophrenic withdrawal. Adolescents who begin to spend more and more time in their rooms and in their fantasy lives and eventually become frankly psychotic are a familiar clinical phenomenon. And schizoid personality and schizophrenia may, in fact, be cousins: Recent research into the schizophrenic disorders has identified genetic dispositions that can be manifested anywhere on a broad spectrum from severe schizophrenia to normal schizoid personality.[5] (On the other hand, there are many people diagnosed with schizophrenia whose premorbid personality could be conceptualized as predominantly paranoid, obsessional, hysterical, depressive, or narcissistic.)

Another possible reason for associating the schizoid with the pathological is that many schizoid individuals feel an affinity for people with psychotic disorders. One colleague of mine, self-described as schizoid, prefers working with psychotically disturbed individuals to treating "healthy neurotics," because he experiences neurotically troubled people as "dishonest" (i.e., defensive), whereas he perceives psychotic ones as engaged in a fully authentic struggle with their demons. Some seminal contributors to personality theory—Carl Jung[6] and Harry Stack Sullivan,[7] for example—not only seem by most accounts to have been characterologically rather schizoid, but may also have had one or more short-lived psychotic episodes that never turned into a long-term schizophrenic condition. The capacity of these analysts to grasp the subjective experience of more seriously disturbed patients may have had a lot to do with their access to their own potential for madness.

Even highly effective and emotionally secure schizoid people may worry about their sanity. A close friend of mine found himself distressed when watching the movie, *A Beautiful Mind*, which depicts the gradual descent into psychosis of the brilliant mathematician John Nash. The film effectively draws the audience into Nash's delusional world and then discloses that individuals whom the viewer had seen as "real" were actually hallucinatory figments of Nash's imagination. It becomes suddenly clear that his thought processes have moved from creative brilliance to psychotic confabulation. My friend found himself painfully anxious as he reflected on the fact that, like Nash, he cannot always discriminate between times when he makes a creative connection between two seemingly unconnected phenomena that are in fact related, and times when he makes connections that are completely idiosyncratic, that others would find ridiculous or crazy. He was discussing this anxiety with his relatively schizoid analyst, whose rueful response to his description of this insecurity about how much he could rely on his mind was "Yeah. Tell me about it!" (In the section on treatment implications, it will become clear why I think this was a responsive, disciplined, and therapeutic intervention, despite its seeming to be a casual departure from the analytic stance.)

Notwithstanding the existence of some connections between schizoid psychology and psychotic vulnerability, I have been impressed repeatedly with the phenomenon of the highly creative, personally satisfied, and socially valuable schizoid individual who seems, despite an intimate acquaintance with what Freud called the "primary process," never to have been at serious risk for a psychotic break. The arts, the theoretical sciences, and the philosophical and spiritual disciplines seem to contain a high proportion of these people—as does the profession of psychoanalysis. Harold Davis (personal communication, August 22, 2002) reports that Harry Guntrip once joked to him that "psychoanalysis is a profession by schizoids for schizoids." Empirical investigations into the personalities of psychotherapists at Macquarie University in Sydney, Australia[8] found that, although the modal personality type among female therapists is depressive, among male therapists, schizoid trends predominate.

I believe that high-functioning schizoid people are not surprised by evidence of the unconscious. That is, they have intimate—and at times uneasy—familiarity with processes that are out of the awareness of most people. This capability makes psychoanalytic ideas more accessible and commonsensical to them than they are to those of us who spend years on the couch hacking through repressive defenses to make the acquaintance of our more alien impulses, images, and feelings. Schizoid people are temperamentally introspective; they like to wander among the nooks and crannies of their minds, and they find in psychoanalysis many evocative metaphors for what they find there. In addition, the professional practice of analysis and the psychoanalytic therapies offers an attractive resolution of the central conflict about closeness and distance that pervades schizoid psychology.[9]

I have always found myself attracted to schizoid people. In recent years, I have realized that most of my closest friends fit this description. My own dynamics, which tilt more toward the hysterical and depressive, are implicated in this attraction, in ways I speculate about later in this chapter. In addition, I have been fascinated by an unexpected response to my book on diagnosis.[10] Although it is not unusual for readers to tell me that they found a particular chapter on a personality type useful, or that the book was helpful in their work with a patient, or even that they recognized in its description some of their own dynamics, something unique occurs when they note the section on schizoid personalities. Several times, after a lecture or workshop, a person has come up to me (often someone who was sitting quietly in the back, closest to the door), checked to be sure he or she was not impinging on me, and said something like "I just want to thank you for your chapter on schizoid personality. You really got us."

In addition to the fact that these readers are expressing personal gratitude rather than professional praise, I am struck by the use of the plural "us." I have been wondering lately whether schizoid people are in a similar psychological position to that of individuals in sexual minorities: They are sensitive to the risk of being considered "deviant" or "sick" or "behavior-disordered" by those of us with more common psychologies simply because they are a minority. Mental health professionals sometimes discuss schizoid themes in a tone similar to the tone in which they once spoke about the gay, lesbian, bisexual, and transgendered populations. We have tended both to equate dynamics with pathology and to generalize about a whole class of people on the basis of individuals who have sought treatment for something problematic about their idiosyncratic version of a particular psychological orientation.

The rest of us may unthinkingly reinforce the stigmatization of schizoid individuals through our common belief that our more mainstream psychology is normative and that exceptions to it must therefore constitute psychopathology. Obviously, another possibility is that there are significant internal differences among people, expressing psychodynamic factors as well as others (e.g., constitutional, experiential, and contextual) that are neither better nor worse in terms of mental health. The human propensity to rank differences along some hierarchy of value runs deep, however, and minority groups are typically relegated to the lower rungs of these hierarchies.

Consider further the significance of the term "us." Schizoid people recognize each other. They feel like members of what one reclusive friend of mine called "a community of the solitary." Like homosexually oriented people with "gaydar," many schizoid individuals can spot each other in a crowd. They describe a sense of deep and compassionate kinship with one another, despite the fact that these relatively isolative people rarely verbalize such kinship or approach each other for explicit recognition. I have noted, however, that there is starting to be a genre of popular books[11] that normalize and even valorize many schizoid themes as extreme sensitivity,[11] introversion,[12] and preference for solitude.[13] A schizoid man described walking through a hall with several classmates on the way to a seminar with a teacher he suspected of having a similar psychology. On the way to the instructor's office, they passed a photo of Coney Island on a hot day, a beach scene with people crowded together so tightly that the sand was hardly visible. The teacher made eye contact with this man, nodded toward the picture, and made a wincing gesture indicating dread and avoidance. The schizoid man opened his eyes wider and nodded. They understood each other.

Defining the Schizoid Personality

I am using the term "schizoid" as it was used by the British object-relations theorists,[14-17] rather than as it appears in the DSM.[1] The DSM, arbitrarily and without empirical basis, differentiates between schizoid and avoidant psychology, postulating that avoidant personality disorder includes a wish to be close despite the taking of distance, while schizoid personality disorder represents an indifference to closeness. However, I have never seen a person, among mental health patients or otherwise, whose reclusiveness was not originally the product of conflict.[18] Recent empirical literature supports this clinical observation.[19] We are animals who seek attachment. The detachment of the schizoid person represents, among other things, the defensive strategy of withdrawal from overstimulation, traumatic impingement, and invalidation. Most experienced psychoanalytic clinicians know not to take it at face value, however severe and off-putting it may appear.

Before the discovery of the neuroleptics, when pioneering analysts used to work with unmedicated psychotic patients in facilities such as Chestnut Lodge, there were many reports of even catatonically withdrawn men and women who emerged from their isolation when they felt safe enough to reach out for human contact. One famous case, for which I can find no written account, involves Frieda Fromm-Reichmann. She is said to have sat quietly next to a catatonic schizophrenic patient for an hour a day, making occasional observations about what was happening on the ward and what the patient's feelings about it might be. After almost a year of these daily meetings, the patient abruptly turned to her and stated that he disagreed with something she had said several months previously.

The psychoanalytic use of the term "schizoid" derives from the observations of "schisms" between the internal life and the externally observable life of the schizoid individual.[20] For example, schizoid people are overtly detached, yet they describe in therapy a deep longing for closeness and compelling fantasies of intimate involvement. They appear self-sufficient, and yet anyone who gets to know them can attest to the depth of their emotional need. They can be absent-minded at the same time that they are acutely vigilant. They may seem completely nonreactive, yet suffer an exquisite level of sensitivity. They may look affectively blunted, while internally coping with what one of my schizoid friends calls "protoaffect," the experience of being frighteningly overpowered by intense emotion. They may seem utterly indifferent to sex while nourishing a sexually preoccupied, polymorphously elaborated fantasy life. They may strike others as unusually gentle souls, but may nourish elaborate fantasies of world destruction.

The term may also have been influenced by the fact that the characteristic anxieties of schizoid people concern fragmentation, diffusion, or going to pieces. They feel all too vulnerable to uncontrollable schisms in the self. I have heard numerous schizoid individuals describe their personal solutions to the problem of a self that is experienced as dangerously fissiparous. These solutions may include wrapping oneself in a shawl, rocking, meditating, wearing a coat inside and outside his home and office, retreating to a closet, and other means of self-comfort that express the conviction that other people are more upsetting than soothing. Annihilation anxiety is more common than separation anxiety in schizoid people; even the healthiest schizoid person may occasionally suffer psychotic terrors such as the sense that the world could implode or flood or fall apart at any minute, leaving no ground beneath one's feet. The urgency to protect the sense of a core, inviolable self can be profound.[21,22]

Having been originally trained in an ego-psychology model, I have found it useful to think of the schizoid personality as defined by a fundamental and habitual reliance on the defense mechanism of withdrawal. This withdrawal can be more or less geographical, as in the case of a man who retreats to his den or to some remote location whenever he is feeling overwhelmed, or internal, as illustrated by a woman who goes through the motions of being present while attending mostly to internal fantasies and preoccupations. Theorists in the object-relations movement emphasized the presence in schizoid people of a core conflict with interpersonal closeness versus distance in which physical (not internal) distance usually wins out.[17,23]

In more severely disturbed schizoid people, withdrawal can look like an unremitting state of psychological inaccessibility, whereas in those who are healthier, there is a noticeable oscillation between connection and disconnection. Guntrip[17] coined the phrase "in and out programme" to describe the schizoid pattern of seeking intense affective connection followed by having to distance and re-collect the sense of self that is threatened by such intensity. Although this can be particularly visible in the sexual realm, it seems to be equally true of other instances of intimate emotional contact. One of the reasons that I find people with central schizoid dynamics appealing is that withdrawal is a relatively "primitive," global, encompassing defense,[24,25] which can make it unnecessary to use the more distorting, repressing, and putatively more "mature" defensive processes. A woman who simply goes away, either physically or psychically, when she is under stress, does not need to use denial, displacement, reaction formation, or rationalization. Affects, images, ideas, and impulses that nonschizoid people tend to screen out of their consciousness are consequently freely available to her, making her emotionally honest in a way that strikes me, and perhaps other not particularly schizoid people, as unexpectedly and even breathtakingly candid.

A related characteristic of schizoid individuals (one that may be misunderstood either negatively as perversity, or positively as strength of character) is an indifference to, or outright avoidance of, personal attention and admiration. Although they may want their creative work to have an impact, most schizoid people would rather be ignored than celebrated. Their need for space far outweighs their interest in the usual sort of narcissistic supplies. Colleagues of my late husband—esteemed among his students for his originality and brilliance—have frequently lamented his tendency to publish his writings in oddly marginal journals, with no apparent concern for building a broad reputation in the mainstream of his field. Fame per se did not motivate him; being understood by those who mattered to him personally was far more important. Similarly, when I told a schizoid friend that I had heard him described as "brilliant, but frustratingly reclusive," he looked worried and asked, "Where did they get 'brilliant'?" "Reclusive" was fine with him, but "brilliant" might have sent somebody in his direction.

Origins of Schizoid Dynamics

I have written previously about the possible etiology of schizoid dynamics,[10] but in this chapter, I will focus on its phenomenology. However, let me make a few summary statements about the complex etiologies of schizoid versions of personality structure. I have become increasingly impressed with the centrality of a constitutionally sensitive temperament, noticeable from birth. One of the expressions of this presumably genetic disposition. One of the expressions of this genetic heritage is a level of sensitivity, in all its negative and positive meanings,[26] far more extreme and painful than that of most nonschizoid people. This acute sensitivity manifests itself from birth in behaviors that reject experiences that are felt as too overwhelming, impinging, or penetrating.

I have heard a number of schizoid individuals describe their mothers as both cold and intrusive. For the mother, the coldness may be experienced as coming from the baby. Several self-diagnosed schizoid people have told me their mothers said that they rejected the breast as newborns or complained that when they were held and cuddled, they pulled away as if overstimulated. A friend confided to me that his internal metaphor for nursing is "colonization," a term that conjures up the exploitation of the innocent by an intrusive imperial power. Related to this image is the pervasive concern with poisoning, bad milk, and toxic nourishment that commonly characterizes schizoid individuals. One of my more schizoid friends once asked me as we were having lunch in a diner, "What is it about straws? Why do people like to drink through straws?" "You get to suck," I suggested. "Yucch!" she exclaimed as she shuddered.

Schizoid individuals are frequently described by family members as hypersensitive or thin-skinned. Doidge[15] emphasizes their "hyperpermeability," the sense of being skinless, of lacking an adequately protective stimulus barrier, and notes the prevalence of images of injured skin in their fantasy life. After reading an early draft of this chapter, one schizoid colleague commented, "The sense of touch is very important: We're both frightened of it and want it." As early as 1949, Bergman and Escalona[27] observed that some children show, from infancy on, an acute sensitivity to light, sound, touch, smell, taste, motion, and emotional tone. More than one schizoid person has told me that their favorite childhood fairy tale was "The Princess and the Pea." Their sense of being easily overwhelmed by invasive others is frequently expressed in a dread of engulfment; a fears of spiders, snakes, and other devourers; and an Edgar Allen Poe-like preoccupation with being buried alive.

Complicating their adaptation to a world that overstimulates and agonizes them is the experience of invalidation by significant others. Most of my schizoid patients recall being told by exasperated parents that they were "oversensitive," "impossible," "too picky," or that they "make mountains out of molehills." Their painful experiences are repeatedly disconfirmed by caregivers who, because their temperament differs from that of their child, cannot identify with his or her acute sensitivities and consequently treat the child with impatience, exasperation, and even scorn. Khan's[28] observation that schizoid children show the effects of "cumulative trauma" is one way of labeling this recurring disconfirmation. Withdrawal becomes their preferred adaptation: Not only is the outer world too much for them sensually, it invalidates their experience, demands behaviors that are excruciatingly difficult, and treats them as crazy for reacting in ways that they cannot control.

Referring to Fairbairn's work,[23] Doidge[15], in a fascinating analysis of schizoid themes in the movie *The English Patient*, summarizes the childhood predicament of the schizoid person:

> Children . . . develop an internalized image of a tantalizing but rejecting parent . . . to which they are desperately attached. Such parents are often incapable of loving, or are preoccupied with their own needs. The child is rewarded when not demanding and is devalued, or ridiculed as needy for expressing dependent longings. Thus, the child's picture of "good" behavior is distorted. The child learns never to nag or even yearn for love, because it makes the parent more distant and censorious. The child may then cover over the resulting loneliness, emptiness, and sense of ineptness with a fantasy (often unconscious) of self-sufficiency. Fairbairn[23] argued that the tragedy of schizoid children is that . . . they believe it is love, rather than hatred, that is the destructive force within. Love consumes. Hence the schizoid child's chief mental operation is to repress the normal wish to be loved.[15]

Describing the central dilemma of such a child, Seinfeld[29] writes that the schizoid individual has "a consuming need for object dependence, but attachment threatens the schizoid with the loss of self." This internal conflict, elaborated in countless ways, is the heart of the psychoanalytic understanding of schizoid personality structure.

Some Seldom-noted Aspects of Schizoid Psychology

Reactions to Loss and Separation

Nonschizoid people often conclude that, because schizoid individuals resolve their closeness/distance conflicts in the direction of distance and seem to thrive on being alone, they are not particularly attached and therefore are not reactive to separation. Yet, internally, schizoid people may have powerful attachments. In fact, their attachments may be more intensely invested with emotion than are the attachments of people with much more obviously "anaclitic" psychologies. Because schizoid individuals tend to feel safe with comparatively few others, any threat to or loss of their connection with these people can be devastating. If there are only three individuals by whom one feels truly known, and one of these is lost, then one third of one's support system has vanished.

Thus, a common precipitant of a schizoid person's seeking treatment is loss. A related concern is loneliness. As Fromm-Reichmann[30] noted, loneliness is a painful emotional experience that remains curiously unexplored in the professional literature. The fact that schizoid people repeatedly detach and seek solitude does not mean that they are immune to loneliness, any more than obsessive individuals' avoidance of affect means that they are indifferent to strong emotion, or depressive persons' clinging denotes the absence of wishes for autonomy. Schizoid individuals may seek treatment because, as Guntrip[17] notes, they have retreated so far from meaningful relationships that they feel enervated, futile, and internally dead. Or they may come to therapy with a specific goal: to go on a date, to become more social, to initiate or improve a sexual relationship, or to conquer what they have been told is "social phobia."

Sensitivity to the Unconscious Feelings of Others

Possibly because they are undefended against their own more primal thoughts, feelings, and impulses, schizoid individuals can be remarkably attuned to unconscious processes in others. What is obvious to them is often invisible to less schizoid people. I have had many experiences of thinking that I was behaving relatively inscrutably, or no differently from how I behaved on any other day, only to have a schizoid friend or patient confront me about my "obvious" state of mind. In my book on psychotherapy,[31] I told the story of a schizoid client, a woman whose most passionate attachments were to animals, who was the only one of my patients to pick up on the fact that something was bothering me in the week after I was diagnosed with breast cancer, when I was trying to keep that fact private pending further medical intervention. Another schizoid patient once arrived for her session on an evening when I was looking forward to a weekend with an old friend, took one look at me acting in what I thought was a thoroughly ordinary, professional way as I sat down to listen to her, and teased, "Well! Aren't we happy tonight!"

One seldom-appreciated quandary in which interpersonally sensitive schizoid individuals often find themselves involves the social situation in which they perceive, more than others do, what is going on nonverbally. They are likely to have learned from a painful history of parental disapproval and social gaffes that some of what they see is conspicuous to everyone, and some is emphatically not. Because all of these undercurrents may be equally visible to schizoid people, it is impossible for them to know what is socially acceptable to talk about and what is either unseen or unseemly to acknowledge. Thus, some of the withdrawal of the schizoid individual may represent not so much an automatic defense mechanism as a conscious decision that avoidance is an effective adaptation to their dilemma.

This is inevitably a painful situation for schizoid people. If there is a proverbial elephant in the room, they start to question the point of having a conversation in the face of such silent disavowal. Because schizoid individuals lack ordinary repressive defenses and therefore find repression hard to understand in others, they are left to wonder, "How do I go forward in this conversation not acknowledging what I know to be true?" There may be a paranoid edge to this experience of the unspoken/unspeakable: Perhaps the others are aware of the elephant and have decided not to talk about it. What is the danger they perceive that I do not? Or perhaps they are genuinely unaware of the elephant, in which case their naiveté or ignorance may be equally dangerous. Kerry Gordon (personal communication, June 10, 2004) notes that the schizoid person lives in a world of possibility, not probability. As with most patterns that reenact a theme repeatedly and come to have a self-fulfilling quality, schizoid withdrawal both increases a tendency to live in primary process and creates further withdrawal because of the aversive consequences of living increasingly intimately in the realm of primary-process awareness.

Oneness with the Universe

Schizoid individuals have often been characterized as having defensive fantasies of omnipotence. For example, Doidge[15] mentions a seemingly cooperative patient who "disclosed, only well into treatment, that he always had the omnipotent fantasy that he was controlling everything I said." Yet the schizoid person's sense of omnipotence differs in critical ways from that of the narcissistic, psychopathic, paranoid, or obsessional person. Rather than being invested in preserving a grandiose self-image or maintaining a defensive need for control, schizoid people tend to feel connected with their surroundings in profound and interpenetrating ways. They may assume, for example, that their thoughts affect their environment, just as their environment affects their thoughts. This is more of an organic, syntonic assumption than a wish-fulfilling defense.[32] Gordon (personal communication, March 1, 2004) has characterized this experience more as "omnipresence" than omnipotence and relates it to Matte-Blanco's[33] notion of symmetrical thinking.

I am struck by this feeling of a lack of ontological differentiation or elaboration of self. Schizoid individuals may retain some sense of primary fusion, of Balint's[34] "harmonious, interpenetrating mix-up," rather than omnipotence. The recurring narrative in schizoid psychology concerns how this relatedness has become inharmonious and toxic. In this connection, Doidge[15] mentions the frequent assertion of Samuel Beckett, whose work resounds with schizoid themes, that he had never been born. A therapist in an audience to whom I talked about schizoid psychology voiced the perception that schizoid people are "insufficiently incarnated," existing in a world in which their bodies are no more real to them than their surround.

This sense of relatedness to all aspects of the environment may involve animating the inanimate. Einstein seems to have approached his understanding of the physical universe by identifying with particles and thinking about the world from their perspective. This tendency to feel a kinship with things is usually understood as a consequence of turning away from people. However, it may also represent unrepressed access to the animistic attitude that most of us encounter only in dreams or vague memories of how we thought as a child. Once when we were eating muffins together, a friend of mine commented, "I must be doing well. These raisins aren't bothering me." I asked what it was about raisins that was problematic: "You don't like the taste?" She smiled. "You don't understand. They could be flies!" This anecdote sparked an association in a colleague to whom I told it. She volunteered that her husband, whom she considers schizoid, dislikes raisins for a different reason. "He says they hide."

The Schizoid–Hysterical Romance

My attraction to people with schizoid psychologies—and the frequency with which other heterosexual women with hysterical dynamics seem to be drawn to men with schizoid traits—is not only based on their experience of schizoid people as inspiringly honest; there are dynamic reasons for this resonance. Clinical lore abounds with observations about hysterical–schizoid couples, about their misunderstandings and pursuer–distancer problems, and each party's inability to imagine that the other sees one as powerful and demanding rather than as one sees oneself—that is, as fearful and needy. But despite our recent appreciation of two-person processes, there is surprisingly little professional writing about the intersubjective consequences of specific and contrasting individual psychologies. Wheelis's short story[35] "The Illusionless Man and the Visionary Maid," and Balint's[36] classic depiction of the ocnophil and the philobat, seem more germane to the schizoid–hysterical chemistry than any more recent clinical writing.

The admiration between a more hysterical person and a more schizoid one is frequently mutual. Just as the hysterically organized woman idealizes the capacity of the schizoid man to stand alone, "speak truth to power," contain affect, and tap into levels of creative imagination that she can only dream of, the schizoid man admires her warmth, comfort with others, empathy, grace in expressing emotion without awkwardness or shame, and capacity to experience her own creativity in a relationship. To whatever extent opposites do attract, hysterical and schizoid individuals tend to idealize each other—and then drive each other crazy when their respective needs for closeness and space come into conflict. Doidge[15] memorably compared love relations with a schizoid person to litigation.

I think that the affinity between these personality types goes further, however. Both schizoid and hysterical psychologies can be characterized as hypersensitive, as preoccupied with the danger of being overstimulated. Whereas the schizoid person fears being overwhelmed by external sources of stimulation, the hysterical individual feels endangered by drives, impulses, affects, and other internal states. Both types of personality have also been associated with cumulative or strain trauma. Both are almost certainly more right- than left-brained. Both schizoid men and hysterical women (at least those who regard themselves as heterosexual; my clinical experience is not vast enough for me to generalize about others) tend to see the opposite-sex parent as the locus of power in the family, and both feel too easily invaded psychologically by that parent. Both suffer a consuming sense of hunger, which the schizoid person may try to tame, and the hysterical person may sexualize. If I am right about these similarities, then some of the magic between schizoid and hysterical individuals is based on convergence rather than opposition. Arthur Robbins (personal communication, April 19, 2005) goes so far as to say that inside every schizoid individual is a hysterical one, and vice versa.

Therapeutic Implications

People with significant schizoid dynamics—at least the healthier, more vital and more interpersonally competent individuals—tend to be attracted to psychoanalysis and the psychoanalytic therapies. Typically, they cannot imagine how anyone would want to comply with manualized interventions that relegate individuality and the exploration of the inner life to a minor role in the therapeutic project. If they have the resources to afford it, higher-functioning schizoid individuals are excellent candidates for psychoanalysis proper. They like the fact that the analyst intrudes relatively little on their associative process, they enjoy the inviolable space that the couch can provide, and they appreciate being freed from potential overstimulation by the therapist's corporeality and facial affect. Even in once-a-week and face-to-face arrangements, schizoid patients tend to be grateful for the therapist's careful avoidance of intrusion and premature closure. And because they "get" primary process and know that a training program has acquainted the therapist intimately with it, they believe that their inner life will not evoke shock, criticism, or disdain.

Despite the fact that most high-functioning schizoid patients accept and value traditional analytic practices, their successful treatment is not well captured by Freud's formulation of making the unconscious conscious. Although some unconscious aspects of schizoid experience—most notably the dependent longings that stimulate defensive withdrawal—do become more conscious in a successful therapy, the experience of elaborating the self in the presence of an accepting, nonintrusive, but still powerfully responsive other constitutes most of what is therapeutically transformative to schizoid individuals (Gordon, unpublished paper). The celebrated hunger of schizoid individuals is, in my experience, mostly for the kind of recognition about which Benjamin[37] has so evocatively written, a recognition of their subjectivity. It is their capacity to engage in the struggle to attain such recognition, and to reinitiate that process when it has broken down, that has been most deeply injured in those who come to us for help.

Winnicott, whose biographers[38-40] depict him in ways that suggest a deeply schizoid man, has described development in language directly applicable to the treatment of the schizoid patient. His concept of the caregiver who allows the child to "go on being" and to "be alone in the presence of the mother" is particularly relevant. His appreciation of the importance of a facilitating environment characterized by nonimpinging others, who value the true and vital self over compliant efforts to accommodate to others' defenses, might be a recipe for psychoanalytic work with schizoid patients. Because the analytic frame supplies the essential ingredients of a nonimpinging atmosphere, relatively conventional technique is well suited to high-functioning schizoid patients. Unless the analyst's narcissism expresses itself in a need to bombard the analysand with interpretations, classical analytic practice gives the schizoid person room to feel and talk at a tolerable pace.

Still, there has been some attention in the clinical literature to the special requirements of those schizoid patients who need something that goes beyond standard technique. First, because speaking from the heart can be unbearably painful for the schizoid person, and being spoken to with emotional immediacy may be comparably overwhelming, a therapeutic relationship may be furthered by transitional ways to convey feeling. One woman I worked with, who struggled every session to talk at all, finally called me on the telephone, weeping. "I want you to know that I do want to talk to you," she said, "but it hurts too much." We were eventually able to make therapeutic progress in a highly unconventional way, by my reading to her from the more accessible and less-pejorative psychoanalytic literature on schizoid psychology and asking her if the descriptions fit her experience. My hope was to spare her the agony of formulating and giving voice to feelings she regarded as incomprehensible to others and symptomatic of a profound, lone madness. She reported that it was the first time she had known that there were other human beings like her.

A schizoid person who cannot directly describe the anguish of isolation can probably talk about this state of mind as it appears in a film, poem, or short story. Empathic therapists working with schizoid clients often find themselves either initiating or responding to conversations about music, the visual arts, the dramatic arts, literary metaphors, anthropological discoveries, historical events, or the ideas of religious and spiritual thinkers. In contrast to obsessional patients, who avoid emotion by intellectualizing, schizoid patients may find it possible to express affect once they have the intellectual vehicle in which to do so. Because of this transitional function, the art therapies have long been seen as particularly suited to this population.

Observant clinical writers have noted that schizoid individuals are sensitive to evasion, role playing, and false notes. For this reason, one may need to be more "real" with them in therapy. Unlike analysands who eagerly exploit information about the therapist in the service of intrusive demands, or the fueling of idealization or devaluation, schizoid patients tend to accept the analyst's disclosures with gratitude and continue to respect his or her private, personal space. Writing under a pseudonym, an Israeli patient notes that:

> People with schizoid personality . . . tend to feel more comfortable with people who are in touch with themselves, who do not fear to reveal their weaknesses and appear mortal. I refer to an atmosphere that is relaxed and informal, where it is accepted that people err, may even lose control, behave childishly or even unacceptably. In such surroundings a person who is very sensitive by nature may be more open and expend less energy on hiding his/her differences.[41]

In a case report exemplifying both a sensitivity to transitional topics and the awareness of the patient's need for him to be real, Robbins[42] describes a schizoid woman who came to him devastated by the sudden death of her analyst and yet unable to talk about her pain. The image she evoked in him of a stranger on a lonely island, simultaneously contented and crying out for rescue, seemed potentially too frightening to share with her. The therapy began to deepen, however, when the two participants talked about an ostensibly trivial topic:

> One day she came in and mentioned that she had just had a quick bite at a local pizza shop. . . . We started to talk about the wide variety of pizza places on the West Side, both agreeing that Sal's was by far the best. We continued to share our mutual interest, now extending throughout Manhattan, in pizza shops. We traded information and seemed to take mutual pleasure in the exchange. Certainly, quite a deviation from standard analytic procedure. On a far subtler level, both of us started to learn something very important about the other though I suspect her knowledge was largely unconscious. Both of us knew what it meant to eat on the run, to hungrily grab something that filled an inexplicable dark hole but which at best was a temporary palliative to an insatiable appetite. This hunger, of course, was kept to oneself, for who could bear to reveal the intensity of such rapaciousness. . . . The pizza discussions became our bridge to a union, the re-experiencing of a shared relatedness that ultimately became the starting point for the patient to give form and shape to her past and present. Our pizza connection served as a haven, a place where she felt understood. [42]

A therapist's willingness to reveal personal experiences catalyzes the therapy with schizoid clients because, even more than other individuals, these patients need to have their subjective experience acknowledged and accepted. Reassurance feels patronizing to them, and interpretation alone, however accurate, may fall short of conveying that what has been interpreted is unsurprising and even positive. I have known many people who spent years in analysis and emerged with a detailed understanding of their major psychodynamics, yet experienced what they uncovered as shameful admissions rather than as expressions of their essential humanity in all its ordinary depravity and virtue. The willingness of the analyst to be "real"—to be flawed, wrong, mad, insecure, struggling, alive, excited, authentic—may be the most believable route to fostering the schizoid person's self-acceptance. This is why I view the quip of my friend's analyst—the "Yeah, tell me about it!" response to his anxieties about losing his mind—as both quintessentially psychoanalytic and deeply attuned.

Finally, there is the danger with schizoid patients that—as they become more comfortable and self-revealing in therapy—they will make the professional relationship a substitute for the satisfactions they could be pursuing outside the consulting room. Many a therapist has worked with a schizoid client for months or years, feeling increasingly gratified in their engagement, before remembering with a jolt that the person originally came for help to develop an intimate relationship that has so far shown no signs of happening. Because the line between being an encouraging presence and an insensitive nag can be thin, it is a delicate art to embolden the patient without being experienced as impatient and critical in ways reminiscent of early love objects. When the therapist inevitably fails to be perceived differently, it takes discipline and patience to contain the patient's hurt and outrage about once more being pushed into toxic relatedness. Review a summary of therapeutic implications in the treatment of schizoid individuals in Box 17.1.

Concluding Comments

In this chapter, I have found myself feeling a bit like an ambassador for a community that prefers not to be involved in public relations. It is interesting which aspects of psychoanalytic thinking enter the public professional domain, as it were, and which aspects remain relatively arcane. On its own merits, the work of Guntrip should have done for schizoid psychology what Freud did for the Oedipus complex or Kohut did for narcissism: expose

---

Box 17.1 Summary of Therapeutic Implications for the Treatment of Schizoid Individuals

- Higher-functioning schizoid individuals, who are interpersonally competent individuals with significant schizoid dynamics, tend to be attracted to psychoanalytic therapies and can be excellent candidates for psychoanalysis proper.
- Conscious awareness of dependent longings that stimulate defensive withdrawal and a hunger for the recognition of their subjectivity, and elaborating the schizoid self in the presence of an accepting, nonintrusive, but still powerfully responsive therapist may be achieved in a successful psychotherapy.
- Because schizoid individuals are sensitive to evasion, role playing, and false notes, psychotherapists may need to be more "real" with these patients when conducting psychotherapy.
- A therapist's willingness to reveal personal experiences can catalyze the therapy with schizoid clients because it validates their need to have their own subjective experience acknowledged and accepted.
- Patients with schizoid dynamics can make the professional psychotherapy relationship a substitute for the satisfactions they want to pursue outside the consulting room. Therapists may need to remind them that they came for help seeking to develop intimate relationships in their daily life.

its presence in many domains, and detoxify and destigmatize our relationship to it. Yet even some experienced psychoanalytic therapists are relatively unfamiliar with or indifferent to analytic thinking about schizoid subjectivities. I suppose that, for obvious reasons, writers who understand schizoid psychology from personal experience lack the urge that a Freud or Kohut had to start a movement touting the universality of the themes that pervade their own subjectivity.

I also find myself wondering if some large-scale parallel process is at work in the lack of general attention to psychoanalytic knowledge about schizoid issues. George Atwood once commented to me that the controversy over whether or not multiple personality (dissociative-identity disorder) "exists" is strikingly parallel to the ongoing, elemental internal struggle of the traumatized person who develops a dissociative psychology: "Do I remember this right or am I making it up? Did it happen or am I imagining it?" It is as if the mental health community at large—in its dichotomous positions about whether there really are dissociative personalities or not—is enacting a vast, unacknowledged countertransference that mirrors the struggle of these patients. In comparison, we might wonder whether our marginalizing of schizoid experience parallels the internal processes that keep schizoid individuals on the fringes of engagement with the rest of us.

I think that we in the psychoanalytic community have both understood and misunderstood the schizoid person. We have been privy to some brilliant writing about the nature of schizoid dynamics, but—in parallel to what can happen in a psychotherapy that produces insight without self-acceptance—the discoveries of the most intrepid explorers in this area have too often been translated into the language of pathology. Many of the patients who come to us for help do have quite pathological versions of schizoid dynamics. Many others, including countless schizoid individuals who have never felt the need for treatment, exemplify highly adaptive versions of similar dynamics. I have tried to explore some ways in which schizoid psychology differs from other self-configurations, emphasizing that this differentness is neither inherently worse nor inherently better, neither less nor more mature, neither a developmental arrest nor a developmental achievement. It just is what it is and needs to be appreciated for what it is. Review Box 17.2 for resources for patients, families, and clinicians.

Box 17.2 Resources for Patients, Families, and Clinicians

- Mayo Clinic
  https://www.mayoclinic.org/diseases-conditions/personality-disorders/symptoms-causes/syc-20354463?page = 0&citems = 10.
- Mind for Better Mental Health; Personality Disorders
  https://www.mind.org.uk/media-a/4256/personality-disorders-2020-pdf-download.pdf.
- How to Help Someone with Schizoid Personality
  https://www.therecoveryvillage.com/mental-health/schizoid-personality-disorder/related/how-to-help-someone-with-schizoid-personality-disorder/#gref.
- Portrait of Schizoid Personality Disorders in the Movies
  https://tariq-thowfeek-2g43.squarespace.com/movies/2015/12/8/the-english-patient.

Acknowledgments

The author wishes to thank George Atwood, Michael Eigen, Kerry Gordon, Ellen Kent, Sarah Liebman, Arthur Robbins, Deborah Thomas, and the late Wilson Carey McWilliams for their contributions to this essay.

Conflict of Interest/Disclosure: The author of this chapter has no financial conflicts and nothing to disclose.

References

1. American Psychiatric Association, *Diagnostic and Statistical Manual of Mental Disorders: DSM-IV*. Washington, DC: American Psychiatric Association; 1994.

2. Steiner J. Psychic Retreats: *Pathological Organizations in Psychotic, Neurotic and Borderline Patients*. New York, NY: Routledge; 2003.

3. Klein M. Notes on some schizoid mechanisms. *Int J Psychoanal*. 1946;27: 99–110.

4. Sass LA. *Madness And Modernism: Insanity in the Light of Modern Art, Literature, and Thought*. New York, NY: Basic Books; 1992:21.

5. Weinberger DR. Genetics, neuroanatomy, and neurobiology: New findings in schizophrenia: an update on causes and treatment. *Clin Psychiatry News*. 2004; 32 (Suppl.).

6. Hirsch I. Discussion of interview with Otto Will: interpersonal psychoanalysis then and now. *Contemp Psychoanal*. 1998; *34*(2): 305–322.

7. Zinken L. "Your self: did you find it or did you make it?" *J Anal Psychol*. 2008; *53*(3): 396–397.

8. Hyde, J. Fragile narcissists or the guilty good. What drives the personality of the psychotherapist? Doctoral dissertation, Macquarie University, Sydney, Australia; 2009.

9. Wheelis A. The vocational hazards of psychoanalysis. *Int J Psychoanal*.1956; 37: 171–184.

10. McWilliams, N. *Psychoanalytic Diagnosis: Understanding Personality Structure in the Clinical Process*. 2nd ed. New York, NY: Guilford; 2004.

11. Aaron EN. *The Highly Sensitive Person: How to Thrive When the World Overwhelms You*. New York, NY: Harmony; 1996.

12. Laney MO. *The Introvert Advantage: How to Thrive in an Extrovert World*. New York, NY: Workman Publishing; 2002.

13. Rufus AR. *Party of One: The Loner's Manifesto*. New York, NY: Avalon; 2003.

14. Akhtar S. *Broken Structures: Severe Personality Disorders and Their Treatment*. Lanham, Maryland: Rowman & Littlefield; 1992.

15. Doidge N. Diagnosing *The English Patient*: Schizoid fantasies of being skinless and of being buried alive. *JAPA*. 2001; 49: 279–309.

16. Gabbard GO. *Psychodynamic Psychiatry in Clinical Practice: The DSM-IV Edition*. Washington, DC: American Psychiatric Press; 1994.

17. Guntrip HJS. *Schizoid Phenomena, Object-Relations and the Self*. New York, NY: International Universities Press; 1969.

18. Kernberg O. *Severe Personality Disorders: Psychotherapeutic Strategies*. New Haven, CT: Yale University Press; 1989.

19. Shedler J, Westen D. Refining personality disorder diagnosis: Integrating science and practice. *Am J Psychiatry*. 2004; 161: 1350–1365.

20. Laing RD. *The Divided Self: An Existential Study in Sanity and Madness*. London, England: Penguin; (1960) 1965.

21. Eigen M. Abstinence and the schizoid ego. *Int J Psychoanal*. 1973; 54: 493–498.

22. Elkin H. On selfhood and the development of ego structures in infancy. *Psychoanal Rev*. 1972; 59: 389–416.

23. Fairbairn WRD. Schizoid factors in the personality. In Kegan P., ed. *Psychoanalytic Studies of the Personality*. New York, NY: Routledge; (1940) 1994: 3–27.

24. Laughlin HP. *The Ego and Its Defenses*. 2nd ed. New York, NY: J Aronson; 1979.

25. Vaillant GE, Bond M, Vaillant CO. An empirically validated hierarchy of defense mechanisms. *Arch of Gen Psychiatry*. 1986; 43: 786–794.

26. Eigen M. *The Sensitive Self*. Middletown, CT: Wesleyan University Press; 2004.

27. Bergman P, Escalona K. Unusual sensitivities in very young children. *Psychoanal Study Child*. 1949; 3:333–352.

28. Khan MM R. (1963). The concept of cumulative trauma. *Psychoanal Study Child*. 1963; 18: 286–306.

29. Seinfeld, J. *The Empty Core: An Object Relations Approach to Psychotherapy of the Schizoid Personality*. New York, NY: Jason Aronson; 1991.

30. Fromm-Reichmann F. Loneliness. *Contemp Psychoanal*. 1990: 26; 305–330.

31. McWilliams N. *Psychoanalytic Psychotherapy: A Practitioner's Guide*. New York NY: Guilford Press; 2004.

32. Khan M. Role of phobic and counterphobic mechanisms and separation anxiety in schizoid character formation. *Int J Psychoanal*.1966: 47; 306–312.

33. Matte BI. *The Unconscious as Infinite Sets: An Essay in Bi-Logic*. New York, NY: Routledge; 1975.

34. Balint M. *The Basic Fault: Therapeutic Aspects of Regression*. London, England: Tavistock Publications; 1968.

35. Wheelis A. (1966). The illusionless man and the visionary maid: In Wheelis A, ed. *The Illusionless Man: Some Fantasies and Meditations on Disillusionment*. New York, NY: Other Press; 1966: 13–44.

36. Balint M. Friendly expanses—Horrid empty spaces. *Int J Psychoanal*. 1945; 36; 225–241.

37. Benjamin J. Intersubjective distinctions: Subjects and persons, recognitions and breakdowns: Commentary on paper by Gerhardt, Sweetnam, and Borton. *Int J Psychoanal*. 2000; 10: 43–55.

38. Kahr B. *D. W. Winnicott: A Biographical Portrait*. New York, NY: International Universities Press; 1996.

39. Phillips A. *Winnicott*. Cambridge, MA: Harvard University Press; 1989.

40. Rodman FR. *Winnicott: Life and Work*. Cambridge, MA: Perseus Publishing; 2003.

41. Mitmodedet. Living with a schizoid personality. *Isr J Psychiatr Rel*. 2002; 39: 189–191.

42. Robbins A. Filling the void on the run: A case study of a schizoid patient. In Thorne, E, Schaye, SH, eds. *Psychoanalysis Today: A Casebook*. Springfield, IL: Charles C. Thomas; 1991: 223–232.

18

Antisocial Personalities

Glen O. Gabbard

Key Points

- Antisocial personalities exist on a spectrum from antisocial behavior in narcissists to pure psychopathy.
- Longitudinal studies suggest that some individuals on this continuum may have symptomatic improvement with aging, but the antisocial nature persists.
- Diagnosis of these patients is challenging because of the ubiquity of deception and misinformation provided by the patient.
- Both biological genetic factors and psychosocial issues contribute to the development of antisocial personalities.
- Clinicians who are treating these patients should carefully monitor countertransference and consult with a knowledgeable colleague.
- No randomized controlled trials of psychotherapy of antisocial persons have been conducted.

Introduction

Antisocial personalities can be conceptualized as a group of disorders that reside on a continuum from least pathological to most disturbed. At the top of this continuum is the phenomenon of antisocial features in other personality disorders. The next step down on this spectrum would consist of the many cases of narcissistic personality disorder that feature antisocial behavior as a major problem.[1] These individuals can be ruthlessly exploitative of others but have the capacity to experience guilt and concern. Moreover, their difficulty making commitments to others may appear as deceptiveness that results in hurting others. Further down this continuum, one would encounter malignant narcissists who have a paranoid orientation and ego-syntonic sadism. However, they differ from true antisocial personality disorder patients and cases of psychopathy in that they have some capacity for loyalty and concern for others. Finally, one encounters true psychopathy, featuring individuals who cannot imagine altruism of any sort and who are incapable of investing themselves in nonexploitative relationships.

The epidemiology of these disorders, including their life course, will be discussed as well as the common comorbidities found with people who have antisocial personalities. Diagnostic considerations are complicated in this cohort of patients because of the propensity of these individuals to falsify their histories. In this overview, the full spectrum of antisocial behavior will be considered with relevant differential diagnostic material that helps the clinician differentiate what sort of disorder is being treated and the nature of the individual with the diagnosis. The biological/genetic underpinnings of these disorders will be discussed as well as the psychosocial contributions. Typical countertransference reactions will also be covered. A section on treatment strategies will suggest a general approach designed to help manage the spectrum of antisocial features and various kinds of difficulties presented by patients who may not be seriously invested in treatment. There are no rigorous controlled trials of antisocial patients.

Epidemiology of Antisocial Personality Disorders

Despite the treatment difficulty characteristic of antisocial personality disorders (ASPDs), a considerable amount of effort has been invested in understanding and treating persons with this condition. ASPD has a 3.6 percent lifetime prevalence in the US population.[2] Many of those on the antisocial continuum will manifest a downward drift as they fail repeatedly, and some appear to "burn out" at some point in their lives. While many of these individuals have been debilitated by severe alcoholism or drug abuse, others have managed to thrive despite their dishonest behavior by moving from town to town or city to city as needed. Impulsivity may decrease with aging, but most continue to have struggles with work, parenting, and romantic partners.[3]

Some data exist on the life course of antisocial individuals. Robins, in her groundbreaking and compelling research, was able to locate 90 percent of a cohort of 524 subjects an average of 30 years after they had been identified as delinquents in a child guidance center between 1922 and 1932.[4] The average age at that time was 13. When they were interviewed by Robins's team, 94 were identified as antisocial in adulthood, and 82 of them were interviewed in their 30s and 40s. Only 12 percent had remitted. There was no improvement in 61 percent of the sample, while 27 percent were improved but still engaged in antisocial behavior.

Black studied the outcome of 45 antisocial individuals (from an original sample of 71) who had been hospitalized many years earlier and were in their mid-50s at the time of follow-up.[2] Of this group, 31 percent had improved, and 27 percent had remitted. However, the largest group—42 percent—revealed no improvement whatsoever. Studies suggest that there is some degree of burnout in the older individuals who are diagnosed with ASPD, but Black notes that it is a lifelong disorder even if the most striking symptoms dissipate.[2]

It has long been known that there is a significant correlation between antisocial character pathology and substance abuse.[5] However, this comorbidity may be deceptive. Many clinicians will focus exclusively on treating the drug problem while not paying attention to the psychopathy and deceptiveness. In fact, criminal activity is intimately tied to their substance abuse. Among felons, 52–65 percent have been found to be drug abusers.[6] Studies of the comorbidity of substance abuse and ASPD range from 42–95 percent.[6] Other comorbid illnesses include depression, anxiety, attention deficit hyperactivity disorder (ADHD), sexual deviancy, and pathological gambling.[2]

The majority of patients with ASPD are male, and the male-to-female ratio for this spectrum of disorders is approximately 4:1.[2] However, psychopathy does occur in female patients despite the fact that it is much more common among males.[2] It is easy for clinicians to overlook the diagnosis in females based on sex-role stereotypes. Indeed, a manipulative and seductive woman who exhibits considerable antisocial activity is still much more likely to be labeled histrionic or borderline than psychopathic.

A Case of Antisocial Personality Disorder and Psychopathy

A 19-year-old female, whom we will call Jenny, was admitted to the hospital after allegedly murdering a man with a gun. She explained that he was trying to rape her, and it was self-defense. Once she was in the hospital, she was involved in stealing, lying, and undermining the treatment of other patients. At one point during the hospital stay, Jenny talked two young male patients into taking a crowbar to her window to help her escape. They fled the hospital with her. After flying across the country using her parents' credit card, they landed in the airport. Jenny told her two companions that she had to use the restroom and then disappeared. The two young men didn't know what to do. These two male accomplices called the hospital, and their parents became involved, allowing their credit cards to be charged for the return flight.

Eventually, Jenny was located, and she agreed to go back to the hospital for further treatment. Shortly after arriving back in her hospital room, her treatment reached a turning point when she started a fire in her room that threatened the safety of everyone on the hospital unit. In fact, the unit had to be abandoned, leading to a situation in which all patients were standing outside on the grass under the supervision of the staff. Because she was charming and compelling in her storytelling, some treaters believed her when she said she was trying to burn her hand and she accidentally started a fire. She explained that she felt so guilty about shooting the man who tried to rape her that she was trying to punish herself by burning the hand in which she held the gun. Some staff believed her and supported her, while others viewed her as a psychopath, reflecting a form of splitting that is common in the treatment of antisocial patients. It is important in this regard to note that she met the criteria for antisocial personality disorder and psychopathy. Her older male psychotherapist in the hospital was convinced that she was *not* antisocial and became angry when other staff members referred to her in that way.

Diagnostic Considerations

In attempting to understand the complex diagnostic features of people who are thought to be antisocial, one must begin with the recognition that a variety of terms are used to describe them: "psychopaths," "sociopaths," "character disorders," and, of course, "antisocial personalities." Moreover, Kernberg has stressed that the exact point at which antisocial personality disorder transitions into narcissistic personality disorder is difficult to identify.[7] Kernberg's category of "malignant narcissism" is a category that is one step up on the continuum from ASPD.[7] He characterizes this entity as having a paranoid orientation and ego-syntonic sadism. However, these individuals differ from the antisocial or psychopathic individual in an important respect: They have concern for others and the capacity for loyalty. They are also able to imagine that other people have moral convictions and concerns.

Kernberg also noted that there is some degree of antisocial behavior in many patients with narcissistic personality disorder who are not consider malignant narcissists.[7] These individuals lack the paranoid and sadistic qualities of a malignant narcissist but would still be capable of exploiting other people to meet their own needs. These cases of narcissistic personality disorder with some degree of antisocial behavior, however, are able to experience concern and guilt while also struggling with making commitments to in-depth relationships. Hence, many clinicians and researchers share Kernberg's view that there is a spectrum that begins at the highest level with varying degrees of narcissistic organization, shading into antisocial behavior and thinking, and ends in psychopathy. Robert Hare has focused his attention on "true psychopathy," which he conceptualizes as lower on the spectrum than antisocial personality disorder.[8] Hare developed his Psychopathy Checklist-Revised (PCL-R)[9] in an effort to differentiate true psychopathy from the more broadly conceptualized diagnosis of ASPD. In his research, he applied the criteria of his psychopathy checklist to incarcerated offenders and found that only 15–25 percent would qualify as true psychopaths.[8]

As a result of the rigorous research of Hare and others, the term *psychopath* has once again gained popularity as a diagnostic term after having fallen out of favor in the late 20th century. Psychopathy is now regarded as much more severe, both in its clinical manifestations and in its treatment-resistance, compared to ASPD. Patients with psychopathy appear to have more substantial neuropsychological problems compared to non-psychopathic ASPD individuals; they are more ruthless and more incapable of any type of emotional attachment, with the exception of sadomasochistic interactions based on power.

Moreover, there is a growing body of research suggesting that certain personality traits observable in children may be linked to psychopathy. For example, callous-unemotional traits are defined by reduced guilt and empathic concern, and fewer displays of appropriate emotion.[10] These children and adolescents with callous-unemotional traits are typically viewed as less responsive to interventions than adolescents without such traits, perhaps reflecting a distinct neurobiology associated with callous-unemotional traits. There is generally a history that, as children, they showed a lack of fear of consequences for their actions and did not feel uncomfortable in any respect if they hurt someone or broke their parents' rules. Individuals with callous-unemotional traits show reduced bonding with others and lack significant attachments.

Callous-unemotional traits are also associated with greater gun violence.[10] They predict both the frequency of gun carrying at first arrest and the use of a gun during the commission of a serious crime in the 48 months after arrest.[10] Individuals with this distinct biological profile are less likely to be inhibited from acting aggressively, with a gun or other weapon, by the aversive emotional reactions typical of most healthy individuals when contemplating actions that will bring harm to others. Adolescents with callous-unemotional traits are actually less responsive to current interventions than youths with conduct problems who do not have these traits.[10] Research has also demonstrated that individuals with these traits show atypical social affiliation.[11] In other words, they have reduced bonding with others and are less influenced by others in their behavioral choices.

These recent findings contribute to a major effort in the field to clarify the specific differences between antisocial personalities and true psychopathy. For example, mood and anxiety disorders are rarely present with psychopathy, although they do appear in antisocial patients who are not psychopathic.[12] The lack of amygdala reactivity due to the structural deficits in that area of the brain seems to prevent psychopathic individuals from developing mood or anxiety disorders.[12]

A recent prototypicality analysis asked 57 forensic mental health professionals to rank the 20 items in the PCL-R in terms of their relevance to the diagnosis of psychopathy.[13]

The results from this study confirmed that a callous lack of empathy, a tendency toward conning and manipulation, and lack of remorse or guilt were judged to be of most importance and were rated as being of greater significance than nearly all other items. In this study, the interpersonal-affective items were clearly judged to be of more significance than the antisocial-lifestyle items. The fact that the callous lack of empathy and the absence of remorse were highly rated reflects the chilling characteristics of many psychopaths who have no sense of human relatedness or caring.

Biological and Psychological Underpinnings of Antisocial Personalities

The continuum of ASPD and psychopathy provides a compelling example of the interface of biological/genetic factors with early environmental experiences in the pathogenesis of these spectrum disorders. Family studies of antisocial personality disorder suggest that children who have one antisocial parent have approximately a 16 percent likelihood of developing the disorder.[2] However, in addition to genetic factors, environmental neglect and abuse appear to be part of the pathogenic picture. In the Dunedin Multidisciplinary Health and Development Study, investigators followed a birth cohort of 137 children prospectively from ages 3–26.[14] Between the ages of 3 and 11, 8 percent of the sample experienced "severe" maltreatment, 28 percent experienced "probable" maltreatment, and 64 percent experienced no maltreatment.[14] Maltreatment was defined as maternal rejection, repeated loss of a primary caregiver, harsh discipline, physical abuse, and sexual abuse.

When the investigators reviewed their findings, they determined that a functional polymorphism in the gene responsible for the neurotransmitter metabolizing enzyme monoamine oxidase-A (MAO-A) was found to moderate the effect of maltreatment.[14] In other words, males who had high MAO-A activity did not have elevated antisocial scores even when they had experienced childhood maltreatment. Males with low MAO-A activity genotype who were maltreated in childhood had elevated antisocial scores. Those males who had both low MAO-A activity genotype and severe maltreatment demonstrated an 85 percent rate of antisocial behavior.[14] A Swedish study involving a randomized sample of 81 male adolescents replicated the Dunedin study but also provided additional intriguing data.[15] The MAO-A genotype appeared to have no effect on adolescent criminal activity if the genotype were considered alone, that is, without the adverse environmental factors. These findings suggest that the genotype may moderate a child's sensitivity to environmental stressors, and the combination of genetic vulnerability and adverse experience may produce the appearance of antisocial behavior. Reiss et al. studied 708 families with at least two same-sex adolescent siblings involving multiple variations.[16] Ninety-three families had monozygotic twins, 99 had dizygotic twins, 95 had ordinary siblings, 181 had full siblings in stepfamilies, 110 had half-siblings in stepfamilies, and 130 were characterized by genetically unrelated siblings in stepfamilies. Data on parenting styles were collected by video recordings and by questionnaire. Approximately 60 percent of the variance in adolescent antisocial behavior could be accounted for by negative and conflictual parental behavior directed specifically at the adolescent. The investigators suggested that certain heritable characteristics of the children, including ADHD, temper outbursts, physical violence, and verbal contempt, may evoke harsh and inconsistent parenting. Siblings without those heritable characteristics did not evoke negative parental behavior, and they seemed to experience a protective effect when harsh parental behavior was directed at the other sibling.

The researchers in this impressive study found that family response to these heritable characteristics tended to take one of four forms: they (1) exacerbate troublesome aspects of the child; (2) enhance desirable features of the child; (3) protect the child from the negative outcomes related to difficult behavior; or (4) lead parents to back off from the difficult child in an attempt to protect the sibling with better prospects. These data were further analyzed with the intention of determining whether latent genetic factors and measured parent–child relationships interacted in predicting adolescent antisocial behavior and depression.[17] The investigators found that an interaction of genotype with both parental negativity and low warmth predicted overall antisocial behavior, but not depression. In other words, the genetic influence was greater for adolescent antisocial behavior when parenting lacked warmth and showed greater negativity.

As previously noted, another consistent finding in the research on the subject is that psychopathy appears to have strong biological origins, as seen in the importance of callous-unemotional traits, lack of empathy, and an absence of guilt.[12] When boys with these traits are compared with control subjects of the same age, they have much less amygdala reactivity to fearful faces. In short, children who grow up to be psychopaths show no indication of having had the kind of learning that leads to an increase in anxiety and participatory fear when an antisocial act is contemplated.

A Brazilian study attempted to link the different types of childhood trauma and parental bonding with antisocial traits in adulthood.[18] They identified 357 abstracts, and 18 of the studies met the inclusion criteria. The investigators then attempted to determine what types of trauma and bonding characteristics were specifically related to antisocial personality traits. Their major instruments were the Childhood Trauma Questionnaire (CTQ)[19] and/or the Parental Bonding Instrument (PBI).[20] The data from the CTQ suggested a clear linkage between physical abuse/neglect and antisocial traits. Sexual abuse was the variable least related to antisocial traits. Regarding the PBI, the data were more heterogeneous. Maternal variables most associated with antisocial traits were low maternal care and high overprotection. Regarding paternal variables, the only consistent variable associated with antisocial traits was a low level of care.

Raine has stressed that antisocial personality disorder should be regarded as a neurodevelopmental disorder that may be recognized early in childhood.[21] Fronto-limbic brain abnormalities are a key feature of antisocial personality disorder. Raine emphasizes three main brain regions that are affected: the prefrontal cortex, the amygdala, and the striatum. These regions correlate with the findings regarding psychopathic features associated with antisocial youth, such as callous-unemotional traits.

Countertransference Reactions to Antisocial Patients

The profession of psychiatry has long known that patients in the antisocial-psychopathic continuum are not likely to respond to treatment. Yet the stories of failed attempts are plentiful. The profession does not have rigorous data that would allow clinicians to discern which patients are likely to be responsive to treatment and which are undoubtedly hopeless. A feeling of hope about the patient's amenability to treatment may itself be an example of countertransference in the therapist. In fact, one of the principal pitfalls is for psychotherapists to have higher expectations of the patient than are realistic. When treatment is attempted in general psychiatric hospital units, these patients are known to steal from other patients and staff members, sexually exploit patients, lie to staff and patients, and even assault those who are in their way on the same unit. Antisocial patients are also notorious for smuggling alcohol and drugs into the hospital or treatment center.

There is a broad consensus that true psychopaths do not belong on general psychiatry units because they will not benefit from the treatment and are likely to disrupt the treatment of others. There are anecdotes suggesting that specialized units may be helpful. Often they are in prison settings where there is a high degree of control and observation of those incarcerated. However, one never knows for sure if the patient who is improving is a good actor or a sincerely concerned individual wanting to change. Moreover, we do not have rigorous and systematic data on whether such patients benefit from high-intensity prison programs.

In addition to the overestimation of the patient's capacity to use treatment, another intense countertransference reaction is often evoked by antisocial patients. Many people who have chosen to work in the mental health professions are inclined to be charitable, generous, big-hearted, and overly optimistic. They tend to give patients the benefit of the doubt, and this may lead treaters to downplay the extent of sadism and cruelty in patients who are on the antisocial to psychopathic spectrum.

Another variation of countertransference is the tendency for hospital staff members to regard themselves as capable of treating the "untreatable" patient. They may "run the extra mile" to connect with a patient who has no interest in meaningful human relationships. A principle form of countertransference is the therapist's denial that patients are as ill as they seem. In other words, they are often underdiagnosed by zealous staff members. One manifestation of this underdiagnosis is for the treatment staff to conceptualize them as narcissistic rather than psychopathic, or as simply an immature person who needs to grow up.[22]

Countertransference Unfolding in the Hospital

Frank was a 21-year-old male patient who was hospitalized for "high suicide risk" on the psychiatry unit of a general hospital. He had been "in love" with a young woman whom he said had abandoned him. He couldn't live without her, so he tried to cut his wrists with a kitchen knife he got from his mother's house. Frank reported that his mother found him bleeding and took him to the emergency room, where she dropped him off. His bleeding was minimal, but he continued to cry and maintain that he was "heartbroken." He said he saw no reason to continue living. He was polite and charming, despite his "desperate" state of mind, and Alice, an attentive nurse on the unit, tried to console him. He kept saying that he had lost his one and only love and would never be the same. Alice was worried about him, and she told him, "Any time you want to talk, just let them know at the front desk, and I'll be happy to chat with you." He thanked her but said he was inconsolable.

Alice saw him each day and tried to engage him in an optimistic view of the future with no success. He always thanked her but continued to grieve. One evening when she came to work and checked in on him, she found him trying to hang himself with his belt. She was extremely worried, but he promised he wouldn't do it again, and he begged her not to tell anyone because he would "get in trouble." She reluctantly agreed. He continued to tell her about his former girlfriend and how it was all his fault that she had left him. Alice tried to buoy his spirits by saying, "I'm sure it wasn't all your fault. It takes two to tango. She must have had problems also." He kept saying that she was perfect, and the problem stemmed from his selfishness. He spent a good deal of time telling her how awful his childhood had been. He described repeated beatings by his stepfather, and cried as he explained that his mother would never come to his aid. Alice told him to tell all this to the treating psychiatry resident on his unit. He replied, "I can't talk to him. He only spends 5 minutes with me and just talks about the medication."

One evening when Alice was trying to cheer him up, she said she wished there was something she could do for him. He replied that actually there *was* something she could do. He told her tearfully and seemingly reluctantly that he had to come up with $20,000 or some "evil dudes" were going to kill him. He asked if there was any way she could help him out. Alice became alarmed and said she couldn't come up with that much money. He then asked her if she could at least get her hands on $10,000. He explained with intensely gripping desperation that they might find out that he was in the hospital and come after him. Alice took some money from her savings and gave him $7,000, explaining that she shouldn't be doing this, and Frank could never tell anyone. He promised that he wouldn't and said he would definitely repay her. He then hugged her, and said "you saved my life."

The next day when she came to work, he was gone. She never heard from him again, and she felt like a fool for believing him. The resident assigned to him did some checking and found out that he had an outstanding warrant for his arrest for assault and battery in a neighboring city.

This vignette involving Frank and Alice depicts two of the most common countertransference reactions with antisocial patients: disbelief and collusion.[23] Disbelief often arises as a form of denial that the patient is seriously disturbed or antisocial. Collusion is perhaps the most problematic form of countertransference. The antisocial patient will corrupt one or more staff members, who then in turn commits an illegal act or behaves unethically in the service of "helping" the patient. Staff members have lied on behalf of such patients; they have falsified records; they have engaged in sexual relations with the patient; and some staff members have even assisted patients in their "escape" from the hospital.

Further Manifestations of Countertransference

There are other common forms of countertransference that are well known to experienced clinicians. One is to conceptualize the patient's antisocial behavior as growing out of the influence of drugs and alcohol, so that the diagnosis is one of substance abuse rather than character pathology. A common countertransference is for a treating professional to argue with other staff members that the patient's substance abuse is the main focus of treatment, followed by a statement like "If he gets clean, the antisocial stuff is going to disappear." Treaters should be aware that "gut feelings" about antisocial patients are notoriously unreliable.

Antisocial patients who are suffering from a clear major depressive episode or an anxiety disorder may be treated for those conditions, although the therapist must have a high index of suspicion about the potential that the patient is faking the illness. There are many case examples in which a psychopathic patient has decided to seek hospital treatment as an alternative to prison, but the treatment responses are almost always poor because the patient is not truly motivated to change. Many patients will use the hospital to "hide out" from an unresolved legal situation that might require a court appearance.

Yet another common countertransference is the fear that staff feel unsafe. This may lead a staff member to try to please the antisocial patient as a way of placating the patient and managing his/her own anxiety. Of course, it could be argued that such fear is not truly countertransference, but is a realistic reaction to someone who is dangerous. Clinicians should carefully note such feelings and take them seriously.

Meloy and Yakeley note that one of the most problematic countertransferences is the assumption of psychological complexity in a psychopathic individual.[6] The most difficult issue for treatment staff is to accept that a psychopath is fundamentally *different* than them. Such individuals interact with treatment staff only in the service of exploiting them for their own purposes. Hence, psychopaths can use this countertransference blind spot by presenting themselves as identical to the treaters. They may tell a clinician that they have similar taste in music, food, sports, or whatever will win over the person treating them. Those involved in the treatment must accept the notion that most of the time the patient is "playing" them.

Treatment Strategies with Antisocial Patients

Because we have no convincing data that antisocial patients respond to psychiatric treatment, one must be cautious in recommending specific strategies. However, some patients at the higher end of the continuum, who have malignant narcissism or antisocial traits, *may* be treatable under certain circumstances. Comorbid conditions may also make the prognosis somewhat better. One study of hospitalized patients with antisocial features but not true psychopathy identified three predictors of a reasonably positive treatment outcome for these patients: the presence of anxiety; the presence of depression; and a treatable psychotic diagnosis.[24] Even in these instances, professionals involved in the treatment must recognize that medication may help with psychotic elements of the clinical picture, but will not treat antisocial personality disorder.

Moreover, short-term hospitalization for antisocial patients is unlikely to treat the underlying personality pathology, even if it helps depression or psychotic elements. Hence the general consensus in the field has been that only long-term hospital treatment has a chance of dealing with the deceptiveness, impulsivity, violence, theft, substance abuse, lack of mentalizing, and sexual exploitation that characterize this diagnostic picture. The structure of the treatment must be clearly laid out for the patient, and there must be clear consequences for the breaking of the structure. If the patient is a known drug abuser, all mail must be opened in front of staff members. At the beginning of treatment, patients must be told that they will be accompanied by staff members whenever they leave the unit and that cash and credit cards must be restricted. One of the most important principles is to make it clear to patients that they are being given a *trial of treatment only.* The treatment should be considered an evaluation to determine if the patient is suitable for treatment. The stipulations of treatment can be written out as a *contract* at the time of admission.

When patients begin their treatment, a heavy emphasis should be given to faulty thought processes.[25] Holding patients accountable for their actions, the principal of agency, must be repeated again and again. Many antisocial patients will maintain that they are the victim of what others are doing to them, rather than seeing their own role in what happens to them. Staff members can make a point to the patient that his/her repeated failures revolve around not taking the time to think through the consequences of the action being contemplated. Treatment staff must also deal with the tendency of antisocial patients to go directly from impulse to action. When a patient has an impulse, staff members must encourage the patient to think through the consequences *before* acting on the impulse. Many antisocial patients have no sense of an internal life where feelings and thoughts motivate action. Hence groups that emphasize mentalizing and internal awareness may be helpful.

Hospital staff members must also be alert to the potential for impulsive suicide attempts. Verona et al. conducted a survey of 4,745 subjects and found that antisocial behavior was linked to suicide risk in both men and women.[26] When addressing suicidality or impulsive behavior, staff members must focus their strategies on the here and now. Focusing on childhood determinants of the suicidality is rarely helpful for antisocial patients. Staff members must also keep in mind that antisocial patients who lack true empathy for others may nevertheless be skilled at discerning a staff member's internal state and exploiting it for their own benefit. They may try to pull a role reversal where they ask the staff member, "What is wrong? You look worried." Such inquiries may catch treaters off guard, and they may suddenly find themselves in a role reversal with the patient.

Guidelines for Psychotherapy

The first, and perhaps the least controversial, guideline for psychotherapy of antisocial patients is simple: be extremely wary of outpatient treatment. The therapist will have no way of knowing what the patient is doing between sessions and cannot resort to checking with other members of a treatment team in the way one can in an inpatient setting. The chances of helping the patient are most likely in a hospital-like setting where a team is involved and oversight of the patient is feasible.

The patient who is a pure psychopath with a callous-unemotional profile will not respond to psychotherapy. Many hours have been spent in attempts to change such patients in group and individual therapy, with no measurable success. However, some patients on the continuum with narcissistic personality and antisocial behavior may benefit from psychotherapy in certain situations.[1] A careful assessment is necessary to determine if the patient has the capacity to form some semblance of a psychological attachment to others as well as some primitive form of superego functioning. The presence of true depression may be a sign of potential to use psychotherapy. In fact, one study of opiate addicts found that the presence of depression indicated suitability for psychotherapy even if there were some behavioral signs of antisocial/psychopathic features.[27] In this study, those antisocial patients who did not have depression did not do well. In fact, the absence of relatedness to others was the most negative predictor of psychotherapy response.

When clinicians are evaluating the feasibility of psychotherapy with a potential patient, they must feel comfortable if they reach a conclusion that treatment is not recommended. Therapists are prone to overestimate who may respond to therapy and may take on "heroic" cases. Therapists should follow their impressions and not feel that they are acting in a punitive or depriving way toward a patient who is unlikely to be able to use therapy.

Therapists who decide to treat an antisocial spectrum patient should probably follow 14 time-honored principles:

1. Before starting the therapy, one should make sure that there are no legal complications to the treatment. It is wise to remember that few antisocial patients actually come on their own for therapy. If they insist that they are there by their own volition, clinicians should carefully screen for pending court actions or lawsuits that may be the "real" reason that they are signing up for therapy. Their main motive for therapy may be to "look good" in the eyes of a jury or a judge.

2. When making the decision to start psychotherapy, therapists should use a colleague as a consultant so that they have a second opinion from the beginning. A wise and trusted consultant who is *not* involved in the evaluation or treatment may have an objectivity that the therapist lacks because of the therapeutic relationship. Ideally, the consultant should periodically meet with the therapist for candid discussions about countertransference and other issues.

3. Therapists should not make a decision to start a treatment unless they feel safe in the treatment context. It is difficult to think clearly about the patient if one is afraid. In some settings, such as prisons or hospitals, it may be helpful to have an attendant sitting outside the therapy room.

4. Therapists must not have excessive expectations for improvement. Antisocial patients will detect this *furor therapeuticus*, and will take great delight in thwarting their therapist's wishes to change them.

5. The therapist must be stable, persistent, and thoroughly incorruptible. One will feel pulled in various directions by the patient, but more than with any other patient group, the therapist must be absolutely scrupulous about maintaining normal procedures in therapy. Deviating from the structure and usual context of the hours is inadvisable. These patients will do whatever they can do to corrupt the therapist into unethical or dishonest conduct.

6. Countertransference must be rigorously monitored to avoid acting out by the therapist. Any collusion must also be carefully avoided, despite the tendency to "take the path of least resistance."

7. The therapist must repeatedly confront the patient's denial and minimization of antisocial behavior. Pervasive denial even infiltrates the antisocial patient's choice of words. If the patient says, "I ripped off this guy," the therapist needs to clarify, "So, you are saying you are a thief." This technique of repeated confrontation about what the patient is saying may help patients become aware of their tendency to externalize all responsibility, and they can therefore begin to acknowledge and accept responsibility for their antisocial behavior.

8. The therapist must help the patient connect actions with internal states of thoughts and feelings.

9. Confrontations of here-and-now behavior are likely to be more effective than interpretations of unconscious material from the past. In particular, the patient's

denigration of the therapist and contemptuous devaluation of the process must be repeatedly challenged.

10. Therapists should be alert to comorbidities. Depression and substance abuse may be diagnosed and treated in conjunction with the psychotherapy.

11. Mentalization and empathy in the patient should be promoted. This group of patients has been motivated by self-interest for their entire lives, and often do not stop and think about the ultimate impact of what they say and do on others. Hence, trying to develop a capacity for mentalizing associated with compassion for the victim may be worth a systematic effort in the psychotherapy. A pilot project of mentalization-based therapy for violent men with a diagnosis of antisocial personality disorder found that treatment led to a reduction in aggressive acts.[28]

12. Therapists cannot expect to maintain a neutral position regarding the patient's antisocial activities. If one attempts to do so, it can easily be seen as a tacit endorsement of or collusion with the patient's actions. Moreover, the therapist's moral outrage will be evident in myriad nonverbal communications and vocal intonations, so the patient will view any effort at neutrality as hypocritical. It is perfectly reasonable to say to the patient that one is shocked at the patient's antisocial behavior.

13. The therapist must be prepared that the patient will quit the therapy, undermine it, or deceive the therapist. Competent therapists who are able to avoid being destroyed by the patient's "tricks" may evoke envy and competitiveness in the patient. A negative therapeutic reaction may be the result. The patient's contempt toward the therapist, as well as the denigration of the therapist in the process, must be challenged by the therapist. Ultimately, therapists cannot *make* patients collaborate in a meaningful therapeutic process, and we must all be prepared for that outcome.

14. Finally, the therapist must emphasize the need for honesty and the unacceptability of lying or withholding information. Without honesty, there is no treatment.

Conclusion

Antisocial patients reside on a spectrum beginning with severe malignant narcissism through varying degrees of antisocial pathology and ending at the dead end of psychopathy, where there is little hope for improvement. They may have comorbidities with substance abuse that create tremendous upheaval in their lives, and they may be unable to work successfully because of their incapacity to be engaged, honest, and punctual. There is often a downward drift in their life course. The antisocial spectrum is one that is characterized by a combination of biological and genetic influences along with psychosocial contributions. Clinicians must remember that attempted treatment strategies are unlikely to make major changes no matter how much patients may pretend that they are using the treatment or benefiting from it. There is no persuasive evidence that treatment is effective with patients in the antisocial spectrum, and more rigorous controlled studies are needed. See Box 18.1, p. 471 for resources for patients, families, and clinicians.

Conflict of Interest/Disclosure: The authors of this chapter have no financial conflicts and nothing to disclose.

Box 18.1 Resources for Patients, Families, and Clinicians

- Mayo Clinic; Antisocial Personality Disorder. https://www.mayoclinic.org/diseases-conditions/antisocial-personality-disorder/symptoms-causes/syc-20353928.
- Nation Health Service: Antisocial Personality Disorder. https://www.nhs.uk/conditions/antisocial-personality-disorder.
- Web MD: Antisocial Personality Disorder. https://www.webmd.com/mental-health/antisocial-personality-disorder-overview#1.
- Mental Health.gov: Antisocial Personality Disorders. https://www.mentalhealth.gov/what-to-look-for/personality-disorders/antisocial-personality-disorder.
- Fox DJ. *Antisocial, Borderline, Narcissistic and Histrionic Workbook: Treatment Strategies for Cluster B Personality Disorders.* Eau Claire, WI: PESI Publishing; 2015.
- Black DW. *Bad Boys, Bad Men: Confronting Antisocial Personality Disorder (Sociopathy).* New York, NY: Oxford University Press; 2013.
- Anderson D. *Dealing with a Sociopath: How to Survive the Antisocials, Narcissists and Psychopaths in Your Life.* Eau Claire, WI: PESI Publishing; 2015.

References

1. Kernberg OF. Pathological narcissism and narcissistic personality disorder: theoretical background and diagnostic classification In: Ronningstam ER, ed. *Disorders of Narcissism: Diagnostic Clinical, and Empirical Implications.* Washington DC: American Psychiatric Press; 1998:29–51.

2. Black DW. *Bad Boys, Bad Men: Confronting Antisocial Personality Disorder (Sociopathy).* New York: Oxford University Press; 2013.

3. Paris J. Personality disorders over time: precursors, course, and outcome. *J Pers Disord.* 2003; 17: 479–488.

4. Robbins LN. *Deviant Children Grown Up.* Baltimore, MD: Williams & Wilkins; 1966.

5. Walsh Z, Allen LC, Cosson DS. Beyond social deviance: Substance abuse disorders and the dimensions of psychopathy. *J Pers Disord.* 2007; 21: 273–288.

6. Meloy JR, Yakeley J. Antisocial personality disorder. In Gabbard, GO, ed. *Gabbards Treatments of Psychiatric Disorders.* 5th Ed. Washington, DC: American Psychiatric Publishing; 2014:132–143. doi:10.1176/appi.books.9781585625048.gg69

7. Kernberg OF. Overview of the treatment of severe narcissistic pathology. *Int J Psychoanal.* 2014; 95: 865–888.

8. Hare RD. Psychopathy: A clinical and forensic overview. *Psychiatr Clin North Am.* 2006; 29: 709–724

9. Hare RD. *The Hare Psychopathy Checklist-Revised.* Toronto, Ontario: Multi-Health Systems; 1991.

10. Blair JR. Callous-unemotional traits and gun violence. *A J Psychiatry.* 2020; 177: 797–798.

11. Viding E, McCrory E. Towards understanding atypical social affiliation in psychopathy. *Lancet Psychiat.* 2019; 6: 437–444.

12. Blair JR. Cortical thinning and functional connectivity in psychopathy. *A J Psychiatry.* 2012; 169: 684–668.

13. Verschuere V, te Kaat L. What are the core features of psychopathy? A prototypicality analysis using the Psychopathy Checklist-Revised (PCL-R). *J Pers Disord.* 2020; 34: 410–419.

14. Caspi A, McClay J, Moffitt TE, et al. Role of genotype in the cycle of violence in maltreated children. *J Sci.* 2002; 297: 851–854.

15. Nilsson KW, Sjoberg RL, Damberg M, et al. Role of monoamine oxidase-A genotype and psychosocial factors in male adolescent criminal activity. *Biol Psychiatry.* 2006; 59: 121–127.

16. Reiss D, Neiderhiser JM, Heatherington EN, Plomin R. *The Relationship Code: Deciphering Genetic and Social Influences on Adolescent Development.* Cambridge, MA: Harvard University Press; 2003: Volume 1.

17. Feinberg ME, Button TM, Neiderhiser JM, Reiss D, Hetherington EM. Parenting and adolescent antisocial behavior and depression: evidence of genotype X parenting environment interaction. *Arch Gen Psychiatry.* 2007; 64: 457–465.

18. Schorr MT, Tietbohl-Santos B, Mendes de Oliveira L, Terra L, Borbatellis LE, Hauck S. Association between different types of childhood trauma and parental bonding with antisocial traits in adulthood: A systematic review. *Child Abuse & Negl.* 2020; 107: 111–220.

19. Bernstein DP, Fink L, Handelsman L, et al. Initial reliability and validity of a new retrospective measure of child abuse and neglect. *A J Psychiatry.* 1994; 151: 1132–1136.

20. Parker, G, Tupling H, Brown, LB. A parental bonding instrument. *Br J Med Psychol.* 1979; 52: 1–10.

21. Raine, A. Antisocial personality as a neurodevelopmental disorder. *Ann Rev Clin Psychol.* 2018; 14: 259–289.

22. Gabbard GO. *Psychodynamic Psychiatry in Clinical Practice.* 5th ed. Washington, DC: American Psychiatric Publishing; 2014.

23. Symington N. The response aroused by the psychopath. *Rev of Psychoanal.* 1980; 7: 291–298.

24. Gabbard GO, Coyne L. Predictors of response to antisocial patients to hospital treatment. *Hosp Community Psychiatry.* 1987; 38: 1181–1185.

25. Yochelson S, Samenow SE. *The Criminal Personality, Vol 1: A Profile for Change.* New York: Jason Aronson; 1976.

26. Verona E, Sachs-Ericsson N, Joiner TE. Suicide attempts associated with externalizing psychopathology in an epidemiological sample. *Am J Psychiatry.* 2004; 161: 444–451.

27. Woody GE, McLellan AT, Luborsky L, O'Brien CP. Sociopathy and psychotherapy outcome. *AMA Arch Gen Psychiatry.* 1985; 42: 1081–1108.

28. McGauley G, Yakeley J, Williams A, Bateman A. Attachment, mentalization and antisocial personality disorder: The possible contribution of mentalization-based treatment. *Eur J Psychother Couns.* 2011; 13: 1–22.

19

Borderline Personality Disorder

Curtis C. Bogetti and Eric A. Fertuck

Key Points

- Borderline personality disorder (BPD) is characterized by identity disturbance, unstable relationships, emotional instability, and impulsivity.
- BPD was first included as a discrete mental disorder in the DSM in 1980.
- Categorical models of BPD have received criticism due to the heterogeneity and co-occurrence of the diagnosis with other mental disorders, with most experts advocating for a transition toward a dimensional or hybrid conceptualization of the disorder.
- Approximately 2.7 percent–5.9 percent of the general population meet the criteria for BPD at some point in their lives.
- BPD commonly co-occurs with several other mental disorders, including major depressive disorder, bipolar disorder, anxiety disorders, post-traumatic stress disorder, and substance use disorders.
- Few genome-wide association studies with large enough sample sizes have been performed to pinpoint specific genetic risk variants, but gene-based analysis suggests that dihydropyrimidine dehydrogenase and plakophilin-4 may be implicated.
- Individuals with BPD may have brain abnormalities in areas involved in emotion regulation, including the amygdala and insula, and frontal brain areas involved in regulatory control and social cognition.
- Reduced amounts of the neuropeptide oxytocin and a dysregulated hypothalamic-pituitary-axis may also be associated with BPD.
- Environmental risk factors for BPD are childhood adversity, early trauma and neglect, and insecure and disorganized attachment styles.
- Clinical care of patients with BPD involves thoroughly assessing patient functioning and symptoms, attending to the implications of possible co-occurring mood and other disorders, and assessing prognostic factors (e.g., antisocial features) and severity of illness.
- Individuals with BPD may exhibit a number of transference types and may, in turn, engender a number of countertransference reactions that can influence clinical care if not managed by the clinician.
- Evidence-based psychosocial treatments are front line interventions for BPD. The most robust support is for specialized psychodynamic treatments and dialectical behavior therapy, among other efficacious therapies.
- Pharmacological treatments are adjunctive to psychosocial, evidence-based treatment for BPD. No single pharmacological agent has emerged as the treatment of choice, although atypical antipsychotics and SSRIs may help to alleviate specific symptoms.

Introduction

Borderline personality disorder (BPD) is a mental disorder characterized by instability in interpersonal relationships, affective lability, intense and inappropriate aggressivity and hostility, identity disturbance, and impaired impulse control.[1] BPD commonly co-occurs with a number of other mental disorders, including mood disorders, anxiety disorders, and substance use disorders. BPD is also characterized by relatively high levels of psychosocial impairment relative to other mental disorders.[2] Individuals with BPD are 50 times more likely to die by suicide than those in the general population.[3,4]

History, Phenomenology, and Diagnostic Systems

Three distinctive time periods—late 19th to early 20th century, 1950–2000, and 2000–present—provide a structured way of examining the evolving conceptualizations of BPD.[5]

Phenomenological Description: Late 19th to Early 20th Century

Phenomenological descriptions of likely individuals with BPD date back to the late 19th and early 20th centuries.[6] These individuals were often described by clinicians as having milder forms of psychosis. Kraepelin, for example, described patients with dementia praecox (psychosis) and manic-depression, but also described patients with milder symptoms of each who were somewhere between these two conditions.[7] However, the term "borderline personality" was not used until 1938, when Adolph Stern described a group of patients fitting "neither into the psychotic nor into the psychoneurotic group in terms of symptoms."[8] This label did not appear in either the *Diagnostic Statistical Manual of Mental Disorders* (DSM) I[9] or the DSM II,[10] but began gaining popular use by psychoanalysts after Stern's description of borderline appeared. Helene Deutsch, while not using the term "borderline," published a paper in 1942 describing "as-if" personalities characterized by a lack of warmth and a mild depersonalization that appear to fit a subset of individuals with BPD, including one patient who remarked "I am so empty! . . . I have no feelings."[11]

Kernberg updated Stern's use of the term "borderline" by proposing the term "borderline personality organization", characterized by a specific constellation of symptoms and clinical features including intact relationship to reality, use of defense mechanisms (e.g., splitting and idealization),[12,13] and identity diffusion (e.g., object relations; see Chapter 2 on Levels of Personality Organization). In terms of a specific assessment, borderline personality organization was also considered to include intact general intelligence but disturbed and primitive object relations;[14] support for this conceptualization is mixed.[15,16] Gunderson and Singer[17] conducted a pivotal diagnostic review of the empirical indicators of the "borderline type" of PDs, which eventually led to the construction of the seminal DSM-III BPD criteria. Even at this early stage, their review noted the heterogeneity of descriptions depending on the context for this type. Six distinguishing symptom dimensions were identified that had sensitivity and specificity for the BPD diagnosis: intense affect; history of impulsive behavior; social maladaptiveness; brief, stress-induced psychotic experiences; disorganized thinking in unstructured situations; and relationships that vacillated between superficial and dependent.

DSM-III: 1950–2000

The beginning of a new phase in the conceptualization of BPD was marked by the publication of the DSM-III in 1980.[18] This was characterized by a shift in psychiatry toward observable traits for diagnosis, emphasizing reliability and validity in the assessment. BPD was first included as a distinct disorder in the DSM-III, and began to receive more attention from clinical researchers. The publication of the DSM-III led to increasing standardization of the diagnosis of BPD and the use of semi-structured clinical interviews such as the International Personality Disorder Examination (IPDE).[19] BPD was also included in the DSM-IV in 1994, with only minor changes made to its diagnostic criteria.[20] This conceptualization of BPD is characterized by the use of semi-structured interviews as the gold standard method of identifying BPD in research and some clinical settings, rather than unstructured clinical interviews.[21–23]

Current Understanding: 2000 to Present

Despite the evolution of the scientific literature and conceptualization of PDs since 1980, BPD was maintained without any changes from DSM-IV to DSM-5[1] as a discrete categorical diagnosis. The APA Committee of the DSM-5 deemed newer, dimensional models proposed by the Personality Disorder Task Force to be worthy of further study, but not yet validated. In the current polythetic, categorical formulation, individuals must meet five of the nine listed criteria for a sustained period of time, and the symptoms must cause significant psychosocial distress or functional impairment. The current DSM-5 criteria for BPD involve disruption and dysregulation in the domains of personal relationships, emotions, identity, and impulsive behavior. Disturbances in these areas must be observable in a number of different contexts in order to meet the diagnostic criteria.

As noted by Kendell and Jablensky,[24] the diagnostic criteria used by the DSM allows clinicians and researchers to have some homogeneity in BPD patients across studies and clinics. While diagnostic systems may be useful in providing a common language to describe categorical types of psychopathology, a number of taxometric analyses suggest that disorders such as BPD have a dimensional structure.[25,26]

Hybrid Dimensional-Categorical Taxonomy of BPD

The current understanding of BPD is defined by an evolution from a polythetic, categorical taxonomy of BPD toward a dimensional or hybrid dimensional-categorical taxonomy of BPD and related PDs. Dimensional and hybrid of models of BPD have gained promise for several reasons. First, within the diagnosis of BPD, there is considerable heterogeneity (as exemplified by the 256 ways of meeting the DSM-5 criteria for BPD). Second, there is no clear cut-off point in symptom severity, suggesting a non-binary range of severity rather than discrete PDs. Third, BPD commonly co-occurs with a number of other mental disorders including mood, substance use, post-traumatic stress, and other personality disorders.[27,28] Although the DSM-5 conceptualizes BPD and other personality disorders as categorical, the extensive comorbidities between personality disorders at least suggest a common underlying structure.[29]

DSM-5 Alternate Model of Personality Disorders

In response to growing empirical evidence questioning the DSM-5's categorical conceptualization of BPD, the DSM-5 Personality Disorders Work Group proposed an alternate model to diagnose BPD and other personality disorders. This hybrid model retains a categorical diagnosis while adding supplemental dimensional ratings of specific traits. Section III of the DSM-5 includes an Alternative Model for Personality Disorders, requiring an assessment of impairment level in personality functioning (Criterion A) and an evaluation of 25 dimensional trait facets (Criterion B). In this model, individuals with BPD must experience impairment in at least two of four areas of personality functioning, which include identity, self-direction, empathy, and intimacy. Individuals must also have at least four of seven pathological personality traits, which include impulsivity, emotional lability, and hostility.[1] This hybrid conceptualization of BPD is influenced by trait and psychodynamic object-relations theory approaches to psychopathology. However, Trull et al.[30] have criticized the Work Group's proposed revision for broadening the construct of BPD, citing lack of research on diagnostic validity and inadequate attention to BPD's high comorbidity with other disorders.

International Classification of Diseases, 11th Edition

Alongside the DSM-5, the *International Classification of Diseases* (ICD), 11th edition, is the latest revision of the World Health Organization's taxonomy for mental disorders. The previous version of the ICD, the ICD-10, used a categorical approach similar to that of the DSM-5, describing "emotionally unstable personality disorder," which consisted of an impulsive type, characterized by emotional instability and a lack of impulse control, and a borderline type, which involves identity disturbance, chronic feelings of emptiness, and involvement in intense and unstable relationships.[31] The ICD-11,[32] in contrast, has adopted a dimensional approach to classifying personality disorders, using a global scale of severity as well as specific trait qualifiers (Negative Affectivity, Detachment, Dissociality, Disinhibition, and Anankastic). This approach aligns the ICD-11 with the Five-Factor Model[33] (see Current Models of Personality Disorder section) and the DSM-5's Alternative Model of Personality Disorders, in that it requires clinicians to focus on the overall presence of a personality disorder rather than diagnosing based on heterogeneous sub-types. However, the ICD-11 also allows practitioners to select an optional Borderline Pattern Qualifier, which requires an individual to meet five of the nine diagnostic criteria from the DSM-5. Bach et al.[34] obtained trait domain scores in a sample of psychiatric outpatients with both the ICD-11 and the DSM-5 criteria, and found substantial overlap between the two models. However, the ICD-11 was found to better capture obsessive-compulsive personality disorder, while the DSM-5 was found to better capture schizotypal personality disorder.

Current Models of Personality Disorder

In addition to the ICD-11, other current models of BPD and PDs have been proposed including the Five-Factor Model, G-Factor model,[29] and the Hierarchical Taxonomy of Personality (HiTOP)[34,35] model. Detailed descriptions of these models are beyond the scope of this chapter, but they are important areas of future research as understandings of the structure of BPD continue to evolve. Each of these models attempt to address the limitations of categorical models, such as heterogeneity of diagnoses and excessive comorbidities with other disorders.

Briefly, the Five-Factor Model of personality (FFM) provides a model of both abnormal and normal personality functioning.[33] In this model, personality disorders are understood as maladaptive variants of five factors of personality. Another model, the G-Factor model, is analogous to theoretical models of intelligence. The G-Factor model accordingly considers a PD in terms of both general ("g") and specific ("s") factors.[29] In the G-Factor model, a general factor "g" may underlie all personality disorders, while unique aspects of specific disorders may be explained by other distinct factors ("s"). Finally, the hierarchical taxonomy of psychopathology, or HiTOP model, addresses the limitations of categorical models by grouping related symptoms dimensions together (as derived via statistical factor analysis) into syndromes, to reduce diagnostic heterogeneity.[35]

Epidemiology, Gender, and Ethnicity

Studies of the prevalence of BPD have used a number of different sampling and assessment methods, leading to an estimated range of prevalence and incidence for the disorder. Gunderson[36] calculated the range for the two-year to five-year prevalence of BPD across a number of studies using structured clinical interviews as being between >1 percent and 4.5 percent, with a median of 1.7 percent and a mean of 1.6 percent.[37-40] This prevalence rate would make BPD the fourth most prevalent of the ten DSM-5 personality disorders.

Studies indicate that between 2.7 and 5.9 percent of the general population have met the diagnostic criteria for BPD at some point during their lifetimes.[30,41] In terms of prevalence rates for BPD in clinical populations in the healthcare system, Gross et al.[42] found a lifetime prevalence of 6.4 percent in an urban primary care practice.

The prevalence rate of BPD in psychiatric clinical populations appears to be much higher than both the point prevalence and the lifetime prevalence of community and population samples. Gunderson et al. report the point prevalence of BPD in psychiatric clinics and hospitals to be 15–28 percent across a number of studies of psychiatric patients.[43-45] Similarly, Ellison et al. report a point prevalence for BPD of about 10–12 percent for outpatient clinics, and 20–22 percent among inpatient psychiatric settings.[46]

Remission Rate of BPD

At a 16-year follow-up assessment of individuals with BPD, Zanarini et al.[47] found an eight-year remission rate of 78 percent and a two-year remission rate of 99 percent for BPD criteria. In this unique longitudinal study, remissions occurred more rapidly among other PDs than among individuals diagnosed with BPD. Gunderson[48] reported a remission rate of 85 percent for individuals diagnosed with BPD after ten years; in this study, all criteria of BPD remitted at a similar rate, but social functioning scores failed to improve significantly. A third study showed that symptoms of anger and self-destructive behavior in BPD remit over time, while older adults with BPD remain impaired in terms of emotion regulation, impulsivity, and social functioning.[49]

Gender and Ethnicity Differences

In terms of gender differences in rates of BPD, the long-standing conventional wisdom is that there are higher rates of BPD in women than in men. However, while there are higher rates of women with BPD than men in clinical settings, the prevalence appears to be equal between men and women in several population-based epidemiologic studies.[50] In the National Epidemiologic Survey on Alcohol and Related Conditions (NESARC), Grant et al.[41] found no significant gender differences in BPD rates between women (6.2 percent) and men (5.6 percent). Tomko et al.[51] found slightly higher rates of BPD in women (3.0 percent) than in men (2.4 percent), while also finding that men in the lowest income bracket had higher levels of BPD than women in the same bracket. In terms of gender differences in presentation of the disorder, Silberschmidt et al.[52] found that women diagnosed with BPD reported greater levels of hostility, relationship disruption, symptoms of depression, anxiety, and somatization, than men.

In terms of race, ethnicity, and sexual identity, the NESARC study found an interaction between gender and ethnicity, such that BPD was more prevalent in Native American men, and less prevalent among Asian women. A study of sexual minority individuals found that they were more likely to be diagnosed with BPD than heterosexuals, but this may be the result of clinician bias.[53] While there have been intriguing preliminary results in the area, there is a need for more studies investigating the relationships between BPD and race, ethnicity, gender, and sexual identity.[54]

Self-Injury, Suicidal Ideation, and Suicide

Individuals with BPD complete suicide more often than individuals in the general population.[4] Individuals with BPD may account for between 9–33 percent of all completed suicides.[54-56] The rate at which individuals with BPD complete suicide has been estimated at almost 50 times greater than in the general population.[57] This is especially concerning considering the relatively high prevalence rates of BPD: around three times higher than that of schizophrenia, which is often considered to be a diagnosis with one of the most debilitating clinical courses.[58] Rates of non-suicidal self-injury in BPD are also very high, estimated to be as high as 90 percent.[59] Taken together, the high rates of both suicidality and non-suicidal self-injury in individuals with BPD indicate the severity of the distress experienced by many of those diagnosed.

Common Co-occurring Disorders

Individuals with BPD commonly meet criteria for other co-occurring conditions, including depressive disorders, bipolar disorder, anxiety disorders, post-traumatic stress disorder, substance use disorder, and eating disorders.

BPD and Major Depressive Disorder

Approximately 75 percent of those with a lifetime BPD diagnosis also have met the criteria for a lifetime mood disorder.[41] In terms of specific mood disorders, major depressive disorder (MDD) is the most common. Lifetime rates of experiencing a major depressive episode or another depressive disorder in those with BPD ranges between 70–90 percent.[28,60-62] BPD co-occurs for 25 percent of those with MDD[63] or dysthymia.[64] Despite these high rates of co-occurrence, BPD cannot be reduced to a subtype of MDD, because they each exhibit distinct phenomenology, course of illness, treatment response, and biomarkers.[65,66] However, the co-occurrence of BPD and MDD is clinically significant both in terms of treatment planning and the course of the illnesses. Those with both MDD and BPD are more likely to attempt suicide than those with MDD without BPD;[67] co-occurring BPD and MDD are also associated with both longer major depressive episodes as well as shorter length of time between depressive episodes.[61,68]

BPD and Bipolar Disorder

Reviews performed by Zimmerman and Morgan[69] and Frías et al.[70] indicate that around 20 percent of those with BPD also have bipolar disorder, either type I or type II. These moderate rates of co-occurrence between BPD and bipolar disorder, and the similarities in the disorders such as features of impulsivity and mood instability, have led to some reviewers to suggest that BPD should be conceptualized as belonging to the bipolar spectrum.[71,72] Others, such as Paris[73] and Dolan-Sewell et al.[74] argue that the evidence does not support this conclusion. Prospective studies have not shown BD to occur in BPD patients at higher rates than other psychiatric disorders.[75,76] Imaging studies indicate that the two disorders may exhibit differences in hippocampal morphology.[77] Regardless of the exact nature of the relationship between BPD and BD, their co-occurrence is associated with negative outcomes such as more suicide attempts than those who only have BD[72,78] and prolonged unemployment.[79]

BPD and Anxiety Disorders

Anxiety disorders are nearly as common as mood disorders in those with BPD. The lifetime prevalence of anxiety disorders found in a community sample of those with BPD was 74 percent.[41] The prevalence ranges from 0–35 percent for generalized anxiety disorder, 2–48 percent for panic disorder, 3–46 percent for social phobia, and 0–20 percent for obsessive- compulsive disorder.[80] These anxiety disorders may be intermittent, however, as a longitudinal study performed by Silverman et al.[81] found that after a period of ten years, prevalence rates of anxiety disorders in treated BPD reduced from approximately 80 percent pre-treatment to 38 percent post-treatment. The relationship between anxiety sensitivity and BPD suggests that anxiety disorders and BPD may have shared underlying trait anxiety.[82]

BPD and Post-traumatic Stress Disorder

Grant et al.[41] found that 31.6 percent of BPD patients in a national comorbidity study met the criteria for post-traumatic stress disorder (PTSD). However, similar to the co-occurrence between BPD and mood disorders, BPD and PTSD appear to be distinct disorders with unique patterns of symptoms.[83] Due to symptomatic similarities between the two disorders—including irritability, dissociation, and inability to tolerate emotional extremes[84]—clinicians can often have difficulty differentiating BPD from PTSD.[85] The symptomatic similarities may be due in part to the mutual influence of childhood trauma on both BPD and PTSD. However, childhood trauma does not occur in all those with BPD.[86] Individuals with co-occurring BPD and PTSD may engage in more non-suicidal self-injury than those with only one of these disorders[87] (see Chapter 3 for further discussion about trauma and the relationship to BPD).

BPD and Attention-deficit Hyperactivity Disorder

Attention-deficit hyperactivity disorder (ADHD) often co-occurs with BPD.[88,89] One study using a structured clinical interview found that 27 percent of adults with ADHD met criteria for co-occurring BPD.[90] Overlapping features between BPD and ADHD include impulsivity[91] and emotion dysregulation.[92,93] Further studies are needed to compare the use of ADHD medications to treat those with co-occurring ADHD and BPD.

BPD and Substance Use

A review by Trull et al.[94] found that approximately half of those with BPD have a co-occurring substance use disorder (SUD), most often alcohol use disorder, and that approximately 25 percent of those with a current SUD meet the criteria for BPD. Approximately 73 percent of those with a lifetime BPD diagnosis meet the criteria for a SUD.[39] Similar to ADHD, theorists have suggested that both impulsivity and emotion regulation play a role in the development of both disorders.[95,96]

BPD and Eating Disorders

A meta-analysis of eating disorders found rates of personality disorders including BPD ranging from 0–58 percent among individuals with anorexia nervosa and bulimia nervosa.[97] BPD and other personality disorders may be associated with poorer outcomes for individuals with eating disorders.[98,99]

BPD and Other Personality Disorders

Substantial overlap exists between BPD and other personality disorders, which may result from issues with the categorical model discussed in the section on history, phenomenology, and diagnostic systems. In a large epidemiological study, the majority of patients diagnosed with any personality disorder were diagnosed with more than one.[100] Grant et al.[41] found that BPD was strongly associated with schizotypal and narcissistic personality disorders.

BPD and Other Psychiatric and Medical Disorders

Recent studies have begun to examine the co-occurrence of BPD and other disorders with which it has been less commonly linked. One study found that 40 percent of individuals with BPD had co-occurring psychotic disorders, especially of the Not Otherwise

Specified subtype, which may relate to the DSM-5 criterion of "transient, stress-related paranoid ideation" for BPD.[101]

BPD is also associated with health conditions such as cardiovascular disease, stroke, diabetes, obesity, gastrointestinal disease, arthritis, chronic pain, venereal disease, HIV infection, and sleep disorders.[102] Accordingly, medical service utilization is high among those with BPD.

Genetic, Biologic, and Neural Underpinnings

Both genetic and environmental factors interact in the development of BPD.[103] Twin studies examining BPD suggest a mean heritability of approximately 40 percent.[104] However, larger sample sizes are needed in order to conduct genome-wide association studies (GWAs) with enough statistical power to detect the contribution of specific genetic risk variants. While GWAs for schizophrenia have used tens of thousands of subjects, the largest such study for BPD had only 1,075 participants.[105] No genetic variants in this GWA reached significance using single-marker analysis, but gene-based analysis yielded significance for two genes: dihydropyrimidine dehydrogenase (DPYD) and plakophilin-4 (PKP4).[106] The paucity of significant associations found between BPD and specific risk genes may be explained in part by the small sample sizes of studies conducted, BPD's heterogeneous diagnostic presentation, interactions between multiple genes, and the complex interaction between genetic and environmental factors.

Individuals with BPD appear to have abnormalities in areas of the brain involved in social-emotional processing, including the amygdala and the insula, as well as frontal brain regions involved in regulatory control, including the anterior cingulate cortex, medial frontal cortex, orbitofrontal cortex, and dorsolateral prefrontal cortex.[107] A meta-analysis by Schulze et al.[108] found reduced gray matter volume along with hyperactivity of the left amygdala in individuals with BPD, relative to controls. Amygdala hyperactivity was moderated by individuals' medication status. Individuals with BPD also exhibit impaired amygdala habituation when presented a series of negative affect inducing images.[109] A meta-analysis of neuroimaging studies by Yang et al.[110] found that individuals with BPD have reduced gray matter in areas of the brain associated with the frontolimbic circuit, including the right insular cortex, the left hippocampus, and the left medial orbitofrontal cortex.

Studies using diffusion tensor imaging to examine white matter integrity in individuals with BPD have yielded mixed results. One study found lower axial diffusivity in the cingulum and the inferior occipital and the inferior fasciculus.[111] Others studies have found decreased fractional anisotropy in the corpus callosum, corona radiata,[112] dorsal anterior cingulate cortex,[113] uncinate fasciculus,[114] cingulum, and fornix.[115]

Processing of social stimuli such as faces and other nonverbal cues are negatively biased in BPD, leading to impairments in accurately appraising the trustworthiness of others.[116] Impaired appraisal of trustworthiness is associated with less frontal activation relative to controls, suggesting impaired top-down decision-making with regard to trustworthiness appraisal specifically. Those with BPD were comparable behaviorally and neurologically when appraising fear in others.[117] The neuropeptide oxytocin may play an important role in the rejection sensitivity and attachment difficulties of individuals with BPD.[118] Women with BPD were found to have reduced oxytocin concentrations, with a negative relationship between their levels of plasma oxytocin and the number of traumatic childhood experiences they reported.[119]

The hypothalamic–pituitary–adrenal (HPA) axis has been implicated in BPD due to its role in stress responses.[120] Results have been mixed in terms of cortisol concentrations in patients with BPD. Some studies report increased levels and other studies report no differences.[121] Corniquel et al.[122] have proposed an animal model of BPD in which early life stress affects the maturation of the hypothalamic–pituitary–adrenal axis, and later mild stress in early adulthood results in increased impulsivity and issues with habituation and social interactions.

Psycho-social-cultural Risk Factors

Several studies have found that individuals with BPD are more likely to report adverse childhood experiences.[123,124] A meta-analysis of case-control studies found that individuals with BPD with emotional abuse and neglect are 13.91 times more likely to report childhood adversity than controls.[125] Hengartner et al.[126] found that childhood sexual abuse had a small but significant association with BPD. Dysregulation of the HPA axis, as previously mentioned, has been associated with childhood trauma experiences.[127] This may help explain the relationship between genetic factors and environmental factors such as childhood trauma in BPD. Cohen et al.[128] found that low socioeconomic status is also associated with the development of BPD.

BPD has been associated with insecure and disorganized attachment styles, which develops from a childhood marked by erratic or inconsistent caregiving.[129] One study found that BPD individuals with a disorganized attachment style have lower plasma levels of oxytocin than BPD patients with an organized attachment style.[130] A disorganized attachment style in individuals with BPD has also been associated with increased amygdala activation as measured by fMRI in response to the administration of the Adult Attachment Projective Picture System.[131]

A number of cultural factors have been identified that may play a role in the diagnosis of BPD, particularly in Asian cultures. Ronningstam et al.[132] describe how the diagnosis of BPD has been met with skepticism in the Chinese psychiatric community due to the focus of several criteria on interpersonal relationships, which may not translate to the collectivistic values of Chinese culture. Despite this skepticism, prevalence rates of BPD in China and other Asian countries appear to be comparable to those reported in North America and Europe.[133] A study in Singapore of BPD using the McLean Screening Instrument suggested that the factor structure of BPD symptoms may differ from that measured in Western cultures, such that behavioral and interpersonal dysregulation are more tightly intertwined in collectivistic cultures like that of Singapore.[134] In Western studies using the McLean Screening Instrument, by contrast, behavioral and interpersonal dysregulation appear to be more independent factors.[135]

Interviewing, Assessment, Case Formulation, and Treatment of BPD

This section reviews several dimensions related to the assessment and treatment of BPD, including symptom assessment, personality assessment, differential diagnosis, prognosis, case formulation, and the role of transference and countertransference.

Assessment of BPD

A thorough assessment of BPD is crucial for treatment planning and requires several steps.[136,137] After gathering identifying information (demographics, race/ethnicity, relationship status, sexual orientation, occupation, education level, physical appearance, etc.), the clinician should clarify the presenting problem(s) including the "chief complaint" and an initial mental status examination. A comprehensive assessment of the current life of someone potentially with BPD should not just focus on symptoms, but also functioning in life more generally. This is because individuals with BPD are often struggling in multiple spheres of functioning. In addition, the clinician should ascertain functioning in three spheres of life functioning: (1) love and sexual relations; (2) work, career, and vocation; and (3) creative pursuits and leisure activity. For most individuals with BPD, it is essential to consult with former treaters and close family members to get a full clinical picture due to the possibility that the patient is a poor historian, unable to convey a coherent biography due to identity diffusion, or dishonesty if antisocial features are prominent.[138] Finally, suicidality, including history of suicide attempts, their precipitants and motivations, and history of other self-destructive behaviors is essential, with a particular focus on current suicidality.[3,139]

Only after a thorough assessment of present life should the clinician then focus on the background to the problem, including a history of the disorder, symptoms, history of mental health treatment, and evaluation of both psychopharmacologic and previous psychosocial treatments. Finally, a relevant developmental and family history is required, including any relevant developmental delays, early adversity, and socio-emotional difficulties. A family history of mental health and substance abuse diagnoses and treatment can point toward patient vulnerabilities in these areas. The Structured Interview for Personality Organization[140] provides the clinician concrete questions that facilitate diagnosis of levels of personality organization and major character types with relevance for prognosis and treatment course (i.e., pathological narcissism).

Diagnosis and Comorbidities for BPD

Most individuals with BPD exhibit some form of depressive symptomatology. Analogous to a fever in a medical diagnosis, however, depressive symptoms alone are insufficient for differential diagnosis and effective treatment recommendations. With regard to depressive disorders, clinicians tend to engage in two primary pitfalls.[141] The first is accurately diagnosing a mood disorder, but not thoroughly assessing a personality disorder like BPD. This issue is particularly common for clinicians diagnosing bipolar disorder without considering BPD. This concerning practice often leads to ineffective polypharmacy and the delay in the implementation of evidence-based treatment for BPD. Moreover, suicidality and hospitalization that could be prevented is more likely if a BPD diagnosis is mistaken for a bipolar disorder. Importantly, for individuals with both depressive disorders and BPD, treatment of BPD symptoms leads to improvements in mood disorder symptoms.[60] This finding is contrary to conventional clinical wisdom that one cannot treat BPD until depression is first treated.

The second common pitfall for clinicians is accurately diagnosing BPD, while neglecting a co-occurring mood disorder. The consequence of this missed diagnosis could be an unnecessary delay in treatment for moderate to severe depressive symptoms or manic symptoms, and an untreated mood episode. The consequence of untreated mood episodes in BPD are increased risk for preventable suicidality and hospitalization.[3,139]

After the completion of the assessment, the clinician should be able to formulate an initial diagnosis (or, revised diagnosis, if the diagnosis changed during the course of the treatment). A descriptive, phenomenological (DSM-5) diagnosis should include any medical conditions and a thorough differential diagnosis of mood disorders, anxiety disorders, PTSD, SUD, learning disability, and eating disorders. Some clinicians avoid disclosing the BPD diagnosis, citing concerns about stigma or inducing hopelessness in patients. However, reviewing the symptoms and problems actively with the patient and discussing how they support a BPD diagnosis sets the stage for ensuring that the clinician and patient have a shared understanding of the clinical presentation and facilitates the recommendation of appropriate evidence-based treatment. Individuals with BPD deserve clarity why they are not being recommended other non-indicated treatment options such as polypharmacy or other standard treatments for non-BPD diagnoses that have common symptoms (e.g., exposure therapy for PTSD or cognitive-behavioral therapy for depression).[142]

Personality Organization Assessment and BPD

In addition to a phenomenological diagnosis, a diagnosis of psychodynamically in-formed personality organization and character style can greatly aid in evaluating prognosis, treatment planning, and anticipating predominant transference and countertransference dynamics.[136,137] Facets of personality functioning that can greatly aid assessment and treatment planning include: assessment of identity (the coherence and continuity of one's self-concept and understanding of others and investment in goals); quality of object relations (the maturity of internalized mental representations of significant others and capacity for intimacy); defensive operations (the adaptability versus rigidity/maladaptiveness of psychological defenses in the face of internal and external stressors); moral functioning (the capacity for an ethical and consistent set of values that one lives by); aggression (the capacity to adaptively tolerate and express anger, hostility, and aggressive behavior versus inhibiting and "acting out" impulsively with aggressive impulses); and reality testing (the capacity to differentiate shared perceptions of social reality from perceptual distortions unique to the patient).

Those with borderline personality organization exhibit rapidly shifting, polarized, and rigid mental representations of self and others. Identity diffusion is a consequence of these "split" mental representations. Additionally, these individuals have a superficial understanding of the mental life of self and others and poor capacity to reason about mental states. Except under psychosocial stress, individuals exhibit intact reality testing, which distinguishes them from individuals with psychotic personality organization. By contrast, patients with a healthier neurotic personality organization have a relatively consolidated identity, adaptive repression-based defenses, and more mature object relations including a capacity for intimacy and healthy dependency on significant others (see Chapter 2 Levels of Personality Organization).

Case Formulations

While an assessment of descriptive phenomenology and relevant bio-psychosocial context is common to all treatment approaches for BPD, each treatment approach has a particular framework and emphases for case formulation based on their model of BPD. For instance, transference-focused psychotherapy (TFP)[137] considers the patient's person-ality structure as driving symptoms and functioning, and thus requires careful formula-tion of personality levels and object relations in case formulation. By contrast, dialectical behavior therapy (DBT)[143] considers deficits in emotion regulation as the core driver of ineffective behaviors (e.g., suicidality and non-suicidal self-injury); a case formulation identifies areas of weakness and skills that the patient might develop to bolster emotion regulation. (More details on case formulation, based on different theories, are offered throughout the book.)

Transference and Countertransference

Individuals with BPD can elicit intense and polarized transference dynamics[136,144] and countertransference reactions.[145] Transference is often emotionally intense, conscious, and either negative (i.e., paranoid) or positive (i.e., idealizing) from the earliest first clin-ical encounters in individuals with BPD. In contrast to individuals with a neurotic per-sonality organization, who can often express transferential sentiments verbally, those with BPD often express transference most robustly through nonverbal channels (facial expression, tone of voice, posture, behaviors, etc.) and enactments. Clinicians' intense negative countertransference to individuals with BPD are common and are often diffi-cult to manage without adequate training and supervision.

Typical Transferences in Patient with BPD
There are several predominant transference types in clinical work with BPD patients.[144] A paranoid transference is present when an individual with BPD fears that if they are open with their clinician about their problems, the clinician will be critical, rejecting, or cruel toward the patient. This type of transference is typical at the beginning of psycho-therapy for BPD as the patient begins to be more forthcoming with their difficulties.

A narcissistic transference is dominant when patients expresses depreciation of the therapist and a corresponding entitlement and inflated self-worth in relation to the ther-apist. The patient in a narcissistic transference experiences the realistically helpful atti-tude of the therapist as a threat. This is because the patient has an underlying fear that being in a dependent role with the therapist will be a humiliating weakness. The skill and benevolence of the therapist also stimulates intolerable envy in the narcissistic pa-tient. Often, a rivalry or competition between the patient and clinician around who is more powerful in the relationship is enacted in a narcissistic transference. The patient's attempt to control the session and appropriate the therapist's insights as their own are also common in this transference.

An erotic transference is apparent when sexual interest or desires emerge toward the therapist, or the patient attributes sexual desire to the therapist. In some instances, an individual with BPD may engage in risky sexual encounters as a reaction to feeling frustrated by the therapist. Other difficulties with the treatment can emerge if a patient attempts to destroy the therapy by inducing a sexual relationship with the therapist. In other instances, a more benign erotic transference can emerge as part of a working-through of sexual inhibitions or traumas that the patient has not resolved.

Depressive transference, although less common in the early stages of therapy with BPD, may emerge as the individual with BPD begins to work through the loss of "ideal-ized" images of others. These unrealistic idealizations are rooted in early, infantile wishes for ideal and perfect caregivers. Feelings of sadness, loss, regret, and guilt toward the therapist and others may be associated with this type of transference. A more realistic view of the therapist as an authentic but imperfect ally in the patient's life can emerge, and a more collaborative atmosphere can develop in the transference.

Countertransference to Patients with BPD

Distressing countertransference feelings that arise when working with individuals with BPD can confuse therapists and disrupt their ability to empathize with their patients and communicate effectively with them. These emotional reactions in the therapist can develop rapidly, feel "alien" to the therapist, be unstable, and compel the therapist to act rather than reflect. Individuals with BPD express, in nonverbal behavior and in interpersonal dynamics, what they cannot symbolize and articulate. Accordingly, the dominant affects and conflicts can be "felt" in the countertransference or experienced as enactment within the treatment. Therefore, a clinician working with an individual with BPD would do well to recurrently ask, "How do I feel with this person, and what might that tell me about what is going on between us?" A full range of countertransference feelings— including the urge to avoid the patient, feelings of disgust, and other negative effects— need to be tolerated by the therapist. Countertransference reactions, if reflected upon by the clinician, can facilitate assessment and treatment of BPD. Countertransference can be a "third channel" (alongside verbal and nonverbal channels) of communication that is an indispensable source of raw material regarding the object relations of the individual with BPD as activated in the transference.

There are several classes of countertransference reaction common to BPD and other Cluster B personality disorders.[145] An overwhelmed/disorganized countertransference is experienced by a clinician as feeling dread toward or threatened by a patient, leading to feeling overwhelmed and confused (as opposed to competent, helpful, and curious). If the feeling is unique to one particular BPD patient, then the potential importance of this countertransference increases. Inexperienced clinicians may have a difficulty tolerating this countertransference, as it can dovetail with their own doubts about their competence.

A special/overinvolved countertransference is experienced by the clinician with a feeling that a patient is special and perhaps a "favorite." This can lead to difficulties in maintaining professional boundaries ranging from excessive self-disclosure to getting involved in the patient's life outside of sessions. Therapist feelings of guilt or pity related to an image of the patient as vulnerable and the victim of external forces can cloud the clinician's clinical judgment and disturb the maintenance of a therapeutic treatment structure.

A sexualized countertransference is experienced when a clinician develops erotic feelings or desires toward the patient, or experiences sexual tension in the therapeutic relationship.

A criticized/mistreated countertransference is experienced when a clinician feels undervalued, helpless, criticized, inadequate, and incompetent with regard to a patient (often in contrast to other patients).

A parental countertransference may occur when a therapist takes on a maternal or paternal, nurturing role that goes beyond the typical genuine warmth that one might feel for a patient. The clinician may fantasize of re-parenting the patient, often in compensation for some perceived poor parenting in the patient's actual life.

A study examining clinicians' perceptions of their Cluster B personality disorder patients using a countertransference questionnaire identified a number of factors associated with clinical work with this patient population.[145] Clinicians with individuals with BPD as patients tended to endorse the "special/overinvolved" countertransference. More broadly, patients with Cluster B personality disorders (which also include antisocial personality disorder and narcissistic personality disorder) were also associated with the factors "overwhelmed/disorganized," "helpless/inadequate," and "sexualized."[145] In summary, knowledge and tolerance of countertransference reaction is particularly useful when treating individuals who have BPD, because it is a window into their interpersonal experience that they cannot articulate and express in another way at the outset of treatment.

Treatment Recommendations and Plan

The current state of the treatment and patient's functioning and response to current and prior treatment should also inform a treatment recommendation and plan. While there are several evidence-based options for the treatment of BPD, there are several factors that predict poor treatment response. Negative prognostic signs include high levels of antisocial features (dishonesty, ego-syntonic aggression, exploitation of others), investment in the sick role, somatization, active substance use, and a history of severe suicide attempts.[146,147] With regard to predicting suicidality, a multi-site study of personality disorders found that identity disturbance, frantic efforts to avoid abandonment, and chronic feelings of emptiness were the strongest predictors of suicidality over a ten-year period.[148]

Evidence-based Treatment for BPD

Until about the early 2000s, clinicians were taught to consider BPD as largely untreatable with a negative long-term prognosis. With the evolution of specialized, manualized form of psychotherapy and targeted medications, clinicians now have reason for optimism in the treatment of BPD.[149–151] Furthermore, the long-term prognosis for most with BPD is more positive than previously appreciated.[152] Recent meta-analyses suggest that specialized theory- based psychotherapies for BPD are effective, with psychodynamic treatments and DBT evidencing robust effects.[150,151] However, the magnitude of therapeutic effects are moderate, the long-term stability of improvement is not rigorously documented for most interventions, and there is some evidence of biases in publication and interpretation of outcomes. With regard to the Strength of Recommendation Taxonomy (SORT),[153] treatments subsequently described in the next section for BPD would likely receive a "A" grade, indicating acceptability to patients, support from at least two well-conducted clinical trials, and support from systematic review or meta-analysis. At this point, there is no "treatment of choice" for BPD, because meta-analytic studies have not found one treatment that has emerged as superior in clinical efficacy to others. Therefore, the clinician must make treatment recommendations based predominantly on the prognostic signs, case severity, and the presence and availability of specialized clinicians or treatment programs.

There are now several psychosocial treatments for BPD that have some empirical support from randomized control trials (RCTs).

Dialectical Behavior Therapy (DBT)

DBT is a cognitive-behavioral treatment that balances "acceptance" and "change" strategies to help individuals with BPD improve emotion-regulation capacities. It has two components: individual therapy and weekly group-skills training. The therapist functions as a coach in teaching patients emotion-regulation skills, and supports the patient in applying them in everyday life. DBT also recommends weekly group supervision and consultation among therapists. The individual treatment focuses on a hierarchy of target behaviors that the patient tracks on a daily basis using diary cards. DBT has been found to be efficacious in reducing suicidality and several symptom dimensions in many RCTs.[150,151] See Chapter 11 for a detailed description of DBT for BPD.

Cognitive-behavioral Therapy (CBT)

CBT is a structured, time limited, individual treatment that focuses on altering core dysfunctional beliefs specific to BPD. CBT plus treatment as usual for BPD had better outcomes in suicide prevention and other symptom domains compared to treatment as usual without CBT.[154] See Chapter 10 for a detailed description of CBT for BPD.

Schema Therapy (ST)

ST posits the existence of schema modes (conceptions of self in relation to significant others) common and specific to BPD. Schemas are expressed in enduring and chronic patterns of thinking, feeling, and behaving. The putative mechanism of change in ST is to help the patient become less influenced by these pervasive schemas. This therapy has demonstrated efficacy in multiple domains of symptoms and functioning in one RCT.[155] See Chapter 12 for a detailed description of ST treatment of BPD.

Mentalization-based Treatment (MBT)

MBT for BPD is a based on psychodynamic and attachment theories and neuroscience in partial hospital and other outpatient settings. MBT focuses on increasing "mentalization" in BPD. Mentalization entails making sense of the actions of oneself and others on the basis of intentional mental states, such as desires, feelings, and beliefs. MBT has been found to be efficacious and cost-effective compared to treatment as usual and other treatments.[156] See Chapter 9 for a detailed description of MBT treatment of BPD.

Transference-focused Psychotherapy (TFP)

TFP is a psychoanalytic treatment rooted in object-relations theory that addresses disturbance in identity and conceptions of self and significant others in patients with BPD. It aims to reduce suicidality and aggressive behaviors, increase the coherence of identity, and to improve vocational and social functioning. TFP has received empirical support in RCTs,[157] and there is preliminary support for TFP specific mechanisms of change in BPD.[158] See Chapter 8 for a detailed description of TFP treatment of BPD.

Dynamic Supportive Psychotherapy (DSP)

DSP[159] provides emotional support and advice on the daily problems of living for individuals with BPD. The therapist follows and manages the therapeutic relationship but, unlike treatments such as TFP, does not primarily utilize an understanding and reappraisal of the therapeutic relationship to engender clinical change. Instead, DSP aims to bolster the use of healthy coping strategies and defenses rather than more primitive and "acting out" defenses. DSP has empirical support in one RCT.[160]

Good Psychiatric Management (GPM)

GPM is a group of psychosocial interventions that integrate case management with supportive psychotherapy for individuals with BPD.[161,162] The GPM therapists eclectically apply psychodynamic and cognitive-behavioral techniques and strategies; however, extensive training in either of these approaches is not required to implement GPM. The case management component provides concrete support and problem-solving assistance for present challenges in the patient's life. The psychotherapy component aims to improve self-concept and adaptation to life stressors. See Chapter 13 for a detailed description of GPM treatment of BPD.

Efficacy of Medication in BPD

The use of medication(s) as a first-line or solo interventions for BPD is not supported. No single pharmacologic agent has emerged as the treatment of choice for BPD.[163,164] Atypical neuroleptics show promise for reducing quasi-psychotic symptoms and the other dimensions of BPD.[165] Placebo-controlled studies provide debatable preliminary support for the efficacy of selective serotonin reuptake inhibitors (SSRIs) on mood dysregulation, irritability and hostility, and anxiety.[166] Mood stabilizers may be efficacious in the treatment of dimensions of BPD such as impulsive-aggression.[167] There is also limited support for the use of omega-3 fatty acids in the treatment of BPD,[164] with better compliance, fewer side effects, and less stigma than conventional mood stabilizers. Review Chapter 15, Psychopharmacology of Personality Disorders, for a very detailed review.

Conclusion

This chapter provides an overview of BPD, describing its historically evolving conceptualization. BPD is a relatively common condition in both clinical settings and in the general population. Complicating assessment and treatment planning, BPD frequently co-occurs with major depressive, bipolar, anxiety, post-traumatic stress, and substance use disorders. Both genetic and environmental factors contribute in the development of BPD.

Box 19.1 Relevant resources for Patients, Families, and Clinicians

---

- The National Education Alliance for BPD (NEA BPD). https://www.border-linepersonalitydisorder.org.
- Emotions Matter. https://emotionsmatterbpd.org/
- Treatment and Research Advancements for BPD (TARA4BPD). https://www.tara4bpd.org/.
- National Institute of Mental Health Information on BPD. https://www.nimh.nih.gov/health/topics/borderline-personality-disorder/index.shtml.
- Project Air Strategy for Personality Disorders. https://www.uow.edu.au/project-air/.

Neuroanatomical findings suggest abnormalities in regions of the brain involved in social-emotional processing and regulation control. Childhood adversity appears to be associated with BPD, which often coincides with an insecure or disorganized attachment style. Diagnosis, case formulation, and treatment planning for BPD requires careful assessment. There are now several psychosocial treatments with some promise. Understanding and tolerance for common transferences and countertransference observed in individuals with BPD can facilitate clinical work with this underserved and high-risk population. Review Box 19.1 for relevant resources for patients, families, and clinicians.

Conflict of Interest/Disclosure: The authors of this chapter have no financial conflicts and nothing to disclose.

References

1. *Diagnostic and Statistical Manual of Mental Disorders.* 5th ed. Washington, DC: American Psychiatric Association; 2013.

2. Skodol AE, Gunderson JG, McGlashan TH, et al. Functional impairment in patients with schizotypal, borderline, avoidant, or obsessive-compulsive personality disorder. *Am J Psychiatry.* 2002; 159: 276–283.

3. Fertuck EA, Makhija N, Stanley B. The nature of suicidality in borderline personality disorder. *Prim Psychiatry.* 2007; 14: 40–47.

4. Pompili M, Girardi P, Ruberto A, Tatarelli R. Suicide in borderline personality disorder: a meta-analysis. *Nord J Psychiatry.* 2005; 59: 319–324.

5. Fertuck EA, Lenzenweger MF, Hoerman S, Stanley B. Executive neurocognition, memory systems, and borderline personality disorder. *Clin Psychol Rev.* 2006; 26: 346–375.

6. Stone MH. *Essential Papers on Borderline Disorders: One Hundred Years at the Border.* New York, NY: NYU Press; 1986.

7. Kraepelin, Emil. "Dementia praecox and paraphrenia." (1921): 384.

8. Stern A. Psychoanalytic investigation of and therapy in the border line group of neuroses. *Psychoanal Q.* 1938; 7: 467–489.

9. *Diagnostic and Statistical Manual of Mental Disorders.* 1st ed. Washington, DC: American Psychiatric Association; 1952.

10. *Diagnostic and Statistical Manual of Mental Disorders*. 2nd ed. Washington, DC: American Psychiatric Association; 1968.

11. Deutsch H. Some forms of emotional disturbance and their relation to schizophrenia. *Psychoanal Q*. 1942; 11: 301–321.

12. Kernberg OF. Borderline personality organization. *J Am Psychoanal Assoc*. 1967; 15: 641–685.

13. Kernberg OF. Technical considerations in the treatment of borderline personality organization. *J Am Psychoanal Assoc*. 1976; 24: 795–829.

14. Rapaport D. *Diagnostic Psychological Testing*. Vol. 1. Chicago, IL: Year Book Publishers; 1945.

15. Gartner J, Hurt SW, Gartner A. Psychological test signs of borderline personality disorder: a review of the empirical literature. *J Pers Assess*. 1989; 53: 423–441.

16. Widiger TA. Psychological tests and the borderline diagnosis. *J Pers Assess*. 1982; 46: 227–238.

17. Gunderson JG, Singer MT. Defining borderline patients: an overview. Am J Psychiatry. 1975; 132: 1–10.

18. *Diagnostic and Statistical Manual of Mental Disorders*. 3rd ed. Washington, DC: American Psychiatric Association; 1980.

19. Loranger AW, Janca A, Sartorius N. *Assessment and Diagnosis of Personality Disorders: The ICD-10 International Personality Disorder Examination (IPDE)*. Cambridge, England: Cambridge University Press; 1997.

20. *Diagnostic and Statistical Manual of Mental Disorders*. 4th ed. Washington, DC: American Psychiatric Association; 1994.

21. McDermutt W, Zimmerman M. Assessment instruments and standardized evaluation. In: Oldham, JM, Skodol, AE, Bender, DS, eds. *The American Psychiatric Publishing Textbook of Personality Disorders*. Arlington, VA: American Psychiatric Publishing; 2005: 89–101.

22. Samuel DB, Caroll KM, Rounsaville BJ, Ball SA. Personality disorders as maladaptive, extreme variants of normal personality: borderline personality disorder and neuroticism in a substance using sample. *J Pers Disord*. 2013; 27: 625–635.

23. Hopwood CJ, Morey LC, Edelen MO, et al. A comparison of interview and self-report methods for the assessment of borderline personality disorder criteria. *Psychol Assess*. 2008; 20: 81–85.

24. Kendell R, Jablensky A. Distinguishing between the validity and utility of psychiatric diagnoses. *Am J Psychiatry*. 2003; 160: 4–12.

25. Arntz A, Bernstein D, Gielen D, et al. Taxometric evidence for the dimensional structure of cluster-C, paranoid, and borderline personality disorders. *J Pers Disord*. 2009; 23: 606–628.

26. Haslam N, Holland E, Kuppens P. Categories versus dimensions in personality and psychopathology: a quantitative review of taxometric research. *Psychol Med*. 2012; 42: 903–920.

27. Zanarini MC, Frankenburg FR, Dubo ED, et al. Axis I comorbidity of borderline personality disorder. *Am J Psychiatry*. 1998; 155: 1733–1739.

28. Zimmerman M, Mattia JI. Axis I diagnostic comorbidity and borderline personality disorder. *Compr Psychiatry*. 1999; 245–252.

29. Sharp C, Wright AGC, Fowler JC, et al. The structure of personality pathology: both general ('g') and specific ('s') factors? *J Abnorm Psychol*. 2015; 124: 387–398.

30. Trull T, Distel M, Carpenter R. DSM-5 borderline personality disorder: at the border between a dimensional and a categorical view. *Curr Psychiatry Rep*. 2011; 13: 43–49.

31. *The ICD-10 Classification of Mental and Behavioral Disorders*. Geneva, Switzerland: World Health Organization; 1993.

32. *International Classification of Diseases for Mortality and Morbidity Statistics*. 11th ed. Geneva, Switzerland: World Health Organization; 2018.

33. McRae RR, Costa PT. The five-factor model of personality: theoretical perspectives. In: McCrae, RR, Costa, PT, Jr., eds. *Toward a New Theory of Personality Disorders: Theoretical Contexts for the Five-factor Model*. New York, NY: Guilford Press; 1996: 51–87.

34. Bach B, Sellbom M, Skjernov M, Simonsen E. ICD-11 and DSM-5 personality trait domains capture categorical personality disorders: finding a common ground. *Aus N Z J Psychiatry*. 2018; 52: 425–434.

35. Kotov R, Krueger RF, Watson D. The Hierarchical Taxonomy of Psychopathology (HiTOP): a dimensional alternative to traditional nosologies. *J Abnorm Psychol*. 2017; 126: 454–477.

36. Gunderson JG, Herpertz SC, Skodol AE, Torgersen S, Zanarini MC. Borderline personality disorder. *Nat Rev Dis Primers*. 2018; 4: 1–20.

37. Torgersen S, Kringlen E, Cramer V. The prevalence of personality disorders in a community sample. *Arch Gen Psychiatry*. 2001; 58: 590–596.

38. Johnson JG, Cohen P, Kasen S, Skodol AE, Oldham JM. Cumulative prevalence of personality disorders between adolescence and adulthood. *Acta Psychiatr Scan*. 2008; 118: 410–413.

39. Samuels J, Eaton WW, Bienvenu OJ, Brown CH, Costa PT, Nestadt G. Prevalence and correlates of personality disorders in a community sample. *Br J Psychiatry*. 2002; 180: 536–542.

40. Crawford TN, Cohen P, Johnson JG, et al. Self-reported personality disorder in the children in the community sample: convergent and prospective validity in late adolescence and adulthood. *J Pers Disord*. 2005; 19: 30–52.

41. Grant BF, Chou SP, Goldstein RB. Prevalence, correlates, disability, and comorbidity of DSM-IV borderline personality disorder: results from the Wave 2 National Epidemiologic Survey on Alcohol and Related Conditions. *J Clin Psychiatry*. 2008; 69: 533–545.

42. Gross R, Olfson M, Gameroff M. Borderline personality disorder in primary care. *Arch Intern Med*. 2002; 162: 53–60.

43. Zanarini MC, Frankenburg FR, Hennen J, Silk KR. Mental health service utilization by borderline personality disorder patients and Axis II comparison subjects followed prospectively for 6 years. *J Clin Psychol*. 2004; 65: 28–36.

44. Zimmerman M, Chelminski I, Young D. The frequency of personality disorders in psychiatric patients. *Psychiatr Clin North Am*. 2008; 31: 405–420.

45. Korzekwa MI, Dell PF, Links PS, Thabane L, Webb SP. Estimating the prevalence of borderline personality disorder in psychiatric patients using a two–phase procedure. *Compr Psychiatry*. 2008; 49: 380–386.

46. Ellison WD, Rosenstein L, Morgan TA, Zimmerman M. Community and clinical epidemiology of borderline personality disorder. *Psychiatr Clin North Am*. 2018; 41: 561–573.

47. Zanarini MC, Frankenburg FR, Reich DBF, Fitzmaurice G. Attainment and stability of sustained symptomatic remission and recovery among patients with borderline personality disorder and Axis II comparison subjects: a 16-year prospective follow-up study. *Am J Psychiatry*. 2012; 169: 476–483.

48. Gunderson JG. Ten-year course of borderline personality disorder: psychopathology and function from the collaborative longitudinal personality disorders study. *Arch Gen Psychiatry*. 2011; 68: 827–837.

49. Martino F, Gammino L, Sanza M, et al. Impulsiveness and emotional dysregulation as stable features in borderline personality disorder outpatients over time. J Nerv Ment Dis. 2020; 208: 715–720.

50. Lenzenweger MF. Epidemiology of personality disorders. *Psychiatr Clin North Am.* 2008; 31: 395–403.

51. Tomko RL, Trull TJ, Wood PK, Sher KJ. Characteristics of borderline personality disorder in a community sample: comorbidity, treatment utilization, and general functioning. *J Pers Disord.* 2014; 28: 734–750.

52. Silberschmidt A, Lee S, Zanarini M, Schulz SC. Gender differences in borderline personality disorder: results from a multinational, clinical trial sample. *J Pers Disord.* 2015; 29: 828–838.

53. Rodriguez-Seijas C, Morgan TA, Zimmerman M. Is there a bias in the diagnosis of borderline personality disorder among lesbian, gay, and bisexual patients? *Assessment.* 2020; 1073191120961833.

54. De Genna NM, Feske U. Phenomenology of borderline personality disorder. J Nerv Ment Dis. 2013; 201: 1027-1034.

55. Runseson B, Beskow J. Borderline personality disorder in young Swedish suicides. *J Nerv Ment Dis.* 1991; 179: 153–156.

56. Kullgren G, Renberg E. An empirical study of borderline personality disorder and psychiatric suicides. *J Nerv Ment Dis.* 1986; 174: 328–331.

57. American Psychiatric Association. Practice guideline for the treatment of patients with borderline personality disorder. *Am J Psychiatry.* 2001; 158: 1–52.

58. Saha S, Chant D, Welham J, McGrath J. A systematic review of the prevalence of schizophrenia. *PLoS Med.* 2005; 2: 141.

59. Zanarini MC, Frankenburg F, Reich DB, Fitzmaurice G, Weinberg I, Gunderson JG. The 10-year course of physically self-destructive acts reported by borderline patients and Axis II comparison subjects. *Acta Psychiatr Scand.* 2008; 117: 177–184.

60. Gunderson JG, Morey LC, Stout RL, et al. Major depressive disorder and borderline personality disorder revisited: longitudinal interactions. *J Clin Psychiatry.* 2004; 65: 1049.

61. Skodol AE, Grilo CM, Keyes KM, Geier T, Grant BF, Hasin DS. Relationship of personality disorders to the course of major depressive disorder in a nationally representative sample. *Am J Psychiatry.* 2011; 168: 257–264.

62. Zanarini MC, Frankenburg FR, Hennen J, Silk KR. The longitudinal course of borderline psychopathology: 6-year prospective follow-up of the phenomenology of borderline personality disorder. *Am J Psychiatry.* 2003; 160: 274–283.

63. Pfohl B, Stangl D, Zimmerman M. The implications of DSM-III personality disorders for patients with major depression. *J Affect Disord.* 1984; 7: 309–318.

64. Pepper CM, Klein DN, Anderson RL, Riso LP, Ouimette PC, Lizardi H. DSM-III-R Axis II comorbidity in dysthymia and major depression. *Am J Psychiatry.* 1995; 152: 239–247.

65. Gunderson JG, Phillips KA. A current view of the interface between borderline personality disorder and depression. *Am J Psychiatry.* 1991; 148: 967–975.

66. New AS, Triebwasser J, Charney DS. The case for shifting borderline personality disorder to Axis I. *Biol Psychiatry.* 2008; 64: 653–659.

67. Corbitt EM, Malone KM, Haas GL, Mann JJ. Suicidal behavior in patients with major depression and comorbid personality disorders. *J Affect Disord.* 1996; 39: 61–72.

68. Grilo CM, Stout RL, Markowitz JC, et al. Personality disorders predict relapse after remission from an episode of major depressive disorder: a six-year prospective study. *J Clin Psychiatry*. 2010; 71: 1629–1635.

69. Zimmerman M, Morgan TA. The relationship between borderline personality disorder and bipolar disorder. *Dialogus Clin Neurosci*. 2013; 15: 155–169.

70. Frías A, Baltasar I, Birmaher B. Comorbidity between bipolar disorder and borderline personality disorder: prevalence, explanatory theories, and clinical impact. *J Affect Disord*. 2016; 202: 210–219.

71. Smith DJ, Muir WJ, Blackwood DHR. Is borderline personality disorder part of the bipolar spectrum? Harv Rev Psychiatry. 2004; 12: 133–139.

72. Perugi G, Angst J, Azorin J-M, Bowden C, Vieta E, Young AH. The bipolar-borderline disorders connection in major depressive patients. *Acta Psychiatr Scand*. 2013; 128: 376–383.

73. Paris J. Borderline or bipolar? Distinguishing borderline personality disorder from bipolar spectrum disorders. *Harv Rev Psychiatry*. 2004; 12: 130–145.

74. Dolan-Sewell RT, Krueger RF, Shea MT. Co-occurrence with syndrome disorders. In: Livesley WJ, ed. *Handbook of Personality Disorders: Theory, Research, and Treatment*. New York, NY: Guilford Press; 2001: 84–104.

75. Links PS, Heslegrave RJ, Mitton JE, van Reekum R, Patrick J. Borderline psychopathology and recurrence of clinical disorders. *J Nerv Ment Dis*. 1994; 183: 582–586.

76. Zanarini MC, Frankenburg FR, Hennen J, Reich DB, Silk KR. Axis I comorbidity in patients with borderline personality disorder: 6-year follow-up and prediction of time to remission. *Am J Psychiatry*. 2004; 161: 2108–2114.

77. Rossi R, Lanfredi M, Pievani M. Volumetric and topographic differences in hippocampal subdivisions in borderline personality and bipolar disorders. Psychiatry Res Neuroimaging. 2012; 203: 132–138.

78. Gonda X, Pompili M, Serafini G, et al. Suicidal behavior in bipolar disorder: epidemiology, characteristics and major risk factors. *J Affect Disord*. 2012; 143: 16–26.

79. Zimmerman M, Galione JN, Ruggero CJ, et al. Screening for bipolar disorder and finding borderline personality disorder. *J Clin Psychiatry*. 2010; 71: 1212–1217.

80. Shah R, Zanarini MC. Comorbidity of borderline personality disorder: current status and future directions. *Psychiatr Clin North Am*. 2018; 41: 583–593.

81. Silverman MH, Frankenburg FR, Reich DB, Fitzmaurice G, Zanarini MC. The course of anxiety disorders other than PTSD in patients with borderline personality disorder and Axis II comparison subjects: a 10-year follow-up study. *J Pers Disord*. 2012; 26: 804–814.

82. Gratz KL, Tull MT, Gunderson JG. Preliminary data on the relationship between anxiety sensitivity and borderline personality disorder: the role of experiential avoidance. *J Psychiatr Res*. 2008; 42: 550–559.

83. Bolton E. Symptom correlates of posttraumatic stress disorder in patients with borderline personality disorder. *Compr Psychiatry*. 2006; 47: 357–361.

84. Herman JL, van der Kolk BA. Traumatic antecedents of borderline personality disorder. In: van der Kolk BA, ed. *Psychological Trauma*. Washington, DC: American Psychiatric Publishing; 1987: 111–126.

85. Woodward HE, Taft CT, Gordon RA, Meis LA. Clinician bias in the diagnosis of posttraumatic stress disorder and borderline personality disorder. *Psychol Trauma*. 2009; 1: 282-290.

86. Zanarini MC, Frankenburg FR, Reich DB, et al. Biparental failure in the childhood experiences of borderline patients. *J Pers Disord*. 2000; 14: 264–273.

87. Harned MS, Rizvi SL, Linehan MM. Impact of co-occurring posttraumatic stress disorder on suicidal women with borderline personality disorder. *Am J Psychiatry*. 2010; 167: 1210–1217.

88. Biederman J. Impact of comorbidity in adults with attention deficit/hyperactivity disorder. *J Clin Psychiatry*. 2004; 65: 3–7.

89. Wilens TE, Biederman J, Kwon A, et al. Risk of substance use disorders in adolescents with bipolar disorder. J Am Acad Child Adolesc Psychiatry. 2004; 43: 1380–1386.

90. Jacob CP, Ramonos J, Dempfle A. Co-morbidity of adult attention-deficit/hyperactivity disorder with focus on personality traits and related disorders in a tertiary referral center. *Eur Arch Psychiatry Clin Neurosci*. 2007; 257: 309–317.

91. Van Dijk FE, Lappenschaar M, Kan CC, Verkes RJ, Buitelaar JK. Symptomatic overlap between attention-deficit/hyperactivity disorder and borderline personality disorder in women: the role of temperament and character traits. Compr Psychiatry. 2012; 53: 39–47.

92. Moukhtarian TR, Mintah RS, Moran P, Asherson P. Emotion dysregulation in attention-deficit/hyperactivity disorder and borderline personality disorder. Borderline Personal Disord Emot Dysregulation. 2018; 5: 1–11.

93. Philipsen A. Differential diagnosis and comorbidity of attention-deficit/hyperactivity disorder (ADHD) and borderline personality disorder (BPD) in adults. *Eur Arch Psychiatry Clin Neurosci*. 2006; 256: 42–46.

94. Trull TJ, Freeman LK, Vebares TJ, Choate AM, Helle AC, Wycoff AM. Borderline personality disorder and substance use disorders: an updated review. *Borderline Personal Disord Emot Dysregulation*. 2018; 5: 1–12.

95. Littlefield AK, Sher KJ. *Personality and Substance Use Disorders*. Oxford, UK: Oxford University Press; 2016.

96. Gunderson JG, Fruzzetti A, Unruh B, Choi-Kain L. Competing theories of borderline personality disorder. *J Pers Disord*. 2018; 32: 148–167.

97. Cassin SE, von Ranson KM. Personality and eating disorders: a decade in review. *Clin Psychol Rev*. 2005; 25: 895–916.

98. Lilenfeld L, Wonderlich S, Riso L, Crosby R, Mitchell J. Eating disorders and personality: a methodological and empirical review. *Clin Psychol Rev*. 2006; 26: 299–320.

99. Rosenvinge JH, Mouland SO. Outcome and prognosis of anorexia nervosa: a retrospective study of 41 subjects. *Br J Psychiatry*. 1990; 156: 92–97.

100. Zimmerman M, Rothschild L, Chelminski I. The prevalence of DSM-IV personality disorders in psychiatric outpatients. *Am J Psychiatry*. 2005; 162: 1911–1918.

101. Slotema CW, Blom JD, Niemantsverdriet MBA, Deen M, Sommer IEC. Comorbid diagnosis of psychotic disorders in borderline personality disorder: prevalence and influence on outcome. *Front Psychiatry*. 2018; 9: 84.

102. Doering S. Borderline personality disorder in patients with medical illness: a review of assessment, prevalence, and treatment options. *Psychosom Med*. 2019; 81: 584–594.

103. Carpenter RW, Trull TJ. Components of emotion dysregulation in borderline personality disorder: a review. *Curr Psychiatry Rep*. 2013; 15: 335.

104. Amad A, Ramoz N, Thomas P, Jardri R, Gorwood P. Genetics of borderline personality disorder: systematic review and proposal of an integrative model. *Neurosci Biobehav Rev*. 2014; 40: 6–19.

105. Perez–Rodriguez MM, Bulbena-Cabré A, Nia AB, Zipursky G, Goodman M, New AS. The neurobiology of borderline personality disorder. *Psychiatr Clinics*. 2018; 41: 633–650.

106. Witt SH, Streit F, Jungkunz M, et al. Genome-wide association study of borderline personality disorder reveals genetic overlap with bipolar disorder, major depression, and schizophrenia. *Transl Psychiatry*. 2017; 7: 1155.

107. Krause-Utz A, Winter D, Niedtfeld I, Schmahl C. The latest neuroimaging findings in borderline personality disorder. *Curr Psychiatry Rep*. 2014; 16: 438.

108. Schulze L, Schmahl C, Niedtfeld I. Neural correlates of disturbed emotion processing in borderline personality disorder: a multimodal meta-analysis. *Biol Psychiatry*. 2016; 79: 97–106.

109. Koenigsberg HW, Denny BT, Fan J, et al. The neural correlates of anomalous habituation to negative emotional pictures in borderline and avoidant personality groups. *Am J Psychiatry*. 2014; 171: 82–90.

110. Yang X, Hu L, Zeng J, Tan Y, Cheng B. Default mode network and frontolimbic gray matter abnormalities in patients with borderline personality disorder: a voxel–based meta-analysis. *Sci Rep*. 2016; 6: 1–10.

111. Ninomiya T, Oshita H, Kawano Y, et al. Reduced white matter integrity in borderline personality disorder: a diffusion tensor imaging study. *J Affect Disord*. 2018; 225: 723–732.

112. Gan J, Yi J, Zhong M, et al. Abnormal white matter structural connectivity in treatment-naïve young adults with borderline personality disorder. *Acta Psychiatr Scand*. 2016; 134: 494–503.

113. Rüsch N, Bracht T, Kreher BW., et al. Reduced interhemispheric structural connectivity between anterior cingulate cortices in borderline personality disorder. *Psychiatry Res Neuroimaging*. 2010; 181: 151–154.

114. Lischke A, Domin M, Freyberg H, et al. Structural alterations in white-matter tracts connecting (para-)limbic and prefrontal brain regions in borderline personality disorder. *Psychol Med*. 2015; 45: 3171–3180.

115. Whalley HC, Nickson T, Pope M, et al. White matter integrity and its association with affective and interpersonal symptoms in borderline personality disorder. *Neuroimage Clin*. 2015, 7: 476–481.

116. Fertuck EA, Fischer S, Beeney J. Social cognition and borderline personality disorder: splitting and trust impairment findings. *Psychiatr Clin*. 2018; 41: 613–632.

117. Fertuck EA, Grinbad J, Mann JJ, et al. Trustworthiness appraisal deficits in borderline personality disorder are associated with prefrontal cortex, not amygdala, impairment. *Neuroimage Clin*. 2019; 21.

118. Herpertz SC, Bertsch K. A new perspective on the pathophysiology of borderline personality disorder: a model of the role of oxytocin. *Am J Psychiatry*. 2015; 172: 840–851.

119. Bertsch K, Gamer M, Schmidt B, et al. Oxytocin and reduction of social threat hypersensitivity in women with borderline personality disorder. *Am J Psychiatry*. 2013; 170: 1169–1177.

120. Zimmerman DJ, Choi-Kain LW. The hypothalamic–pituitary–adrenal axis in borderline personality disorder: a review. *Harv Rev Psychiatry*. 2009; 17: 167–183.

121. Ruocco AC, Carcone D. A neurobiological model of borderline personality disorder: systematic and integrative review. *Harv Rev Psychiatry*. 2016; 24: 311–329.

122. Corniquel MB, Koenigsberg HW, Likhtik E. Toward an animal model of borderline personality disorder. *Psychopharmacology (Berl)*. 2019; 236: 2485–2500.

123. Zanarini MC. *Role of Sexual Abuse in the Etiology of Borderline Personality Disorder.* Washington, DC: American Psychiatric Press; 1997.

124. Afifi TO, Mather A, Boman J, et al. Childhood adversity and personality disorders: results from a nationally representative population-based study. *J Psychiatr Res.* 2011; 45: 814–822.

125. Porter C, Palmier-Claus J, Branitsky A, Mansell W, Warwick H, Varese F. Childhood adversity and borderline personality disorder: a meta-analysis. *Acta Psychiatr Scand.* 2020; 141: 6–20.

126. Hengartner M, Ajdacic-Gross V, Rodgers S, Müller M, Rössler W. Childhood adversity in association with personality disorder dimensions: new findings in an old debate. *Eur Psychiatry.* 2013; 28: 476–482.

127. Maniam J, Antoniadis C, Morris MJ. Early life stress, HPA axis adaptation, and mechanisms contributing to later health outcomes. Front Endocrinol. 2014; 5: 73.

128. Cohen P, Chen H, Gordon K, Johnson J, Brook J, Kasen S. Socioeconomic background and the developmental course of schizotypal and borderline personality disorder symptoms. Dev Psychopathol. 2008; 20: 633–650.

129. Buchheim A, Diamond D. Attachment and borderline personality disorder. *Psychiatr Clin.* 2018; 41: 651–668.

130. Jobst A, Padberg F, Mauer M-C, et al. Lower oxytocin plasma levels in borderline patients with unresolved attachment representations. *Front.* 2016; 10: 125.

131. Buchheim A, Erk S, George C, et al. Neural response during the activation of the attachment system in patients with borderline personality disorder: an fMRI study. Front Hum Neurosci. 2016; 10: 389.

132. Ronningstam EF, Keng SL, Ridolfi ME, Arbabi M, Grenyer BF. Cultural aspects in symptomatology, assessment, and treatment of personality disorders. *Curr Psychiatry Rep.* 2018; 20: 1–10.

133. Yang J, McRae RR, Costa PT, Yao S, Dai X, Cai T, Gao B. The cross-cultural generalizability of Axis-II constructs: an evaluation of two personality disorder assessment instruments in the People's Republic of China. *J Pers Disord.* 2000; 14: 249–263.

134. Keng SL, Lee Y, Drabu S, Hong RY, Chee CY, Ho CS, Ho RC. Construct validity of the McLean Screening Instrument for borderline personality disorder in two Singaporean samples. *J Pers Disord.* 2019; 33: 450–469.

135. Selby EA, Joiner TE Jr. Ethnic variations in the structure of borderline personality disorder symptomatology. *J Psychiatr Res.* 2008; 43: 115–123.

136. Caligor E, Kernberg OF, Clarkin JF, Yeomans FE. *Psychodynamic Therapy for Personality Pathology: Treating Self and Interpersonal Functioning.* Washington, DC: American Psychiatric Publishing; 2018.

137. Yeomans FE, Clarkin JF, Kernberg OF. *Transference-focused Psychotherapy for Borderline Personality Disorder: A Clinical Guide.* 1st ed. Washington, DC: American Psychiatric Publishing; 2015.

138. Kernberg OF, Yeomans FE. Borderline personality disorder, bipolar disorder, depression, attention deficit/hyperactivity disorder, and narcissistic personality disorder: practical differential diagnosis. *Bull Menninger Clin.* 2013; 77: 1–22.

139. Kernberg OF. The suicidal risk in severe personality disorders: Differential diagnosis and treatment. *J Pers Disord.* 2001; 15: 195–208.

140. Stern, BL, Caligor, E, Clarkin, JF, et al. Structured Interview of Personality Organization (STIPO): preliminary psychometrics in a clinical sample. *J Pers Assess.* 2010; 35–44.

141. Fertuck EA, Chesin MS, Johnston B. *Borderline personality disorders and mood disorders.* In: Stanley B, New A, eds. *Borderline Personality Disorders.* Oxford, UK: Oxford University Press; 2017.

142. Lequesne, ER, Hersh, RG. Disclosure of a diagnosis of borderline personality disorder. *J Psychiatr Pract.* 2004; 10: 170–176.

143. Linehan MM. *Skills Training Manual for Treating Borderline Personality Disorder.* New York City: Guilford Press: 1993.

144. Kernberg OF. Therapeutic implications of transference structures in various personality pathologies. *J Am Psychoanal Assoc.* 2019; 67: 951–986.

145. Betan E, Heim AK, Zittel Conklin C, Westen D. Countertransference phenomena and personality pathology in clinical practice: an empirical investigation. *Am J Psychiatry.* 2005; 162: 890–898.

146. Black DW, Blum N, Pfohl B, Hale N. Suicidal behavior in borderline personality disorder: prevalence, risk factors, prediction, and prevention. *J Pers Disord.* 2004; 18: 226–239.

147. Wedig MM, Silverman MH, Frankenburg FR, Reich DB, Fitzmaurice G, Zanarini MC. Predictors of suicide attempts in patients with borderline personality disorder over 16 years of prospective follow-up. *Psychol Med.* 2012; 42: 2395–2404.

148. Yen S, Peters JR, Nishar S, et al. Association of borderline personality disorder criteria with suicide attempts: findings from the collaborative longitudinal study of personality disorders over 10 years of follow-up. *JAMA Psychiatry.* 2021 Feb 1;78(2):187–194. doi:10.1001/jamapsychiatry.2020.3598

149. Gabbard O. *Do All Roads Lead to Rome? New Findings on Borderline Personality Disorder.* Washington, DC: American Psychiatric Association; 2007.

150. Cristea IA, Gentili C, Cotet CD, Palomba D, Barbui C, Cuijpers P. Efficacy of psychotherapies for borderline personality disorder: a systematic review and meta-analysis. *JAMA Psychiatry.* 2017; 74: 319–328.

151. Størebo OJ, Stoffers-Winterling JM, Völlm BA, et al. Psychological therapies for people with borderline personality disorder. *Cochrane Database Syst Rev.* 2020 May 4;5(5):CD012955. doi:10.1002/14651858.CD012955.pub2

152. Temes CM, Zanarini MC. The longitudinal course of borderline personality disorder. *Psychiatr Clin.* 2018; 41: 685–694.

153. Ebell MH, Siwek J, Weiss BD, Woolf SH, Susman J, Ewigman B, Bowman M. Strength of recommendation taxonomy (SORT): a patient–centered approach to grading evidence in the medical literature. *J Am Board Fam Pract.* 2004; 17: 59–67.

154. Davidson KM, Tyrer P, Norrie J, Palmer SJ, Tyrer H. Cognitive therapy v. usual treatment for borderline personality disorder: prospective 6-year follow-up. *Br J Psychiatry.* 2020; 197: 456–462.

155. Sempértegui GA, Karreman A, Arntz A, Bekker MHJ. Schema therapy for borderline personality disorder: a comprehensive review of its empirical foundations, effectiveness and implementation possibilities. *Clin Psychol Rev.* 2013; 33: 426–447.

156. Vogt KS, Norman P. Is mentalization-based therapy effective in treating the symptoms of borderline personality disorder? A systematic review. *Psychol Psychother.* 2019; 92: 441–464.

157. Clarkin JF, Cain NM. Advances in transference-focused psychotherapy derived from the study of borderline personality disorder: clinical insights with a focus on mechanism. *Curr Opin Psychol.* 2018, 21: 80–85.

158. Kivity Y, Levy K, Wasserman R, Beeney J, Meehan K, Clarkin J. Conformity to prototypical therapeutic principles and its relation with change in reflective functioning in three treatments for borderline personality disorder. *J Consult Clin.* 2019; 87: 975.

159. Rockland LH. *Supportive Therapy for Borderline Patients: A Psychodynamic Approach.* New York, NY: Guilford Publications; 1992.

160. Clarkin JF, Levy KN, Lenzenweger MF, Kernberg OF. Evaluating three treatments for borderline personality disorder: a multiwave study. *Am J Psychiatry.* 2007; 164: 922–928.

161. Gunderson J, Masland S, Choi-Kain L. Good psychiatric management: a review. *Curr Opin Psychol.* 2018; 21: 127–131.

162. McMain SF, Links PS, Gnam WH, et al. A randomized trial of dialectical behavior therapy versus general psychiatric management for borderline personality disorder. *Am J Psychiatry.* 2009; 166: 1365–1374.

163. Starcevic V, Janca A. Pharmacotherapy of borderline personality disorder: replacing confusion with prudent pragmatism. *Curr Opin Psychiatry.* 2018; 31: 69–73.

164. Stoffers JM, Lieb K. Pharmacotherapy for borderline personality disorder: current evidence and recent trends. *Curr Psychiatry Rep.* 2015; 17: 534.

165. Bogenschutz MP, Nurnberg HG. Olanzapine versus placebo in the treatment of borderline personality disorder. *J Clin Psychiatry.* 2004; 65: 104–109.

166. Silva H, Iturra P, Solari A, et al. Serotonin transporter polymorphism and fluoxetine effect on impulsiveness and aggression in borderline personality disorder. Actas Esp Psiquiatr. 2007; 35: 387–392.

167. Hollander E, Swann AC, Coccaro EF, Jiang P, Smith TB. Impact of trait impulsivity and state aggression on divalproex versus placebo response in borderline personality disorder. *Am J Psychiatry.* 2005; 162: 621–624.

20

Histrionic Personality Disorder

Michelle Magid and Isadora Fox

Key Points

- Histrionic personality disorder (HPD) is characterized by a pervasive pattern of excessive emotionality and attention-seeking behaviors, developed by early adulthood across multiple life domains. The HPD patient is characterized by the following: dramatic or theatrical behavior to gain attention; discomfort in situations when not the center of attention; engagement in inappropriate seductive or provocative behavior; shallow, excessive, emotional expressions.
- The patient lacks judgment in interpersonal relationships, is easily influenced, and misinterprets intimacy cues.
- Millon describes six subtypes of HPD which include appeasing, vivacious, tempestuous, disingenuous, theatrical, and infantile varieties.
- HPD may present on its own, occur along with another personality disorder, or present as embedded within an affective disorder.
- HPD is predominantly diagnosed or over-diagnosed in women and gender-diverse men and is underdiagnosed in heterosexual men, secondary to a cultural gender bias.
- HPD has genetic, moderate heritability in classic twin studies.
- Early-life invalidating experiences or overvaluing parenting styles contribute to the development of HPD.
- Patients may present in treatment as entertaining or dramatic and focus on seducing the clinician rather than engaging in meaningful connections and doing the work of psychotherapy.
- It is important to treat physical or psychiatric comorbidities with HPD prior to treating the personality disorder.
- Psychodynamic psychotherapy (PDP) for patients with HPD predominately focuses on interpretation of characteristic defenses, coping styles, emotionality, and behavioral dysregulation, and the impacts these have on patients' interpersonal relationships and other aspects of their lives. The goal of PDP is to consolidate a healthier identity, develop secure attachments, a mature sex life, meaningful relationships, and improved interpersonal relationships.
- Transference to therapists is commonly seductive or competitive.
- Therapists need to be aware of countertransference, which can be difficult and disruptive and may lead the therapist to feeling overinvolved, overwhelmed, disengaged, or sexualized.

- Cognitive behavioral therapy focuses on restructuring cognitive thoughts, such as "If I am not the center of attention, then I won't be accepted, cared for, or loved," and changing maladaptive sexualized, dissociated, or regressive behaviors into more adaptive ones.
- Supportive therapy combined with psychodynamic and cognitive approaches, marital therapy, or group therapy are other clinically viable treatment options.
- Psychopharmacology should primarily be directed at treating disorders which are comorbid with HPD.
- Current non–FDA approved psychopharmacology strategies for HPD are possible treatments. These include the use of antidepressants and mood stabilizers to help with underlying anxiety and mood lability, respectively.

Introduction

"Hysteric" and "histrionic" may sound alike, but diagnostically speaking, they are far from synonymous. Both terms describe patients as loud, disruptive, with emotional dysregulation akin to a sexually interested teenager searching for love while having a temper tantrum when they can't find it. A simple way to better understand their differences is revisiting their respective languages of origin. "Hyster" means "womb" in Greek. The Greeks and Egyptians believed hysteria—wildly emotional responses that presumably only occurred in women—to be the result of a displaced womb.[1] "Histro," on the other hand, means "actor or acting."[1] Hysteria is a time-limited, emotional response; histrionic behavior is a lifetime of enduring traits and dramatic performances.

Histrionic traits such as attention-seeking behavior, shallow affect, and seductive appearances or behaviors often stem from family trauma, emotional abuse, parental neglect or inconsistent discipline, and inherited genetic factors.[2] Histrionic patients are also likely to report somatic symptoms, such as headaches, with no clear underlying medical pathology. They may exaggerate their experiences to family or friends, as well as hop from one medical provider to another looking for answers in the form of attention.[3]

What's the difference between a person who likes to be the life of the party and one with HPD? When the party's over, the average bon vivant dials down attention-seeking behavior and conforms to the social norms of the individual's work, family, and social circles. For example, a corporate lawyer can present as quiet and reserved in the law office, but talkative and gregarious in a social setting with friends. These disparate behaviors are ego-syntonic and may not result in problems in living when the patient understands the unspoken but defined boundaries of behavior within different settings.

Unlike the bon vivant, the person with HPD is either unaware of social boundaries or chooses to ignore them because the drive for attention is simply greater than the drive to adhere to social norms. Patients with a HPD become disturbed when they are internally conflicted or when their ambitions clash with the values, norms, and culture of their respective environments. Features of HPD such as extreme emotional expression, a shallow affect, fear of dependency, and an unstable identity may impact the patient's ability to form long-term relationships because the person's need for attention or drama eclipses the underlying desire for acceptance, deep emotional connections, or love. These dysfunctional symptoms and behaviors can manifest in idealization or fantasies of romantic love associated with someone the patient barely knows—Or, conversely, extreme envy or hatred for others who have what they want. It's difficult to establish an atmosphere of mutual trust with someone who exhibits this type of lability and unpredictability.[2]

Many people with HPD never pursue treatment; in some cases and contexts, their behaviors are ego-syntonic (e.g., do not disturb them). Patients with this disorder seek help when their behavior poses a significant threat to their lifestyle, interpersonal relationships, or at the urging of others; they may lack insight as to why they need help, or they are overwhelmed by the underlying intense hypersensitivity, anxiety, and emotional distress that often drives their behavior.[4]

In the literature and in case review, HPD is often described and presented in a similar fashion to borderline personality disorder. However, Zetzel[5] and Millon[6] both posit that histrionic patients are multilayered, faceted, and have variable levels of psychopathology.

Zetzel's most widely recognized research[5] is exclusively focused on the female hysteric with a neurotic personality organization, whom Zetzel describes as young women who are prepared to be interested and appropriate for psychoanalytic treatment. This patient can maintain functional object relations with herself and others, but experiences post-oedipal ambivalence and thus reacts to interpersonal interactions with fear and anxiety, manifested as hysteric behavior.

Millon[6] posits that HPD is born out of a childhood with multiple caregivers who provide inconsistent attention. When provided, the attention is brief and hyperbolic. This child may also receive little overall discipline and may only receive attention or praise when performing in some manner. Caretakers may be too preoccupied with themselves to care for their children, or are "laissez-faire" in their approach to parenting.

Diagnostic Considerations

According to the *Diagnostic and Statistical Manual of Mental Disorders,* fifth edition (DSM-5), HPD is categorized as Cluster B, the dramatic-emotional subset of personality disorders. HPD is characterized by flamboyant, sexualized, aggressive, and unpredictable behaviors.[7] It usually presents during the teen and early adult years. Classic and easily accessible examples of behavior consistent with the disorder are the antics of celebrities who frequently change their appearance and wear provocative clothing to capture media attention.

To meet DSM-5 criteria for HPD, the patient must demonstrate a pervasive pattern of excessive emotionality and attention-seeking behaviors by early adulthood across multiple life domains, as evidenced by five or more of the characteristics that are outlined in Box 20.1, p. 504. Millon's subtypes, which were conceptualized to add description and dimension to the DSM 5 diagnosis, are featured in Box 20.2, p. 504.[6] It is notable that the subtypes may also be attributed to comorbid affective and other personality disorders; it may be difficult to distinguish where one ends and another begins. The overall treatment philosophy is the same, but the choice of therapy modality may be dictated by presentation and level of psychopathology.

Before diagnosing a patient with HPD, it is necessary to get a thorough medical history including a current and past history of all medications (prescription and over-the-counter). It's important to note that HPD and somatization disorder are often comorbid.[3] Patients with HPD may be poor historians and dramatize minor ailments, so getting an accurate health history may be difficult. Reaching out to family, partners, primary

Box 20.1 Diagnostic Criteria DSM-5: Histrionic Personality Disorder

The patient must demonstrate a pattern of at least five or more specific behaviors by early adulthood across multiple life domains. These include but are not limited to:

- Presents as uncomfortable in situations in which he or she is not the center of attention
- Engages in inappropriate seductive or provocative behavior
- Expresses rapidly shifting, excessive, and shallow emotional expression
- Uses personal appearance and emotional presentation—dramatic, theatrical—to gain attention
- Lacks judgment in perceiving relationships; is easily influenced and misinterprets intimacy cues

Box 20.2 Millon's HPD Subtypes

- *Appeasing:* Attention-seeking behavior coupled with a desperate need for friendship and acceptance driven by fear and anxiety; may engage in abusive or predatory partnerships with codependent traits.
- *Vivacious:* Charming, seductive, but emotionally empty; at times, effervescent to the verge of hypomania; struggles with complex emotional attachment, so relationships are short-lived and shallow, with a lack of empathy consistent with narcissistic behavior.
- *Tempestuous:* Emotionally labile, quick to anger, will engage in conflict if it serves perceived attention needs. Shares several traits with borderline personality disorder and/or bipolar 2 because of excessive mood lability and irritability.
- *Disingenuous:* Attention-seeking behavior is grounded in a desire to manipulate or control others for the patient's personal amusement, particularly in the naïve or unsuspecting; possesses many narcissistic qualities.
- *Theatrical:* Self-promoting and seeks praise and adulation for superficial features such as clothing or appearance. The need for external admiration may exceed the need to maintain strong friendships.
- *Infantile Subtype:* Shares features of its tempestuous counterpart, but behaviors don't match her developmental age. Behaviors may arrange themselves in a borderline fashion; may pout and cry for attention, or present as volatile and respond inappropriately to perceived "injustices"—cancellation of plans due to work commitments, etc.

providers, and other clinicians for collateral history and medical records will provide a clearer picture of the patient's health history.

Another important consideration is onset of behavior and the age of the patient. Personality disorders do not appear in a vacuum; typical age of onset is late teens to early adulthood, and they do not present within days.[8] Some analysts have argued that temperament, which can be identified at a very young age, may be predictive of future histrionics: "the kind of baby who kicks and screams when frustrated, but shrieks with glee when entertained."[9]

When it comes to personality and behavioral perceptions, views of gender and what is traditionally male or female has created a gender bias for this diagnosis. Men who exhibit "feminine" characteristics—homosexual or transgender males, for example—are more likely to receive a diagnoses of HPD or borderline personality disorder (BPD), while men who present as "masculine" may be categorized as antisocial.[10]

If behaviors emerge very suddenly, they may be related to street drug use, such as cocaine, MDMA, methamphetamine, and prescription stimulant abuse.[11] If the patient is older, diagnoses such as early frontotemporal dementia [12] may present with disinhibited behaviors akin to the sexual indiscretions seen in histrionic patients. There are also a number of prescription medications that may cause unusual emotional excitability, such as stimulants[11] and corticosteroids.[13] Substances abuse and excessive use of caffeine[14] or over-the-counter medications (e.g., pseudoephedrine-based decongestants)[15] can cause similar issues of emotional excitability and agitation. If behavioral onset is more gradual, there are several physical ailments, such as hyperthyroidism,[16] that may cause a patient to present with symptoms mimicking HPD, such as hyperactivity and a vivacious manner.

From a psychiatric perspective, hypomania, mania, and some presentations of delusional psychoses may look remarkably like HPD, as these disorders often have hypersexuality as part of their common presentation. There is limited literature on differentiating between bipolar spectrum symptoms and histrionic behavior. Both mania and histrionic disorder can appear with grandiosity, excessive talkativeness, distractibility, and risky behaviors. However, manic patients are more likely to have racing thoughts and a decreased need for sleep. A general guiding principle in teasing out the differences between a personality disorder and bipolar disorder is to ask pointed questions about shifts in mood. Personality disorders are pervasive, whereas mood shifts from bipolar disorders are episodic. Very brief mood swings related to specific triggers are more likely caused by affective instability from a personality disorder, versus mood polarization from a bipolar disorder.[17] Anxiety symptoms and HPD are highly associated as well.[4] This is unsurprising, as the desire for attention-seeking is often driven by anxiety. If anxiety is well-controlled by psychotherapy or pharmacotherapy, the resulting attention-seeking behaviors may diminish.

When contemplating the differential diagnosis with a psychotic disorder, exploring reality testing or disturbances in the sense of reality (e.g., dissociation, derealization, depersonalization, déjà vu) is useful.

Mania and psychoses are psychiatric emergencies that require immediate psychiatric intervention; behavioral histrionics, unless the person is suicidal or homicidal, do not. A 25-year-old female with a 5-year-long history of depression who reports high energy, euphoria, grandiosity, hypersexuality, and sleeplessness that has built up over two weeks is consistent with mania; a 25-year-old female with no reported psychiatric history who describes herself as energetic, popular, is dressed seductively, and reports no past or present neurovegetative symptoms is consistent with HPD.

It's also worth noting that patients with HPD may demonstrate some behaviors and traits that overlap with narcissistic personality disorder (NPD) and BPD, and thus may be misdiagnosed. NPD differs from HPD in that the narcissist's motivation for attention, praise, and power is to reaffirm their grandiosity—that they are superior, more powerful, entitled to special treatments compared to others, despite the fact that patient with NPD may be unconsciously filled with anxiety, self-loathing, and *low* self-esteem. A patient with BPD may seek attention fueled by anxiety and fear, but her need to tether her unstable identity to others and fear of abandonment are the primary motivations.

Histrionic patients may have hyperbolic accounts of their activities, but they're reasonable within the context of their life. "Oh my god, the way Jack proposed was AMAZING, like a Hollywood movie. Brad Pitt couldn't have proposed any better!" The narcissistic patient may turn down the marriage proposal and exclaim, "the only person worthy of marrying me is Brad Pitt." In contrast, the psychotic/manic patient may say, "I had a dream about Brad Pitt. It means he wants to marry me. I will go to Hollywood and find him so he can propose." It is key to get the personality disorders diagnoses versus mood/psychotic/delusional disorders correct, because each require very different treatment responses.

Epidemiology

According to the DSM-5, HPD affects 2–3 percent of the general population and is 1.84 percent more likely to be diagnosed in women than in men.[7,18] It is likely that HPD has equal rates in women and in men, and that the disorder may be *underdiagnosed* in men because of gender bias; men who present as sexually seductive or aggressive may be categorized as antisocial or narcissistic, whereas women presenting with the same behaviors would be categorized as histrionic.[7,18] The exception is homosexual and transgender men, who are frequently diagnosed as histrionic, most likely due to perceived feminine characteristcs.[10] Accounting for prevalence of this disorder is also difficult because these patients only present to treatment when their behavior becomes ego-dystonic (e.g., starts to disturb them or others and is not in line with who they think they are). If they are in a career or environment that values their behavior and appearance, they may not perceive the need for treatment or intervention.[19]

Common Psychiatric Comorbidities

Comorbidities are common and may vary depending upon the subtype. It's not unusual for the patient with HPD to have additional personality disorders that may align with a subtype.[20] For example, Millon's "disingenuous" subtype may have comorbid NPD; the appeasing subtype may have comorbid dependent personality disorder. HPD is also commonly comorbid with BPD.[17]

Cluster B and Cluster C personality disorders are often comorbid with depression and bipolar spectrum disorders.[21] This is important, as even the astute psychiatrist may overlook that unacceptable behaviors might be due to depression or mania and not just personality style. Once a mood disorder is identified, pharmacological treatment may be indicated. Mood stabilizers and/or antidepressants can calm the underlying mood disorder, and often give the histrionic patient the chemical stability necessary to engage in meaningful therapy. Bockian notes that depression comorbid with HPD may arise when the energy required to attract attention and the lack of stable relationships becomes exhausting and subsequently painful.[22]

Biological and Genetic Considerations

According to Reichborn-Kjennerud, from a quantitative genetic standpoint based on twin and family studies, all personality disorders are modestly to moderately heritable. In twin model research of personality disorders, three variance components are considered in an to attempt to tease out genetic phenotypic expression versus environmental exposure and expression.[23]

The baby with a genetically inherited "histrionic" temperament (e.g., throws uncontrollable tantrums when upset, but also laughs uncontrollably when entertained) may be genetically primed for HPD and then be environmentally activated to become a HPD teenager/adult.[9] In one twin study, heritability estimates for HPD were at 63 percent.[23] A more recent population-based twin study reports a 31 percent shared heritability for the disorder.[24]

Psychosocial and Cultural Considerations

When contemplating HPD within the psychosocial realm, context is everything. There are careers and environments in which these personality traits are valued. A fashion designer, Internet influencer, or famous musician can score social media points via attention-seeking behavior, such as making shocking or controversial public comments or wearing outrageous clothing. In this world, such behavior is rewarded with both money and opportunity. There is no reason to seek help if the behavior aligns with the expectations and desires of the audience. This can backfire if the person in question indulges in antics that stray far out of parameters of social acceptability—engaging in activity that isn't intended to, but could potentially harm a child or an animal. If a patient displayed the same kind of behavior as an employee in a medical office, this person could be fired.

Cultural considerations must be nuanced, as levels of emotionality vary widely by culture and country.[25] For example, a provider from a country that scores low on emotionality, such as Russia, may mistake the behavior of a person from a higher scoring country, such as the Philippines, to be histrionic—even though the person's behavior conforms to the social norms of the culture of origin. Similarly, what is considered abnormal behavior in one culture may be perfectly acceptable in another.[26] Perceptions of psychiatry also vary widely from culture to culture, which could also affect a patient's presentation. A patient with bright affect and insistence that life is going well, depending upon its intensity, could present as histrionic rather than as an optimistic person. If someone does have HPD, but symptoms of HPD are culturally perceived as a moral failing, pursuing treatment may be terrifying and change the way a patient interacts with a provider.

Treatment Considerations

Patients with HPD are often unable to sustain deep and meaningful relationships, as their superficial emotional style, attention-seeking behaviors, and dependency often become tiresome to others. The main goal of treatment is usually to improve meaningful interpersonal dynamics, as dysfunctional relationships are typically highly problematic. When choosing treatment, one must consider the individual's expression of the disorder, especially when HPD is comorbid or embedded in another diagnosis.[2] There is no specific evidence-based psychotherapeutic modality that has proven efficacy for the treatment of HPD. However, various forms of psychotherapy, supportive, psychodynamic, and cognitive behavioral therapy (CBT) remain the current clinical standards for treatment.

Supportive Psychotherapy

Supportive psychotherapy aims to reduce the use of maladaptive defenses, bolster self-esteem, and improve coping skills. It can, but does not always, explore family of origin dynamics and deeper influences of trauma. Such therapy may be appropriate for a patient with limited insight or severe disability.

Supportive therapy may help patients with HPD tolerate and name their anxiety which can provide insight into the origins of maladaptive attention-seeking behaviors. For example, feeling unloved or ignored can exacerbate emotionality and anxiety. This, in turn, can lead to an impulsive love affair, somatic symptoms, or acting out in rage. These HPD "coping mechanisms" will reduce anxiety momentarily, but will most likely leave the patient with unwanted long-term life consequences. Pointing out these patterns and supporting the patient as they work on developing less primitive coping mechanisms may be all the therapist can do.

Histrionic patients love to move toward (rather than steering clear of) situations fueled with drama and risk. Supportive therapy can help the patient identify high-risk situations and steer the patient toward more positive choices. For example, if a histrionic patient accidentally overhears a heated fight between a colleague and their spouse, the patient may choose to spread rumors in the workplace. The therapist may encourage the patient to speak directly to the colleague if worried, or "let it go" if escalating the situation serves no purpose. The therapist may also point out that going from crisis to crisis may initially be exciting but may ultimately hurt the patient's ability to form trusting relationships.

When a histrionic patient uses manipulation to control others, a supportive therapist can empathize, stating "It must seem to others that you are trying to control them through your seductive behavior. I don't think you are, at your core, a bad person. I think you are feeling unsafe and unaccepted and perhaps using manipulation to gain some sense of acceptance, stability, control over the situation. I wonder if we can find better ways to make you feel safe."

The supportive therapist may also point out that the histrionic patient may have low self-esteem and feel dependent on others for care. They might use dramatic behaviors as a way to gain attention from the room, or seductive behaviors as a way to procure acceptance, help, and love. The supportive therapist would empathize and help the patient find other strategies to feel worthy, that would help them get what they need and create less discomfort for others. The therapist may end up "reparenting" the unloved, neglected child.

The histrionic patient values superficial beauty above inner beauty. As such, getting old can be a major blow to maintaining self-worth. The supportive therapist can empathize with the difficulties of getting old and highlight other characteristics that make the patient valuable (i.e., their relationships, love of children, or their strong work ethic).

Psychodynamic Therapy

Psychodynamic therapy also aims for similar improvements, but rests on a basic architecture of psychoanalysis to reveal unconscious thoughts and explore how they are affecting the patient's present life.[2] Psychodynamic psychotherapy for HPD may focus on the need for love and approval, dependency needs, and how sexuality was viewed, experienced, and used to create attachments. It may uncover emotional deprivation or invalidation, childhood neglect or abuse, and a longing to be helped, cared for or nurtured, and seen.

As with supportive therapy, showing genuine interest is essential. Using confrontation, clarification, and here-and-now and historical interpretation of the patient's emotions, thoughts, and interpersonal behaviors are the mainstay of good therapeutic technique. Psychodynamic psychotherapy places more emphasis on the transference (what is going on in the room), continually bringing patients back to what they are feeling, thinking, and how they are behaving with the therapist as a way to understand their interpersonal relationships. Countertransference experiences of helpless/inadequate and sexualized responses are common when treating patients with HPD.[27]

In addition, psychodynamic psychotherapy may uncover unconscious defense mechanisms: Patients with HPD and a borderline personality organization (BPO) frequently use the splitting and dissociative defenses, sexualization, regression, and acting out as a way to handle conflicts. Patients with the healthier hysteric configuration and a neurotic personality organization (NPO) may use repression-based defenses, sexualization, and regression. A main goal in the therapeutic process is interpreting maladaptive defenses, which may reduce their use and/or permit the use of more mature defenses.

A patient with HPD and BPO may use splitting, which can lead to: a minimization of the gravity of the situation into all good or all bad; false memories; severe conversion disorders including pseudo-seizures, pseudo-pregnancy, and fugue states; somatic memories of traumatic events not recalled; and cognitively dissociative behaviors, such fits of anger, binge eating, or even violent attacks.[9] Patients may be so dissociated in their behavior that they don't even remember doing something. This can happen when a child is given the message that the needs of others (i.e., the mother or the father) must always come before the needs of the self. When a HPD patient is put into a situation where they must choose between the needs of the other or the needs of the self, the conflict may cause dissociation simply to get through the situation. For example, a histrionic college student may want the attention and love from her professor, but she may not want to sleep with him. She may feel obligated to have sex because his needs come first and may dissociate during the sexual encounter to get through it.

A hysteric patient with NPO may have had repressed sexual desires while growing up. Her sexuality may have been both noticed, admired, and prohibited by her father. Her mother might have felt competitive or overly protective of her daughter, either of which could lead to an inhibition and/or shaming of sexual desire and the fear of sex. When re-pression of these early life experiences becomes activated in a current romantic relation-ship, the patient may become sexually impulsive. Under these circumstances, the sexual encounter may not be gratifying, as it is plagued with conflict. The psychodynamic ther-apist would openly discuss the conflict over love versus sex and how repression has actu-ally led to acting out. The enactment is how the patient may behave seductively, seeking love and affection, when she actually dreads sex. This can lead to traumatic or dissocia-tive sexual acting out.

Regression is often seen in both HPD and hysteric patients in the form of helpless and childlike behavior. The patient may have been brought up in a household where disobedience or normal teenage defiance was met with rage, and regressing, becoming childlike, was effective at reducing anger and could disarm potential abusers.[9] Once the meanings of the defensive use of repression are interpreted, there will be less need to rely on this defense and more access to a better coping style of appropriate assertiveness.

Another common psychotherapy issue is the focus on physical appearance as the main style for fostering attachments. Hysterically organized women may frequently seek reassurance that their appearance is cherished. This may be in contrast to their up-bringing, in which they were chronically unnoticed or neglected or, alternatively, when their physical beauty was praised and over-valued. Either extreme can lead to a preoc-cupation with appearance. Psychodynamic psychotherapy can explore the patient's early experiences with physical appearance, how insecurity is most likely fueling this present-day preoccupation, and how physical appearance was used as the main style to obtain love and acceptance.

Transference and Countertransference

Utilizing the transference and countertransference is the crux of the psychodynamic psychotherapy for HPD.

Transference

Recognizing and discussing with a patient the possibility of a sexualized transference, and the likelihood that this may play out in the initial stages of therapy, may actually improve therapeutic alliance and prevent early therapy dropouts. For example, the ther-apist may interpret that the patient has a pattern of acting sexually seductive when they feel slighted, unaccepted, or rejected; this can create much anxiety and the desire to flee. The therapist may propose that if that happens during therapy, it can be used as an op-portunity to explore the precipitant and the interpersonal interactions which activated the sexualized behaviors. The therapist could encourage the patient to "work through" the situation. The therapist can "warn" the HPD patient that both negative and positive feelings will be felt toward the therapist, and encourage the patient to express these feel-ings whenever they arise.

Transference may vary by the subtype of HPD. As garnering attention, help, accept-ance, and love are the patient's guiding needs, the patient may present as surprisingly en-tertaining, flattering, eager to please, and as "the perfect patient." She may also present as seductive or try to paint herself as a victim. Productive interpretation of transference is a delicate process when treating HPD. For example, a person who has developed the disorder as a response to a cold and distant attachment to her father may enact childhood attention-seeking behaviors with her therapist.[28] Given their often fragile self-state, patients with HPD may initially benefit from a less threatening supportive psychotherapy; when the alliance is stronger, progress to more exploratory forms of psychodynamic psychotherapy may be helpful. The patient must have capacity for insight as to how her needs and behavior affect her life,[29] and there needs to be a strong alliance for the patient to benefit from a psychodynamic approach.

Countertransference

The countertransference felt between the HPD patient and the therapist can be tumultuous and derailing, especially if the therapists feels overwhelmed, anxious, or frightened. The heterosexual female patient may be aroused, intimidating, or seductive with a male therapist. She may be aggressive and competitive with a female therapist. With any therapist, she may regress to childlike behavior as a defense against feeling unloved or rejected, or to disarm the perception of the therapist's sexual interest or aggression.[9] The therapist may utilize their countertransference reactions to help the patient realize that their childhood fears of being rejected and having unmet needs may cause the patient to want to flee.[9]

Even though histrionic patients can be deceptively entertaining and serve as a refreshing distraction from the damp weight of listening to depressed and anxious patients, when it comes to countertransference, Cluster B patients can be particularly tricky. Colli and colleagues report that in patients with Cluster B characteristics, the lower functioning the patient, the higher the level of negatively charged countertransference responses.[30] Patients with HPD are also highly likely to elicit disengagement, feelings of mistreatment, and inadequacy in therapist, or lead toward a sexualized countertransference. Therapists need to be aware that sexualized countertransference can lead vulnerable therapists into damaging sexual encounters with their patients and other boundary or ethical violations.

A common countertransference pitfall is responding to the patient's need for attention, acceptance, dependent care, and love, is to offer the patient special privileges, care, or excessively "parental involvement." For example, the histrionic patient may ask permission to bring her emotional support animal into the therapy session, as she "simply cannot think" without it. She may ask the therapist to follow her blog and leave comments, or she may ask for direct help with managing finances or negotiating problematic work relationships. It is important not to be seduced into doing such things with a histrionic patient. In these instances, therapists may need to discuss their countertransference feelings and interactions with a supervising clinician and/or seek their own treatment, as needed.

Cognitive Behavioral Therapy

Using a CBT approach, a therapist would focus on: identifying triggering situations that may invoke the maladaptive thoughts, emotions, or behaviors; educating a patient about their core beliefs (e.g., patients' views of themselves, others, and the world); and developing behavioral change strategies.

A common triggering situation for histrionic patients is being in a work relationship with a powerful boss or colleague. These work relationships may trigger seductive behaviors with a powerful member of the opposite sex or opposite gender identity, or can trigger competitive behaviors with bosses or work colleagues of the same sex or same gender identity. Simply identifying triggers can create awareness and prevent maladaptive behaviors from developing. Common core beliefs in patients with HPD are that "I need to impress and be dramatic to get acceptance and love,"[31] and "to be happy, I need people to pay attention to me."[32]

Once a repetitive maladaptive thought or behavior is identified, the therapy may entail cognitive restructuring of the thoughts and recognizing maladaptive behaviors. Cognitive strategies are designed to replace automatic thoughts with less distorted and irrational ones, and are designed to help patients replace maladaptive core beliefs with more accurate and realistic views of themselves and others. Behavioral strategies often include replacing maladaptive behaviors (e.g., having a temper tantrum) with a more adaptive, societally acceptable one (e.g., asserting one's needs). In the process, the patient will need to focus on changing core beliefs to more balanced ideas. For example, therapy might replace an automatic thought such as "I'm only likeable if I'm pretty," to "being pretty is an asset, but I have other strengths that make me likeable."[32] It may focus on changing a core belief to a new one: "I don't need to be dramatic, exciting, or impressive all the time . . . as I deserve to be accepted, cared for, and loved because I am a good person."[31,33]

Angela, who dresses provocatively at work, may falsely believe that her behavior improves her chances of promotion by getting the attention of her superiors. Angela may believe that "the only way to get ahead is to get noticed at any cost." Using CBT, the therapist may point out that her dress has caused discomfort and complaints at work, which ultimately reduces her chances of promotion. The therapist may challenge her core belief in various ways: asking if others who were promoted dressed seductively; challenging what happened to the guy at the Christmas party who drank too much and thereby "got noticed at any cost." The therapist may then suggest wearing different clothes for two weeks and collecting evidence to see if this helps or harms work dynamics.

CBT can also be useful in challenging the communication style and information offered by a patient with HPD. The histrionic patient speaks superficially, emotionally, using a lot of words, but may not really be communicating any new facts, ideas, or solutions. The idea that "I need to impress and entertained to be successful" could be replaced with "Better to offer the steak (substance) instead of just the sizzle (emotional style)."

An identified trigger might also elicit a maladaptive behavior. When feeling rejected by a boss, a patient with HPD might regress into childlike behavior and speak even more superficially to avoid further hurt or embarrassment. Using CBT, the therapist may challenge the patient to say something that is hard but important to say to someone in power: tell the boss an idea or solution to improve workflow. The patient and therapist would then use the evidence gathered from these scenarios to determine if the new way of verbal expression and offering substance makes the patient feel better or worse. More likely than not, having authentic conversations and making real contributions, over time, would improve self-esteem and success. If the patient is too scared to engage in a genuine meaningful conversation, the therapist could role-play several scenarios (e.g., where the patient apologizes to friend for a having a fit) to gain confidence in developing relationships. In time, the hope is that the automatic thought will change to something more balanced, such as, "In certain situations, speaking up and saying something meaningful and important can actually be more attractive."

Combined Therapies

Using an eclectic approach—merging several therapy modalities—may also be helpful in treating HPD. Livesley[34] observes that the interplay of internal identity conflict, external interpersonal conflict, and the subsequent behavioral responses may require a combination of therapies to assist the patient with HPD with different elements of the patient's problems in living. One could use a psychodynamic approach as a foundation modality, and then use CBT techniques to assist the patient in managing their emotions. If the patient is able to identify a behavior, its psychodynamic origins, how it expresses itself, how it may be perceived, and how it makes them feel, the patient and the therapist can then use a CBT approach to change the behavior. For example, a young woman may be experiencing conflict with her husband because she is extremely seductive and provocative toward other men when her husband is nearby. She may dynamically understand she uses this strategy to get back at her husband when he is absorbed in his work and does not pay her much attention. She may reflect that her mother used a similar strategy with her father. She may also recognize the undesirable consequences and complications she creates for herself when she sends seductive messages to other men. With these insights, her therapist could help her design some solutions. A psychodynamic solution might entail helping her mentalize the hurt feelings her behaviors engender in her husband, and the arousal her behaviors create in other men. From CBT, she might do a chain analysis, writing down what triggers her behaviors (e.g., insecurity); what happens (the conflict with her husband and complication from other men); and then examine the consequences of her behaviors (loss of her own self-regard, marital discord, interpersonal problems with other men). Intervening in any part of this chain might lead to behavioral change. Identifying the fallacy of her core belief ("I need to seduce to get attention, care, and love") and challenging this belief may also bring about change.

Group Therapy

Psychodynamic group therapy can be extremely helpful with higher functioning hysteric/histrionic patients.[32] Group members tend to confront these patients, sometimes too harshly but often appropriately. Group members may call out the HPD patient's attention-seeking behaviors (such as flamboyant storytelling which lacks significant content useful to others), distorted self-perceptions, and a tendency to monopolize conversations. Groups can also provide an opportunity for a patient with HPD to gain insight into what others really think of them and to feel genuine caring from others who can really see her for who she is, not just as a person who gets attention for behaving badly. Hearing and interacting with others can also challenge maladaptive core beliefs and give her insight and practice in developing more meaningful interpersonal relationships.

For the patient whose attention-seeking behaviors are too disruptive or become unmanageable in a psychodynamic group, a skills-training group might be more beneficial. In this setting, the patient can focus on developing specific skills such as emotional regulation, frustration tolerance, interpersonal effectiveness, and stress reduction. (See Chapter 14 on group therapy for personality disorders for additional information.)

Marital Therapy

Histrionic patients can be overly dependent in a marriage, as they are constantly looking toward their spouse for validation, unconditional love, and gratification of their dependency needs. They are often attracted to a spouse who has an obsessive-compulsive style, as their own emotional, dramatic, and explosive personality can be tempered by the obsessive's rational, logical, stable approach, and control over emotions, which is common in men with an obsessive-compulsive style.[35] The attraction between the couple is often unconsciously based on recognizing that they both have similar dependency needs.[35] These initial attractions can devolve into criticisms of each other, withholding of gratifying dependency needs, and withdrawal from each other. This can lead a patient with HPD to multiple revenge affairs, or to upping the ante to suicidal gestures as demands for more attention and love.

In addition, if the patient with HPD regresses, becomes more dependent and helpless over time, this can leave the obsessive husband to assume increasing responsibility for the relationship. This under-functioning of the HPD and over-functioning of the obsessive husband can leads to significant marital distress.[32,35]

Competition can also develop within this couple. Her exhibitionism may be perceived as controlling and "taking over," and the spouse may begin to feel that he is living in her shadow, which can bring about rivalry and jealousy.[35]

Sexual conflicts in a marriage may also arise, as the patient with HPD may be seductive but actually suffer with low sexual desire or arousal, and anorgasmia, due to conflicts about care, sex, and love.

Marital therapy may be helpful and is usually sought out after a patient with HPD has an affair, a public embarrassment, or an excessive rage response to a mild offense. Marital therapy often focuses on addressing the dynamic between the couple: behavioral acting out when the histrionic patient feels ignored, unloved, and not cared for; or the withdrawal of the husband when he feels hurt and his needs are not satisfied. As the dynamics are unmasked, the therapist can work on de-escalating strategies. Generally, the goal of therapy is to break the vicious cycle of attention-seeking and spousal withdrawal that leads to marital discord, and to change the over-functioning/under-functioning dynamic and figure out new ways to mutually and reasonably gratify each other's reasonable dependency needs.

Medications

Treatment of comorbid psychiatric or substance abuse disorders impacting HPD is often needed as the first step to clear the pathway to treatment. There is no FDA approved pharmacological treatment for HPD. However, despite limited evidence for this approach, histrionic patients are sometimes clinically treated with medication that attempts to target specific symptoms related to HPD. Affective symptoms, anxiety, lability, and emotional dysregulation have been treated with selective serotonin reuptake inhibitors (e.g., fluoxetine, escitalopram).[36] Mood stabilizers such as lamotrigine and oxcarbazepine are sometimes used, and may assist with affective lability. If the patient's cognitive perceptions suggest breaks with reality (rare), severe dissociation, or agitation, antipsychotics such as quetiapine and olanzapine may help manage these symptoms.[2,36,37]

Case Study: Angela

Angela is a 35-year-old married white female naïve to psychiatric or psychotherapeutic treatment. She self-identifies as a cisgender, heterosexual female. She works in the marketing department of a large technology corporation. She presents to treatment with a full face of carefully applied makeup, elaborately styled hair, and tight, revealing clothing. When asked why she came to treatment, she tearfully states that she is "totally panicked and freaking out" over recent negative feedback from her manager about her behavior at work and online. She reports that she did not pursue treatment on her own, as she believes she is "more than fine." Specific problems include her manner of dress—she likes tight, revealing clothing—and overtly flirtatious behavior with male clients. She admits that she may present seductively at times, but winks and states, "Hey, we all know that sex sells." She giggles when she relays that at a recent company happy hour, she jumped up on the bar and did a strip tease, but states that she was wearing a camisole under her blouse, "so it wasn't a big deal."

She is also trying to develop an Internet business as a beauty and lifestyle influencer. As a result, she posts long, personal videos about her life, including when she is drunk. She thinks her boss is unreasonable. She pursues her second business/career on her own time and believes it has nothing to do with her job. Her boss states that employees are "ambassadors to the brands of the company and of the company itself" and insists that her online behavior should reflect that. Angela wants to keep her job and has agreed to try treatment but isn't entirely sure it's warranted. She thinks that there is probably another company out there who would appreciate her fun-loving personality.

Angela describes herself as vivacious, outgoing, and fun-loving; she enjoys curating a unique and interesting external appearance. She reports that beauty is especially important to her, so she spends a lot of time and money on gym workouts and beauty regimens. She has been married for seven years. Her first description of the relationship involved describing how "amazing" her wedding was and how big her diamond ring is compared to other women's. Prior to meeting her husband, she had several boyfriends in high school and college. One was a "very serious," relationship lasting 18 months. They met during their senior year of college. She characterizes this relationship as, "we were the beautiful, popular couple." Angela broke it off because she wanted to get engaged, and her partner at the time stated that he was not ready. She states that he probably didn't really love her, because if he did, he would have proposed.

She met her husband at a bar where many "young, successful financial guys" hung out. She was drawn to him by his looks, confidence, rational style, and the fact that they seemed to have many common interests, such as going to bars and parties, shopping, and beach vacations. Currently, she is concerned about their quite different visions of their future as a couple. She wants to leave the corporate world and pursue her online career, which would involve a reduction in work hours and an investment in props, clothing, and software. He is supportive of this as a hobby, but not as a career. She states that over the years, he has become increasingly "stable and boring"—he is less interested in going out and wants to start a family, as they have been married for seven years. He also has some "jealousy issues" around her Internet presence, as she dresses provocatively on camera. She wants her online career established before she takes the risk of altering her body with a pregnancy.

She has female friends with whom she socializes, but she states that a lot of women are jealous of her looks and overall confidence, so she gets along better with men. She endorses engaging in some "dysfunctional dieting" intermittently in her adolescent years and early 20s, but states that her current strict diet and exercise regimen keeps her "on track." Her current BMI is 19.2, in the low-normal range. She also endorses binge drinking in college and states that she usually has two to three glasses of wine a night with dinner and several cocktails on the weekends. She considers this to be an appropriate alcohol intake. She denies past or present street drug or prescription drug use or abuse.

She describes her family of origin as suburban working middle class and "unsophisticated." Neither parent started nor completed college. Her mother stayed at home, and her father had a contracting business. Angela stated that her father was very quiet and worked many hours in his contracting business. He was estranged from his family of origin. Angela had few details, but states that she stopped seeing his side of the family when she was about eight years old. All extended family interaction and events were with her maternal relatives. Even then, her father preferred not to socialize with them; at family events, he would usually just watch TV.

Angela describes her mother as beautiful, lively, and "the classic movie mother" cooking great meals, keeping a spotless house, keeping her father "happy" by catering to the needs of Angela and her brother and socializing with other parents from school. Because her mother did such a good job meeting his needs, he bought her nice jewelry, and they would go on a cruise once a year; they did not socialize with other couples. Her father also made sure that Angela's material needs and wants were always indulged; though they were not wealthy people, she had expensive, trendy clothes and a new car in high school. She states, "You would never know that we didn't have a lot of money."

Angela reports that her maternal grandfather had "issues" with alcohol and did not interact much with the family, even though they all had dinner together at least once a month and on holidays. She says that he was generally extremely quiet, but would occasionally make loud, negative comments about her mother, such as, "Your food is awful. Can't someone make a decent meal?" or, "You look okay now, but watch yourself in a few years. Men don't like fat girls." Her mother encouraged her to avoid him because he was a "silly old man who didn't know what he was saying." Growing up, Angela's mother did not provide much information about her childhood.

Psychiatric Presentation

Angela denies any past diagnosed psychiatric history, engagement with a therapist, or history of physical, emotional, or sexual trauma. She denies past or present affective symptoms or mood lability, nor does she endorse premenstrual syndrome. She denies past or present anxiety, excessive worry, or ruminations. She states that she has a regular sleep routine and sleeps a full eight hours per night without interruption, as well as a normal appetite. She denies issues managing anger or excessive irritability that has impacted any relationships. Focus, energy, motivation, and concentration are reportedly satisfactory. She denies psychotic or obsessive-compulsive symptoms. She denies past or present passive or active suicidal ideation and has no plans or intent, no suicide attempt, nor a history of self-mutilation or desire to harm others. She has never been hospitalized for a psychiatric illness. She denies any recent bingeing, purging, or restricting of food apart from some "mild restricting" in her early 20s. She endorses being sexually active, starting at age 14, when she slept with a star baseball player at her high school as a way to increase her popularity. She describes sex as a means to an end, and has not ever been truly satisfied by any of her sexual encounters. She thinks she has had an orgasm "once, maybe twice before."

Mental Status

She presents as healthy, awake, alert to person, place, time, and situation, well groomed, and in no acute distress. Her behavior is pleasant and cooperative, but she interacts excitedly, with excessive hand posturing and facial expressions. She also uses hyperbolic language to relay information. Gait and station are intact. She presents with a very bright affect with mood congruency in full range. She is hyperverbal, speaks loudly, with linear and goal-directed speech. She presents as lucid, logical, and reality based. She does not respond to internal stimuli or present as guarded or grandiose. Her recent and remote memory are intact, as is her concentration. Her fund of knowledge is appropriate to her education. She appears to have appropriate judgment and insight within certain contexts, such as the need for her to hold down a job, pay her bills, and get appropriate medical care. In other areas, her judgment is impaired in relation to appropriate workplace behavior within the context of her job, behavioral boundaries with coworkers and clients, and how her appearance and presentation is perceived by others. She perceives herself as attractive and fun-loving (i.e., her symptoms are ego-syntonic) and does not understand why others would not feel the same way.

Medical History and Status and Review of Symptoms

Angela presents as alert, fully developed, and relatively well nourished, despite a low BMI. Her face and body are symmetrical and free of features that may belie any genetic disorders. She has access to medical care and has a medical home with a local primary care physician, whom she sees once a year for a physical and lab work, which had no significant abnormalities. She denies any childhood chronic or acute illnesses and does not take any medications. She had an abortion in college, when she "slept with the football coach at her school," but has had no other pregnancies. She has an IUD x 5 years which has prevented pregnancy but has caused minor menstrual irregularities. She has no known allergies to substances, such as nuts or latex, and no known drug allergies. Her vital signs were normal. Review of symptoms, with the exception of minor menstrual irregularities from her IUD, are all negative.

Differential Diagnosis

Angela's history, behavior, and presentation meet criteria for HPD. She is uncomfortable in situations in which she is not the center of attention; engages in inappropriate seductive or provocative behavior; expresses rapidly shifting, excessive, and shallow emotional expression; uses personal appearance and emotional presentation to gain attention; and lacks judgment in perceiving relationships. She is naïve to both psychotherapy and medications. She has no significant medical history, nor any chronic or acute illnesses.

In session, she answered questions in a very glib and shallow manner, indicative of HPD, and was reticent to provide any significant details of a deeper emotional inner life, past or present. She was excited to share performative details of her life where she received a great deal of praise and attention. Her eating and drinking behaviors warranted further investigation to rule out alcohol abuse and an eating disorder. Given her needs for attention and recognition, comorbid generalized anxiety disorder (GAD) should also be ruled out. This is important as the need for recognition may be indicative of anxiety over performance expressed as GAD. She appeared anxious when she alluded to friction in her marriage secondary to being unable to pursue her Internet ambitions. She was also visibly anxious about the negative feedback she received from her manager. Comorbid Cluster B personality disorders, such as narcissistic PD and BPD should be ruled out, given her grandiose sense of self-importance and potential lack of a fully cohesive identity, respectively.

She presents as lacking insight as to why her manager wanted her to pursue psychiatric help but is willing to admit that she does have concern over losing her job. However, the mere fact that she presented to treatment and expressed valuing her job are a possible indication that her behaviors, consciously or unconsciously, are causing her discomfort.

Biological/Genetic Considerations

The patient denies any significant psychiatric family history, diagnosed or observed. Her description of her mother indicates possible personality traits consistent with HPD or BPD, so her behaviors are likely both learned and with a genetic diathesis.

Her family of origin provided reinforcement for attention-seeking behavior. Her mother received what the patient describes as praise and material rewards for being beautiful and living up to traditional feminine ideals. These signals were communicated positively by Angela's father through trips and jewelry. Correspondently, Angela's grandfather underscored these ideas by outlining the consequences of being average—no adulation equals no attention. Culturally speaking, Angela's family adhered to traditional gender norms. Women were both domestic and ornamental, so Angela's issues are a mosaic of biological, environmental, and cultural factors.

Treatment

Angela agreed to "try a few sessions" of "some kind of therapy" but flatly refused any medication of any kind for fear of gaining weight. She stated that she might be open to learning some coping skills but had no interest in being "psychoanalyzed."

Angela's initial evaluation and subsequent treatment was provided by a female clinician. From a transference perspective, Angela's use of sexualized behavior as both a means of communication and a way to reinforce her perception of herself as an object of male desire might have been reenacted if she were seeing a male therapist. However, because Angela was seeing a female, different transferences regarding competitiveness and envy were inevitable for her.

Initially, she tried to engage the clinician in an overly friendly, gossipy dialogue of avoidance. As Angela stated that she sometimes had trouble connecting with women, she felt that "keeping the conversation light and playful" would improve the chances of the therapist liking her. The clinician responded by asking her about her goals. She encouraged Angela that therapy was a chance to "talk about meaningful issues" and that Angela didn't need to keep things "light and playful" to seek acceptance. Angela thanked her, but remained glib for most of the first session.

Angela's treatment included a combination of psychodynamic therapy and CBT. This combination would provide her with some insight as to the origins and unconscious drives of her behavior, coupled with concrete skills to manage it. Exploring the origins of her behavior, her interpersonal relationship with women and men, her capacity to be in love, to mentalize others, and examining her relationship with alcohol and food help provide her insight as to what motivates her.

In subsequent sessions, Angela utilizes several defenses and coping styles. When the therapist challenged Angela on her coping style of using sex to hide the anxiety she was feeling about not being as successful as her husband, Angela acted out by telling her therapist that she couldn't understand using sex as a coping mechanism, as the therapist had "no sex appeal whatsoever." She became competitive with the therapist, stating that when her business took off, she would be making twice as much money as the therapist. The therapist took this in stride, as she had "warned" Angela of having strong feelings of "competition and envy" toward the therapist. It was worked though, and Angela became aware that when she felt insecure or inadequate, she became "competitive" toward women and "seductive" toward men. When therapy focused on Angela's past relationship with her father, Angela started complaining of headaches and stomach aches. The somatization was pointed out as a defense mechanism used to avoid a painful topic. Several times during the therapy, Angela said in a childlike voice, "I don't know, what do you think? Please just tell me what to do." The therapist interpreted that Angela was a very capable woman who knew what she wanted, and that this type of regression may be a way to "stop people from challenging her about some of her decisions." Angela admitted that being challenged made her feel defensive and unliked. By becoming childlike and deferential, Angela hoped to get "back into the therapist's good graces." The therapist interpreted that becoming childlike does not always equate to becoming more likeable. The therapist commended Angela for her awareness of this coping style. They then made it a goal not to regress when being challenged, but rather to become introspective and problem-solve.

Angela labored under significant cognitive distortions as to how she is perceived by others. For example, "If I'm not perfectly made up, then people will think I'm ugly and will forget about me," and "sex is the only way to get positive attention from anyone." She minimized her boss's and husband's concerns about her dress and behavior and characterized their concerns as a form of "flattery."

When the clinician tried to explore why maintaining her behavior was so important to her, her insecurity and lack of a stable identity emerged. She struggled, using splitting defense: if what she believes to be true isn't real, she no longer exists. She used splitting to minimizes others' negative responses to her behavior, only recognizing their approving responses. Losing her job, her Internet presence, and approval from her husband would further reinforce a loss of identity, a sense of meaninglessness, a life without purpose, a profound sense of emptiness, and could prove to be devastating.

To tie Angela's fears to a meaningful goal, and to help her see therapy as productive rather than mere "psychoanalyzing," she was asked what she wanted to accomplish. She laughed and responded, "Whatever gets people off my back." Together, she and the therapist identified a specific helpful behavior—saving her revealing shirts for non-work weekend activities. When asked how she felt about changing this behavior, she said that she felt kind of anxious and scared. When asked to share more, she stated that she didn't want to be "invisible" at work. She went on to say that she grew up in a household where no one gave her any feedback unless she was "over the top." The only kind of positive feedback, in jobs or relationships, was the attention she received from her outlandish behavior or appearance. At subsequent sessions, the therapist gently challenged Angela if the current work feedback she was getting was "positive."

Angela attended 10 CBT sessions, sprinkled with psychodynamic interpretations. Her stated goals were to be more aware of how her appearance may be perceived, separate recreational behavior and appearance from workplace appearance, and to observe and identify anxiety and depressive moods when external supplies were not forthcoming, and feelings of being invisible and how they affected her. She was not willing to delve deeper into her family of origin at the time, nor was she open to examining eating or drinking behaviors, but left therapy with some tools to assist in being more aware of herself and others.

Conclusion

HPD is in the Cluster B DSM 5 grouping of personality disorders, marked by attention-seeking behaviors and shallow affect. It has six distinct subtypes and is often comorbid with other personality disorders, as well as affective disorders and anxiety. It is more commonly diagnosed in females. The age of diagnosis is typically late adolescence to early adulthood. It may be forged in family trauma or a modeling of parental behavior. The disorder is modestly to moderately genetically heritable, depending upon the study. A medical work-up, such as hyperactive thyroid and stimulant abuse, should be considered before formal diagnosis. If the patient in question is engaged in a culture that values and rewards his or her behavior, he or she may never present to treatment. Psychotherapy is the preferred treatment modality; there is no FDA approved medication regimen, though traditional treatments for affective symptoms, such as antidepressants and mood stabilizers, are used for symptom control. Personality perception varies widely by culture, so groups with higher levels of emotionality and expressiveness may interpret so-called "histrionic" behavior as a cultural norm. Review Box 20.3 for additional resources.

Conflict of Interest/Disclosure: The authors of this chapter have no financial conflicts and nothing to disclose.

Box 20.3 Resources for Patients, Families, and Clinicians

- *Psychology Today*. https://www.psychologytoday.com/us/conditions/histrionic-personality-disorder.
- The Mayo Clinic. https://www.mayoclinic.org/diseases-conditions/personality-disorders/symptoms-causes/syc-20354463.
- National Institutes of Mental Health. https://www.nimh.nih.gov/health/statistics/personality-disorders.shtml.
- Massachusetts General Hospital Psychiatry Academy. Advanced Psychotherapy for Challenging Cases (for clinicians). https://mghcme.org/courses/advanced-psychotherapy-strategies-cbt-dbt-and-dynamic-concepts-for-use-with-challenging-cases-december-2021.
- WebMd. https://www.webmd.com/mental-health/histrionic-personality-disorder#1.

References

1. Novais F, Araújo A, Godinho P. Historical roots of histrionic personality disorder. *Front Psychol.* 2015;6. doi:10.3389/fpsyg.2015.01463

2. French J, Shrestha S. Histrionic Personality Disorder. Published 2021. Statpearls.com. https://www.statpearls.com/articlelibrary/viewarticle/38407/.

3. Morrison J. Histrionic personality disorder in women with somatization disorder. *Psychosomatics.* 1989;30(4):433–437. doi:10.1016/s0033-3182(89)72250-7

4. Vergés A, Kushner M, Jackson K et al. Personality disorders and the persistence of anxiety disorders: evidence of a time-of-measurement effect in NESARC. *J Anxiety Disord.* 2014;28(2):178–186. doi:10.1016/j.janxdis.2013.09.012

5. Zetzel ER. The so called good hysteric. *Int J Psychoanal.* 1968;49(2):256–260. PMID: 5685197.

6. Millon T, Grossman S. *Personality Disorders In Modern Life.* Hoboken, NJ: Wiley; 2004.

7. *Diagnostic And Statistical Manual Of Mental Disorders: DSM-5.* 5th ed. Washington, DC: American Psychiatric Publishing; 2013

8. de Girolamo G, Dagani J, Purcell R, Cocchi A, McGorry P. Age of onset of mental disorders and use of mental health services: needs, opportunities and obstacles. *Epidemiol Psychiatr Sci.* 2011;21(1):47–57. doi:10.1017/s2045796011000746

9. McWilliams N. Hysterical (histrionic) personalities. In: McWilliams N. *Psychoanalytic Diagnosis: Understanding Personality Structure in the Clinical Process,* 2nd ed. New York, NY: Guilford; 2011: 311–331.

10. Klonsky E, Jane J, Turkheimer E, Oltmanns T. Gender role and personality disorders. *J Pers Disord.* 2002;16(5):464–476. doi:10.1521/pedi.16.5.464.22121

11. Rawson RA. How stimulants affect the brain and behavior. In: *Treatment for Stimulant Use Disorders: Treatment Improvement Protocol.* (TIP) Series 33. Rockville, MD: US Department of Health and Human Services; 1999:13–32. https://www.ncbi.nlm.nih.gov/books/NBK64328/.

12. Manoochehri M, Huey E. Diagnosis and management of behavioral issues in frontotemporal dementia. *Curr Neurol Neurosci Rep.* 2012;12(5):528–536. doi:10.1007/s11910-012-0302-7

13. Warrington T, Bostwick J. Psychiatric adverse effects of corticosteroids. *Mayo Clin Proc.* 2006;81(10):1361–1367. doi:10.4065/81.10.1361

14. Cappelletti S, Daria P, Sani G, Aromatario M. Caffeine: cognitive and physical performance enhancer or psychoactive drug? *Curr Neuropharmacol.* 2015;13(1):71–88. doi:10.2174/1570159x13666141210215655

15. Tinsley J, Watkins D. Over-the-counter stimulants: abuse and addiction. *Mayo Clin Proc.* 1998;73(10):977–982. doi:10.4065/73.10.977

16. Hyperthyroidism (Overactive Thyroid) | NIDDK. National Institute of Diabetes and Digestive and Kidney Diseases. Published August 2016. https://www.niddk.nih.gov/health-information/endocrine-diseases/hyperthyroidism.

17. Sanches M. The limits between bipolar disorder and borderline personality disorder: a review of the evidence. *Diseases.* 2019;7(3):49. doi:10.3390/diseases7030049

18. Schulte Holthausen B, Habel U. Sex differences in personality disorders. *Curr Psychiatry Rep.* 2018;20(12). doi:10.1007/s11920-018-0975-y

19. Nestadt G, Romanoski A, Chahal R, et al. An epidemiological study of histrionic personality disorder. *Psychol Med.* 1990;20(2):413–422. doi:10.1017/s0033291700017724

20. Smith SF, Lilienfeld SO. Histrionic personality disorder. In: Stein J, ed. *Reference Module in Neuroscience and Biobehavioral Psychology*. Amsterdam: Elsevier; 2017:312–315. doi:10.1016/B978-0-12-809324-5.06447-6.

21. Friborg O, Martinsen E, Martinussen M, Kaiser S, Øvergård K, Rosenvinge J. Comorbidity of personality disorders in mood disorders: a meta-analytic review of 122 studies from 1988 to 2010. *J Affect Disord*. 2014;152–154:1–11. doi:10.1016/j.jad.2013.08.023

22. Bockian N. Depression in histrionic personality disorder. In N Bockian, ed. *Personality-Guided Therapy for Depression*. Washington, DC: American Psychological Association; 2006: 169–186.

23. Reichborn-Kjennerud T. The genetic epidemiology of personality disorders. *Dialogues Clin Neurosci*. 2010;12(1):103–114. doi:10.31887/DCNS.2010.12.1/trkjennerud

24. Torgersen S, Lygren S, Oien PA, et al. A twin study of personality disorders. *Compr Psychiatry*. 2000;41(6):416–425. doi:10.1053/comp.2000.16560

25. Rossier J, Ouedraogo A, Dahourou D, Verardi S, de Stadelhofen FM. Personality and personality disorders in urban and rural Africa: results from a field trial in Burkina Faso. *Front Psychol*. 2013 March 11;4:79. doi:10.3389/fpsyg.2013.00079

26. Lim N. Cultural differences in emotion: differences in emotional arousal level between the East and the West. *Integr Med Res*. 2016;5(2):105–109. doi:10.1016/j.imr.2016.03.004

27. Betan E, Heim AK, Zittel Conklin C, Westen D. Countertransference phenomena and personality pathology in clinical practice: an empirical investigation. *Am J Psychiatry*. 2005;162(5):890–898. doi:10.1176/appi.ajp.162.5.890

28. Gabbard GO. Hysterical and histrionic personality disorders. In Gabbard GO, ed. *Psychodynamic Psychiatry in Clinical Practice*. Washington, DC: American Psychiatric Publishing; 2014: 545–576.

29. Ogrodniczuk JS, Piper WE. Use of transference interpretations in dynamically oriented individual psychotherapy for patients with personality disorders. *J Pers Disord*. 1999;13(4):297–311. doi:10.1521/pedi.1999.13.4.297

30. Colli A, Tanzilli A, Dimaggio G, Lingiardi V. Patient personality and therapist response: an empirical investigation. *Am J Psychiatry*. 2014;171(1):102–108. doi:10.1176/appi.ajp.2013.13020224

31. Beck JS. *Cognitive Therapy for Challenging Problems: What to Do When the Basics Don't Work*. New York, NY: Guilford Press; 2005.

32. Sperry L, Sperry J. *Cognitive Behavior Therapy of DSM-5 Personality Disorders: Assessment, Case Conceptualization, and Treatment*. New York, NY: Routledge; 2015.

33. Sungur MZ, Gunduz A. Histrionic personality disorder. In: Beck AT, Davis DD, Freeman A, eds. *Cognitive Therapy of Personality Disorders*. 3rd ed. New York, NY: Guilford Press; 2015: 325–345

34. Livesley WJ, Dimaggio G, Clarkin JF. *Integrated Treatment for Personality Disorder: A Modular Approach*. New York, NY: Guilford Press; 2015.

35. Barnett J. Narcissism and dependency in the obsessional-hysteric marriage. *Fam Process*. 1971;10(1):75–83. doi:10.1111/j.1545-5300.1971.00075.x

36. Silk KR, Feurino III L. Psychopharmacology of personality disorders. In: Widiger TA, ed. *The Oxford Handbook of Personality Disorders*. New York, NY: Oxford University Press; 2012. doi: 10.1093/oxfordhb/9780199735013.013.0033.

37. Sulz S. Hysteria I. [Histrionic personality disorder. A psychotherapeutic challenge]. *Nervenarzt*. 2010;81(7):879–888. 879–888. doi:10.1007/s00115-010-3016-6

21

Narcissistic Personality Disorder

Alyson A. Gorun, Benjamin A. Scherban, and Elizabeth L. Auchincloss

Key Points

- NPD is defined in DSM-5 as "a pervasive pattern of grandiosity, need for admiration, and lack of empathy . . . " and lists traits including: a grandiose sense of self-importance; a preoccupation with fantasies of unlimited success; a belief that one is special; and an envy of, exploitative use of, and arrogance toward other people.
- NPD is difficult to define diagnostically, making its prevalence difficult to measure.
- Twenge has argued that there is an increase in narcissism using the Narcissistic Personality Inventory (NPI) which measures adaptive and maladaptive narcissistic traits. It is debatable whether the NPI truly carries over into pathological narcissism.[8]
- There is general consensus that there are three different types of NPD: (1) the thick-skinned, grandiose/malignant, or the oblivious type described in the DSM-5; (2) the thin-skinned, fragile type is basically equivalent to the DSM-5 hypervigilant or vulnerable type; and (3) a high-functioning/exhibitionist type,[1] which is outgoing and energetic, interpersonally adept, and often highly charming.
- Otto Kernberg espouses the "defense model" while Heinz Kohut supports the "deficit model" for the development of NPD. Mentalization models have also been used to describe the development of NPD.
- There is limited research supporting the heritability of NPD, though temperament, attachment, and environmental factors including parenting also contribute the development of NPD.
- Adaptive narcissism versus pathological narcissism continues to be an area of debate.
- Typical transferences and countertransferences that can arise include idealization/devaluation, feeling bored, hostility, or a lack of transference, among others.
- There are no randomized controlled trials for the treatment of NPD, though several manualized psychotherapies are currently being investigated.
- Psychotherapy is recommended as first-line treatment over psychopharmacology.
- Psychopharmacology can be used to treat comorbidities.
- Some general principles that can guide the treatment of narcissistic spectrum disorders are described.

Introduction

This chapter will give an overview of narcissistic personality disorder (NPD) using clinical guidelines and experience, anecdotal reports, and the limited evidence-based research on this disorder. The topics covered include the epidemiology, common comorbidities, diagnostic considerations, psycho-social and cultural contributions, developmental origins and theories of narcissistic pathology, and biologic, neuropsychiatric, and genetic underpinnings of NPD. Typical transference and countertransference reactions that can occur during the treatment of NPD will also be discussed. Recommendations for various treatment approaches, and different treatment modalities for NPD will be reviewed.

Epidemiology

NPD is difficult to define and thus difficult to measure. Estimates of prevalence of NPD in the community vary depending on the study. A systematic review of seven non-clinical samples utilizing *Diagnostic and Statistical Manual of Mental Disorders* (DSM-5) criteria and using structured or semi-structured interviews found a mean prevalence of 1.06 percent with the range between 0 to 6.2 percent.[1,2] This is the range of prevalence that is cited in DSM-5 as well.[1] It is worth noting, however, that most studies of the prevalence of NPD in clinical samples tend to be higher, although this also varies by the study.[3] It has been pointed out that in the clinical population, patients with narcissistic pathology are likely to be of the "vulnerable" subtype (see "Diagnostic Considerations" below), while in the general population, the proportion of "overt" narcissists—who, it is thought, are less likely to seek treatment—is likely to be proportionally higher.[4]

In terms of male versus female, the DSM-5 says that of those diagnosed with NPD, 50–75 percent are male.[1] This is supported by recent studies. For example, a large epidemiological study, the National Epidemiological Survey on Alcohol Related Disorders (NESARC) which found the overall prevalence of NPD to be 6.2 percent), found 7.7 percent of men had NPD but only 4.8 percent of women.[5] Again, this is using DSM criteria for NPD, and it is worth noting that this view is not universal. Gabbard, for instance, suggests that "the assumption that men are more likely to be narcissistic than women does not hold up to scrutiny."[6] Interestingly, when the NPD construct was first created in psychodynamic theory, although early descriptions were often of men, it was often thought to be more associated with women.[7]

One question of increasing interest is whether NPD is on the rise. Twenge has argued that there is an increase in narcissism, although her work uses the Narcissistic Personality Inventory (NPI), which measures narcissistic traits (adaptive as well as maladaptive); it is debatable whether the NPI truly carries over into pathological narcissism.[8]

Interestingly, at least one epidemiological study found NPD to be inversely related to age; in other words, it was more prevalent in younger groups of people than in older groups.[9]

Diagnostic Considerations

When we say that someone is a "narcissist," we mean that they have an exaggerated sense of self-importance and are very self-involved. However, there is no agreement among clinicians or scientists as to how to formally diagnose NPD.

The DSM-5 defines NPD as a "pervasive pattern of grandiosity, need for admiration, and lack of empathy . . ." and lists some traits including: a grandiose sense of self-importance; a preoccupation with fantasies of unlimited success; a belief that one is special; and an envy of, exploitative use of, and arrogance toward other people.[1] One group on the APA's DSM-5 task force wanted to eliminate the disorder completely, arguing that there was a paucity of research evidence in support of the diagnosis. Another group, fueled by clinician protest that such a disorder was highly prevalent among real-world patients, argued that this diagnosis should be included. Ultimately, the clinical group prevailed.

However, NPD defies diagnostic categories that are based on a checklist for several reasons:

1. NPD is confused with those aspects of narcissism that are considered "healthy." Everyone has some narcissism, just as everyone has satisfaction in a job well done or some sensitivity to criticism.[10]
2. Cultural factors confuse the diagnosis. Cultural factors play a role in the diagnosis of all personality disorders, but in NPD they are especially relevant. For example, what is considered "healthy" self -esteem and what is considered too much or not enough?[10]
3. Life stage has a lot to do with diagnosis. For example, what is the role of self-centeredness and fluctuating self-esteem in adolescence? Can NPD be diagnosed in all age groups?[10]
4. There appears to be a paucity of research on NPD compared to other personality disorders.

Rosenfeld, a well-known psychoanalyst, delineated two types of NPD: the "thick-skinned" narcissist (analogous to the type described in the DSM-5) and the "thin-skinned" narcissist.[11] Gabbard wrote that there were two types of NPD: the oblivious or grandiose type (analogous to Rosenfeld's thick-skinned narcissist), and the hypervigilant or vulnerable type (analogous to Rosenfeld's thin-skinned narcissist). However, to avoid the self-report, prevalent in much research, Russ's research group used the Shedler-Westen Assessment Procedure-II (SWAP-II) to see how the diagnosis was actually made by clinicians. They were able to identify three subtypes of NPD that are in use today: (1) the grandiose/malignant[12] or the oblivious type largely described in the DSM-5; (2) the fragile type[12] that is basically equivalent to the DSM-5 hypervigilant or vulnerable type (in this type, the grandiose defenses of the oblivious type have been punctured, leaving a pervasive sense of inadequacy or low self-esteem, negative affect, and loneliness/emptiness); and (3) a high-functioning/exhibitionist type,[12] which is outgoing and energetic, interpersonally adept, and often highly charming.[6,10,12-14] These three types are not rigidly constructed but often have permeable borders based on context.[6]

Social-personality psychology research using the NPI[15] conceptualizes NPD as a "normative personality trait" which can be adaptive or maladaptive. However, the NPI has been criticized for assessing adaptive components as well as maladaptive components of personality. The cognitive behavioral therapy (CBT) literature is relatively sparse but emphasizes social learning of core beliefs or self-schemas.[16] Many have proposed that early experiences ranging from parental abuse and neglect to parental overindulgence lead to NPD.[17]

Common Comorbidities and Mixed Personality Disorders

Major depressive disorder (MDD), bipolar I disorder, anxiety disorders, and substance use disorders are frequently comorbid with NPD.[9] One epidemiologic survey estimates that there is a 49.5 percent comorbidity rate for mood disorder, with MDD at 20.6 percent and bipolar I disorder at 20.1 percent.[5] Anxiety disorders were comorbid 54.7 percent of the time, and substance use disorders are present a striking 64.2 percent of the time.[5] Patients frequently present for treatment for one of these co-occurring disorders and not for NPD. A comprehensive diagnostic assessment is thus essential, especially since the presence of narcissism may worsen prognosis of other psychiatric illnesses.[18]

NPD can also be comorbid with other personality disorders. NPD is most often found along with histrionic personality disorder and antisocial personality disorder (ASPD).[17] Borderline personality disorder (BPD) is also frequently present and has an estimated comorbidity of 37 percent.[5] Clinicians describe that comorbid BPD and NPD can be particularly difficult to treat, above and beyond BPD on its own.[18] A 2018 study found that male patients with BPD had higher narcissistic scores than female patients with BPD, as well as evidence that vulnerable narcissism may be more highly associated with BPD than grandiose narcissism.[19]

Other comorbidities include the masochistic-narcissistic personality style described by Cooper[20] (See Chapter 25 on masochistic/self-defeating personality styles for additional information) or a mix of NPD and obsessive-compulsive personality disorder that can be found in higher functioning professionals.[21] Of all of these personality disorders, comorbid ASPD has the most negative impact on prognosis.[17,22] Indeed, Otto Kernberg has characterized the syndrome of "malignant narcissism," which consists of NPD and severe antisocial behaviors, paranoid trends and ego-syntonic aggression, at the most severe end of the narcissism spectrum.[22]

Biologic, Neuropsychiatric, and Genetics of NPD

Structural and functional brain imaging have identified differences in the brain regions of individuals with NPD. In these patients, the left anterior insula as well as other fronto-limbic structures have a smaller gray matter volume in comparison to non-clinical controls.[23] These areas have been identified as related to emotional empathy,[23] as well as low self-esteem, empathic processing, anxiety producing stimuli, and social rejection.[24] Additionally, the anterior insula, along with the anterior cingulate cortex, are important to the salience network which helps switch between an internal state and an external state, as well as integrating sensory and emotional stimuli.[24] The salience network thus would be important for the ability to empathize. Dysfunction in this area could lead to a focus on internal processes rather than the outside world, and the relative lack of empathy, an observation seen clinically in narcissistic patients.[24] The anterior insula and fronto-limbic structures have consistent empirical support from neuroimaging studies implicating their role in narcissism.[24]

Skin conductance studies, which measure the level of physiological arousal in humans, have shown that individuals with high levels of narcissism as measured by the

NPI have similar responses to those of psychopathic individuals when expecting an aversive stimulus in a laboratory setting. This response is characterized by low physiological activity[24] and may be suggestive of impaired ability to inhibit their behaviors or impulsivity.[24] One study found larger cortisol output following social stressors for men with high levels of narcissism on the NPI as compared to men with low levels of narcissism.[24] In a different study, secretion of cortisol and alpha-amylase in response to negative emotions was correlated with levels of narcissism (measured by the NPI) in women.[24] These findings are suggestive of hypoathalmic-pituitary-adrenal axis hyperreactivity associated with levels of narcissism, which would be consistent with sensitivity to stressful events.[24]

There are a limited number of studies looking at the genetic basis for NPD. A number of different twin studies have given estimates of heritability for NPD as falling between 24 percent and 79 percent.[10,17,23] One twin study using a structured DSM interview for personality disorders in addition to self-report questionnaires (differing from other studies that only used the DSM criteria) found a heritability of 71 percent for NPD.[23] After finding significant correlations of father–daughter levels of narcissism in 36 biological family groups, but not for other parent–offspring dyads, one study cautiously suggested that there may not only be a genetic component to levels of narcissism, but also possible X chromosome involvement.[17] Although the degree of heritability varies widely between studies, there is evidence to suggest that the trait of narcissism is heritable.

It is important to mention that although narcissism appears to have a heritable component, the role of attachment and shared environmental influence also have an important role in the etiology of pathological narcissism. NPD has both constitutional and environmental origins, but the relevant contribution of each is not yet known.[6] This remains an ongoing area of investigation that requires further research.

Cultural and Psycho-social Considerations

In 1979, both Lasch and Stern wrote about the rise of narcissism in America and cultural contributions to this, including the impact of the media and its centrality to American culture.[25,26] More recently, Twenge and Campbell, using NPI as a measure of narcissistic personality traits in the general population, describe increasing levels of narcissism and an increasing sense of entitlement among those born after 1982. They posit this rise as related to changes in parenting to a more permissive style and the increased use of social media.[8,27] Permissive parenting leads to young people feeling entitled to things without actually accomplishing what is necessary to do to attain them, and social media encourages them to seek out superficial affirmation of their self-worth without engaging in real relationships. Because they used NPI and not NPD from the DSM-5, they may overestimating the level of narcissism because they are capturing healthy self-esteem and more adaptive components of narcissism such as leadership in addition to NPD traits such as grandiosity.[6,17]

Other studies also show evidence of increasing NPD. A survey done in 2008 showed that people ages 20–29 are almost three times more likely than people over 65 to meet criteria for NPD as defined by DSM-5.[9]

Other writers propose a different view of narcissism, such as Lunbeck in her book, *The Americanization of Narcissism*; she emphasizes the positive and normative qualities of these traits.[7] The role of healthy narcissism versus pathological narcissism in society continues to be debated and written about today.

Developmental Origins and Theories of Narcissistic Pathology

Psychoanalysis had much to say about NPD, as Freud was very concerned with exploring the psychology of narcissism, although he never wrote about NPD per se. From the psychoanalytic perspective, one theme that runs across all types of NPD is a concern about being seen by others and a wish to avoid the consequent shame and humiliation.[28-30] This wish to avoid shame at all cost leads to a pursuit of perfection.[29] Modell used the metaphor of the cocoon to describe the narcissist's feeling of non-relatedness to his or her environment.[31]

Much controversy surrounding the concepts of pathological narcissism centers on the difference between the views of Heinz Kohut's deficit model[32-34] versus Otto Kernberg's defense model.[35,36] Kohut saw NPD as reflecting a developmental delay or deficit due to environmental factors, namely a failure in empathic mirroring by caregivers. Kernberg distinguishes between the normal narcissism of childhood and NPD. In contrast to Kohut, Kernberg sees NPD as reflecting a pathological structure of the self, deformed by defensive operations, which results in a type of object relations characterized by apparent self-sufficiency and the devaluing of others.[35,36] Kohut believed that slights or threats to the self often result in what he called "narcissistic rage," where Kernberg believed that the rage often seen in these individuals results from inborn wishes.

Some see this dispute between Kohut and Kernberg as reflecting different patient populations. Kernberg was writing about the grandiose/malignant or oblivious narcissist who devalues others and fears dependency; Kohut was writing about the fragile/vulnerable narcissist who has low self-esteem and is in search of people to idealize, so as to shore up their low self-esteem. Which comes first, the grandiose self or the deflated self, is the great "chicken or the egg" riddle of narcissistic pathology.[29] See Table 21.1 for a comparison.

Table 21.1. Kernberg versus Kohut Models of Narcissism

Kernberg	Kohut
"Defense model": The grandiose self is a *defense* against dependency on others. The self is comprised of a pathological grandiose structure. Aggression is inborn and results in significant envy. Idealization is a defense against aggression. This model typically reflects the malignant grandiose or oblivious narcissist.	"Deficit model": The grandiose self is the result of a *deficit* originating from empathic failures of caregivers. The grandiose self is nondefensive, "normal," and developmentally appropriate given caregiver deficits in empathic mirroring from childhood. Aggression is secondary to empathic failures of caregivers. Idealization is a "normal" process given their arrested developmental phase. This means their need for an exalted or admiring object is necessary in order to bolster their own development of their self. This model typically reflects the vulnerable narcissist.

Parental Styles and NPD

Empiric research has sought to validate both Kernberg's and Kohut's theoretical ideas, including the impact on the development of NPD of parental style, versus the temperamental predisposition of a child. A majority of these studies look at the participant's own experience retrospectively, which may impact the reliability of these findings.[4] Parental coldness, overvaluation, and overindulgence have been looked at as potentially impacting the development of narcissism.[6,17] One prospective study showed that between the ages of 7–12 years, parental overvaluation predicted narcissism, but not lack of parental warmth. Positive self-esteem, however, was predicted by parental warmth but not by parental overvaluation.[6] Based on this study, it seems that an accurate assessment of a child's strengths, in addition to parental warmth, are important contributors to a nonpathological view of the self. Further studies have attempted to differentiate which parental styles result in grandiose versus vulnerable narcissism, with some studies suggesting that parental coldness may be more associated with vulnerable narcissism, while parental overindulgence/overvaluation may contribute to both kinds of NPD.[4,17] A review of studies looking at the influence of parenting on the development of pathological narcissism does suggest that parental styles can influence its development in adulthood.[17,37] Other influences, such as childhood adversity, have also been associated with the development of NPD.[38]

Attachment and NPD

Attachment theory has also been used to describe how narcissism can develop in an individual, although research is limited. A study by Diamond et al. showed that patients with NPD and BPD were more likely to have dismissive or cannot-classify attachment style, as compared to a group of patients with BPD without NPD, who were categorized as having a preoccupied attachment style base on unresolved loss and abuse. There were no differences in mentalization, although both BPD and NPD scored low.[39] Dickinson and Pincus used the NPI to attempt to differentiate grandiose and vulnerable subtypes of narcissism as related to attachment styles and found that grandiose subtypes were more likely to have secure or dismissive attachment styles, rather than fearful or preoccupied attachment styles. Vulnerable subtypes were more likely to have fearful or preoccupied attachment styles.[40] This and other studies suggest that both dismissing and preoccupied styles of attachment are associated with pathological narcissism.[17] Overall, research points to a bi-directional interaction between a child's temperament and inadequate parental style, leading to a development of narcissistic disturbances in a child.

The Relationship, Transference, and Countertransference with Narcissistic Patients

Overview and History

In addition to particular challenges in developing a therapeutic alliance with narcissistic patients, there are also typical transference and countertransference reactions that can arise at the beginning and over the course of treatment. Originally, early psychoanalytic theory posited that narcissistic patients did not establish a transference.[29] While patients we would today classify as narcissistic were described in the early clinical literature, truly narcissistic patients were felt to be untreatable because they did not establish a transference neurosis. Two analysts who pioneered new theories and treatment strategies for narcissistic disturbances were Kernberg and Kohut. Kernberg tended to focus on the envious and devaluing aspects of narcissistic transferences.[35,36] Kohut meanwhile conceptualized transferences as distinct "self-object transferences" meaning that the analyst is being utilized by the patient to perform functions that the patient (due to inadequate nurturing in development) now recreates as an adult.[32–34] Kohut outlined a mirror transference, where the patient seeks admiration; an idealizing transference, where the patient idealizes the therapist; or twinship transference, where the therapist is felt as similar. Clinicians today often find using both Kohut and Kernberg's theories useful; both of their theories lie underneath much of what has followed and what clinicians have posited as some of the most consistent transferences and countertransferences experienced with narcissistic patients.[6]

That said, it is true that nowadays we tend to think of psychotherapy within the framework of a "two person psychology." From a postmodern point of view, therapists do have their own subjectivities that they bring to the therapeutic dyad, meaning that every dyad is unique. However, there is empirical data for shared countertransferences when working with NPD patients as discussed in the "Countertransference and NPD"[41] section. Furthermore, there are increasingly other ways to conceptualize some of the ways narcissistic patients relate and establish a transference. While in some ways these are similar to Kernberg and Kohut's models, they are theoretically distinct. For instance, inspired by Fonagy's understanding of mentalizing deficits in patients with NPD (as opposed to BPD, where Fonagy originated this work), some have recently sought to explain narcissistic transferences from the mentalizing perspective.[42] Drozkeh and Unrah hypothesized that due to the caregiver's incongruent mirroring of the child's affective experience, for example of overvaluation of a child's abilities while not mirroring feelings of insecurity or vulnerbaility, a child will start to internalize the caregiver and begin to project self-enhancement onto themselves. This is in contrast to a patient with BPD, who addresses a lack of congruent mirroring by projecting badness onto others. For narcissistic patients, this ultimately leads to a sense of discontinuity and fragmentation, and creates a "narcissistic alien self" of the caregivers' overvalued conceptualization represented onto a child's actual affective experience. This requires them to utilize others to project "good" onto their own selves in order to ensure self-coherence.[42]

From a contemporary clinical point of view, the type of transference and countertransference that develops within a therapeutic relationship will likely depend at least in part on the specific type of narcissist one is treating, (e.g., the more oblivious/grandiose subtype, vulnerable subtype, or the high-functioning type), which can lead to the narcissistic dynamics being missed at first. A caveat about these subtypes must be kept in mind. Despite utilizing these subtypes as a useful schematic, a given patient may oscillate between how these subtypes present and relate during the treatment. This most commonly occurs between the oblivious/grandiose and the vulnerable subtype. Thus, a patient's way of relating toward the therapist, and the therapist's own corresponding countertransference, may change over the course of treatment. Therefore, although this section will sketch out classic reactions of both patient and therapist, ultimately each therapeutic dyad is unique.

Therapeutic Relationship

Creating a good working alliance is a challenge from the first when working with a narcissistic patient, regardless of the subtype. From the very beginning of the first clinical encounter, a narcissistic patient, whether grandiose or vulnerable, is often struggling with profound shame and humiliation at needing assistance and feelings of dependency toward another person—in this case the therapist.[43] They may not want to admit that they need help, whether to themselves or to someone else. Even if they are able to admit it, they may also be concerned that the therapist doesn't really care about them, and feel they need to be on the lookout for exploitation. Conversely, some narcissistic patients may begin therapy with the goal of trying to "perfect" themselves rather than seeking insight or realistic change.[29] Some higher functioning narcissists may seem charming and may even be seductive, and their goal may be to try to win over the therapist and to become the favorite patient. They may not actually be interested in the therapist's thoughts, having an actual relationship, or doing therapeutic work; but this may not be obvious at first.[6] Given all that has been mentioned, the construction of a true therapeutic alliance is a difficult but essential task. It is important to pay attention to this both at the beginning of treatment and throughout. In fact, poor attendance and the sudden termination of treatment can often be seen when treating narcissistic patients.[18]

Transferences and NPD

As the therapy gets underway, typical patterns tend to emerge, usually depending on the subtype. The oblivious/grandiose narcissist may seem to ignore the therapist almost entirely, and spends the session arrogant and self-centered, name-dropping, and difficult to interrupt. This type of patient seems not to care what the therapist has to say. Conversely, the vulnerable narcissist may present as self-loathing, full of shame, and trying to avoid feeling slighted in some way.[6] In fact, rather than ignoring the therapist as the oblivious narcissist seems to, these vulnerable narcissistic patients often seem to be carefully sizing up the therapist and appear exquisitely sensitive to the therapist's words or behavior, whether positive or negative.[43] Again, though some patients seem to behave more like one or the other, they can oscillate between these two presentations. For example, while a seemingly grandiose narcissistic patient may seem oblivious to the therapist, they can also—at times suddenly—be incredibly sensitive to the therapist's perceived lack of interest, or to comments that the therapist makes that they find hurtful or insufficiently empathetic.

Meanwhile, there are a number of transferences patients often experience regardless of their subtype. Idealization and devaluation are frequently utilized by narcissistic patients, and can be expressed either from a grandiose stance or vulnerable one. Idealization can be the patient's way of shoring up their own self-esteem by creating a connection to an admired object. However, this idealization is fragile and can be quickly turned into contempt. Devaluation may be a way of inflating their self-esteem by putting down the other, or it may be a response to perceived slights or insults.[29] Especially in grandiose patients, narcissistic rage can be a response to a feeling of shame or inferiority caused by the therapist's perceived slight. The vulnerable narcissist may also erupt when slighted, although they might also retreat further into a depression. Kernberg has pointed out that while the patient may idealize or devalue the therapist, ultimately narcissistic patients feel that either the patient or the therapist is ultimately superior. Thus, they want to maintain their own superiority over the therapist, even if they are also defensively idealizing the therapist at the same time.[22]

In addition, narcissistic patients of all types often experience tremendous shame, which can lead to the patient using various strategies to avoid their feelings of shame such as the use of avoidance in the context of the therapy and the therapeutic relationship.[18] They also seek to avoid humiliating dependency, in this case on the therapist, and therefore may try to control the treatment and the frame, and demonstrate a strong sense of entitlement.[43] Envy toward the therapist may emerge, whether for the therapist's ability to be insightful about their difficulties or the therapist's ability to have a relationship with others.[22] Additionally, there can be a range of a lack of empathy in narcissistic patients, especially in those with antisocial traits or comorbid psychopathy.

One typical observation by therapists about narcissistic patients, in general, is their lack of interest in actually exploring the therapeutic relationship. Thus, regardless of the actual transference, narcissistic patients often don't see the point in discussing it. If the therapist actually does try to bring it up, the patient may be confused or even annoyed.[29]

Countertransference and NPD

Grandiose/oblivious narcissists generate classic countertransference reactions such as feeling bored, tired, or uninterested in what the patient is saying.[29] This boredom may be because the therapist feels that rather than being a participant in an actual conversation or relationship, they are merely "an appreciative audience."[43] It is theorized that this occurs due to a patient projecting only their devalued or idealized part of self onto the therapist, rather than a whole, discrete object. This leads the therapist to be a vehicle for self-esteem regulation rather than a full person.[29] Additionally, more grandiose narcissists may elicit in the therapist feelings of competition, annoyance, or frustration.[18] Of course, one must be careful that these countertransference reactions are due to the patient rather than to the therapist actually being tired or in an unsympathetic mood from something in their personal life. Time, clinical experience, and outside consultation, if needed, can help a therapist gain a sense of what is coming from a patient and what is coming from the therapist.

Vulnerable narcissistic patients may cause the therapist to feel an identification with the patient's suffering and become more invested. While this sometimes can be dangerous (if it leads to a boundary violation or enactment), Gabbard points out that in and of itself, this is not necessarily a bad thing, as it can also allow clinicians to build a sense of connection and caring for these patients.[6] Vulnerable narcissistic patients may also attempt to elicit in the therapist a very specific empathic response, wanting admiration and praise for their specialness. Some therapists might find this rewarding if they can actually discern and provide the empathy and mirroring the patient needs. Others may find this controlling, coercing, and even irritating. No matter what, it can be very emotionally draining.[6]

As previously noted, both grandiose/oblivious and vulnerable narcissistic patients may idealize or devalue the therapist. The corresponding countertransference in the therapist is often, unsurprisingly, feeling idealized or devalued. McWilliams has noted that perhaps therapists early in their career feel more frequently devalued rather than idealized.[29] Ultimately, it is important to remember that either way, devaluation and idealization are the flip sides of a coin and can switch to the opposite quickly. This ideali- zation and devaluation can feel to the therapist as if the patient is not relating to the ther- apist as a real person, and that neither the idealization or devaluation is truly merited.[29]

Additionally, narcissistic patients may also seek to control the treatment; oblivious narcissists perhaps more obviously, vulnerable narcissists sometimes more subtly. Either way, the therapist may feel the desire to exert their own power in return, leading to power struggles and enactments.[18]

Another countertransference reaction often cited is that therapists may feel that nothing is actually happening in the treatment, and no progress is being made. Sometimes, this may, in fact, be the case; other times, it may not actually be the case, but may be due to the therapist feeling frustrated in response to contempt and devaluation from the patient who claims no progress is being made.[6,29]

There have been studies that attempted to look at countertransference reactions more empirically. Earlier studies often looked at DSM personality clusters, showing for instance that cluster B personality disorders tended to evoke intense reactions in cli- nicians.[41] More recently there have been studies that have attempted to study therapist reactions to narcissistic patients specifically, and for the most part, these corroborate many of the statements above. However, hearkening back to the difficulties in defining narcissism, although the results do tend to converge, it is worth noting that these studies are not all defining narcissistic patients in the same way and are thus not necessarily looking at the exact same patient populations.

For instance, in a 2005 study, Betan and colleagues had therapists complete a number of scales for randomly selected patients in their care, including a countertransference questionnaire.[44] For patients who met *Diagnostic and Statistical Manual of Mental Disorders*, 4th ed. (DSM-IV)[45] criteria of NPD, clinicians in the Betan study reported feelings "anger, resentment, and dread," feeling devalued and criticized; and finding themselves "distracted, avoidant, and wishing to terminate the treatment."[45] They did not find therapists felt inadequate or incompetent. As Betan et al. pointed out, however, DSM-IV NPD is more associated with obvious grandiose narcissism than with the vul- nerable subtype.[41]

Another recent study by Tanzilli et al. in 2017 also looked at countertransfer- ence responses to patients with DSM-IV NPD. This study found that therapists treat- ing these patients reported the following countertransference patterns: (1) criticized/ devalued, wherein therapists felt "devalued, unappreciated, demeaned, or belittled"; (2) hostile/angry, which indicated feelings of "anger, resentment, and irritation"; (3) disen- gaged, characterized by feelings of "distraction, distance, indifference, withdrawal, or boredom"; and (4) helpless/inadequate, where clinicians felt "incompetent, ineffective, invisible, insecure, anxious, and less confident."[46] In general, NPD patients tended to evoke less positive countertransference than other patients. The only clinician variable found that seemed to influence these countertransference patterns was clinician experi- ence. They described their "empirically derived prototype . . . (as) remarkably similar to theoretical and clinical accounts."[46]

A study by Colli et al. in 2014 had clinicians use the SWAP-200 (Shedler-Westen Assessment Procedure, an empirically derived personality diagnostic test scored by the clinician) rather than the DSM-IV criteria to diagnose the personality disorder popula- tion it studied. The SWAP-2000 uses diagnostic prototypes, which are based for the most part on DSM-IV axis II disorders. They again assessed therapist countertransference by questionnaire, and the narrative description they found associated with narcissistic patients was again similar to what was previously described: "Clinicians tend to feel bored, distracted, and annoyed in sessions with these patients. They do not feel engaged when working with them and often feel frustrated. Therapists also sometimes feel interchangeable, as if they could be anyone to the patient. They can feel ineffectual, invisible, and deskilled."[47]

Gazzillo and colleagues' 2015 study of therapist countertransference has studied the broadest possible narcissistic population. They had clinicians diagnose the patients in the study with personality disorders as codified in the 2006 *Psychodynamic Diagnostic Manual* (PDM).[48] The clinicians used empirical instruments that were developed based on the PDM, which is "generally more centered on inner psychological dynamics than on their explicit features," and in its narcissistic prototype includes (in their words) both "arrogant/entitled" and "depressed/depleted" subtypes. They found that the two factors that distinguished the therapist relationship to narcissistic patients were the "overwhelmed" factor ("desire to avoid the patient, along with strong negative feelings, including dread, repulsion, and resentment") and the "parental" factor ("a desire to protect and nurture the patient"). The latter attribute would be different than the "disengaged" factor earlier studies have tended to find with narcissistic patients. As they pointed out, these two aspects may be the therapist responding to the two opposing sides of idealization and devaluation. But they point out it could also be because actually the vast majority of their narcissistic patients had a "depressed/depleted" subtype, as opposed to earlier studies which use the DSM or SWAP-200, which tend to select for more classically oblivious narcissistic patients, and perhaps it was these "vulnerable" patients who were eliciting the more parental countertransferances.[49]

Thus, even in these empirical studies, we see that defining narcissism is difficult to do comprehensively and consistently. Nevertheless, there are some consistent countertransference responses that are empirically frequently experienced by clinicians with a range of patients being diagnosed as narcissistic. These responses for the most part correspond to what has been clinically described in the literature, even if there is more work to be done in further validating the more vulnerable population from an empirical perspective.

Ultimately, at least in part due to these complex and often negative countertransference reactions, narcissistic patients can be extremely challenging patients with whom to work. It is key, therefore, that while the therapist may feel bored, or like an audience, or that they don't have a separate existence, or even are devalued, the therapist needs to try not to become demeaning of the patient (even in one's mind), but rather to appreciate this feeling as a window into the patient's negative affects and inner suffering.[43] Indeed, enactments generated by giving way to the countertransference can be one reason treatments with narcissistic patients go poorly, as the therapist may be too harsh, compete with the patient, distance him or herself from the patient, or even end the treatment itself.[18] If a patient is idealizing, the therapist may also be tempted to enjoy the positive feeling; conversely, if the patient is devaluating, the therapist may feel pressured to try to demonstrate insight or power to the patient. Again, the therapist may become caught in these enactments, doing these behaviors due to their own countertransference rather than thinking through what is best for the patient.[6] Thus, it is extremely important to try to pay attention to one's countertransference when working with narcissistic patients. In complex situations, or when a therapist feels he/she is in the midst of enactment, consultation with a senior colleague can be helpful.

Treatment of Narcissistic Personality Disorder

Given the various diagnostic difficulties described earlier in this chapter, evaluating treatments for NPD has proven to be challenging. Despite this, clinicians and researchers have more recently sought to investigate this disorder, given its high prevalence, functional impairment, and comorbidity with other disorders. Manualized therapies that have successfully been used for treatment of BPD are now being adapted for NPD. These therapies include Transference-Focused Psychotherapy (TFP), Mentalization-Based Therapy (MBT), Dialectical Behavioral Therapy (DBT), and Schema Therapy, and will be discussed.

There are no randomized controlled trials evaluating these therapies for NPD. Besides, these treatments are often difficult to find due to lack of clinicians who are trained in the specific modalities. Supportive psychotherapy and psychodynamic principles, although not supported by any systemic empirical research, anecdotally are widely used and useful in treatment.[6] Overall, there is a lack of empiric evidence supporting one psychotherapy over another, although psychotherapy is consistently recommended instead of medication.

General Principles for the Treatment of NPD

Several general principles have been recommended in the treatment of NPD based on clinical experience, falling into the categories of setting the frame, fostering a therapeutic alliance, and discussing the diagnosis.

Setting the Treatment Frame
Setting the treatment frame and adhering to it is especially critical for patients with NPD given their sense of entitlement, grandiosity, and difficulty with mentalization. The treatment frame sets up the parameters needed in order for treatment to occur, and includes both patient and therapist responsibilities. Patient responsibilities include elements that are common across diagnostic categories, such as paying fees, coming on time, and engaging meaningfully with the therapist by free associating and reflecting on their and the therapist's comments and interactions.[50] Therapist responsibilities can include maintaining a regular schedule, setting limits with the patient as appropriate, and helping the patient in their psychotherapeutic goals.[50] Transference-focused psychotherapy (TFP), which is subsequently discussed, also recommends specifically for narcissistic patients that they engage in a meaningful activity and that they be truthful with the clinician.[51] This is done because narcissistic patients often have difficulty working or even volunteering due to their hypersensitivity and overall fragility. This also attempts to limit any possible secondary gain, such as not being able to work or financially support themselves because of their symptoms.[52] The clinician should be aware that the NPD patient is likely to attempt to deviate from the frame by making special requests, and that can be an opportune moment to refer back to the frame and then discuss the feelings that come up when the clinician does not comply with the patient's demands. For example, because of their feelings of specialness and entitlement, narcissistic patients may expect that the clinician is available at all times of the day, or that the patient can cancel the appointment five minutes beforehand without any consequences. The contract will allow the clinician to address treatment-interfering or unsafe behaviors as they arise, such as suicidal

behaviors, not paying for therapy, or disengagement through devaluation.[18] Also, the treatment frame fosters the patient's own responsibility for how their behaviors affect treatment, and encourages the patient to play an active role in their progress.

Fostering a Therapeutic Alliance

Fostering a therapeutic alliance is another challenging aspect of treatment with NPD patients. Part of a therapeutic alliance is developing mutual treatment goals and referring back to these as the treatment progresses.[18] If the patient chooses grandiose and unrealistic goals, this is a useful opening to discuss more realistic goals and explore what negative effects, such as shame or fear of failure, the patient may be attempting to defend against. As discussed in the transference and countertransference sections, attending to these processes are especially important due to the propensity for devaluing, envy, and competition that may arise and contribute to a difficult alliance.

Discussing the Diagnosis of NPD

Discussing the diagnosis of NPD is controversial given the fear that this will lead patients to leave treatment due to the pejorative way the diagnosis is used colloquially. Additionally, patients told they have NPD already have fragile self-esteem and are sensitive to perceived criticism and thus may feel especially humiliated or ashamed to receive this diagnosis when named as NPD. However, discussing the diagnosis using different names, such as a you have a "self-confident style" or "your self-esteem fluctuates" may actually provide a cohesive and integrated explanation of the patient's experience and allow the clinician to provide a treatment that is targeted to their diagnosis.[51] A clear and comprehensive formulation can be given to the patient using the patient's own words and experience-near terms. Focusing on how the patient's symptoms may be adaptive, or discussing the patient's positive attributes, may be a good way to begin. A clinician can also discuss the patient's distress and core symptoms of narcissism, such as feelings of emptiness or entitlement, rejection sensitivity, or difficulties with self-esteem, which can lay the groundwork for a deeper discussion of the diagnosis.

Possible Treatments for NPD

Transference-focused Psychotherapy

Although there is no specific empiric evidence for using TFP for the treatment of NPD, some of the studies showing that TFP is an evidenced-based therapy for BPD had patients that had co-occurring NPD, ranging from 10 percent to 70 percent.[52] One group of patients with comorbid NPD and BPD were more likely to show an improvement in reflective functioning with TFP as compared to DBT or supportive psychotherapy, although the sample size was too small for any firm conclusions.[53] TFP explicitly includes setting a specific treatment frame, describes the roles of the therapist and patient, and discusses the diagnosis and treatment plan with the patient. As previously described, the contract also goes into contingencies specific to TFP for NPD such as doing some kind of activity, plus contingencies for suicidal thoughts and self-harm, substance use, or other dangerous behaviors that may be treatment-interfering.[52] Since TFP is based on an object-relations theory, it also highlights the importance of defining the dominant dyad in the treatment. This will help improve the self and other internalized mental representations of the patient's. A typical dyad for the narcissistic patient is one of a superior self versus a devalued other, often manifesting as the therapist being devalued while the patient acts as if they are superior.[52] Helping the patient to integrate the projected devalued self into themselves, and vice versa, can improve their difficulties in interpersonal functioning as well as affective dysregulation related to their sense of self, among other targets.[51] Review Chapter 8 on TFP for more information.

Mentalization-based Treatment

MBT is based on attachment theory and address difficulties in NPD patients' mentalization. Specifically, patients improve their own self-reflection and then learn to recognize the different mental states in others and how these influence behavior. Although it has not been looked at systematically for NPD, it has been used for patients with narcissistic traits.[17] MBT may be especially interesting to investigate for NPD because of its ease in implementation and flexibility, as well as the significant difficulty patients with NPD have with accurately perceiving (and being empathic with) the minds of others. Review Chapter 9 on MBT for more information.

Other Psychotherapies and Treatment of NPD

Other therapies that have been described as potentially being useful in NPD include cognitive behavioral therapy (see Chapter 10), schema therapy (see Chapter 12), and metacognitive psychotherapy.[17,18] These cognitive therapies use techniques such as cognitive reframing and behavioral modification and have shown some benefit in increasing adherence to therapy.[17] Dialectical behavioral therapy (DBT) and good psychiatric management (GPM) were originally designed for BPD but have been described as useful for patients with NPD as well.[17,18,] Review Chapters 11 and 13 on DBT and GMP, respectively, for more information.

Group psychotherapy as the sole treatment can be difficult due to a narcissistic patient's desire for specialness in the group, as well as their tendency to focus on others' problems instead of their own. However, with those caveats, it still can be useful.[10] Individual psychotherapy in combination with group psychotherapy, however, has been suggested as more useful because other patients can help diffuse the negative transference. The group setting also allows these patients to reflect on others' experiences, as well as to experience the reality that they cannot be special in the group.[10]

Pharmacotherapy for NPD

There is little evidence supporting the use of psychopharmacology in the treatment of NPD. Specifically, there are no FDA-approved medications for NPD, and there are no clinical trials evaluating its effectiveness or efficacy. There are limited studies looking at treating psychiatric comorbidities in patients with BPD, but no specific studies looking at treating comorbidities in patients with NPD. However, it is still clinically indicated to use medications in patients with NPD who suffer with common comorbid disorders such as MDD, anxiety disorders, bipolar disorder, and substance use disorders. Differentiating between MDD and the chronic dysthymic reaction of narcissistic patients is important. However, it is important to be clear that treatment for MDD or other clearly defined comorbidities may help, but no medications will resolve a narcissist's core sense of inadequacy and/or emptiness. Additionally, the significant countertransference generated by NPD patients can lead the clinician to undertreat or overtreat the comorbidities. A narcissistic injury can result from either the suggestion that the patient needs a medication or that a medication will not help what the patient is suffering from. When a patient with NPD displays a suicide risk related to depression, or risk secondary to substance abuse, medication use may be warranted. Similar to the pharmacology of treating BPD, apart from targeting specific symptom clusters such as impulsivity and irritability, affective instability, and cognitive-perceptual disturbances, is not likely to be useful. Review Chapter 15 on the psychopharmacology of personality disorders.

Clinical Pearls

Therapists who decide to treat patients on the narcissistic spectrum might want to follow some of these time-honored clinical principles:

1. Setting the frame of treatment is a critical part of therapy for NPD and should be collaboratively developed with the patient. The therapist's and patient's responsibilities should be clear, and the therapist should closely monitor for deviations. A narcissistic patient's difficulty with mentalization and, at times, tendency to exploit others means that challenges to the frame should be anticipated. Any deviations should be addressed immediately and in a straightforward way, referring back to the mutually agreed-upon treatment frame and goals. The frame can be changed as new information emerges in the treatment that the patient may not have initially disclosed, or as treatment-interfering behaviors arise.
2. Consider discussing the diagnosis of NPD with the patient, although be aware that it may be experienced as a slight and make a therapeutic alliance more fragile. If you choose to not discuss the specific NPD diagnosis, discuss in clear and experience-near terms what the patient's difficulties are and what the treatment goals will be (e.g., issues with self-esteem, hypersensitivity to slights, prominent feeling of shame). Try to use the patient's own words, and also emphasize the positive aspects of their personality traits including any successes in their lives.
3. If the patient was encouraged to come to therapy at the urging of someone in their life and claims no insight into their difficulties, starting with what others see can be useful.
4. Discuss with the patient the limits of medication use (if applicable), in order to set achievable and realistic treatment goals. Although medication can be used to treat comorbidities, it will not treat the narcissistic patient's core feelings of emptiness and shame.
5. Begin the therapy by clarifying the patient's experience, including their experience of the therapist as being ineffective or incompetent if relevant, prior to more confrontational techniques. At the beginning, the therapist may need to tolerate a long period of empathic listening.
6. Avoid early interpretations of the split-off devalued or inferior self, as this may lead to a strengthening of the patient's defensive processes.

7. Although you do not want to directly challenge the patient's grandiosity at first, you also don't want to ignore it. A patient's grandiosity is better engaged by exploring the function it serves for the patient and how this positively or negatively effects the patient or others.

8. Address negative transference and countertransference head on, and anticipate this may be difficult but will inevitably emerge.

9. Look for common countertransference responses in a therapist, including feelings of being devalued, irritated, bored, distracted, ineffective, or incompetent.

10. Seek outside consultation if needed and consider regular peer supervision to manage this countertransference.

11. Don't let the patient assume a "passive" role in the therapy; encourage collaboration, and curiosity about the patient's efforts to externalize the responsibility for change onto the therapist.

12. Avoid power struggles with the patient, including who is "right" and who is "wrong." Patients may claim that the mutually agreed-upon treatment goals were imposed by the therapist. This should be explored rather than challenged. A power struggle may take the form of treatment-interfering behaviors such as refusing to talk or engaging only superficially with the therapist. Patients do this in order to maintain control of the treatment, and this should be explored.

13. Narcissistic patients may initially over-idealize the therapist, leading the therapist to feel charmed or seduced. This may make the therapist believe that they are connecting with the patient and that the treatment is progressing well. Be aware that underneath idealization is devaluation, including the narcissistic patient feeling that they no longer need the therapist or that the therapist is actually quite useless. Be on the lookout for this developing in the treatment, since this may lead to an abrupt termination or withdrawal from therapy.

Conclusion

This chapter discusses some of the many challenges associated with the diagnosis and treatment of patients with NPD. NPD is difficult to diagnostically characterize, difficult to treat, and presents with significant functional impairments in patients. There is general consensus that there are three different types of NPD: (1) the thick-skinned, grandiose/malignant, or the equivalent oblivious type which is described in the DSM-5; (2) the thin-skinned, fragile type, that is basically equivalent to the DSM-5 hypervigilant or vulnerable type; and (3) a high-functioning/exhibitionist type. NPD appears to be highly prevalent and with significant comorbidity in patients when using current DSM-5 diagnostic categories. There are ongoing efforts to further characterize NPD, along with more clearly defining what is pathological narcissism and what is healthy or adaptive narcissism. Heinz Kohut and Otto Kernberg both contributed major theories to the development and treatment of NPD, in addition to more recent theories stemming from relational or mentalization frameworks. Researchers are looking at the contribution of genetics, parenting, attachment, and other variables to further understand NPD's development and presentation. A variety of transferences and countertransference can arise in the treatment of a patient with NPD, including idealization and devaluation, feelings of boredom, and hostility. Although there are no evidence-based treatments specific to NPD, there are many promising and emerging psychotherapies (e.g., TFP, MBT, DBT,

---

Box 21.1   Relevant Resources for Patients, Families, and Clinicians

---

- Sheppard Pratt Narcissistic Personality Disorder. https://www.sheppard-pratt.org/knowledge-center/condition/narcissistic-personality-disorder/.
- Mclean Narcissistic Personality Disorder. https://www.mcleanhospital.org/video/narcissistic-personality-disorder.
- Narcissistic Abuse Support Groups. https://narcissistabusesupport.com/narcissist-abuse-support-groups/.
- Kernberg, O. *Narcissism: A Defense Against an Underlying Borderline Structure.* https://www.youtube.com/watch?v = DlopY4DfFV4.
- Yeomans, F. *What is Personality (and Personality Disorder)?* https://www.youtube.com/watch?v = bM11wlL25-c.

CBT and others) currently used to treat other personality disorders that a clinician can use to treat NPD. Psychotherapy is the first-line treatment, though psychopharmacology may be useful in select patients to treat significant comorbidities. While psychiatry has made significant progress in being able to delineate more clearly what NPD is and how best to treat it, there remain many unknowns for helping this challenging patient population. Review Box 21.1 for relevant resources for patients, families, and clinicians.

Conflict of Interest/Disclosure: The authors of this chapter have no financial conflicts and nothing to disclose.

References

1. *Diagnostic and Statistical Manual of Mental Disorders (DSM5).* 5th ed. Arlington, VA: American Psychiatric Association; 2013: 669–672.

2. Dhawan N, Kunik ME, Oldham J, Coverdale J. Prevalence and treatment of narcissistic personality disorder in the community: A systematic review. *Compr Psychiatry.* 2010;51(4):333–339.

3. Zimmerman M. Chelminski I, Young D. The frequency of personality disorders in psychiatric patient. *Psychiatr Clin North Am.* 2008;31(3):405–420, vi. doi:10.1016/j.psc.2008.03.015.

4. Miller JD, Lynam DR, Hyatt CS, Campbell WK. Controversies in narcissism. Annu Rev Clin Psychol. 2017;13:291–315.

5. Hasin DS, Grant BF. The national epidemiologic survey on alcohol and related conditions (NESARC) waves 1 and 2: review and summary of findings. *Soc. Psychiatr Epidemiol.* 2015;50(11):1609–1640.

6. Gabbard GO, Crisp H. *Narcissism and its Discontents: Diagnostic Dilemmas and Treatment Strategies with Narcissistic Patients.* Washington, DC: American Psychiatric Press; 2018.

7. Lunbeck E. *The Americanization of Narcissism.* Cambridge, MA: Harvard University Press; 2014.

8. Twenge JM. *Generation Me: Why Today's Young Americans Are More Confident, Assertive, Entitled—and More Miserable Than Ever Before.* New York, NY: Free Press; 2006/2014.

9. Stinson FS. Dawson DA, Goldstein RB, et al. Prevalence, correlates, disability, and comorbidity of DSM IV NPD: Results from the WAVE 2 National Epidemiologic Survey on Alcohol and Related Conditions. *J Clin Psychiatry.* 2008;69(7):1033–1045.

10. Gabbard GO. *Psychoanalytic Psychiatry in Clinical Practice*. 5th ed. Washington, DC: American Psychiatric Press; 2014.

11. Rosenfeld H. On the psychopathology of narcissism: a clinical approach. *Int J Psychoanal*. 1964;45:332–337.

12. Russ E, Shedler J, Bradley R, Westen D. Refining the construct of narcissistic personality disorder: diagnostic criteria and subtypes. *Am J Psychiatry*. 2008;165(11):1473–1481.

13. Caligor E, Levy KN, Yeomans FE. Narcissistic personality disorder: diagnostic and clinical challenges. *Am J Psychiatry*. 2014;172(5):415–422.

14. Caligor E, Stern B. Diagnosis and classification and assessment of narcissistic personality disorder within the framework of object relations theory. *J Pers Disord*. 2020;34:104–121.

15. Raskin R, Terry H. A principal-components analysis of the Narcissistic Personality Inventory and further evidence of its construct validity. *J Pers Soc Psychol*. 1988;54(5):890–902.

16. Millon T, Grossman S, Millon CM, Meagher S, and Ramnath R. *Personality Disorders in Modern Life*. 2nd ed. Hoboken, NJ: Wiley; 2004.

17. Yakely P. Current understanding of narcissism and narcissistic personality disorder, *B J Psych Advances*. 2018;24(5):305–315.

18. Weinberg I, Ronningstam E. Dos and don'ts in treatments of patients with NPD. *J Pers Disord*. 2020;34:122–114.

19. Euler S, Stöbi D, Sowislo J, et al. Grandiose and vulnerable narcissism in borderline personality disorder. *Psychopathology*. 2018;51(2):110–121.

20. Cooper AM. Narcissism and masochism: the narcissistic-masochisticcharacter. *Psychiatr Clin North Am*. 1989;12(3):541–552.

21. Crisp H, Gabbard GO. Principles of psychodynamic treatment for patients with narcissistic personality disorder. *J Pers Disord*. 2020;34(Supplement):143–158.

22. Kernberg OF. The almost untreatable narcissistic patient. *J Am Psychoanal Assoc*. 2007;55(2):503–539.

23. Roepke S, Vater A. Narcissistic personality disorder: an integrative review of recent empirical data and current definitions. *Curr Psychiatry Rep*. 2014; 6(5): 445.

24. DiSarno M, DiPierro R, Madeddu F. The relevance of neuroscience for the investigation of narcissism: a review of current studies. *Clin Neuropsychiatry: J Treat Eval*. 2018;15(4):242–250.

25. Lasch C. *The Culture of Narcissism: American Life in an Age of Diminishing Expectations*. New York, NY: Norton; 1979.

26. Stern A. *Me: The Narcissistic American*. New York, NY: Ballentine; 1979.

27. Twenge JM, Campbell WK. *The Narcissism Epidemic: Living in the Age of Entitlement*. New York, NY: Free Press; 2010.

28. Lingiardi V, McWilliams N, eds. *Psychodynamic Diagnostic Manual*. 2nd ed. New York, NY: Guilford Press; 2017: 46–48

29. McWilliams N. *Psychoanalytic Diagnosis: Understanding Personality Structure in the Clinical Process*. New York, NY: Guilford Press; 1994.

30. Steiner J. Seeing and being seen: narcissistic pride and narcissistic humiliation. *Int J Psychoanal*. 2006;87:939–951.

31. Modell AH. "The holding environment" and the therapeutic action of psychoanalysis. *J Am Psychoanal Assoc*. 1976;24:285–307.

32. Kohut H. Forms and transformations of narcissism. In: Ornstein P, ed. *The Search for the Self.* Vol 1. New York, NY: International Universities Press; 1965/1978:243–272.

33. Kohut H. *The Analysis of the Self: A Systematic Approach to the Treatment of Narcissistic Personality Disorders.* New York, NY: International Universities Press; 1971.

34. Kohut H, Wolf ES. Disorders of the self and their treatment: an outline. In: Ornstein P, ed. *The Search for the Self.* Vol. 3. Madison, CT: International Universities Press; 1978/1990: 359–386.

35. Kernberg OF. *Borderline Conditions and Pathological Narcissism.* New York: Jason Aronson; 1975.

36. Kernberg OF. *Aggression in Personality Disorders and Perversions.* New Haven: Yale University Press; 1992.

37. Horton RS, Parenting as a cause of narcissism: empirical support for psychodynamic and social learning theories. In: Campbell WK and Miller JD, eds. *The Handbook of Narcissistic Personality Disorder.* Hoboken, NJ: Wiley; 2011:181–190.

38. Afifi TO, Mather A, Boman J, et al. Childhood adversity and personality disorders: results from a nationally representative population-based study, *J Psychiatr Res.* 2011;45(6):814–822.

39. Diamond D, Levy K, Clarkin J, et al., Attachment and mentalization in female patients with comorbid narcissistic and borderline personality disorder. *Pers Disord.* 2014;5(4):428–433.

40. Dickinson K, Pincus AL. Interpersonal analysis of grandiose and vulnerable narcissism. *J Pers Disord.* 2003; 17(3):188–207.

41. Betan EJ, Westen D. Countertransference and personality pathology: development and clinical application of the countertransference questionnaire. In: Levy, RA, Ablon, S, eds. *Handbook of Evidence-based Psychodynamic Psychotherapy.* New York, NY: Springer; 2009:179–198.

42. Drozek RP, Unruh BT. Mentalization-based treatment for pathological narcissism. *J Pers Disord.* 2020;34(Supplement):177–203.

43. Mackinnon RA, Michels R, Buckley PJ, *The Psychiatric Interview in Clinical Practice.* 3rd ed. Washington, DC: American Psychiatric Press; 2016.

44. Betan E, Heim AK, Zittel Conklin C, Westen D. Countertransference phenomena and personality pathology in clinical practice: an empirical investigation. *Am J Psychiatry.* 2005;162(5):890–898

45. *Diagnostic and Statistical Manual of Mental Disorders (DSM-IV).* 4th ed. Washington, DC: American Psychiatric Association;1994

46. Tanzilli A, Muzi L, Ronnigstam E, Lingiardi V. Countertransference when working with narcissistic personality disorder: an empirical investigation. *Psychotherapy.* 2017;54(2):184–194.

47. Colli A, Tanzilli A, Dimaggio G, Lingiardi V. Patient personality and therapist response: an empirical investigation. *Am J Psychiatry.* 2014;171(1):102–108.

48. American Psychoanalytic Association, Alliance of Psychoanalytic Organizations. *Psychodynamic Diagnostic Manual (PDM).* Washington, DC: American Psychoanalytic Association; 2006.

49. Gazzillo F, Lingiardi V, Del Corno F, et al. Clinicians' emotional responses and Psychodynamic Diagnostic Manual adult personality disorders: a clinically relevant empirical investigation. *Psychotherapy (Chic).* 2015;52(2):238–246.

50. Yeomans F, Clarkin J, Kernberg O. *Transference-focused Psychotherapy for Borderline Personality Disorder*. Washington, DC: American Psychiatric Publishing; 2015.

51. Oldham J, Morris L. *The New Personality Self-Portrait: Why You Think, Work, Love and Act the Way You Do*. New York: Bantam Books; 1995.

52. Diamond D, Hersh R. Transference-focused psychotherapy for narcissistic personality disorder: an object relations approach. *J Pers Disord*. 2020;34:159–176.

53. Diamond D, Yeomans F, Stern B, et al. Transference focused psychotherapy for patients with comorbid narcissistic and borderline personality disorder. *Psychoanal Inq*. 2013;33(6):527–551.

54. Bernanke J, McCommon B. Training in good psychiatric management for borderline personality disorder in residency: an aid to learning supportive psychotherapy for challenging-to-treat patients. *Psychodyn Psychiatry*. Summer 2018;46(2):181–200.

22

Avoidant Personality Disorder

Len Sperry and Gerardo Casteleiro

Key Points

- AVPD is characterized by shyness, low self-esteem, and rejection sensitivity wherein these individuals avoid others even though they crave human contact.
- The avoidant personality style is more flexible and causes less distress and impairment than the AVPD.
- Its optimal DSM-5 criterion is avoidance of work activities that involve significant interpersonal contact because of fear of rejection.
- A structured interview using the DSM-5 criteria is a common, quick, and accurate means of diagnosing this disorder.
- Five common models for conceptualizing this disorder are: psychodynamic; biosocial; cognitive-behavioral; interpersonal; and integrative.
- Five effective psychotherapy approaches for treating this disorder are: psychodynamic therapy; cognitive-behavioral therapy; schema therapy; interpersonal psychotherapy; and combined/integrated treatment.
- Four other clinically useful treatment modalities are: group therapy; marital and family therapy; medication; and combined/integrated treatment.

Introduction

Avoidant personality disorder (AVPD) is a psychiatric condition characterized by shyness, hypersensitivity, loneliness, rejection sensitivity, and low self-esteem. Although individuals who suffer from it are desperate for human contact, they avoid involvement with others out of fear of disapproval and sensitivity to rejection.[1] Individuals with this disorder present with a unique number of treatment challenges for the therapist. Nevertheless, treatment can be highly effective.

Descriptors of AVPD

Several descriptors of AVPD are identified in the professional literature. The seven most relevant to clinical practice are triggering event(s), behavioral styles, interpersonal styles, cognitive styles, affective styles, attachment style, and optimal diagnostic criterion.

Triggering Event(s)

The demands for close interpersonal interactions or social and public appearances is the most common circumstance, or event, that triggers or activates the maladaptive response in individuals with AVPD.[1] This is noted in their behavioral, interpersonal, cognitive, and affective styles.

Behavioral Style

Common characteristics of avoidant personalities include chronic tenseness and self-consciousness, controlled speech and behavior, and awkward or apprehensive appearances. Individuals with avoidant personality tend to be self-critical and play down or discount their own achievements.

Interpersonal Style

Individuals with AVPD are keenly sensitive to rejection. Although they desire others' acceptance, they distance themselves from others and require unconditional approval before "opening up" to others. They guardedly "test" others to determine who can be trusted.

Cognitive Style

AVPD patients' cognitive style can be described as hypervigilant. They continually scan the environment for potential threats; that leads to distracted thinking and hypersensitivity to perceived criticism, disapproval, or rejection. They also tend to overemphasize their shortcomings while downplaying their triumphs, resulting in low self-esteem.

Affective Style

AVPD sufferers' affective or feeling style is characterized by shyness and apprehensiveness. Given that unconditional approval from others is rarely achievable, experiences of sadness, loneliness, and tension are routine. When experiencing marked distress, they report feelings of lability, emptiness, and depersonalization, which are symptoms shared with borderline personality disorder (BPD). In a study that used experience-diary sampling methods over 21 days to assess groups of individuals diagnosed with BPD, AVPD, and a healthy control group, results showed that individuals with AVPD had significantly lower lability than the BPD group, but also significantly higher lability than the control group.[2]

Attachment Style

Individuals with a negative self-view and a view of others that vacillates between positive and negative tend to exhibit an attachment style that is both preoccupied and fearful. Their avoidance reflects their desire to be liked and accepted by others while fearing abandonment and rejection. Accordingly, the preoccupied-fearful attachment style is common in individuals with AVPD.[3] A study that compared the attachment styles in individuals with AVPD to those of individuals diagnosed with social phobia found higher levels of anxiety for abandonment, separation, and frustration in avoidant individuals.[4]

Optimal Diagnostic Criterion

The optimal diagnostic criterion for a personality disorder refers to the single *Diagnostic and Statistical Manual-5* (DSM-5)[5] diagnostic criteria that most accurately predicts the disorder. It is derived from research with the Structured Interview for Diagnosing Personality Disorders.[6] Of the seven DSM-5 criteria for AVPD, the optimal criterion is avoidance of occupational activities that involve significant interpersonal contact for fear of criticism, disapproval, or rejection.

Avoidant Style versus AVPD

Personality can be defined as one's consistent and distinctive pattern of perceiving, thinking, feeling, acting, and coping. When personality is conceptualized on a continuum ranging from healthy to disordered, personality style represents the healthy and adaptive end of the continuum while personality disorder represents the disordered end, namely pathological, impaired, and maladaptive. The avoidant personality spans this continuum with the avoidant personality style at one end and AVPD on the other. The clinical value of viewing personality on such a continuum is twofold. First, the continuum assists the therapist in assessing style versus disorder and planning treatment accordingly. For example, a patient who exhibits avoidance and meets fewer than five of the seven DSM-5 criteria for AVPD would not merit the diagnosis of AVPD. Nevertheless, effective treatment planning could anticipate the unique ways in which avoidance dynamics influence treatment engagement and compliance. Second, the continuum can serve as a metric of progress; in other words, movement from the disordered end of the continuum to the style end represents positive therapeutic change.

Two case examples illustrate the difference between the avoidant style and the personality disorder.

Case Study: Avoidant Personality Style

Dr. A. is a 32-year-old vascular surgeon who was recently hired by an outpatient surgery center. He had recently completed residency training and, being new, good looking, and single, was quickly noticed by the female staff. His specialty was laser surgery, for which he was exquisitely skilled and respected by his patients. Although courteous, he was somewhat emotionally distant and shy. Dr. A seldom participated in staff parties, and if he did make an appearance, he would politely excuse himself after his beeper sounded; this seemed to occur all the time, and he would not return. His social life seemed to be a mystery. He had little contact after hours with his male colleagues, except for one. Dr. L.

had run into Dr. A. at a hobby convention in another city, and to his surprise, he learned of Dr. J's long-standing collection of *Star Wars* memorabilia. In time the two became very good friends, spending considerable time together. Although he had his own apartment, Dr. A. spends most of his free time at home with his parents. Dr. L. soon became a regular guest at the A. home, and initially Dr. L. was surprised at how warm, cordial, and comfortable Dr. A. was in this small setting as compared to the surgery center.

Case Study: AVPD

Ms. R. is a 24-year-old female student who went to the university's counseling center seeking relief from "difficulty concentrating." She indicated that the problem started when her roommate of two years precipitously moved out to live with her boyfriend. Ms. R. says she was "emotionally crushed" by this. She reported no close friends and described herself as "being really shy my whole life" and having had only one date since middle school. Since then, she avoided efforts by anyone trying to date her, explaining that she had been rejected as a high school sophomore by a senior who had dated her once and never contacted her again. She was unable to maintain eye contact with the staff therapist and appeared painfully shy and self-conscious.

DSM-5 Criteria

The DSM-5 identifies specific behaviors for this disorder.[5] These are unremitting patterns of social inhibition, feelings of inadequacy, and oversensitivity to negative evaluations from others. Patients with AVPD are likely to view themselves as socially inept, unappealing, and inferior to others. They predictably avoid work activities that require close interpersonal contact that they fear will lead to criticism or rejection. Unless they have high certainty that they will be accepted, they will not engage or get involved with others. In ongoing relationships, they are uncomfortable and often act with restraint for fear of being ridiculed or shamed. Similarly, they are likely to feel inhibited and inadequate in new interpersonal situations. Accordingly, they avoid activities that involve personal risk or may prove to be embarrassing.[5]

Prototypic Description of AVPD

A brief description capturing the essence of a particular disorder's most common presentation is known as a prototype. Therapists will use prototypic descriptions because they are convenient, rather than rely on lists of behavioral criteria or core beliefs. A common prototypic description of AVPD is: These individuals tend to be frightened and interpersonally awkward, and experience extreme sensitivity to rejection and criticism. Fear of humiliation and embarrassment surfaces with the prospect of meeting someone new. Therefore, it is simpler to avoid different or new work, social engagements, or responsibilities that could threaten their established sense of interpersonal safety. On the other hand, they crave interpersonal connections, especially to those with whom they have established trust. They may have one or a few special friends or relatives whom they can trust and with whom they feel safe.[7] See Chapter 1 for more details about this prototype description.

Prevalence of Avoidant Personality Disorder

Estimates of the prevalence of this disorder have been 2.4 percent in the general popula-tion.[6] However, it is estimated that 5.1 to 55.4 percent of the clinical population have this disorder, making it the most frequently occurring personality disorder in three epidemi-ological studies.[8]

AVPD versus Social Anxiety Disorder

Distinguishing between this personality disorder and social anxiety disorder (SAD) has been problematic until recently. There are two opposing views when it comes to differ-entiating between the two. One view is that AVPD is a *personality disorder* that differs from *symptom disorders* such as SAD and other phobias. The other view is that AVPD is on a spectrum of severity between SAD on the less severe end and AVPD at the most severe end. There is empirical evidence to support each hypothesis.[9] For instance, a study that measured the fear of being laughed at in samples of SAD and AVPD found that the criterion did not differentiate between the two conditions.[10] However, a recent study found evidence that a continuum of severity does not explain the differences between the two disorders, as there were no global severity index differences in SAD groups when compared to AVPD groups.[11] Moreover, researchers have found other marked differ-ences between the disorders, such as higher deficits in metacognitive skills for individ-uals with AVPD.[12] The major differences between the disorders seem to be accounted for in components such as avoidant behavior, early attachment, attachment styles, and self-concept,[9] which are further described in the conceptualization section. Finally, drawing from findings from factor analytic and biometric studies, Welander-Vatn and colleagues[13] concluded that AVPD and SAD are related but separate constructs. They also presented empirical evidence to support that, in terms of personality traits, individ-uals with AVPD and SAD differed in terms of extraversion, agreeableness, and openness to experience.

Conceptualizations of AVPD

There are multiple theories useful for conceptualizing and treating AVPD, which include psychodynamic, biosocial, cognitive-behavioral, and schema therapy, interpersonal, combined, and integrated treatment approaches.

Psychodynamic Case Conceptualization

Psychodynamically, avoidance, shyness, and shame are understood as defense mech-anisms (e.g., avoidance/withdrawal, inhibition, and fantasy) against humiliation, embarrassment, rejection, and failure.[14] The fear of exposure of the self to others is in-terconnected with shame. This shame stems from self-perceptions of weakness, incom-petence, defectiveness, disgust, and inability to control bodily functions. Developmental experiences throughout the childhood years influence these feelings of shame. Added to the constitutional predisposition toward avoidance, this shame in avoidant patients is reactivated upon being exposed to individuals who matter a great deal to them.[14] Psychodynamic theorists also contend that problematic behaviors of individuals with AVPD can be conceptualized as motivated by shame of failure to live up to the ego ideal.[15] This results in a low self-esteem that prompts avoidant individuals to protect themselves by misreading others' neutral reactions and restricting social experience to avoid situations that might reveal their perceived inadequacies.

Biosocial Case Conceptualization

The etiology and development of AVPD is believed to represent a constellation of biogenic environmental factors.[16] Researchers have hypothesized that the characteristic vigilance of this personality is explained by a combination of a dominant sympathetic nervous system and lowered autonomic arousal threshold. This could allow for the intrusion of irrelevant impulses on logical association, diminishing control and direction of cognitive processes and memory. These processes could logically result in marked obstruction with normal cognitive processes. Millon and Davis[16] cite research suggesting that shyness traits are of genetic-constitutional origin that require environmental experiences to progress into a fully-fledged pattern of timidity and avoidance.

Two critical and prevalent environmental influences are parental and peer group rejection. Parental rejection seems to be particularly high in intensity and frequency. When peer group rejection mirrors and reinforces parental rejection, the child's self-competence and self-worth can be severely impacted, leading to self-critical attitudes and behavior. As a result, avoidant individuals tend to restrict social experiences and peer group interactions. They become increasingly introspective and hypersensitive to rejection. The restriction of social interaction further limits their social development and competence, which may actually foster the ridicule and negative reactions of others. Given their hypersensitivity, even when no rejection is intended, minor snubs tend to be interpreted as evidence of rejection. Finally, because of excessive introspection, avoidant individuals tend to over-analyze their ongoing circumstances and conclude that that they are not deserving or worthy of others' acceptance.

Cognitive-Behavioral and Schema Therapy Case Conceptualizations

According to Beck,[17] those with AVPD maintain the core belief of rejection. This explains their fearfulness when they attempt to initiate relationships, as well as their fearful response when others attempt to relate to them. In essence, social rejection is so intolerable that they resort to avoidance of social situations. They also engage in cognitive and emotional avoidance by attempting to reduce thoughts and internal experiences that could cause discomfort or dysphoria.

Maladaptive schemas or long-standing dysfunctional beliefs about self and others also underlie these avoidance patterns. They tend to view themselves as socially inept and incompetent in both academic and vocational settings. Their view of others is characterized as critical, indifferent, and disparaging. Schemas about self are comprised of themes such as being different, inadequate, defective, and unlikeable, whereas schemas about others include themes of indifference and rejection.

These individuals make predictions that are likely interpreted as solely caused by personal deficiencies. That is, extraneous contextual or environmental influences may be misinterpreted or missed altogether. These ongoing predictions of rejection result in dysphoria. Finally, avoidant individuals lack internal criteria to form positive self-judgments. Therefore, they heavily rely on their perception. They are more likely to misread neutral or positive reactions as negative, which creates a compounding effect that heightens their sensitivity toward rejection and avoidance. Essentially, their negative schemas result in avoidance of the very behaviors that could prove to be a solution for their ongoing problems (i.e., social interaction). They also avoid other tasks or behaviors that could result in feelings of discomfort or potential dysphoria. Instead, they engage in excuses and rationalization as a result of their low tolerance for dysphoria.

This disorder has also been described as primarily anxiety-based, characterized by timidity and anxiety based on negative evaluation, rejection, and humiliation. Fortunately, this disorder is responsive to behavioral interventions. These include anxiety management and exposure methods that target the fear of rejection, negative evaluation, and criticism.

Interpersonal Case Conceptualization

Individuals with AVPD begin their sequence of development with appropriate social bonding, attachment, and nurturance. Thus, they continue to desire this social bonding throughout their development. However, as they are subjected to relentless parental control toward creating a certain social image, visible flaws become the subjects of humiliation and embarrassment, especially within the family. Despite their appeals to be admirable, these individuals experience mockery and social retribution for shortcomings and failures. The consequence that follows is that as an adult, these individuals are expected to perform flawlessly and avoid any potential for humiliation or embarrassment. The typical association to humiliation for these individuals was that of banishment and rejection. Therefore, the anticipation of rejection is internalized, and they resort to isolation from others. Nevertheless, they still crave relationships and social contact, while being extremely sensitive to rejection or dejection.

Even though rejection and ridicule from their families were rampant, they internalized the belief that their family was their main source of support. Therefore, they remain thoroughly loyal to their families but harbor fear toward others. Essentially, the main fears are rejection and humiliation. In order to avoid these experiences, avoidant individuals withdraw from others and restrain themselves, while simultaneously craving social interaction and acceptance. Once they establish trust with an individual, through a series of highly stringent safety tests, they can reach high levels of intimacy. However, they can at times lose control and react with indignation and rage.[18]

Integrative Case Conceptualizations

The following integrative formulation is provided to illustrate how a biopsychosocial approach explains the development and maintenance of this personality. In terms of biology, these individuals were commonly hyperirritable, fearful, and demonstrating a "slow to warm" temperament as infants. It is also likely that these individuals experienced considerable colic and were difficult to soothe as infants. These plus their hyperirritability are attributed to increased sympathetic discharge of the autonomic nervous system.[19]

Psychologically, individuals with AVPD typically hold self-views of "I am inadequate and scared of being rejected." They are likely to hold worldviews, such as "Life is unjust—people are critical and rejecting of me—and still I want to be accepted and liked." Accordingly, they are likely to conclude, "Therefore, I must stay vigilant, demand reassurance from others, and when all else fails, I will have to imagine in my mind some fantasy about what life should be." Fantasy is a common defense mechanism for the avoidant personality. It is no surprise that they are avid consumers of soap operas and romance novels.

Socially, predictable patterns of parenting are noted in avoidant individuals. It is highly likely that these individuals experience parental ridicule and rejection. It is likely that the parental injunction was, "You are unacceptable to us and probably to others as well." Their parents may have had high standards, and therefore they worried that they could not meet these standards and were unworthy and unlovable. It is also worth noting the influence of culture and level of acculturation, because families may have specific expectations for certain family members that impact the expression of certain avoidant and dependent behaviors. For example, a father in a paternalistic culture spends more time with his sons and much less with his daughters. The impact of this cultural norm is that his daughter may feel rejected. Yet, her experience can be greatly amplified if the rejection sensitivity dynamic of AVPD is operative.

A sense of personal inadequacy and fear of rejection that leads to hypervigilance and restricted social experiences are all individual and systemic factors that confirm, reinforce, and perpetuate the avoidant pattern. These experiences, added to cognitive patterns of catastrophizing, also result in hypervigilance and hypersensitivity. The self-pity, anxiety, and depression that results from these patterns further confirm the style and beliefs of avoidance.[19]

Assessment of AVPD

Supplementing the patient's self-report, information stemming from observation, collateral sources, and psychological testing are all useful for establishing the diagnosis and treatment plan for personality disorders. This section will provide a brief description of some observations and the nature of typical rapport that develops between therapists and patients with AVPD during initial therapy encounters.

Interview Behavior and Rapport

During the initial interview, patients with AVPD tend be guarded, circumstantial, and typically respond with single-word answers. Some may present as anxious or suspicious, but all will engender hypersensitivity to criticism and rejection. Empathy and reassurance must be employed as a response to guardedness and reluctance. Confrontation will likely be interpreted as condemnation. On the other hand, empathic responses will encourage sharing of past difficulties, pain, and fears. To the extent to which these patients feel that their therapist understands their hypersensitivity and is protective of them, they will become more trusting and cooperative with treatment. As an effective working alliance is achieved, they can relax and begin to describe their hypersensitivity and fear of being misunderstood. To the extent to which the therapist fails to respond with empathy and compassion, they are likely to feel embarrassed and ridiculed and withdraw further.

Treatment Approaches and Interventions

There are general treatment considerations and specific treatment approaches for the treatment of AVPD including individual, group therapy, marital and family therapy, and medications.

General Treatment Considerations

The essential goals of treatment with individuals with AVPD are to expand their capability to tolerate feedback and selectively trust others. Rather than assuming that others intend criticism, rejection, or humiliation, or resorting to a reflexive "test" of others' worthiness, they can be encouraged to take some risks in their social interactions. At times, this may mean assertively communicating their needs, wants, and wishes, or taking the risk of requesting feedback from those who were previously supportive of them.

Avoidant individuals typically have a small number of relationships, often with their relatives, which means that they already know how to relate to some people. It is unlikely that the patient's basic pattern will change if the therapist simply becomes one more of the few. Only through learning to recognize the impact of their own patterns on others, and through taking risks in their relationships, can they succeed in long-term personality change.

Individual therapy can aid avoidant individuals to recognize patterns of avoidance and social withdrawal. A review conducted by Weinbrecht, Shulze, Boettcher, and Renneberg[20] found that CBT and schema therapy are the most empirically supported treatments for AVPD. However, couple's therapy and group therapy allow both the therapist and individual to observe their pattern's impact on others as well as providing an opportunity for individuals to take new interpersonal risks. Group and couple's therapy also provide an opportunity for patients to learn necessary mentalization skills, which is a deficit that has been found as a crucial component differentiating AVPD from other disorders such as SAD.[12]

Triangular patterns are often present if the individual is married or in a long-term committed relationship. For example, an avoidant individual may be married to an individual whose work demands frequent and extensive travel. They may make few, if any, demands on their partner. The avoidance may manifest in a secret extramarital affair. The triangular pattern reveals provisions for some degree of intimacy, protection from embarrassment or humiliation, and also permits interpersonal distance.

In the following sections, we describe several modalities and therapeutic approaches and interventions separately. However, it is not uncommon for therapists to utilize two modalities simultaneously—such as individual psychotherapy and group therapy—and therapeutic interventions from differing individual psychotherapy approaches, for example psychodynamics therapy and exposure, which is a key intervention in cognitive-behavioral therapy.

Individual Psychotherapies

Psychodynamic Psychotherapy

Psychodynamic psychotherapy can be effective in the treatment of individuals with AVPD through its expressive and supportive aspects.[14] Empathic appreciation of the embarrassment, humiliation, and rejection associated with interpersonal circumstances comprise the supportive aspect. Therapists may also assist by prescribing exposure to the situations that patients fear. Firm and supportive encouragement is needed in conjunction with this approach. The actual situations of exposure are more likely to activate anxieties and fantasies rather than a withdrawal and defensive posture. Explaining how and why exposure works can encourage patients to seek out opportunities to confront their fears.

The expressive aspect of the therapy is focused on uncovering the root causes of shame linked to prior experiences of rejection and humiliation, especially during the patient's early development. This therapy is greatly enhanced by the individual's willingness to risk confronting the feared circumstance. In the beginning, individuals may feel a sense of frustration because they may be unsure of who, or what, it is they fear. The tendency will be geared toward vague or general explanations such as "shyness" or "rejection" rather than specific imagined events. Therefore, the therapist must resort to examining specific fantasies within the transference context. Feeling frustrated by the patient's repeated efforts to "test" the therapist's trustworthiness and a sense of helplessness at the patient's resistance to change to a more adaptive pattern of relating are two common countertransferences.

Patients with avoidant personality may have considerable difficulty and anxiety in sharing thoughts and feelings openly. Accordingly, the therapist would do well to explicitly foster the patient's awareness of their nonverbal reactions (i.e., blushing, looking away), and have the patient attend to their feelings and thoughts about embarrassment. Specifically encouraging these disclosures may aid the patient's awareness and access to their feelings of shame.[14] This shame is best exemplified by a quote from qualitative study of the lived experiences of those with AVPD. One participant shared: "I would rather manage on my own so I say that I am fine. I may have difficult days at home, but then when I get to the clinic, I say that I am okay. I do not want to be that kind of person that does not dare to do things."[21(p. 6)]

Exploratory/interpretive techniques are also useful as either the primary intervention or as adjunctive to behavioral and interpersonal approaches. The basic strategy involves interpreting the patient's unconscious fantasies that their fear or impulses will become uncontrollable and harmful to self and others. Not surprisingly, their avoidant behavior maintains a denial of unconscious wishes or impulses.[14] Also, these patients tend to have harsh superegos, and subsequently project their own unrealistic expectations that others take care of them, while instead expecting that others will criticize and reject them. Their solution is to avoid relationships and evade criticism and embarrassment. A complete interpretation identifies the unconscious impulse and the fear, and traces the resulting avoidant defensive pattern in early life experiences, in outside relationships, and in the transference.[14]

Compared to other personality disorders, there is limited research on the effectiveness of long-term psychodynamic treatment for this disorder. In a randomized trial of 40 sessions of cognitive therapy versus psychodynamic therapy within 50 participants diagnosed with Cluster C personality disorders, 31 of them met criteria for a diagnosis of

AVPD.[22] Although results showed that both forms of therapy led to significant favorable changes, only the psychodynamic therapy group showed decreased distress symptoms at the conclusion of the treatment.

Cognitive-behavioral Therapy (CBT)

An in-depth discussion of the CBT approach with individuals diagnosed with AVPD is provided by Beck.[17] The basic CBT strategy and treatment goals for effecting change with these patients is described.

The initial goal of CBT with AVPD patients is to build trust while progressively reducing social anxiety, as well as reducing avoidance of emotions and cognition. From there, therapy can proceed toward correcting social skills deficits through behavioral methods prior to challenging automatic thoughts and schemas. Finally, therapy encourages a safe environment to attempt socially proactive and effective behavior that can improve interpersonal relationships.

Given their avoidance and hypersensitivity to perceived criticism, AVPD patients are difficult to engage in treatment. Accordingly, a therapist must work diligently yet carefully at building trust. Trust "tests" are commonly used by patients in the early stage of treatment. They can include a pattern of canceling appointments or having difficulty scheduling regular appointments. It is important not to prematurely challenge automatic thoughts, as such challenges tend to be experienced as personal criticism. Only after these individuals are solidly engaged in a working alliance should the therapist use cognitive interactions to test patients' expectancies in social situations. To the extent the therapist utilizes collaboration, rather than confrontation and guided discovery and direct disputation, these individuals are more likely to view therapy as constructive and are likely to remain in treatment.

Introducing anxiety management strategies early in treatment is useful, because these patients experience high levels of interpersonal anxiety. In order to reduce unpleasant feelings and increase emotional tolerance, desensitization, exposure, reframing, and mindfulness can be utilized to decrease avoidance of actual exposure and of imaginal emotional and cognitive exposure. Also, structured social-skills training can help patients learn important basics of social interaction that they may have not learned throughout their development.

After patients have achieved some of these short-term treatment goals and established sufficient trust with their therapist, challenging automatic thoughts and restructuring maladaptive schemas may be appropriate. The therapist must maintain a focus on resolving issues around the risks of developing close relationships and intimacy. This will be crucial to preventing catastrophizing of disapproval and rejection. Patients will become more capable and accepting of some disapproval in a close relationship as their self-efficacy increases and they become more effective in their interpersonal relationships. Thus, disapproval gradually loses its devastating impact.

The behavioral management of this personality pattern is relatively straightforward. Increasing social confidence may be achieved through anxiety management procedures and assertiveness, and social-skills training (e.g., role playing, direct instruction, and modeling). However, gradual exposure is the most effective behavioral intervention for reducing avoidant behavior and intolerance of anxiety.

Paradoxical intention is another strategy that may prove useful, particularly if the avoidant patient also presents with some opposition. Using this strategy, the patient is prompted to seek rejection in a predictable and controllable way. For example, a single male who presents with a fear of dating and speaking to women may be prompted to agree to an experiment of being rejected by two women in a given week. If accepted by one of the women, the patient would be able to go out with her, given that he would agree to ask out another and be rejected in either case. Essentially, seeking the rejection would be the goal of the treatment. This intervention would seek to reduce sensitivity toward rejection. The use of a paradoxical intervention is especially effective with oppositional avoidant patients, because they accentuate the patient's need to oppose the clinician by doing the opposite of what is suggested.[23]

Group therapy is a common adjunctive therapy with CBT. After the patient has engaged in treatment, but not before, these patients can learn to practice new attitudes and skills that they learned in individual therapy, in an accepting and supportive group environment. In other words, individual therapy comes first and prepares individuals who have difficulty feeling safe among others to enter a safe setting. Group therapy is particularly important for those with AVPD, so they can develop new relationships within the relatively safe context of other group members, many who have also issues of trust.

CBT with AVPD and SAD

What about the effectiveness of CBT with AVPD and SAD? Brown and colleagues[24] found that CBT was effective with both conditions separately. Because AVPD is considerably more impairing than SAD, it is not surprising that those with AVPD continued to report some continued impairment despite other gains in treatment. Similarly, Osterbaan and colleagues[25] found that individuals with SAD and comorbid AVPD had poorer response to treatment and remained more impaired in the short term than those without AVPD. Regardless, those with the comorbidity showed similar progress to those without it after a span of 15 months.[25]

Schema Therapy

Schema therapy is a specialized form of CBT that focuses primarily on changing core beliefs and schemas. It was specifically developed for personality disorders and other difficult individuals and couple problems.[26] It involves identifying maladaptive schemas and planning interventions and strategies.

Four of 18 maladaptive schemas are typically identified in those with AVPD. They are: (1) defectiveness: the belief that one is defective, bad, unwanted; (2) social isolation: the belief that one is different from others, alienated, and unable to be accepted into any group; (3) self-sacrifice: the belief that one must sacrifice one's needs for the needs of others; and (4) approval-seeking: the belief that the need to belong supersedes all other needs, and one must always be accepted, even at the expense of authenticity.[26]

After identifying the specific maladaptive schemas, therapy involves changing those schemas to more adaptive ones. Cognitive restructuring is a key intervention for making this change. Adjunctive treatments are also utilized with schema therapy. These include the use of imagery exercises, homework assignments, empathic confrontation, and limited reparenting.[26]

Interpersonal Psychotherapy

Interpersonal psychotherapy (IPT) is a brief psychotherapy that focuses on resolving interpersonal problems and leads to symptom reduction. It is highly structured and time-limited approach that usually involves 12–16 sessions. According to Benjamin,[18] interventions with individuals who suffer with AVPD can be planned according to their ability to: (1) enhance collaboration; (2) enable learning about underlying maladaptive patterns; (3) modify or stop these patterns; (4) increase the will to change; and (5) encourage new patterns of responding.

It is fortunate that avoidant individuals already know how to relate to one or a few individuals. Therefore, a supportive therapist can provide a safe space for the therapy. Patients respond well to accurate empathy and support. Their disclosure of feelings of inadequacy, guilt, and shame increase gradually along with their self-acceptance, which is necessary to begin the exploration of maladaptive patterns. Given their extreme sensitivity, early confrontation must be avoided.

Reconstructive, general, and long-lasting changes only occur if these individuals gain a thorough understanding of how their maladaptive patterns affect their lives. Benjamin suggests couple's therapy for individuals with avoidant personality who are married or in long-term relationships. These relationships typically provide interpersonal distance and safety for the avoidant individual. A pattern such as distance has its origin in unrooted loyalty to the family rules, such that the avoidant individual must remain isolated and safe. In couple's therapy, the therapist would provide the needed safety to the avoidant patient by blocking any attempts of criticism or humiliation by their partners that would "justify" their ongoing pattern of withdrawal. The most challenging task is for the avoidant patient to forgo the seemingly "favorable benefits" of their maladaptive pattern and replace it with a more adaptive pattern, namely one in which they feel safer relating to people and situations they previously avoided.

Developing insight about humiliation and loyalty toward their parents or siblings is not sufficient to facilitate long-term change. On the other hand, Benjamin contends that ongoing encouragement and reassurance in a competent and protective context of instruction can foster the favorable change.[18]

In a case study that used metacognitive interpersonal therapy to treat a 48-year-old male computer manager with obsessive-compulsive personality disorder and AVPD, individual and group therapy were used to accomplish modifying perfectionism, reducing avoidance, and acknowledging suppressed desires.[27] After one year of treatment, this patient no longer met criteria for either personality disorder. In another case study, a 24-year-old female graduate student who was treated with interpersonal therapy for AVPD and depression experienced significant improvements in areas of self-confidence, somatic complaints, anxiety, worry, and depression following two years of twice-monthly IPT and skills training for a total of 44 sessions.[28]

Group Therapy

Patients with AVPD are typically apprehensive of group therapy in the same way they are toward other novel and socially challenging circumstances. This explains why group therapy can be especially effective for these avoidant patients if they are persuaded to persist despite their anxiety. Sørensen and colleagues[21] noted that while participants found the group very challenging, they also agreed that it changed them: "It is horrible to be in the group. I just want to cry, my heart beats, I get a lump in my throat like I am going to throw up. It is like everybody is looking at me and thinking . . . but it is interesting to listen because they are there for a reason too. It is like a wake-up call that others might be like me."[21(p. 8)]

The benefits of group therapy can extend not just to overcoming social anxiety, but also to developing interpersonal trust and rapport with peers. It presents avoidant individuals with opportunities to feel a sense of belonging and being wanted, which may challenge previous and rigidly held beliefs. Feedback from other group members may contradict the avoidant individual's negative self-image; the new feedback can also be reinforced in individual therapy settings.[27]

Benjamin[18] likewise contends that a context in which safety is assured by the therapist (e.g., blocking abusive or negative behavior from other members) can greatly benefit the patient's self-acceptance and development of social skills. Additionally, individuals with AVPD often have poor metacognitive functioning;[29] they have difficulty mentalizing their own mind, as well as the minds of others. This capacity to mentalize can be addressed in group therapy, especially in process-oriented interpersonal groups.

Social-skills training seems to be effective in combination with cognitive therapy. Alden[30] incorporated aspects of cognitive therapy in group processes, including: (1) identifying underlying fears; (2) increasing awareness of fear-related anxiety; and (3) shifting the focus of attention from fear-related thinking to behavioral action. The sessions incorporated basic techniques such as psychoeducation, modeling, and role playing. Other researchers have found evidence that brief group therapy focused on social-skills training can improve social skills discrepancies that exacerbate anxiety about social adequacy.

Individuals with avoidant personalities avoid activities that contain risk of exposure or ridicule. This makes it more difficult for them to adapt to a group setting and to participate actively in their treatment. Therefore, it is important that the group therapist manages how much engagement is expected and helps the patient to pace their individual disclosure. Rennenberg found that the avoidance and anxiety in these patients was so pronounced that directly proceeding to behavioral rehearsal and social-skills training was not productive.[31] An alternate approach would be to begin with systematic desensitization and progressive relaxation training. Behavioral rehearsal was used as an exposure technique, which was found effective for social phobia.[32]

Structured activities support efficiency in therapy because they help avoidant individuals organize how they think and behave. Patients can be asked to accomplish specific homework goals in order to generalize treatment-session behaviors into their daily lives. Patients can select several social tasks to try, starting with simple tasks and proceeding to more difficult ones. In a group setting, Alden[30] also introduced interpersonal skills training. Friendship formation processes were presented, and patients were encouraged to practice their interpersonal skills between sessions. The therapists described and modeled four sets of behavioral skills that facilitate relating to others: empathic sensitivity, appropriate self-disclosure, listening and attending skills, and respectful assertiveness.

Rennenberg and colleagues[31] found that improvements through individual therapy and group intervention were stable over one year. However, most patients continued with individual therapy after the conclusion of group treatment. It is likely that continued individual therapy maintained the improvements made during the group therapy program. Group members, as well as their individual therapists, typically report more clinical changes. Participants reported diminished reticence in social settings, less social anxiety interference at work and in social situations, fewer symptoms of social anxiety, and increased satisfaction with social events.

In a study that measured the effectiveness of CBT groups on individuals with personality disorders, most of whom were diagnosed with AVPD, significant improvements were found in those who participated in group therapy as compared to those who did not. Skewes, Samson, Simpson, and van Vreeswijk[33] conducted a short-term group schema therapy pilot study for mixed personality disorders. Five out of the six individuals who were diagnosed with AVPD at the outset no longer met criteria for diagnosis at a six-month follow-up.

Marital and Family Therapy

It is important for patients with avoidant personalities to recognize how their dysfunctional patterns were developed. However, they also need to focus on their ongoing and current interpersonal experiences with others. Individuals with AVPD may characteristically provide vague descriptions of their interpersonal experiences. Therefore, it can undoubtedly be helpful to meet with other individuals who can fill in the gaps of information. Couple's and family treatments may be indicated. This can allow family structures to have more room for interpersonal exploration outside a tightly closed circle of family. Benjamin[18] advocates couple's therapy for individuals with avoidant personality who are married or in a long-term relationship, because there will likely be a pattern of avoidance and interpersonal distance within that relationship. It has been noted that those with AVPD may experience a sense of being disloyal to their family of origin, even if they experienced family humiliation or abuse. This may create an obstacle for the family to participate in the therapy. Even with agreed participation, the family may exacerbate issues by attacking the therapist, mocking the patient, or ridiculing any desire for change, making matters worse.

Medication

Currently, there are no specific psychotropic medications indicated for treating AVPD.[34] However, specific symptoms associated with the disorder such as problems with sleep, anxiety, and depression can be treated with medications. Medications are generally used in conjunction with psychotherapy and skills training. Given that associated troubling symptoms are responsive to medication faster than psychological interventions, medications are typically prescribed at the beginning of treatment. Unfortunately, research evidence to provide guidelines for the use of such medications is lacking. Given the comorbidity of this disorder to SAD, however, it has been speculated that it may respond well to medications with anxiety-reducing effects, such as serotonergic reuptake inhibitors (SSRIs). There is some evidence from a randomized control trial that individuals with AVPD respond favorably to low doses of sertraline, which is an SSRI medication.[34]

One of the themes from Sørensen and colleagues' qualitative study[21] was that benefits from medications were not attributed to personal gains. That is, patients viewed medication as a tool for suppressing or creating distance between their difficult feelings and thoughts. This distance allowed them to work and move through their daily lives. The caveat is that over the long term, this can essentially become yet another strategy of avoidance and thus result in diminishing returns. This makes a combined/integrated treatment approach paramount.

Combined Treatment Approach

As the basic premise, a single treatment modality such as psychotherapy may be effective for high-functioning personality disordered individuals. However, psychotherapy alone may be less effective for moderate-functioning individuals and essentially ineffective for severely dysfunctional individuals. Lower-functioning patients require combined treatment approaches. Combined modalities include the integration of psychotherapeutic intervention with medication, and group treatments such as group therapy or a support group. Individuals with avoidant personalities will struggle considerably with any groups. Ideally, lower-functioning avoidant patients should maintain involvement in both individual and group therapy. If it is not feasible for the patient to do both, a time-limited, skills-oriented group or a support group may be sufficient. An important focus of individual therapy will be transitioning a patient with avoidant personality into group therapy or a supportive group. Medication may be indicated in the treatment's early stages. It can be particularly useful in reducing distress and self-guarding behavior during the group-treatment transition.

There is considerable comorbidity between personality disorders and substance-use disorders. Some estimates are that as high as 90 percent of personality disorders are present in those treated for multiple addictions.[35] In a case study of a 43-year-old musician with comorbid AVPD and substance-use disorder (heroin), treatment progressed through the following stages: drug therapy to manage withdrawal from heroin; the formation of a therapeutic bond; fostering awareness of triggers and emotions for substance use; exploring maladaptive interpersonal schemas; understanding links between interpersonal events and substance use; acquiring distance from maladaptive schemas; and using adaptive skills instead of resorting back to substance use.[36]

Novel treatments have been explored in order to overcome the difficulty of treating those with avoidant personality given their social, emotional, and cognitive avoidance. A quasi-experimental study integrating traditional inpatient treatment with a wilderness program reported positive results.[37] The overarching theme of the courage of self-acceptance despite feeling unacceptable was noted in a qualitative study reported by Sørensen and colleagues.[21]

Combined/Integrated Treatment Approach

Poor treatment outcomes with AVPD have been attributed to issues with the therapeutic relationship.[16] Successful treatment requires an open, trusting relationship with the therapist, and developing effective social relationship skills with others. Those with AVPD initially have considerable difficulty forming such a therapeutic relationship, as well as demonstrating such relational skills. Premature termination or limited treatment outcomes are likely, irrespective of whether the therapy offered is primarily psychodynamic, focusing on therapeutic relationship, or primarily cognitive-behavioral focusing on relational skills. Both are required for successful treatment outcomes.

Consequently, an integrative approach may be indicated. Alden[30] describes the integration of both cognitive-behavioral and psychodynamic-interpersonal approaches. The cognitive approach is based on Beck,[17] whereas the psychodynamic-interpersonal approach is derived from Time-Limited Dynamic Psychotherapy, developed by Strupp and Binder.[38]

The cognitive-interpersonal patterns that are characteristic of individuals with avoidant personality are dysfunctional beliefs of being different and biologically defective. These individuals also have beliefs that their defects and feelings are apparent to others, and others will be disgusted, disapproving, or dismissing of them. They engage in significant safeguarding of themselves by looking to the therapist for direction and understanding. Additionally, they may withhold feelings or reactions due to expected disapproval from the therapist. Hence, the therapist's chief objective is to work collaboratively with the patient to modify their cognitive-interpersonal style. This four-step process includes (1) recognizing the treatment process issues, (2) increasing awareness of cognitive-interpersonal patterns, (3) developing alternative strategies, and (4) offering experiments and cognitive evaluation.

The first step in this integrative approach is recognizing the treatment process issues.[30] The therapist must detect that these patients will likely withhold or downplay clinically relevant information. Therapists should also expect common responses such as "I'm not sure" or "I don't know." Such responses function as evasion or avoidance, and they prevent the patients from encoding details about social situations. Unfortunately, therapists may fall into the trap of interpreting this vagueness and lack of focus as resistance. Alternatively, it may be useful to focus on global or vague interpersonal beliefs and behavior as targets for treatment. Either way, both the therapist and the patient will likely experience discouragement, and there will be a deterioration of the potential for favorable treatment outcomes. Additionally, therapists must consider that the patient's "hopelessness" and depression, which can be infectious, are largely influenced by their inability to process favorable information, lack of attentiveness, and their deeply rooted schemas and negative beliefs. It can be useful for therapists to be mindful of characteristically low levels of normative personality traits such as openness to experience, agreeableness, and extraversion in individuals with AVPD.[30] These can potentially account for difficulties in establishing therapeutic rapport and increase the likelihood of premature termination.

The second step is to increase awareness of cognitive-interpersonal patterns. Patients must be encouraged to keep a diary or logs and self-monitor in order to observe their interpersonal encounters outside of the therapy sessions. Alden described four components of the interpersonal pattern: (1) beliefs and expectancy of the other person; (2) behavior that arises from the beliefs; (3) the other's reaction to them; and (4) the conclusions drawn from the experiences.[30] As this process develops, patients begin to realize that their understanding of these problems is incomplete, and common patterns emerge such as the urge to avoid people and situations they consider unsafe or threatening. The role of the therapist is to shine a light on the beliefs that underlie the self-perception leading to self-protective behaviors.

The third step is focused on developing alternative strategies. As patients become more capable of recognizing and understanding their patterns and style, the therapist can foster their motivation to engage in new behaviors. This is achieved by pointing out the conflict between old and new views of self. As patients become able to integrate their current views with earlier experiences, they can begin to understand that their social fears and expectations stem partly from their temperament and partly from early parenting. This increased understanding can result in trying out new behavioral strategies, whether they are prompted by the therapist or emerge on their own.

Finally, step four follows with experiments and cognitive evaluation. These therapeutic strategies are thoroughly outlined by Beck.[17] Assertive communication and friendship formation are two basic interpersonal skills that avoidant patients must expand. Particularly useful interventions in this regard are role playing and directed assignments. Zimbardo's[39] social-skills interventions have been extremely useful to those working with avoidant patients. Assertive communication skills are presented, and patients are gently guided through them. In fact, Beck's text,[17] as a whole, is an invaluable adjunct in treating avoidant personality.

Box 22.1   Resources for Patients, Families, and Clinicians

- TalkSpace.com Blog: Avoidant Personality. www.talkspace.com/blog/avoidant-personality-disorder.
- Amelia's story–Project Air Strategy. https://projectairstrategy.org/mpapersonaljourneys/amelia/index.html.
- Quora: What does it feel like to be in a relationship with someone with severe social anxiety/AVPD? https://www.quora.com/What-does-it-feel-like-to-be-in-a-relationship-with-someone-with-severe-social-anxiety-avoidant-personality-disorder.
- TalkSpace.com Blog: How to Identify an Avoidant Partner and Improve Your Relationship. https://www.talkspace.com/blog/identifying-avoidant-partner-improve-relationship/.
- Meyers, E. *Overcoming Shyness: Break Out of Your Shell and Express Your True Self.* Lewiston, ID: Dom & Eric Fitness; 2017.

Conclusion

AVPD is a common personality disorder that is characterized by shyness, low self-esteem, and rejection sensitivity wherein these individuals avoid others even though they crave human contact. In contrast, the avoidant personality style is more flexible and causes less distress and impairment than the AVPD. The optimal DSM-5 criterion for this disorder is avoidance of work activities that involve significant interpersonal contact because of fear of rejection. A quick and accurate means of diagnosing this disorder is to utilize a structured interview using the DSM-5 criteria. Effective treatment planning begins with an accurate case conceptualization. Five common models for conceptualizing this disorder are offered: psychodynamic, biosocial, cognitive-behavioral, interpersonal, and integrative. Implementing such a treatment plan with this disorder usually involves one or more treatment modalities—group therapy, marital and family therapy, medication, or combined/integrated treatment—and interventions from one or more psychotherapeutic approaches: psychodynamic, cognitive-behavioral, or interpersonal. Review Box 22.1 for relevant resources for patients, families, and clinicians.

Conflict of Interest/Disclosure: The authors of this chapter have no financial conflicts and nothing to disclose.

References

1. Sanislow CA, da Cruz K, Gianoli MO, Reagan EM. Avoidant personality disorder, traits, and type. In: Widiger T, ed. *The Oxford Handbook of Personality Disorders.* New York, NY: Oxford University Press; 2012: 549–565.

2. Snir A, Bar-Kalifa E, Berenson KR, Downey G, Rafaeli E. Affective instability as a clinical feature of avoidant personality disorder. *Personal Disord.* 2017; 8(4): 389–395.

3. Lyddon WJ, Sherry A. Developmental personality styles: an attachment theory conceptualization of personality disorders. *J Couns Dev.* 2001; 79(4): 405–414.

4. Eikenæs I, Pedersen G, Wilberg T. Attachment styles in patients with avoidant personality disorder compared with social phobia. *Psychol Psychother*. 2016; 89(3): 245–260.

5. American Psychiatric Association. *Diagnostic and Statistical Manual of Mental Disorders. Fifth Edition*. (DSM-5). Washington, DC: American Psychiatric Association; 2013.

6. Allnutt S, Links PS. Diagnosing specific personality disorders and the optimal criteria. In: Links P, ed. *Clinical Assessment and Management of the Severe Personality Disorders*. Washington, DC: American Psychiatric Press; 1996: 21–47.

7. Frances A. *Essentials of Psychiatric Diagnosis: Responding to the Challenge of DSM-5*. New York, NY: Guilford Publications; 2013.

8. Torgersen S. Epidemiology. In: Widiger T, ed. *The Oxford Handbook of Personality Disorders*. New York, NY: Oxford University Press; 2012: 186–205.

9. Lampe L, Malhi GS. Avoidant personality disorder: current insights. *Psychol Res Behav Manag*. 2018; 11: 55–66.

10. Havranek MM, Volkart F, Bolliger B, et al. The fear of being laughed at as additional criterion in social anxiety disorder and avoidant personality disorder? *PloS One*. 2017; 12(11): 1–11.

11. Frandsen FW, Simonsen S, Poulsen S, Sørensen P, Lau ME. Social anxiety disorder and avoidant personality disorder from an interpersonal perspective. *Psychol Psychother*. 2020; 93(1): 88–104.

12. Pellecchia G, Moroni F, Colle L, et al. Avoidant personality disorder and social phobia: does mindreading make the difference? *Compr Psychiatry*. 2018; 80(1): 163–169.

13. Welander-Vatn A, Torvik FA, Czajkowski N, et al. Relationships among avoidant personality disorder, social anxiety disorder, and normative personality traits: a twin study. *J Pers Disord*. 2019; 33(3): 289–309.

14. Gabbard, G. *Psychodynamic Psychiatry in Clinical Practice: The DSM-IV Edition*. Washington, DC: American Psychiatric Press; 1994.

15. Eskedal GA, Demetri JM. Etiology and treatment of cluster C personality disorders. *J Ment Health Couns*. 2006; 28(1): 1–7.

16. Millon T, Davis R. *Personality Disorders in Modern Life*. New York, NY: John Wiley & Sons; 2000.

17. Beck AT. Theory of personality disorders. In: Beck AT, Davis DD, Freeman A, eds. *Cognitive Therapy of Personality Disorders*. 3rd ed. New York, NY: Guilford Publications; 2015: 19–62.

18. Benjamin LS. *Interpersonal Diagnosis and Treatment of Personality Disorders*. 2nd ed. New York, NY: Guilford Publications; 2003.

19. Sperry L. Personality disorders. In: Sperry L, Carlson J, Sauerheber JD, Sperry J, eds. *Psychopathology and Psychotherapy: DSM-5 Diagnosis, Case Conceptualization, and Treatment*. 3rd ed. New York, NY: Routledge; 2016: 27–61.

20. Weinbrecht A, Schulze L, Boettcher J, Renneberg B. Avoidant personality disorder: a current review. *Curr Psychiatry Rep*. 2016; 18(3): 1–8.

21. Sørensen K D, Wilberg T, Berthelsen E, Råbu M. Lived experience of treatment for avoidant personality disorder: searching for courage to be. *Front Psychol*. 17 Dec. 2019; 10:2879. doi:10.3389/fpsyg.2019.02879

22. Svartberg M, Stiles TC, Seltzer MH. Randomized, controlled trial of the effectiveness of short-term dynamic psychotherapy and cognitive therapy for cluster C personality disorders. *Am J Psychiatry*. 2005; 161(3): 810–817.

23. Weeks G, L'Abate L. *Paradoxical Psychotherapy: Theory and Practice with Individuals, Couples, and Families*. New York, NY: Brunner/Mazel; 1982.

24. Brown EJ, Heimberg RG, Juster HR. Social phobia subtype and avoidant personality disorder: effect on severity of social phobia, impairment, and outcome of cognitive behavioral treatment. *Behav Ther.* 1995; 26(3): 467–486.

25. Oosterbaan DB, van Balkom AJ, Spinhoven P, de Meij TG, van Dyck R. The influence on treatment gain of comorbid avoidant personality disorder in patients with social phobia. *J Nerv Ment Dis.* 2002; 190(1): 41–43.

26. Young JE, Klosko JS, Weishaar ME. *Schema Therapy: A Practitioner's Guide.* New York, NY: Guilford Publications; 2006.

27. Fiore D, Dimaggio G, Nicoló G, Semerari A, Carcione A. Metacognitive interpersonal therapy in a case of obsessive-compulsive and avoidant personality disorders. *J Clin Psychol.* 2008; 64(2): 168–180.

28. Gilbert SE, Gordon KC. Interpersonal psychotherapy informed treatment for avoidant personality disorder with subsequent depression. *Clin Case Stud.* 2013; 12(2): 111–127.

29. Moroni F, Procacci M, Pellecchia G, et al. Mindreading dysfunction in avoidant personality disorder compared with other personality disorders. *J Nerv Ment Dis.* 2016; 204(10): 752–757.

30. Alden, LE. Cognitive-interpersonal treatment for avoidant personality disorder. In: Vandecreek, L, Knapp, S, Jackson, TL, eds. *Innovations in Clinical Practice: A Source Book.* Sarasota, FL: Professional Resource Press; 1992: 5–22.

31. Renneberg B, Goldstein AJ, Phillips D, Chambless DL. Intensive behavioral group treatment of avoidant personality disorder. *Behav Ther.* 1990; 21(3): 363–377.

32. Stravynski A, Marks I, Yule W. Social skills problems in neurotic outpatients: social skills training with and without cognitive modification. *JAMA Psychiatry.* 1982; 39(12): 1378–1385.

33. Skewes SA, Samson RA, Simpson SG, van Vreeswijk M. Short-term group schema therapy for mixed personality disorders: a pilot study. *Front Psychol.* 2015; 5: 1–9.

34. Silk K, Feurino L. Psychopharmacology of personality disorders. In: Widiger T, ed. *The Oxford Handbook of Personality Disorders.* New York, NY: Oxford University Press; 2012: 713–726.

35. Rentrop M, Zilker T, Lederle A, Birkhofer A, Hörz S. Psychiatric comorbidity and personality structure in patients with polyvalent addiction. *Psychopathology.* 2014; 47(2): 133–140.

36. Dimaggio G, D'Urzo M, Pasinetti M, Salvatore G, Lysaker PH, Catania D, Popolo R. Metacognitive interpersonal therapy for co-occurrent avoidant personality disorder and substance abuse. *J Clin Psychol.* 2015; 71(2): 157–166.

37. Eikenæs I, Gude T, Hoffart A. Integrated wilderness therapy for avoidant personality disorder. *Nord J Psychiatry.* 2006; 60(4): 275–281.

38. Strupp H, Binder JL. *Psychotherapy in a New Key: A Guide to Time-limited Dynamic Psychotherapy.* New York, NY: Basic Books; 1984.

39. Zimbardo PG, Pilkonis PA, Marnell ME. *Shyness: What It Is, What to Do About It.* Reading, MA: Addison-Wesley; 1977.

23

Dependent Personalities

Robert F. Bornstein and Adam P. Natoli

Key Points

- The prevalence rate of dependent personality disorder (DPD) in the general population is about one percent, with women receiving two-thirds of DPD diagnoses. DPD prevalence rates in psychiatric inpatient and outpatient settings are in the range of 5–10 percent and 2–3 percent, respectively.
- DSM-5 DPD diagnostic criteria are: (1) difficulty making decisions without excessive advice and reassurance; (2) needing others to assume responsibility for most major areas of life; (3) difficulty expressing disagreement; (4) difficulty initiating projects or doing things on one's own; (5) going to excessive lengths to obtain nurturance and support; (6) feeling helpless when alone; (7) urgently seeking another source of protection when an important relationship ends; and (8) being preoccupied with fears of being left to care for oneself.
- DPD is comorbid with depression, anxiety disorders, substance use disorders, bulimia, and several other PDs (i.e., avoidant, borderline, narcissistic, OCPD and histrionic).
- Interpersonal dependency is the tendency to rely on other people for nurturance, guidance, protection, and support, even in situations where autonomous functioning is possible.
- About 30 percent of the variance in interpersonal dependency and DPD is attributable to genetic factors. Environmental upbringing including overprotective and authoritarian parenting also contribute to the development of pathological dependency.
- Culture affects the experience and expression of underlying dependency needs: Self-reported dependency is higher in sociocentric cultures (e.g., Japan, India) than in more individualistic cultures (e.g., United States, Great Britain).
- Although interpersonal dependency and DPD are often associated with passivity and submissiveness, evidence suggests that dependent patients can also exhibit active, sometimes even aggressive, behavior when important relationships are threatened.
- Because dependent patients show varying degrees of insight regarding their underlying dependency strivings, multi-method assessment of interpersonal dependency and DPD that integrates self-report and performance-based test data helps set the stage for effective treatment.

> - Evidence supports the effectiveness of cognitive interventions for pathological dependency; evidence regarding the effectiveness of psychodynamic and pharmacological interventions is less strong.
> - Although a common goal in treatment is to reduce dependent thoughts, feelings, and behaviors, it may also be useful to help patients express underlying dependency needs in healthier, more adaptive ways.

Introduction

Case of James Novy

On December 1, 1989, four-year-old James Novy died from injuries sustained over a period of several days. He was covered with bruises, bleeding internally, and his skull had been fractured in two places. On January 12, 1990, James Novy's stepmother, Kimberly Novy, was charged with first-degree murder in the death of her stepson. She was eventually found guilty, but the charge was reduced to involuntary manslaughter based on an unusual mitigating circumstance: Kimberly Novy suffered from dependent personality disorder (DPD), an overreliance on other people for external support, reassurance, and validation. She claimed that as a result of her disorder she was unable to resist her husband's demands that she punish her stepson severely for various offenses, real and imagined. The court held that Kimberly Novy's DPD was sufficient to diminish her culpability for the death of James Novy and shifted much of the accountability to her husband, the boy's father, Keith Novy.

*****

Virtually every mental health professional has encountered patients who are highly dependent. These patients alienate those around them with clinging insecurity, and seem unable to make even the smallest decision on their own. During the past several decades, there have been hundreds of studies examining the antecedents, correlates, and consequences of high levels of interpersonal dependency, and DPD. As is true of several other *Diagnostic and Statistical Manual of Mental Disorders: DSM-5*[1] personality disorders (e.g., avoidant, narcissistic, histrionic, borderline, obsessive-compulsive), there is considerable conceptual and empirical overlap between the more pathological manifestations of dependency (i.e., DPD) and normally distributed interpersonal dependency (sometimes called *trait dependency*) found in these personality disorders (PDs) and in the broader population. As a result, research on interpersonal dependency in clinical and nonclinical samples has helped inform contemporary conceptualizations of DPD. Research on the etiology and dynamics of DPD has also helped shape researchers' understanding of interpersonal dependency. High levels of interpersonal dependency are associated with elevated levels of DPD symptoms and increased likelihood of a DPD diagnosis in a variety of participant groups, including psychiatric inpatients and outpatients, and medical patients.[2,3]

Dependent patients have always presented unique clinical challenges. However, in today's healthcare environment, with its emphasis on time-limited, cost-effective treatment, therapeutic work with dependent patients can be especially difficult. Dependent psychotherapy patients have a greater number of "pseudo-emergencies" than do nondependent patients; they make more requests for after-hours or between-session contact. Dependent psychiatric inpatients receive a greater number of psychotropic medications than do nondependent inpatients with similar demographic and diagnostic profiles; they receive more referrals for consultation from other hospital services, driving up healthcare costs. Evidence also suggests that dependent psychotherapy patients have difficulty ending therapy, even when termination is appropriate, and may sabotage their treatment to delay termination.

Although most clinicians associate interpersonal dependency with passivity and submissiveness, dependent individuals are capable of behaving actively, even downright aggressively, in certain situations; this can further complicate their treatment. Evidence confirms that dependent men are at increased risk for perpetrating partner abuse, with abuse episodes typically triggered by the dependent man's belief that his partner may reject or abandon him.[4] As the case of Kimberly Novy illustrates, dependent parents, women and men alike, are at increased risk for perpetrating child abuse.

This chapter reviews research and clinical writing on interpersonal dependency and DPD. After reviewing evidence regarding the epidemiology of DPD, issues regarding differential diagnosis and comorbidity are discussed. Research documenting biological and environmental antecedents of DPD are described, followed by presentation of an integrative framework, the cognitive/interactionist (C/I) model. This model specifies the core cognitive, motivational, behavioral, and affective components of normal and pathological dependency, and provides an overarching structure for conceptualizing contextual variations in dependency-related responding. A case formulation and discussion of treatment challenges in therapeutic work with dependent patients are presented; major psychosocial and pharmacological treatment approaches are evaluated; and guidelines for maximizing treatment efficacy and a brief case discussion are offered.

Epidemiology of Dependent Personality Disorder

A comprehensive review by Disney[5] indicated that DPD is common in inpatient settings, with researchers reporting prevalence rates of 5–10 percent in psychiatric inpatient units, rehabilitation centers, and long-term care facilities. The base rate of DPD in outpatients tends to be lower, in the range of 2 to 3 percent. In large-scale surveys of community adults in the United States, the prevalence rate of DPD is typically about 1 percent; similar prevalence rates have been found in community samples in several European nations. DPD is diagnosed far more often in women than in men, accounting for about two-thirds of all DPD diagnoses.[6] Evidence suggests that DPD symptoms and diagnoses remain fairly stable through middle and later adulthood, although diagnosis of DPD in older adults is complicated by normative increases in physical (i.e., functional) dependency with increasing age.[7] There has been little research examining ethnic and racial differences in interpersonal dependency and DPD.

Diagnostic Considerations

DPD symptom criteria are virtually identical in *International Classification of Diseases*, 10th edition (ICD-10)[8] and DSM-5.[1] The essential feature of DPD in DSM-5 is "A pervasive and excessive need to be taken care of that leads to submissive and clinging behavior and fears of separation, beginning by early adulthood and present in a variety of contexts."[1(p. 675)] DSM-5 lists eight DPD symptoms, five of which must be present to receive the diagnosis:

1. Difficulty making decisions without excessive advice and reassurance
2. Needing others to assume responsibility for most major areas of life
3. Difficulty expressing disagreement
4. Difficulty initiating projects or doing things on one's own
5. Going to excessive lengths to obtain nurturance and support
6. Feeling helpless when alone
7. Urgently seeking another source of protection when an important relationship ends
8. Being preoccupied with fears of being left to care for oneself

Although the DPD symptom criteria will remain unchanged in DSM-5-TR, it is likely that in ICD-11, categorical PD diagnoses will be replaced with dimensional ratings of pathological personality traits on several core domains of functioning.[9] Initial proposals, derived in part from the DSM-5 Alternative Model of Personality Disorder (AMPD), suggest that in future diagnostic systems, patients manifesting excessive interpersonal dependency will be characterized as being high on anxiousness, submissiveness, and separation insecurity. As Bornstein[3,6] noted, however, evidence only supports the characterization of interpersonal dependency and DPD as reflecting elevated levels of anxiousness and separation insecurity. Dependency-related submissiveness is typically expressed in certain situations (e.g., when attempting to curry favor with figures of authority), whereas in other situations (e.g., when important relationships are at risk) more active social influence strategies are often used.

Differential Diagnosis and Comorbidity

DPD is comorbid with four clinical disorders (formerly labeled Axis I disorders in earlier versions of the DSM): depression, somatization disorder, social anxiety disorder, and agoraphobia.[10,11] It is also comorbid with three other PDs: borderline, avoidant, and histrionic.[10] Some evidence suggests that the DSM-5 comorbidity information for DPD may be overly conservative. In addition to the diagnoses noted, DPD also co-occurs with substance use disorders. Prospective studies show that dependency levels actually increase as substance abuse progresses; dysfunctional dependency may follow rather than precede substance use.[12] In addition, bulimic women show higher than expected rates of DPD, although studies indicate that DPD symptoms often decrease as eating-disorder symptoms remit.[13]

Diagnosing DPD can be challenging, in part because underlying dependency strivings play a role in an array of other syndromes (e.g., borderline PD, histrionic PD, agoraphobia, social anxiety disorder). As a result, the clinician may erroneously assign a DPD diagnosis to a patient when in fact that patient's dependent behavior results from another form of pathology (e.g., clinging insecurity and fear of abandonment resulting from borderline pathology). To minimize the possibility of misdiagnosis, it is important to obtain an accurate personal and clinical history, ascertaining (1) the age of onset of relevant symptoms and diagnoses and (2) the degree to which problematic dependency may be secondary to another syndrome.[14]

Assessing Interpersonal Dependency and DPD

Interpersonal dependency is the tendency to look to others for nurturance, guidance, protection, and support, even in situations where autonomous functioning is possible.[3,15] Assessing interpersonal dependency is complicated by the fact that patients show varying degrees of insight into their underlying and expressed dependency needs. Table 23.1, p. 570 summarizes widely used questionnaire, interview, and performance-based measures of interpersonal dependency and DPD. Evidence bearing on the construct validity and clinical utility of these measures is provided by Bornstein,[3,16] First et al.,[17] Gore et al.,[18] and Krueger et al.[19]

As Table 23.1, p. 570 shows, these measures capture an array of dependency-related thoughts, feelings, and behaviors; in some instances, different measures focus on contrasting manifestations of dependency. As is true of other PDs (and other measurements of pathological personality traits), questionnaire measures typically yield a greater number of false positive diagnoses than do interviews;[24] as a result, the Interpersonal Dependency Inventory (IDI)[20] and the Personality Inventory for DSM-5 (PID-5)[19] are best conceptualized as screening tools that should be followed up with a structured or semi-structured interview to confirm a PD diagnosis.

Self-report scales such as the IDI,[20] PID-5,[19] and Five-Factor Model Dependent Personality Disorder Scale[18] assess *self-attributed dependency needs*, dependency needs that are recognized and openly acknowledged by the patient. Performance-based measures such as the Rorschach Oral Dependency scale (now included in the Rorschach Performance Assessment System as the Oral Dependent Language Scale)[23] assess *implicit dependency strivings*, dependency needs that shape dependent responding indirectly, often with little or no awareness on the patient's part. McClelland et al.[25] provided a useful contrast of implicit and self-attributed motives, noting that:

> Measures of implicit motives provide a more direct readout of motivational and emotional experiences than do self-reports that are filtered through analytic thought and various concepts of self and others [because] implicit motives are more often built on early, prelinguistic affective experiences, whereas self-attributed motives are more often built on explicit teaching by parents and others as to what values or goals it is important for a child to pursue.[25(pp. 698-699)]

Thus, a complete picture of a patient's dependency strivings requires that self-report test data be combined with performance-based test data; evidence confirms that integrating implicit and self-attributed dependency scores provides better predictive power than reliance on one type of score alone.[26,27] Figure 23.1, p. 571 summarizes four possible outcomes when self-report and performance-based dependency test data are collected from the same patient. The upper-left and lower-right panels reflect convergences

Table 23.1. Questionnaire, Interview, and Performance-Based Measures of Interpersonal Dependency and DPD

Measure	Construct(s) Assessed	Length, Format, and Structure
Interpersonal Dependency Inventory[20]	Overall level of self-reported dependency, comprised of three components: Emotional Reliance on Others, Lack of Social Self-Confidence, and Assertion of Autonomy (reverse-scored)	Questionnaire; 48 items, each rated 4-point scale; yields overall dependency score plus three subscale scores
Relationship Profile Test[21]	Destructive Overdependence (DO), Dysfunctional Detachment (DD), and Healthy Dependency (HD)	Questionnaire; 30 items (10 items per subscale), each rated on a 5-point scale; yields separate DO, DD, and HD scores
Five-Factor Model DPD FFM Scale[18]	Degree to which patient reports dependency-related thoughts, feelings, and behaviors, with items derived from an FFM conceptualization of pathological dependency	Questionnaire; 120 items tapping dependency-related variants of domains and facets, with each item on a 5-point scale
Personality Inventory for DSM-5[19]	Degree to which patient reports dependency-related traits and behavioral tendencies, with items derived from the DSM-5 AMPD	Questionnaire; items tap behaviors associated with AMPD trait facets; the PID-5 Brief Form includes 25 items, the Long Form includes 220 items; each item is rated on a 4-point scale
Structured Clinical DSM-5 Personality Disorders[17]	DSM-5 DPD symptoms (along with symptoms of other DSM-5 Interview for PDs)	Structured interview; provides information regarding presence/absence of DPD symptoms and DPD diagnosis (along with symptoms and diagnoses of other PDs)
International Personality Disorder Inventory[22]	DSM-5/ICD-10 DPD symptoms (along with symptoms of other DSM-5 and ICD-10 PDs)	Structured interview; provides information regarding presence/absence of DPD symptoms and DPD diagnosis (along with symptoms and diagnoses of other PDs)
Rorschach Oral Dependency Scale[23]	Level of implicit (underlying) dependency strivings that may not be accessible to verbal report	Performance-based test; open-ended descriptions of Rorschach inkblots are scored for oral and dependent content yielding an overall ROD score

Note. AMPD = DSM-5 Alternative Model of Personality Disorder.[1]

between implicit and self-attributed dependency strivings; the lower left and upper right panels illustrate discontinuities. The lower left cell includes those patients who appear to have high levels of underlying dependency but are unaware of this, or unwilling to acknowledge it when asked. The upper right cell includes patients who appear to have low

SCORE ON
SELF-ATTRIBUTION DEPENDENCY
MEASURE

		LOW	HIGH
SCORE ON STIMULUS-ATTRIBUTION DEPENDENCY MEASURE	LOW	Low Implicit Low Self-Attributed *Low Dependency*	Low Implicit High Self-Attributed *Dependent Self-Presentation*
	HIGH	High Implicit Low Self-Attributed *Unacknowledged Dependency*	High Implicit High Self-Attributed *High Dependency*

Figure 23.1 Continuities and Discontinuities in Implicit and Self-Attributed Dependency Test Scores.

Note: Originally published as Figure 2 in Bornstein RF. From dysfunction to adaptation: An interactionist model of dependency. *Ann Rev Clin Psychol.* 2012;8:291–316. Reprinted with permission from the *Annual Review of Clinical Psychology*, Volume 8, by Annual Reviews, http://www.annualreviews.org.

levels of implicit dependency needs but nonetheless choose to present themselves as being highly dependent.

It is possible that the patient will score high on both types of measures, as illustrated in the upper-left and lower-right quadrants of Figure 23.1. Either of these outcomes would indicate a convergence between that patient's implicit and self-attributed dependency needs and suggest that self-reports are a reasonably accurate reflection of the person's underlying dependency strivings. The other two cells in Figure 23.1 illustrate situations wherein testing has revealed a discontinuity between the patient's implicit and self-attributed dependency needs.

Multimethod Assessment of Interpersonal Dependency: The Case of Kevin

Kevin is a 41-year-old Caucasian male born in Iran. He was admitted to a psychiatric service for the second time due to violent behavior at his group home secondary to psychotic decompensation in the context of medication nonadherence. Upon admission, he presented with labile affect, paranoid thoughts, and impulsive behavior. He was poorly oriented to time, place, and person, and demonstrated limited insight into his mental illness. As his psychosis subsided following psychopharmacological intervention, Kevin showed steady improvement and became more actively engaged in treatment and social interactions. He was referred for psychological testing to obtain a foundational understanding of his cognitive and psychological functioning; the findings of this assessment were used to inform Kevin's continued treatment.

In addition to a cognitive battery, Kevin was administered the Personality Assessment Inventory (PAI)[28] and the Rorschach, from which the Rorschach Oral Dependency (ROD) scores were derived (see Table 23.1, p. 570). Validity indices provided by the PAI indicated that Kevin's response style had a substantial distorting effect on his self-report test responses: There were strong indications that he tended to portray himself in an espe-cially negative or pathological manner by exaggerating his problems and deficits. However, Kevin's performance on the Rorschach showed an appropriate level of effort, and he readily produced a valid number of responses without additional prompting, which offered fur-ther evidence of his good effort during the Rorschach. His intelligence test performance was indicative of full engagement in the various tasks required by the measure.

Kevin's PAI clinical scale scores suggested he was preoccupied with fears of being abandoned or rejected, was indecisive and had difficulty asserting himself, and expected future success to be dependent upon the actions of others. That is, these self-report test data indicated that Kevin was, for all intents and purposes, a dependent individual. As noted, however, PAI validity indices suggested these results may have been the product of an overly negative or pathological self-presentation. Based on this, many assessors would simply regard the results of Kevin's PAI as being invalid and discontinue their in-terpretation. However, Kevin's dependency was evaluated using multiple measurement modalities and his heightened dependency, as indicated by the PAI, was corroborated by his performance on the Rorschach. Kevin obtained consistent results on both self-report and performance-based measures, and was best represented by the lower-right panel of Figure 23.1, p. 571 (high implicit dependency and high self-attributed dependency).

In this case, multi-method assessment allowed for cross-measure confirmation of Kevin's heightened dependency and fostered a more nuanced understanding of his psycho-logical functioning than would have been available from either test alone. Although Kevin did indeed have a tendency to portray himself in an inaccurate and overly negative way, his self-attributed dependency appeared to be genuine and ego-syntonic; he sincerely believed he was inadequate, which understandably contributed to a need to rely on others, and fears of being left to fend for himself. Moreover, he openly endorsed these characteristics and, perhaps in hopes of procuring superfluous care from his treatment team, exaggerated various symptoms on self-report tests. The comprehensive understanding of Kevin's de-pendency afforded by multi-method assessment also highlighted a unique target of inter-vention. Kevin's acceptance of his dependent behaviors, which he saw as ways to maintain nurturing relationships, could be challenged by helping him see the discrepancy between these dependent behaviors and his life goals (e.g., to marry and start a family). With this information, Kevin's treatment team was able to plan and implement interventions that helped him acknowledge difficulties his dependency had caused him while remaining mindful not to invalidate the part of Kevin that valued this aspect of his personality.

The Etiology of Pathological Dependency

During the past several decades, there have been dozens of studies examining the antecedents of pathological dependency in adolescents and adults. Results of these investigations converge to confirm that high levels of interpersonal dependency and DPD are caused by a combination of biological and environmental factors.

Biologic, Neuropsychiatric, and Genetic Underpinnings

Studies indicate that approximately 30 percent of risk for developing DPD can be accounted for by genetic factors, although the pathways that lead from diathesis to disorder have yet to be documented conclusively.[29] The earliest manifestations of interpersonal dependency and DPD are certain infantile temperament variables (e.g., withdrawal, low adaptability, high reactivity). Although some early temperament variables (e.g., low adaptability) may evolve directly into dependency-related traits and DPD symptoms later in life, during early and middle childhood problematic dependency is manifest most prominently as insecure attachments—difficulty tolerating separation from the caregiver, along with an absence of age-appropriate increases in autonomy and self-sufficiency. One consequence of this attachment insecurity is that immersion in an unfamiliar peer group is particularly challenging for highly dependent children; in many cases, the first overt manifestation of excessive dependency during childhood is school refusal.

Psycho-Social-Cultural Contributions

Beyond biological predispositions, several dozen studies confirm that overprotective parenting leads to high levels of dependency in offspring, because overprotective parents inadvertently teach children that they are vulnerable and weak; without a powerful caregiver watching over them they will surely fail on their own (see Bornstein[16] for a review of studies bearing on this issue). Authoritarian parenting is also associated with increased dependency risk, because the authoritarian parent, the rigid, inflexible, rule-oriented parent, teaches the child that the way to get by in life is to accede to others' demands and expectations while simultaneously limiting the trial-and-error learning opportunities that would promote the child's development of autonomy and sense of self-efficacy.[30] When parental overprotectiveness and authoritarianism are both present within the family, DPD is particularly likely to result.[3,31]

Culture plays a key role in the development of dependency as well. People raised in sociocentric cultures, which have traditionally emphasized interpersonal relatedness over individual achievement (e.g., Japan, India), report higher levels of dependency. People raised in more individualistic cultures like America and Great Britain, which emphasize competition and achievement over group harmony, show greater autonomy. Dependency can be adaptive when it is commensurate with the norms and values of an individual's culture, but evidence indicates that when people emigrate from a sociocentric culture to a more individualistic culture they may have difficulty balancing their long-standing values regarding relatedness with the new culture's demand that they compete for prestige and resources rather than putting their own needs aside in the service of the group.[32]

Toward an Integrative Perspective on Normal and Pathological Dependency

In recent years, research and clinical writing on interpersonal dependency and DPD have been facilitated by the emergence of a consensus regarding the core features of pathological dependency. Contemporary definitions of dependency[3,15] emphasize four components. These are:

1. A *motivational* component, characterized by a marked need for guidance, support, and approval from others

2. A *cognitive* component: a perception of oneself as powerless and ineffectual, coupled with the belief that other people are comparatively confident and competent
3. An *affective* (or emotional) component: a tendency to become anxious when required to function autonomously
4. A *behavioral* component: use of a broad array of social influence strategies to strengthen ties to potential caregivers and preclude abandonment

Bornstein[3,16] developed an integrative perspective called the cognitive-interactionist (C/I) model, which makes explicit the interaction of these four core components of interpersonal dependency and DPD. The core elements of the C/I model are summarized in Figure 23.2. As this figure illustrates, dependent personality traits reflect the interplay of cognitive, motivational, emotional, and behavioral features, all of which stem from early learning and socialization experiences within and outside the family. Overprotective and authoritarian parenting play a key role in the development of a dependent personality, because both lead to the construction of a helpless self-concept, which is the core element of a dependent personality style. A perception of oneself as helpless and weak increases dependency-related motives, which in turn set the stage for dependent behavior and affective responding.

A helpless self-concept, coupled with the perception of other people as powerful and potent, is the linchpin of a dependent personality orientation and the psychological mechanism from which all other manifestations of dependency originate. These elements combine to create the motivational component of dependency: If one views oneself as weak and ineffectual, then one's desire to curry favor with potential caregivers and protectors will increase. These dependency-related motivations in turn

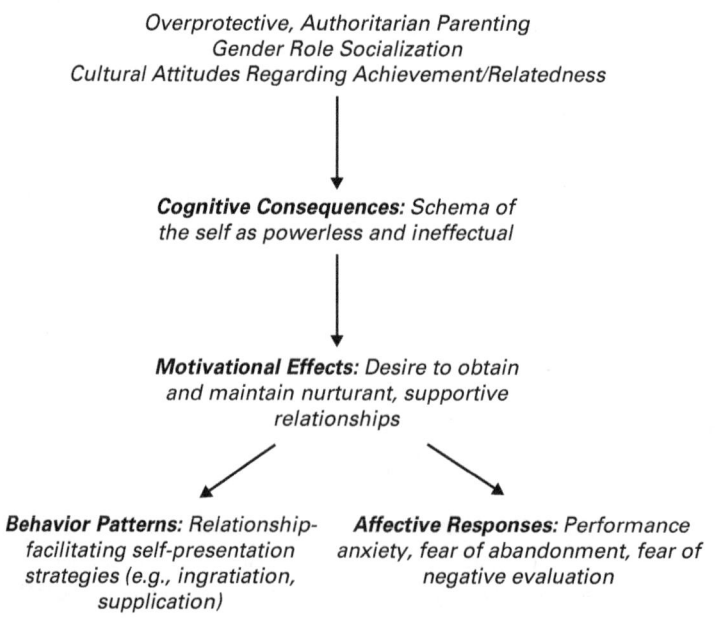

Figure 23.2. A Cognitive/Interactionist Model of Interpersonal Dependency.

Originally published as Figure 1 in Bornstein RF. *Ann Rev Clin Psychol.* 2012;8:291–316. Reprinted with permission from the *Annual Review of Clinical Psychology*, Volume 8, by Annual Reviews, http://www. annualreviews.org.

give rise to dependency-related behaviors (relationship-facilitating self-presentation strategies such as submissiveness and ingratiation) and to affective responses (e.g., fear of negative evaluation) that reflect the dependent person's core beliefs about the self.

Thus, the C/I model conceptualizes dependency-related responding as proactive, goal-driven, and guided by beliefs and expectations regarding the self, other people, and self–other interactions. The C/I model also shifts the locus of stability in dependency from surface situational responding to underlying personality beliefs in thought and motive. Although the behaviors of dependent persons vary considerably from situation to situation, the dependent person's core beliefs (a perception of oneself as powerless and ineffectual) and motives (a desire to strengthen relationships with protectors and caregivers) remain constant. In many situations, dependent patients are passive and compliant, currying favor by acquiescing to others' expectations. That is typically their preferred approach. In other situations (for example, when threatened with relationship disruption or when competing with colleagues for the approval of a supervisor at work), dependent patients can become quite assertive, using whatever behaviors seem necessary to ensure they are not rejected or abandoned. The dependent patient's more active strategies include everything from dramatic emotional displays intended to elicit sympathy from the practitioner, to suicidal gestures (or even serious suicide attempts) aimed at preventing termination of the therapeutic relationship and compelling the clinician to attend to their needs.

Adaptive and Maladaptive Dependency

Psychologists have found that there are substantial differences in the degree to which people express underlying dependency needs in adaptive versus maladaptive ways. Research suggests that in contrast to maladaptive expressions of dependency (which are characterized by intense, unmodulated dependency strivings exhibited across a broad range of situations), more adaptive manifestations are characterized by dependency strivings that, even when strong, are exhibited selectively (i.e., in some contexts but not others) and flexibly (i.e., in situation-appropriate ways). People with a healthy dependent personality orientation show greater insight into their dependency needs, better social skills, more effective impulse control, greater cognitive complexity, and a more mature defense and coping style than do unhealthy dependent persons.[21]

Given the differential impact of unhealthy and healthy expressions of dependency on psychological adjustment and interpersonal behavior, researchers have begun to develop measures that yield separate scores for healthy and unhealthy manifestations of dependency; the most widely used and well-validated measure of healthy and unhealthy dependency is the Relationship Profile Test (RPT).[21] Table 23.2, p. 576 summarizes areas wherein patients who score high on the RPT Destructive Overdependence and Healthy Dependency scale differ (see Abuin & Rivera,[33] Bornstein et al.,[34]; Denckla et al.,[35] Haggerty et al.,[36] Huprich et al.,[37] and Porcerelli et al.[38] for relevant findings). Studies using the RPT confirm that the healthy and unhealthy expressions of dependency summarized in Table 23.2, p. 576 have enduring trait-like qualities, with individual differences in the adaptive versus maladaptive expression of dependency being stable over extended periods in adolescents and adults.

Table 23.2. Contrasting Dynamics of Maladaptive and Adaptive Dependency

Domain	Maladaptive Dependency	Adaptive Dependency
Self-Concept	Separate/Isolated	Relational/Interdependent
Attachment Style	High abandonment fear Anxious/ insecure attachment	Low abandonment fear Secure attachment
Defense Style	Immature/Maladaptive Inflexible	Mature/Adaptive Flexible
Core Personality	High neuroticism	Low neuroticism
Traits	Low extraversion	High extraversion
	Low conscientiousness	High conscientiousness
Alexithymia	High	Low
Affect Regulation	Poor	Good
Resilience Following Relationship Disruption	Weak	Strong
Empathy	Low (rigid self-focus)	High (self- and other-focus)
Well-Being/	Low life satisfaction	High life satisfaction
Quality of Life	Poor relations with parents	Good relations with parents
	Poor self-care	Good self-care
	Low baseline distress	High baseline distress
Risk for Victimization	High	Low
Relations with Health	Frequent requests for help	Adaptive help-seeking
Care Providers	High provider ambivalence	Positive provider attitude

Case Formulation

As Christon et al.[39] noted, the objective of case formulation is to develop "a complete picture of a client by collecting data that are used to generate hypotheses about the causes, antecedents, and maintaining influences for an individual client's problems within a biopsychosocial context."[39(p. 36)] A useful case conceptualization draws upon multiple data sources, integrating the patient's self-reports with clinical observation and inference; psychological test data, archival information (e.g., school records), and reports of knowledgeable informants may enhance case formulation by providing additional, sometimes contrasting, perspectives. Although writers tend to focus on the importance of case formulation in treatment planning, emphasizing its use at the outset of treatment, it is important to conceptualize case formulation as an ongoing process; it is never static, but ever changing. A case formulation should evolve over the course of therapy as the clinician learns more about the patient, and as the patient responds (or fails to respond) to treatment.

Case formulation creates a context for developing and refining treatment goals. In clinical work with dependent patients, a central issue concerns how best to address problematic dependent behaviors. Traditionally, clinical work with dependent patients has emphasized reducing problematic dependency and helping the patient function more autonomously in their personal and professional relationships. However, for some dependent patients, a more realistic and achievable goal is to promote healthy dependency, and help the patient express dependency needs in a way that is more likely to lead to positive outcomes, with fewer relationship conflicts and disruptions. Bockian[10] and

Bornstein[3,16] provided detailed guidelines for ameliorating problematic dependency and strengthening healthy dependency in inpatient and outpatient settings (review the contrasting manifestations of maladaptive and adaptive dependency summarized in Table 23.2, p. 576).

Treatment Challenges

Treatment challenges in clinical work with highly dependent patients include addressing resistance, and risk for harm to self and others. As the dependent patient becomes increasingly attached to the therapist, anxiety regarding rejection and abandonment increase, and behaviors designed to minimize the possibility of relationship disruption begin to dominate and interfere with therapeutic progress. Dependency-related resistance is not limited to the patient, as it can also originate in the therapist. The therapist may fear that the patient's dependency will become increasingly intense over time (the "fantasy of insatiability") and that the patient's dependency will make termination impossible, so therapy can never end (the "fantasy of permanence"). If not managed properly, the patient's and therapist's fears may feed upon each other and become exacerbated as therapy progresses: The patient becomes increasingly anxious about the risks and responsibilities of autonomous functioning, and the therapist becomes increasingly anxious regarding the negative impact of the patient's dependency, fearing that they will be overwhelmed by the patient's insatiable neediness.

One way to prevent dependency-related fears from undermining treatment is to explore the patient's transference reaction and the therapist's countertransference response. Common transference patterns in dependent patients include idealization (maintained through denial of therapist flaws and imperfections); possessiveness (which may have a strong narcissistic component or involve feelings of jealousy and possessiveness); and projective identification (wherein the patient unconsciously adopts the therapist's language and mannerisms in order to secure the attachment). Common countertransference responses include frustration at the patient's insatiable neediness; hidden hostility (sometimes accompanied by passive-aggressive acting out); overindulgence (ostensibly to protect the "fragile" patient); and pleasurable feelings of power and omnipotence (which can, on occasion, lead to exploitation or abuse). Table 23.3 (see p. 578) summarizes key areas of risk for harm to self and others in dependent patients.

As Table 23.3 (see p. 578) shows, these risk-management challenges can be grouped into two domains, with two variants within each domain. Table 23.3 (see p. 578) also describes key precipitants and dynamics of each risk factor. Additional information regarding suicide and parasuicide in dependent patients is provided by Bornstein[16] and Bornstein and O'Neill[40]; information regarding dependency as a factor in partner and child abuse is provided by Bornstein[4] and Kane and Bornstein.[41]

Psychosocial and Pharmacological Interventions

During the past century, there has been a tremendous amount of writing on psychosocial treatment options for dependent patients. Clinical trials have assessed the effectiveness of different forms of psychotherapy in altering dependency-related responding, employing a broad array of outcome measures. The majority of studies have examined

Table 23.3. Risk Management Challenges in Dependent Patients

Domain of Risk	Key Challenges and Vulnerabilities
Self-Harm	
Parasuicide	Increased risk for parasuicide as a strategy for communicating distress and precluding abandonment, often precipitated by relationship conflict or disruption; most common in highly dependent patients with comorbid borderline pathology.
Suicide	Increased risk for suicide, typically precipitated by relationship disruption; dependent patients with comorbid depression are at highest risk.
Harm to Others	
Partner Abuse	High levels of interpersonal/trait dependency are associated with increased risk for perpetration of partner abuse in men, typically precipitated by the man's belief that their partner may abandon them; high levels of DPD are not linked with partner abuse.
Child Abuse	High levels of interpersonal/trait dependency and DPD are associated with increased risk for child abuse in both women and men; the precipitants of dependency-related child abuse have not been documented conclusively.

Note. The absence an association between DPD and partner abuse is likely due to the emphasis on passive features of dependency in the DSM-5 and ICD-10 DPD diagnostic criteria.[4]

the efficacy of insight-oriented therapy and cognitive therapy, and findings generally support the effectiveness of both approaches in ameliorating features of problematic dependency.[3,16] Researchers have also explored the effectiveness of mindfulness-based treatment[42] and clarification-oriented therapy,[43] although additional data are needed to evaluate these interventions.

In addition to psychosocial treatments, about a dozen controlled clinical trials have examined the effectiveness of pharmacological interventions for high levels of interpersonal dependency and DPD. Virtually all controlled clinical trials in this area have focused on tricyclic antidepressants or selective serotonin reuptake inhibitors (SSRIs). Table 23.4 (see p. 579) summarizes the effectiveness of major psychosocial and pharmacological treatment approaches, using Strength of Recommendation Taxonomy (SORT) guidelines.[44]

Psychodynamic Treatment

Psychodynamic treatment models have become increasingly diverse in recent years, incorporating ideas and findings from an array of domains outside psychoanalysis. Despite this diversity, psychodynamic treatment approaches share a core assumption that many psychological symptoms and disorders (including DPD) are rooted in unconscious conflicts, which take two general forms. Some conflicts reflect clashes between incompatible beliefs, fears, wishes, and urges (e.g., a wish to be nurtured and cared for versus an urge to be autonomous and self-reliant). Other unconscious conflicts emerge as compromise formations—the disguised, distorted end products of underlying impulses and defenses against those impulses (e.g., a counterdependent stance that

Table 23.4 Evidence-Based Ratings for Effectiveness of Psychosocial and Pharmacological
Treatments for Pathological Dependency

Treatment	Outcome Measure/Criteria	LOE	SORT
Short-Term Cognitive Therapy	Reduction in self-reported dependency and DPD symptom levels	3	A
Long-Term Psychodynamic Treatment	Reduction in self-reported dependency and therapist ratings of patient dependency	2	B
Tricyclic Antidepressants	Reduction in self-reported dependency	2	B
Selective Serotonin Reuptake Inhibitors	Reduction in self-reported dependency and DPD symptom levels	2	B

Key: Levels of Evidence; Strength of recommendation taxonomy (SORT)*
Level of Evidence A: Good quality patient-oriented evidence.

Level of Evidence B: Limited quality patient-oriented evidence

Level of Evidence C: Based on consensus, usual practice, opinion, disease-oriented evidence, or case series for studies of diagnosis

*Ebell MH, Siwek J, Weiss BD, Woolf SH, Susman J, Ewigman B, Bowman M. Simplifying the language of evidence to improve patient care. *J Fam Pract.* 2004 Feb 1;53(2):111–120.

Level I: Systematic review or meta-analysis of randomized controlled trials

Level II: Randomized controlled trial

Level III: Non-randomized controlled, cohort/follow-up studies

Level IV: Case series or case control

Level V: Mechanism based reasoning

Center for Evidenced based Medicine

https://www.cebm.ox.ac.uk/resources/levels-of-evidence/ocebm-levels-of-evidence

prevents threatening dependent urges from emerging into consciousness). The concept of unconscious conflict is useful in understanding the dynamics of many PDs, and it is particularly relevant for DPD. The myriad rules and restrictions of mid- to late childhood, coupled with society's expectation of increased self-reliance, almost invariably cause girls and boys in individualistic Western cultures to experience some degree of ambivalence regarding dependency, invoking an array of defenses such as denial and reaction formation to manage "unacceptable" dependency-related urges (see Spivak[49] for a discussion of defensive processes that may promote the converse of excessive dependency, "counter-dependency.")

The aim of psychoanalytic therapy with dependent patients is not to ameliorate dependency-related conflicts but to make them accessible to consciousness where they can be examined critically and acted upon mindfully. Thus, one goal of psychoanalytic treatment for problematic dependency is insight: increased awareness of dependency-related thoughts, feelings, and motives that previously operated outside of awareness or on the fringes of consciousness. For many dependent patients, especially those with strong unacknowledged dependency needs, insight is a prerequisite, although insufficient, to create therapeutic change. Although insight by definition must precede working through (that is, the process of applying newfound insights to current relationships), these tasks are not separate but synergistic: Insight is necessary for working through to begin; but as working through proceeds, patients may gain increased insight as well. For most patients, this means moving beyond superficial awareness of how their dependency needs have affected past and present relationships to a more nuanced understanding of how these relationships have influenced (and in some instances, helped propagate) their dependency-related feelings, motives, and fears.[46]

Cognitive Treatment

In contrast to psychodynamic treatment models, which focus on increasing the patient's insight and self-awareness, cognitive approaches share an emphasis on effecting positive change by altering the patient's characteristic manner of thinking about, perceiving, and interpreting the world. To do this, cognitive therapists focus on the dependent patient's *maladaptive schemas*: their self-defeating beliefs about the self and other people (e.g., the belief that disruption of an important relationship will have catastrophic effects).[50,51] In dependent patients these maladaptive schemas can lead them to doubt their abilities, denigrate their skills, and exaggerate the imagined consequences of less-than-perfect performance.[15] Maladaptive schemas not only decrease the dependent patient's self-esteem and increase anxiety, but they also lead to an array of cognitive distortions that strengthen the patient's preexisting negative views (e.g., a perception of oneself as weak and ineffectual; the belief that other people are comparatively confident and competent).

A primary goal of cognitive therapy with dependent patients is *cognitive restructuring*: altering dysfunctional thought patterns that foster self-defeating dependent behavior. Cognitive restructuring often focuses on strengthening the dependent patient's self-efficacy beliefs regarding how much control they have over their environment and their relationships. As part of this process, the therapist tries to help the patient detoxify flawed performance (for example, a less-than-stellar evaluation at work). If the patient can learn to perceive minor errors for what they are, rather than magnifying them into catastrophes, then the patient can respond with less anxiety to adequate but imperfect efforts. In short, the therapist helps the patient practice alternative ways of interpreting negative feedback, so the impact of everyday criticism is less overwhelming.[52]

Psychopharmacological Interventions

Many dependent patients enter outpatient therapy having already begun a regimen of psychotropic medication, often initiated by their primary care physician. For some patients, medication is used as an adjunct to traditional psychotherapy to manage some of the more intrusive symptoms often associated with high levels of interpersonal dependency and DPD (e.g., severe depression or debilitating anxiety). In inpatient settings, dependent psychiatric patients tend to receive more medication prescriptions than do nondependent patients with similar demographic and diagnostic profiles. It may be that the increased number of psychotropic medications received by dependent patients reflects increased symptom severity in these patients (after all, long-standing psychological or physical difficulties often lead to increases in expressed dependency). Alternatively, the dependent patient's generalized help-seeking tendencies may cause physicians to prescribe medications more frequently in response to the patient's persistent complaints. Whatever the cause of dependent patients' increased medication use, it is important that the clinician be aware of the impact of drug treatment on dependent responding.

Although the results of studies examining the efficacy of psychotropic medication in ameliorating problematic dependency and symptoms of DPD have been somewhat inconsistent, findings suggest that both tricyclic antidepressants and SSRIs can diminish self-reported dependency levels in inpatients and outpatients.[45–48] These results dovetail with those of myriad investigations that have shown that dependency and depression levels covary, with dependency levels increasing as depression worsens and decreasing as depression remits.[10] Thus, it may be that the observed effects of antidepressant medications on patients' dependency levels are mediated in part by changes in mood.

Maximizing Treatment Efficacy

Different patients require different interventions, and flexibility on the part of the therapist is essential. In general, dependent patients with significant comorbid character pathology may initially benefit most from more structured problem-focused cognitive interventions, whereas higher-functioning patients often do best in insight-oriented psychodynamic treatment. Clinicians need to keep in mind that different treatment strategies may be required for patients whose problematic dependency preceded the onset of other syndromes and those whose dependency was secondary to one or more clinical disorders (e.g., depression).

It may also be useful for the clinician to help the patient express dependency needs in healthier, more adaptive ways. For example, therapists can reframe things so that the patient can think about asking for help as a way of learning to cope, rather than fleeing responsibility. Therapists, like patients, tend to have many negative stereotypes regarding leaning on others for guidance and support. As a result, in the process of fostering autonomy in dependent patients, many clinicians inadvertently go too far, and actually move the patient toward inflexible independence. Rather than aiming for rigid autonomy, a relationship-facilitating blend of autonomy and connectedness, coupled with situation-appropriate help- and support-seeking, should be a central goal of therapeutic work with dependent patients. Table 23.5 (see p. 582) summarizes five in-session therapeutic strategies that have proven useful in clinical work with dependent patients. As Table 23.5 (see p. 582) shows, these interventions are not tied to a single therapeutic modality, but may be useful for the therapist's overarching therapeutic framework. Detailed discussions of these and other therapeutic strategies are provided by Blatt and Ford,[46] Bornstein,[3,16] Kantor,[53] McClintock et al.,[42] Overholser and Fine,[52] and Sascher and Kramer.[43]

It is important for the clinician using psychosocial interventions to distinguish patients whose problematic dependency preceded the onset of other disorders from those whose dependency was secondary to one or more clinical syndromes (like depression), so interventions can be properly targeted. It is also important for the clinician using psychotropic medications to determine whether the focus of drug treatment is on reducing problematic dependent behavior or symptoms indirectly related to the patient's dependency (like agoraphobia). Given the dependent patient's inclination to ask for help, coupled with the clinician's fears about being overwhelmed by the dependent patient's neediness and insecurity, it is also important that the clinician be wary of over-prescribing psychotropic medication as a way of distancing him- or herself from the patient.

Table 23.5. Helpful In-Session Therapeutic Strategies for Dependent Patients

Treatment Issue/Focus	Strategy
Dysfunctional Relationship Patterns	Explore key relationships from the patient's past that encouraged and reinforced dependent behavior; determine whether similar patterns occur in present relationships
Low Self-Esteem	Examine the patient's helpless self-concept, the key cognitive element of maladaptive dependency and DPD (asking the patient to write an open-ended self-description can be useful in this regard)
Automatic Statements	Make explicit any self-denigrating statements that propagate the patient's feelings of helplessness and vulnerability; challenge these statements as appropriate
Maladaptive Behavior	Help the patient gain insight into the ways they express dependency needs in different situations; explore more flexible, adaptive ways that these needs could be expressed
Coping and Social Skills	Use in-session role-play and between-session homework assignments to help the patient build coping skills that enable them to function more autonomously

Integrative Treatment of Maladaptive Dependency: The Case of Bryce

Bryce is a 22-year-old Mexican-American male who sought out treatment to address his "many problems with family and personal concerns," including difficulty with sleep, procrastination, feelings of depression, and a "feeling that [he could] never do anything right and always need[ed] someone else to help." He reported a previous diagnosis of major depressive disorder, for which he began taking antidepressant medication two months prior (daily SSRI). At intake, Bryce received diagnoses of major depressive disorder and DPD; because his mood had steadily improved with medication, the primary goal of psychotherapy was to gain a better understanding of his interpersonal problems and to work toward enhancing his self-esteem and reducing his self-reported overreliance on others.

Following intake, Bryce and the therapist agreed to meet for 12 sessions. The decision to set a firm termination date at the outset was guided by literature suggesting this boundary could help the patient gain insight into his sense of self as ineffective, and foster enactments of his dependency needs that could then be worked through in sessions within the context of the therapeutic relationship.[54,55] Exploration of Bryce's experience of the therapist setting a firm termination and his associated worries of abandonment assisted Bryce in recognizing his need to make long-term changes in self-efficacy and self-esteem. This acknowledgment initiated a shift toward Bryce engaging in a healthier, more adaptive expression of his underlying dependency needs. Simultaneous skills training helped the patient experience the value of autonomous behavior by offering early, independent behavioral skills (e.g., positive self-affirmations, problem-solving strategies) that he used to make small, immediate changes. Specifically, use of the Socratic method of questioning, instruction on using positive self-affirmations, and problem-solving training resulted in Bryce being more consciously aware of his strengths, and helped him learn how to identify and solve problems independently, which bolstered his sense of competence. At the same time, self-monitoring, self-evaluation, and self-reinforcement skills training allowed him to learn to control specific behaviors that were interfering with and undermining his autonomy (e.g., through self-monitoring, Bryce realized he often minimized his own abilities prior to asking others for help).

Soon thereafter, the focus of treatment shifted to a second element of the cognitive component of interpersonal dependency, Bryce's sense of self as weak and ineffective. Through exploration of the patient–therapist relationship, transference analysis, and continued implementation of cognitive techniques (e.g., self-monitoring, decentering), Bryce and the therapist clarified his impaired sense of self. The therapist then guided Bryce through self-reevaluation, asking him to evaluate how he felt about his sense of self and low self-esteem, which helped him adjust his self-appraisal process. Exploratory techniques, such as the use of Socratic questioning, concurrently offered Bryce opportunities to identify specific aspects of his fears of abandonment and negative self-evaluation. It was only after these fears were made explicit within the therapist–patient dyad that they could be challenged directly, and cognitive and affective changes generalized beyond therapy. Although Bryce was now more aware of his maladaptive dependency strivings, there was still a need to modify his dependent behavior (e.g., his continued avoidance of potential conflict, interpersonal submissiveness, and hesitance to take appropriate risks in his life).

Both psychodynamic and cognitive treatment modalities aim to promote the dependent patient's autonomy by helping the patient take a more active stance within the treatment, which is then extended beyond the therapeutic milieu.[52] In addition to teaching new behavioral skills and working within sessions to help Bryce develop a capacity for healthy dependency, several intervention strategies (e.g., problem-solving training) were utilized to help Bryce avoid self-defeating thoughts that would interfere with autonomous functioning. After 10 sessions, Bryce was able to increase his capacity to adopt a more active stance in interpersonal relations, become more willing to engage in autonomous behavior, and shift his self-perception toward a view of himself as more competent and effective. The final two sessions were devoted to relapse prevention, preparation for termination, and helping Bryce recognize the challenges that would arise after therapy had ended.

Conclusion

DPD is common in outpatient and inpatient treatment settings. At some point, all mental health professionals will work with patients whose difficulties are due in part to high levels of maladaptive dependency. Effective clinical work with dependent patients requires that the clinician incorporate three key principles into case conceptualization and treatment planning. First, contrary to clinical lore, dependent patients are not invariably passive and compliant but may sometimes be active and assertive. Second, patients have varying degrees of insight regarding their underlying dependency strivings; multi-method assessment of interpersonal dependency and DPD is crucial in illuminating these dynamics. Third, treatment need not focus exclusively on reducing dependent behavior, but may also aim to replace unhealthy manifestations of dependency with healthier, more adaptive expressions of dependency. With these principles as context, this chapter presents an integrative overview of interpersonal dependency and DPD, providing evidence-based guidelines for diagnosis, assessment, psychosocial and pharmacological treatment, and risk management. Review Box 23.1 (see p. 584) for relevant resources for patients, families, and clinicians.

Conflict of Interest/Disclosure: The authors of this chapter have no financial conflicts and nothing to disclose.

Box 23.1 Resources for Patients, Families, and Clinicians

Resources for Patients and Families

- Bornstein RF, Languirand MA. *Healthy Dependency: Leaning on Others Without Losing Yourself.* NY: Newmarket Press; 2003. This offers a patient-friendly discussion of the causes and consequences of maladaptive dependency, along with recommendations for strengthening healthy dependency: the ability to ask for help and support in ways that facilitate (rather than impede) autonomous functioning.
- Harvard Mental Health Letter: Dependent Personality Disorder. https://www.health.harvard.edu/newsletter_article/Dependent_personality_disorder. The Harvard Mental Health Letter online overview of DPD is also very informative for patients and their families.

Note: Beyond these, there are few evidence-based resources available for patients and family members. We recommend against obtaining books and other resources that discuss codependency and its consequences, as most are based on conjecture rather than evidence.

Resources for Clinicians

- Bornstein RF. *The Dependent Patient: A Practitioner's Guide.* Washington, DC: American Psychological Association; 2005. This presents a detailed, evidence-based overview of the intra- and interpersonal dynamics of pathological dependency, along with guidelines for diagnosis, assessment, and treatment.
- Nichols WC. Integrative marital and family treatment of dependent personality disorders. In: MacFarlane M, ed. *Family Treatment of Personality Disorders: Advances in Clinical Practice.* Binghamton, NY: Haworth Family Practice Press; 2004:173–204. Nichols's chapter discusses effective strategies for marital and family therapy involving dependent patients.
- Cleveland Clinic guide to Dependent Personality Disorder. https://my.clevelandclinic.org/health/diseases/9783-dependent-personality-disorder#:~:text=Dependentpercent20personalitypercent20disorderpercent20(DPD)percent20is,Dependentpercent20Personalitypercent20Disorderpercent20Menu. A thorough practitioner-focused review of evidence-based DPD treatments, along with discussion of strategies for prevention and risk management.
- PsychCentral: Dependent Personality Disorder. https://psychcentral.com/disorders/dependent-personality-disorder/symptoms/. An excellent clinician-friendly overview of DPD symptoms and dynamics, as well as early antecedents and predictors of pathological dependency.

References

1. *Diagnostic and Statistical Manual of Mental Disorders: DSM-5*. Washington, DC: American Psychiatric Association; 2013.

2. Bornstein RF. Dependent personality disorder: effective time-limited therapy. *Curr Psychiatry*. 2007;6;37–45.

3. Bornstein RF. From dysfunction to adaptation: an interactionist model of dependency. *Ann Rev Clin Psychol*. 2012;8;291–316.

4. Bornstein RF. Synergistic dependencies in partner and elder abuse. *Am Psychologist*. 2019;74;713–724.

5. Disney KL. Dependent personality disorder: a critical review. *Clin Psychol Rev*. 2013; 33:1184–1196.

6. Bornstein RF. Dependent personality disorder. In: Widiger TA, ed. *The Oxford Handbook of Personality Disorders*. 2nd ed. NY: Oxford University Press; 2020:505–526.

7. Baltes MM. *The Many Faces of Dependency in Old Age*. Cambridge, UK: Cambridge University Press; 1996.

8. *International Classification of Diseases, 10th edition (ICD–10)*. Geneva, Switzerland: World Health Organization; 2002.

9. Bach B, First MB. Application of the ICD-11 classification of personality disorders. *BMC Psychiatry*. 2018;18:351.

10. Bockian N. Depression in dependent personality disorder. In: Bockian N, ed. *Personality-guided Therapy for Depression*. Washington, DC: American Psychological Association; 2006:227–246.

11. Ng HM, Bornstein RF. Comorbidity of dependent personality disorder and anxiety disorders: a meta-analytic review. 2005;*Clin Psychol*. 12:395–406.

12. Blatt SJ, Rounsaville B, Eyre SL, Wilber C. The psychodynamics of opiate addiction. *J Nerv Ment Dis*. 1994;172:342–352.

13. Bornstein RF. A meta-analysis of the dependency-eating disorders relationship: Strength, specificity, and temporal stability. *J Psychopathol Behav Assess*. 2001;23:151–162.

14. Borge F, Hoffart A, Sexton H, et al. Pre-treatment predictors and in-treatment factors associated with change in avoidant and dependent personality disorder traits among patients with social phobia. *Clin Psychol Psychother*. 2010;17:87–99.

15. Bornstein RF. An interactionist perspective on interpersonal dependency. *Curr Dir Psychol Sci*. 2011;20;124–128.

16. Bornstein RF. *The Dependent Patient: A Practitioner's Guide*. Washington, DC: American Psychological Association; 2005.

17. First MB, Williams JBW, Benjamin LS, Spitzer RL. *User's Guide for the SCID-5-PD (Structured Clinical Interview for DSM-5 Personality Disorder)*. Arlington, VA: American Psychiatric Association; 2015.

18. Gore WL, Presnall JR, Miller JD, Lynam DR, Widiger TA. A five-factor model of dependent personality traits. *J Pers Assess*. 2012;94:488–499.

19. Krueger RF, Derringer J, Markon KE, Watson D, Skodol AE. Initial construction of a maladaptive personality trait model and inventory for DSM-5. *Psychol Med*. 2012;42:1879–1890.

20. Hirschfeld RMA, Klerman GL, Gough HG, Barrett J, Korchin SJ, Chodoff P. A measure of interpersonal dependency. *J Pers Assess*. 1977;41:610–618.

21. Bornstein RF, Languirand MA. *Healthy Dependency: Leaning on Others Without Losing Yourself*. NY: Newmarket Press; 2003.

22. Loranger AW, Sartorius N, Andreoli A, et al. The International Personality Disorder Examination. *Arch Gen Psychiatry*. 1994;51:215–224.

23. Meyer GJ, Viglione DJ, Mihura JL, Erard RE, Erdberg P. *Rorschach Performance Assessment System: Administration, Coding, Interpretation, and Technical Manual*. Toledo, OH: Rorschach Performance Assessment System; 2011.

24. Rogers R. Standardizing DSM–IV diagnoses: The clinical applications of structured interviews. *J Pers Assess*. 2003;81:220–225.

25. McClelland DC, Koestner R, Weinberger J. How do self-attributed and implicit motives differ? *Psychol Rev*. 1989;96:690–702.

26. Bornstein RF, Hopwood CJ. Evidence based assessment of interpersonal dependency. *Prof Psychol: Res Pr*. 2017;48;251–258.

27. Natoli AP, Bornstein RF. Integrative assessment of interpersonal dependency: Contrasting sex differences in response patterns on self-attributed and implicit measures. *J Projective Psychol Ment Health*. 2011;24: 26–33.

28. Morey LC. *Personality Assessment Inventory Professional Manual*. 2nd ed. Lutz, FL: Psychological Assessment Resources; 2007.

29. Gjerde LC, Czajkowski N, Røysamb E, et al. The heritability of avoidant and dependent personality disorder assessed by personal interview and questionnaire. *Acta Psychiatr Scand*. 2012;126:448–457.

30. McCranie EW, Bass JD. Childhood family antecedents of dependency and self-criticism. *J Abnorm Psychol*. 1984;93:3–8.

31. Head SB, Baker JD, Williamson DA. Family environment characteristics and dependent personality disorder. *J Pers Disord*. 1991;5:256–263.

32. Callies IT, Sieberer M, Machleidt W, Ziegenbein M. Personality disorders in a cross-cultural perspective: impact of culture and migration on diagnosis and etiological aspects. *Curr Psychiatry Rev*. 2018;4:39–47.

33. Abuin MR, Rivera L. Dependency, detachment, and psychopathology in a nonclinical sample: general relations and gender differences. 2015;*Clinica Salud*.2:65–72.

34. Bornstein RF, Languirand MA, Geiselman KJ, et al. Construct validity of the Relationship Profile Test: a self-report measure of dependency-detachment. *J Pers Assess*. 2003;80:64–74.

35. Denckla CA, Bornstein RF, Mancini AD, Bonanno GA. Extending the construct validity of dependency among conjugally bereaved adults. *Assessment*, 2015;22:385–393.

36. Haggerty G, Blake M, Siefert CJ. Convergent and divergent validity of the Relationship Profile Test: investigating the relationship with attachment, interpersonal distress, and psychological health. 2010;*J Clin Psychol*. 66:1–16.

37. Huprich SK, Hsiao WC, Porcerelli JH, Bornstein RF, Markova T. Expanding the construct validity of the Relationship Profile Test: associations with physical health and anaclitic and introjective traits. *Assessment*. 17:81–88;2010.

38. Porcerelli JH, Bornstein RF, Markova T, Huprich SK. Physical health correlates of patholog-
    ical and healthy dependency in urban women. *J Nervous Ment Dis.* 2009;197:761–765.

39. Christon LM, McLeod BD, Jensen-Doss A. Evidence based assessment meets evidence-
    based treatment: an approach to science-informed case conceptualization. *Cog Behav Pract.*
    2015;22:36–48.

40. Bornstein RF, O'Neill RM. Dependency and suicidality in psychiatric inpatients. *J Clin
    Psychol.* 2000;56;463–473.

41. Kane FA, Bornstein RF. Unhealthy dependency in perpetrators and victims of child mal-
    treatment: a meta-analytic review. *J Clin Psychol.* 2018;74:867–882.

42. McClintock AS, Anderson T, Cranston S. Mindfulness therapy for maladaptive interper-
    sonal dependency: a preliminary randomized controlled trial. *Behav Ther.* 46: 2015;856–868.

43. Sasche R, Kramer U. Clarification-oriented therapy of dependent personality disorder. *J
    Contemp Psychother.* 2019;49:15–25.

44. Ebell MH, Siwek J, Weiss BD, et al. Strength of Recommendation Taxonomy (SORT):
    a patient-centered approach to grading evidence in the medical literature. *J Fam Prac.*
    2004;53:111–120.

45. Rathus JH, Sanderson WC, Miller AL, Wetzler S. Impact of personality functioning on
    cognitive-behavioral treatment of panic disorder: a preliminary report. *J Pers Disord.*
    1995;9:160–168.

46. Blatt SJ, Ford RQ. *Therapeutic Change: An Object Relations Perspective.* NY: Plenum
    Press; 1994.

47. Rector NA, Bagby RM, Segal ZV, Joffe RT, Levitt A. Self-criticism and dependency in de-
    pressed patients treated with cognitive therapy or pharmacotherapy. *Cog Ther Res.*
    2000;24:571–584.

48. Zaretsky AE, Fava M, Davidson KG, et al. Are dependency and self-criticism risk factors for
    major depressive disorder? *Can J Psychiatry.* 1997;42:291–297.

49. Spivak N. Subgrouping with psychiatric inpatients in group psychotherapy: linking depend-
    ency and counterdependency. *Int J Group Psychother.* 2008;58:231–252.

50. Lobbestael J, Van Vreezwijk MF, Arntz A. An empirical test of schema mode conceptualiza-
    tions in personality disorders, *Behav Res Ther.* 2008;46:854–860.

51. Nichols WC. Integrative marital and family treatment of dependent personality disor-
    ders. In: MacFarlane M, ed. *Family Treatment of Personality Disorders: Advances in Clinical
    Practice.* Binghamton, NY: Haworth Family Practice Press; 2004:173–204.

52. Overholser JC, Fine MA. Cognitive-behavioral treatment of excessive interpersonal de-
    pendency: a four-stage psychotherapy model. *J Cog Psychother.* 1994;8:55–70.

53. Kantor M. *Diagnosis and Treatment of the Personality Disorders.* St. Louis, MO: Ishiyaku
    EuroAmerica; 1992.

54. Bornstein RF, Bowen RF. Dependency in psychotherapy: toward an integrated treatment ap-
    proach. *Psychotherapy.* 1995;32:520–534.

55. Mann J. *Time-limited Psychotherapy.* Cambridge, MA: Harvard University Press; 1973.

24

Obsessive-compulsive Personality Disorder

Cynthia Playfair

Key Points

- Obsessive-compulsive personality disorder (OCPD) is characterized by pre-occupation with perfectionism, orderliness, and control beginning by young adulthood with other symptoms including: preoccupation with details; excessive devotion to work; over-conscientiousness; fastidiousness; inflexibility/rigidity; stubbornness; difficulty delegating; hoarding; and stinginess.
- OCPD is one of the most common personality disorders. While it can negatively impact the quality of life, it is thought to cause less impairment when compared with other personality disorders.
- OCPD is highly comorbid, often co-occurring and clinically confused with obsessive-compulsive disorder.
- OCPD is also commonly associated with hoarding disorder, major depressive disorder, anxiety disorder, body dysmorphic disorder/eating disorders, autism spectrum disorders, alcohol abuse/dependence, and other personality disorders.
- Studies and observed patterns lend to an etiologic model consistent with an additive genetic effect and unique environmental factors.
- A common clinical psychodynamic in OCPD is outward deference and compliance with the therapist, who is a perceived authority figure, while the treatment process is covertly undermined by unconscious resistance, covert aggression, and avoidance of emotion. The therapist often feels flummoxed, vacillating between countertransference states of numbness and frustration.
- While there is no empirically validated standard for the treatment of OCPD, psychodynamic psychotherapy or CBT are the treatment of choice. Pharmacological treatment is considered adjunctive.

Introduction

Case Vignette

At a party you meet an impeccably dressed man who tells you he is an aerodynamics engineer. He impresses you with extensive knowledge about a recent airplane crash. In a detailed and intellectual, emotionless manner, he describes why the engine failed, how the captain responded, and what the passengers endured for five minutes before the impact. You anxiously comment on the tragedy, but he cuts you off and continues. You excuse yourself, confused that you feel more irritated than sad.

Brief Description of Obsessive-compulsive Personality Disorder

Wilhelm Reich described people with severe obsessive character as being like "living machines," who use thought and action to avoid emotion.[1] Many obsessional people are accomplished, well-adjusted, and enrich the lives of others. Obsessionality exists on a continuum from healthy to neurotic personality organization to borderline personality organization. Individuals with obsessive-compulsive personality disorder (OCPD), not simply those with traits, struggle with their concept of self and others, rigidly adhering to orderliness, perfectionism, and control, at the expense of flexibility, openness, and efficiency.[2] This often results in loss of the meaning or point of the activity altogether. This chapter will focus on an in-depth understanding of OCPD and its treatment.

Diagnostic History of OCPD

The first *Diagnostic and Statistical Manual* (DSM) described Compulsive Personality,[3] which focused on obsessive concern with high standards.[2] DSM-II changed the name to OCPD and added the term "anankastic personality," a historical term that specifically denotes obsessive-compulsiveness, to help differentiate OCPD from obsessive-compulsive disorder (OCD).[3] DSM-III maintained the name OCPD, adding the criteria of reduced emotional warmth and perfectionism.[4] DSM-III-R specified the need for four criteria, adding preoccupation with details, lack of generosity, and hoarding.[5] DSM-IV required that a patient meet at least four of eight criteria,[6] while the DSM-5 requires five criteria.[7] As the diagnostic criteria change, statistical outcome data and their relevance also change.

DSM-5

The DSM-5 places OCPD in the Cluster C (fearful) category of personality disorders. It is defined as a preoccupation with perfectionism, orderliness, and control beginning by young adulthood, with five or more of eight symptoms present, including the preoccupation with details, perfectionism, excessive devotion to work, over-conscientiousness, rigidity and stubbornness, difficulty delegating, hoarding, and stinginess.[2]

The categorical, criterion-based approach of the DSM is an efficient tool for clinical diagnosis. However, the DSM classification system not convey the dimensionality and severity of personality disorders, nor does it account for the predominance or hierarchy of traits. The DSM-5, in Section III on Emerging Measures and Models, added an alternative dimensional hybrid model for diagnosis of personality disorders aimed at addressing shortcomings of the categorical model.

ICD-11

The upcoming International Classification of Diseases-11 (ICD-11) system released by The World Health Organization aims to capture the dimensional aspects of character structure by assessing the severity of suffering (mild, moderate, or severe) and five prominent personality traits: negative affectivity, detachment, disinhibition, antagonism, and anankastia (obsessive-compulsiveness). The ICD-11 was found superior to the DSM-5 in capturing OCPD,[8] likely because obsessive-compulsiveness is one of the trait domains measured.

Epidemiology of OCPD

OCPD is one of the most common personality disorders in the general population, with estimates between 2.1–7.9 percent.[3] OCPD has a lifetime prevalence of 7.8 percent, has no difference in prevalence by gender, income, marital status, or urbanicity, is more common in older and less educated individuals, and is significantly less common in Asians and Hispanics.[9] It is the second most common personality disorder in the general population and inpatient samples,[10] the third most common in outpatient samples,[11] with a steep rise to 26 percent in a clinical sample of Hispanic males.[12] Among patients with a depressive disorder, 30.8 percent suffer from OCPD,[13] and it is one of the highest risk factors for depressive relapse.[14]

OCPD causes long-standing disability and a decrease in life quality, psychosocial functioning,[15] and employment.[16] OCPD has adverse prognostic effects on OCD, agoraphobia, and anxiety disorders.[17] However, OCPD causes less functional impairment as compared with other personality disorders.[18] Interestingly, a community sample found compulsive traits associated with higher status and wealth levels, suggesting a wide range of functioning.[12]

Comorbidity with OCPD

OCPD and OCD

Mixed speculation about the relationship between OCPD and OCD suggests inheritance links,[19] predisposition,[20] and comorbidity,[15] while other data support coincidental co-occurrence. Symptom overlap and the use of different diagnostic criteria distorts statistics. The DSM-5 diagnostic criteria for OCD include intrusive obsessions and compulsions experienced as time-consuming, distressing, or impairing, with an onset in the late teens or early twenties. The thoughts or behaviors are disturbing and ego-dystonic, sometimes described as alien-like, as if injected into one's mind. Unlike psychotic disorders, people with OCD usually have insight (denoted as a specifier in DSM-5) that the obsessions or related compulsions do not have a meaningful purpose, and they are not seen as reality-based.

Comorbidity with Other Associated Conditions

OCPD is highly comorbid with many disorders. In addition to OCD, comorbidities characterized by compulsive behaviors include hoarding disorder (HD),[21] body dysmorphic disorder,[22] eating disorders,[23] and disabling autism spectrum disorder (ASD).[24] HD is newly codified in DSM-5. There is a significant overlap of OCPD in OCD and HD, as depicted in Figure 24.1.[21]

These three disorders share the transdiagnostic trait of perfectionism. However, HD individuals are sentimentally attached to belongings, refusing to give them up. In contrast, OCPD individuals are frugal, while fear and relief of anxiety cause the OCD patient to clean excessively and organize their possessions.

A longitudinal study[25] found comorbidities with OCPD and major depressive disorder (75.8 percent), generalized anxiety disorder (29.4 percent), alcohol abuse/dependence (29.4 percent), anorexia (6.5 percent), and OCD (20.9 percent). OCPD is the most common personality disorder in bipolar affective disorder at 32.8 percent.[26] There is considerable overlap between OCPD and other personality disorders, as listed in Table 24.1 (see p. 593), which includes paranoid, schizotypal, avoidant, narcissistic, passive-aggressive, and dependent personality disorders.

Understanding OCPD

Historical Understanding

Freud described the developmental stages of the infant as oral, anal, and genital. He was the first to associate adult personality difficulties with struggles during childhood developmental phases. In 1908 he described that the obsessional personality style has its origins in the anal stage, developing during the childhood toilet-training years (age 18 months–3 years). Freud believed that control struggles between parent and child

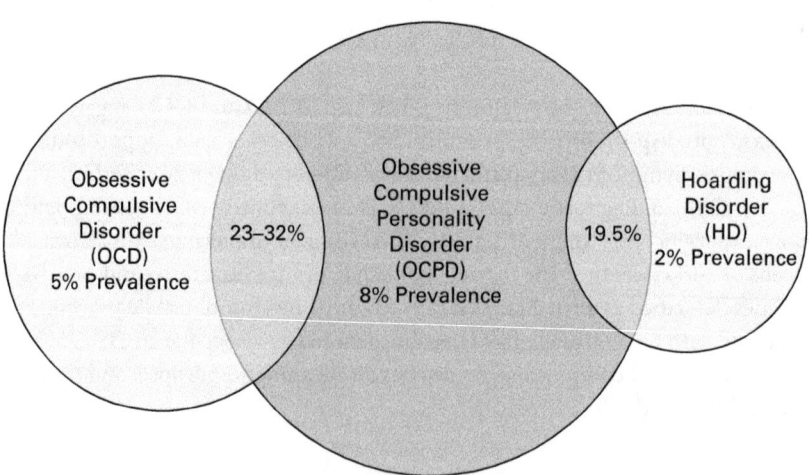

Figure 24.1. Estimates of Prevalence Rates in the General Population and Overlap of Occurrence of OCPD in OCD and HD[21]

Table 24.1. Overlap Between OCPD and Other Personality Disorders

Personality Disorder	Overlap with OCPD in percent
Paranoid	39%
Schizotypal	36%
Avoidant	35%
Narcissistic	32%
Passive-Aggressive	32%
Dependent	31%

contribute to the development of orderliness, parsimony, and obstinacy, which led to defiance, rage, and revengefulness.[27]

Many others have contributed to and expanded upon Freud's ideas about obsessional personality style. While not necessarily inconsistent with Freud, modern psychoanalytic theories progressed from a one-person model to a two-person model, the latter perhaps less pathologizing. In a one-person model, therapy focuses on the patient's distortions as a recapitulation of early child and parent struggles. In contrast, a two-person model explores the relationship between the therapist and patient, as it relates to their childhood but reoccurs in the here-and-now. Problems are contextualized in a relationship with another person rather than within a person. Furthermore, some difficulties are understood as co-created between patient and therapist, even if they are invited. During treatment, both patient and therapist are agents of change.

Biological Understanding

Moderate evidence suggests that cluster C personality disorders are heritable, and that OCPD is etiologically distinct from other cluster C disorders.[28] However, there is no evidence for shared sex or environmental effects.[28] Evidence of genetic links between OCPD and OCD are compelling; one study found OCPD more common in relatives of OCD probands as compared to relatives of control groups.[29] Another study found obsessional personality traits are elevated among relatives of anorexic probands, and found that these two disorders may have shared familial risk factors.[30] OCPD is increasingly conceptualized as a neurocognitive disorder; studies suggest enhanced visual acuity,[31] statistically smaller pineal gland volume compared with normals,[32] and an occurrence rate of 40 percent in Parkinson's disease.[33] OCPD has not yet been studied with systematic brain imaging.

Psychosocial Understanding

On the nurture side of things, patients with OCPD report significantly high parental overprotection and low parental care that likely impact adult attachment style.[34] Likewise, Sullivan suggested that obsessive-compulsive character style is related to a family system that emphasizes compliance and rules in exchange for acceptance and love.[35] Obsessive-compulsive individuals tend to be firstborn,[36] marry histrionic individuals,[37] and display anhedonic temperaments.[38] Sometimes, they present for the first time in midlife, turning on themselves, not having met idealized expectations. Shabad describes the obsessional as a "provocateur" who idealizes stoicism. Enduring chronic, frustrating childhood experiences, day after day, takes on the meaning of trauma and alters personality development.[39] Today, personality is viewed as multi-determined via genetics, early attachment experiences, trauma, family systems, social conditions like war and disease, and cultural influences like sexism and racism.

Theoretical Understanding

"Personality Lane," as seen in Figure 24.2, is a useful theoretical model for the early clinician to conceptualize and diagnose personality disorders. In this model, personality is understood along two dimensions: developmental (the y-axis), and internal or external preoccupation (the x-axis).

The boundary between self and other is established as one travels down the developmental timeline of "Personality Lane." Developmental deficits delineate points of departure from healthy development and distinguish different personality disorders. The development of the boundary between self and other is broken down into three overlapping phases. In the earliest phase, the infant identifies *self from non-self*, literally. Mother is experienced intrinsically, and then slowly as a unique entity. During the

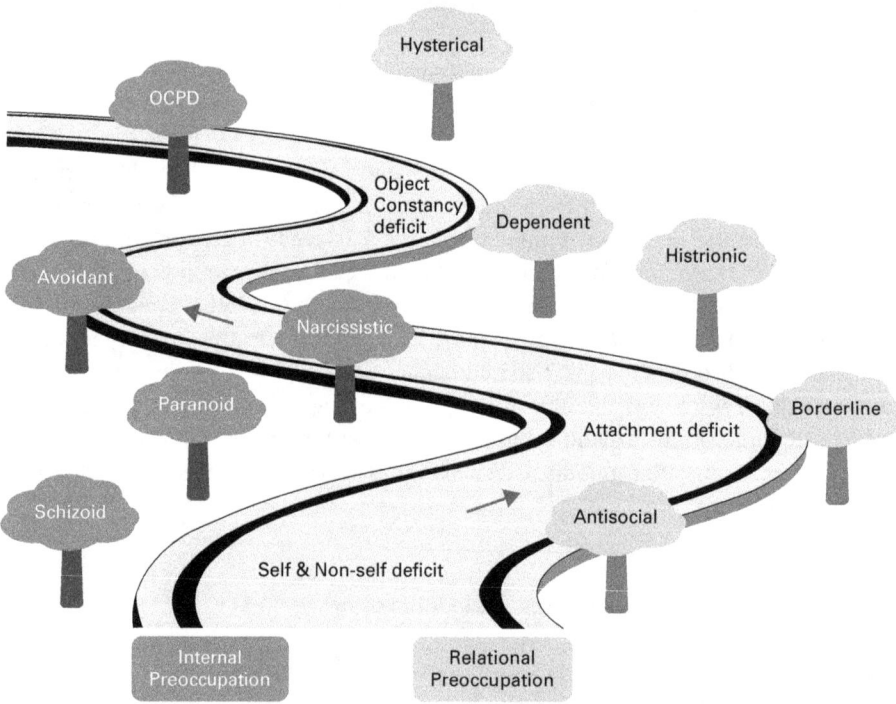

Figure 24.2. "Personality Lane"

second phase, *attachment*, the infant's connection with the mother grows, as does differentiation and autonomy. Lastly, with a safe emotional and physical base, toddlers venture away from mother and back again, until a stable internalized experience of mother is present in her absence. This third phase, culminates in *object constancy* (age 2–3 years), the capacity to know that the attachment with people can remain constant and intact despite separation, setbacks, and conflict. In summary, the severity and type of personality disorder may be a manifestation of an impingement or deficit, in the establishment and health of the boundary between self and other. If one proceeds down "Personality Lane" unimpeded, character disorders are less likely. Biological, interpersonal, and sociocultural influences impact the development of character traits, conceivably producing symptoms of more than one personality disorder in an individual; for example, a patient with OCPD might have narcissistic features if significant earlier attachment disruptions occur. A person without a personality disorder might also appear disordered when stressed.

Illustrating the second dimension, Blatt describes two divergent personality pathways.[40] On the left path, individuals are *internally preoccupied* (e.g., focused on their own thoughts, feelings, and behaviors). On the right path, individuals are *relationally or externally preoccupied* (e.g., excessively focused on interpersonal relationships or concerned with what others think of them). The left side of Figure 24.2 (see p. 594) shows personality disorders with internal preoccupation: schizoid, paranoid, narcissistic, avoidant, and OCPD. The right-side lists personality disorders with relational preoccupation or an overconcern with how people think about and treat them: antisocial, borderline, histrionic, dependent, and hysterical.

Patients with OCPD present at the borderline level of personality organization. They more often present with higher functioning, at the neurotic level of personality organization where self is differentiated from other; however, their internal preoccupation can disrupt healthy attachments. The attachment in the OCPD individual is characterized by remoteness throughout development of object constancy, resulting in (often unconscious) a sense of self as empty and inadequate.

To illustrate, a patient named Mike, whose therapist was running late, says, "I decided to use the time in the waiting room. I see you are overwhelmed, so I went ahead and wrote your check early for next month." This patient's insecurity caused him to feel undesired or even forgotten by the therapist. Instead of feeling annoyed at the therapist, Mike unconsciously projected his feelings of inadequacy into the therapist, implying that the therapist needed help functioning. In addition to being hostile, Mike was also expressing a wish to be liked by the therapist and see more of the therapist.

As treatment progresses for OCPD individuals, the feelings of inadequacy and emptiness become conscious, and depression may arise. The depression or dysthymia is melancholic, they don't mourn a person; instead, they mourn a part of themselves that never developed, the feeling and loving part. They often describe feeling dead inside, and that life feels meaningless, but they are uncertain of what's missing. Even the negative aspects of life become incorporated as though a part of oneself. When confronted with the difficulties they cause themselves and others, individuals with OCPD (operating at a neurotic level of personality organization) cognitively understand that their conflicts arise internally. In contrast, OCPD individuals who operate at borderline levels perceive internal conflicts as if coming from others. As a result, they externalize internal difficulty and blame others.

Clinical Assessment of OCPD

Initial Interview

The initial interview of a patient with OCPD provides a unique window into the individual's internal experience and relations with others and is an opportunity to strengthen the rapport. After introductions, listen and observe. Take in the patient's appearance, body language, and affect. People with OCPD often present meticulously groomed and speak with circumspect detail. They are highly intellectualized, frustrating the early clinician's efforts to get details about their emotional life. The obtuse relational style should aid in the diagnosis and the development of a treatment strategy. Collateral information from family or partners might also be helpful. Rule out other disorders, including but not limited to the obsessive-compulsive and related disorders (OCRDS), ASD, eating disorders, other personality disorders, organic brain disorders such as temporal lobe seizure disorder, and prior brain injury.

Psychometric Tests

In addition to the interview and collateral information, psychometric tests are helpful diagnostic tools for OCPD. The Compulsive Personality Assessment Scale, as seen in Table 24.2, p. 597, has been partially validated and used in clinical and community-based samples in various studies. It provides an observer-rated scale, mirroring the DSM-5 symptoms for both severity and threshold assessment of OCPD.[41]

An abbreviated list of other OCPD assessment tools includes the Minnesota Multiphasic Personality Inventory-2 (MMPI-2),[42] the Shedler-Westen Assessment of Personality (SWAP),[43] the Millon Clinical Multiaxial Inventory (MCMI-IV),[44] the Rorschach Psychodiagnostic Test,[45] and the Thematic Apperception Test.[46] There are multiple subjective questionnaires for OCPD: the Pathological Obsessive Compulsive Personality Scale (POPS);[47] the Frost Multidimensional Perfectionism Scale;[48] and the Hoarding Rating Scale.[49]

Differentiating OCPD from OCD

OCPD and OCD are clinically confused and require vastly different treatment approaches. To help clinicians differentiate between these two disorders, a case study of OCD and a discussion comparing and contrasting the two disorders is provided.

Case Study of OCD: Tom

A respected psychologist referred Tom because he was worsening in therapy. On arrival, he anxiously scanned the office. He appeared unshaven and gaunt. His warm smile quickly faded. He said he was a devout Catholic and a historical theology professor. He was generally happy until recently. He worried his daughter was unsafe. Wincing, he said that after learning his wife was pregnant with their second baby, he began having "disturbing and sinful thoughts." He welled up and said he had repetitive thoughts that he

Table 24.2. Compulsive Personality Assessment Scale[41]

Subject's Name _____ Date of Birth ____ / ____ / _____

Rater's Name _____ Date of Rating ____ / ____ / ____

Items refer to a stable pattern of enduring traits dating back to adolescent or early adulthood. Use the questions listed as part of a semi-structured interview.

For each item circle the appropriate score:
0 = absent; 1 = mild; 2 = moderate; 3 = severe; 4 = very severe

ITEM RATING

1. Preoccupation with details
Are you preoccupied with details, rules, lists, order, organization or 0 1 2 3 4 schedules to the extent that the major aim of the activity is lost?

2. Perfectionism
Would you describe yourself as a perfectionist who struggles with 0 1 2 3 4 completing the task at hand?

3. Workaholism
Are you excessively devoted to work to the exclusion of leisure 0 1 2 3 4 activities and friendships?

4. Over-conscientiousness
Would you describe yourself as over-conscientious and inflexible 0 1 2 3 4 about matters of morality, ethics or values?

5. Hoarding
Are you unable to discard worn-out or worthless objects even when 0 1 2 3 4 they have no sentimental value?

6. Need for control
Are you reluctant to delegate tasks or to work with others unless they 0 1 2 3 4 submit to exactly your way of doing things?

7. Miserliness
Do you see money as something to be hoarded for future catastrophes? 0 1 2 3 4

8. Rigidity
Do you think you are rigid or stubborn? 0 1 2 3 4

TOTAL:

Reprinted with Permission. Fineberg NA, Sharma P, Sivakumaran T, Sahakian B, Chamberlain SR. Does obsessive-compulsive personality disorder belong within the obsessive-compulsive spectrum? *CNS Spectr.* 2007;12(6):467–482. doi:10.1017/s1092852900015340

was a pedophile. He found the thoughts intrusive and exhausting, not sexually arousing. He did not have impulses or plans to touch children. He experienced the thoughts as repulsive and morally reprehensible. He said therapy had increased his guilt and anxiety, causing ritualistic cleaning of clothing and bedding. Each day he methodically moved through the house, washing bedding and selecting clean clothes he feared were dirty. His wife complained he was perfectionistic, worked too much, and didn't enjoy life. She worried he was depressed and thought he should start a medication. He appeared depressed, struggled to maintain eye contact, and reported neurovegetative symptoms of anhedonia, decreased appetite, insomnia, guilt, and psychomotor agitation.

In treatment, Tom learned that OCD is a neuropsychiatric illness that hijacks the mind and is not in his control. This information reduced his guilt and provided hope. With cognitive-behavioral therapy (CBT), Tom separated irrational thoughts about harming children from his compulsions to clean. Within a few weeks, Tom's depression eased with the addition of a selective serotonin reuptake inhibitor (SSRI). However, his disturbing thoughts persisted.

It has been said that "every fear hides a wish," suggesting that a person unconsciously takes issue with something that represents what they want. It makes sense that unacceptable desire provokes opposition, but not always. The line in Shakespeare's Hamlet, "thou dost protest too much" signifies exaggerated objection, and it tips off ambivalence. Like the jilted lover who exclaims, "I hope I never see her again!," then longingly checks his phone. However, in OCD, seemingly meaningless thoughts or impulses arise, like Tom's unnecessary need to do laundry. On occasion, worst-case thoughts manifest as a symptom, often with moralistic irony. In OCD however, a cigar is best left a cigar. These ego-dystonic thoughts are repetitive, as if the defense mechanism of repression is broken. In Tom's case, his mind produced an intolerable idea about himself and put it on a loop. For a father and devout Christian, his obsession was cruel. Without familiarity with OCD, a naive clinician might worry about Tom molesting children and even call the authorities. Tom's well-intended therapist pushed him to understand the possible meanings of why his mind conjured up this thought, which was disorganizing for Tom and only increased his symptoms. Tom's SSRI was increased gradually at two-month intervals to a high dose, and his disturbing thoughts reduced by 90 percent.

There are several clinical distinctions between OCD and OCPD summarized in Table 24.3. In OCD, distressing compulsions occur to quell the anxiety that something terrible will happen related to an intrusive thought or obsession; however, the individual knows that the obsessions, and resulting compulsions, don't make sense. In other words, the obsessions are ego-dystonic, and the individual has insight into the irrational nature of their symptoms. Whereas in OCPD, the connection between thoughts and behaviors is often logical; however, perfectionism and procrastination seen in OCPD still cause dysfunction. In OCD, symptoms are focal, fluctuate over time, and in response to stress. While in OCPD, the traits are pervasive and persistent patterns of thought and behavior, not distressing, are syntonic, and perceived as useful. Understandably, people with OCD, knowing that something is wrong with them, seek professional help. In contrast, people with OCPD tend to present at the insistence of others or because of secondary problems like depression or marital struggles. Lastly, compared with OCD, individuals with OCPD have a greater capacity to delay reward which may be a helpful characteristic.[50]

Table 24.3. Clinical Distinctions between OCD and OCPD

Factors	OCD	OCPD
Symptoms	Focal obsessions and irrationally related compulsions	Pervasive patterns of obsessional thoughts and behaviors
Experience of Symptoms	Distressing/ego-dystonic	Not distressed/ego-syntonic
Perception of Symptoms	Insight that symptoms are irrational	Little insight, does not see problems as symptoms or believes symptoms are reasonable
Other	Seeks help because the symptoms are bothersome	Seeks help because of secondary symptoms or another's insistence

Together, Tom's biological vulnerability and the psychological stress of a growing family triggered the onset of his OCD. His obsessional symptom was isolated to an intrusive and distressing ego-dystonic thought that he was a pedophile. This thought was focal, not diffuse, or integral to his personality functioning. Tom did not find the thoughts about being a pedophile arousing, as would be the case in a person with pedophilia. His ritualized cleaning and avoidance of pleasure might be confused for perfectionism but were born out of an effort to cleanse guilt and reduce his anxiety. Unlike with OCPD, Tom had the insight that something wasn't right with his thinking.

Psychodynamic Treatment Strategies and Clinical Reactions

Opening Phase

People with OCPD often come to treatment at the behest of someone else or because of a related problem, like depression or anxiety. As treatment begins, OCPD patients want to be the "perfect patient," similar to their childhood desire to be a "perfect child." During the early phase of treatment, the therapist's primary role is to build a therapeutic alliance by using active listening, encouragement, reassurance, consistent frame, and being reliable. This vulnerable early phase of treatment is strengthened through the use of clarification and observation, less by confrontation and interpretation. The first treatment approach for OCPD is to foster trust and attachment in a nonjudgmental and genuinely accepting environment.

Transference and countertransference gradually emerge. Classical transference, originating from early life experiences, appears as the patient's distorted ways of relating to and experiencing the therapist. Unaccustomed to the positive regard of the therapeutic stance, a powerful idealized transference forms, a honeymoon of sorts. Eager to please and relieved by the acceptance and empathy, patients arrive on time, pay on time, and offer up copious detail. Gradually, a repetitive transference sets in, as the patient monotonously reports excessively detailed and factual information. Therapists can typically feel numb and perplexed, uncertain how to move the patient's cognition into emotion. The patient's intellectualization often creates an "anesthetizing cloud . . . a smokescreen to mask their feelings."[51] Despite the seeming compliance, another dynamic is afoot. Overtly adhering to the process, OCPD patients covertly and unconsciously commandeer the treatment from a sometimes stupefied "expert." One therapist described digging their fingernail into their thumb to counter the numbing effect of a particularly obsessional patient. These stalemates induce mutual recrimination in both the therapist and the patient. Both parties seemingly try and fail, which becomes the "essence of the transference–countertransference enactment" or the sadomasochistic bind.[52]

Over time, the therapist becomes experienced as a critical parental figure with impossible expectations, and negative condescending transference develops. Early idealization wears thin as patients project feelings of inadequacy onto the therapist. Patients "politely" point out a multitude of flaws in the therapist, inviting negative countertransference. For example, "I notice you don't have a hook in your restroom for coats." or "I see you colored your roots again, but it looks like you missed a spot."

Classical countertransference is the clinician's past mixed with their response to the patient. A "patient-originated countertransference" is the therapist's response to the patient mainly triggered by the patient. However, a "therapist-originated countertransference" occurs when the therapist inadvertently introduces their interpersonal issues into the treatment. Transference, especially when irrational, does not require a therapist's immediate reaction or response. In fact, it is initially best to observe and just experience the transference. Countertransference hazards range from impulses to disengage from the patient, the work of psychotherapy, or to retaliate against the patient for what is commonly a slew of indirect criticism. The clinical challenge is to remain neutral and empathically engaged.

Middle Phase

When the patient is connected, and the transference and countertransference dynamics are underway, the middle phase of the treatment begins. A second treatment strategy at this stage is rigorous confrontation and interpretation of the patient's interpersonal distortions and created sadomasochistic binds.

Josephs describes common patterns of the public and private personas in obsessional character structure,[53] as seen in Table 24.4. Two relational patterns become evident. The first is public deference toward people whom they admire. However, while over-functioning to please, patients privately experience suffering at the perceived superior's hand. Simultaneously, with perceived inferiors, obsessional patients are publicly caring but privately critical and condescending. The oscillation between positions of inferiority and superiority with others plays out in the treatment with the therapist.

Broader than classical transference–countertransference is the *totalistic transference–countertransference* model that encompasses the transference of interpersonal difficulties from the patient's early past, the here-and-now, and the in-the-room experiences. The patient's transference struggles are conceptualized as repetition of old experiences and their actual experiences with the therapist, including in the moment. When the patient and therapist unwittingly collude, in a transference and countertransference dynamic, they recreate or enact the very difficulties that brought the patient to treatment. Enactments, rather than seen as problematic, provide rich opportunities to work through transference–countertransference phenomena in real time, integrating both the patient's and the therapist's contribution to the situation. To illustrate an enactment, we'll return to the case of Mike, whose therapist ran late for his session. Mike had prepaid for his sessions as a defense against feeling both forgotten and angry when his therapist ran late. The therapist, with a classical countertransference response, replied, "Well, unfortunately, your check will be wrong because I will be away a week next month." Rather than understanding that the patient was aggressive because he felt undesired, the therapist identified with a critical figure from his past and unconsciously retaliated, causing Mike to feel more criticized

Table 24.4. Conceptualization OCPD Personas with Perceived Others[51]

Personas	With Perceived Superiors	With Perceived Inferiors
Publicly	Appear as serious, hard workers, obsequious	Appear as caretakers, mentors, thoughtful
Privately	Feels envious, self-doubting, resentful	Feels superior or disgust for others, or acts with condescension
Unconsciously	Suffering or masochistic	Punishing or sadistic toward other

and abandoned. This vignette is an example of *projective identification*. The patient initially projected critical feelings onto the therapist; the therapist, rather than use the experience to inform the work, identified with, and felt controlled by, the patient's critical attitude, and retaliated. In this case, a therapist might realize her/his misstep and say, "Listen, I need to apologize for that response. I think I am feeling guilty about running late and took offense to your paying me for appointments ahead of time, as if you were putting me in my place. Perhaps you felt neglected and abandoned in the waiting room, and I owe you an apology."

Patients with OCPD are exquisitely sensitive to criticism and benefit from therapists who are not critical. If the therapist manages not to react critically while addressing negative aspects of the patient's behavior, the patient is able to separate out his/her role in causing their struggles. During the middle phase, the therapist helps the patient expand her/his story, and patients become aware of the losses in how they were treated and how they treat others.

Termination Phase

The final phase of treatment is often filled with grief related to loss. This might be mistaken for depression, but it is more about mourning what never happened and how life might have been different. Through this long grief process, the therapist's presence allows powerful new feelings of affection and gratitude to emerge in the treatment and in the patient's life.

The Psychodynamic Case of Albert, OCPD

Albert, a 50-year-old man, arrived early for his initial appointment. He briskly took a seat, raised his chin, and declared, "The reason I'm here is to maintain an intact family." He wore an expensive suit with scuffed shoes. After a forced smile from filmy dry lips, he began loudly, "My wife is chronically depressed, especially since ending her affair." The therapist asked, "What was her affair like for you?" He said, "As long as it's over, I think we have a perfect life." The therapist commented that most people would be disturbed by an affair. Albert winced, "I guess I skip over the emotional parts of life." He talked about the investment firm where he worked and the "important" work of the partners. His days were long, and he arrived home late to eat dinner alone at his computer. He said his childhood was, "Just fine. They did what parents do, clothed, and fed us." Albert filled weekly sessions with repetitive intellectual and technical descriptions of his marital difficulties, as a lawyer might lay out two sides of a case. His wife experienced him as critical and cold.

The therapist empathized and listened, sometimes interjecting that Albert sounded angry or appeared upset, to which Albert would pause briefly, then robotically plow ahead. The therapist suggested increasing the session frequency to three times a week in an effort to mobilize Albert's affect. Albert became both excited and distressed. Sitting forward, he spoke louder and faster and said, "It's difficult for me to say it's the least bit pleasurable in here. You recognize my discomfort and empathize with me. I feel guilty." Albert observed his repetition and worried he was a bad patient. He scolded himself but could think of nothing else to say. Sessions fell silent, the therapy seemingly at a standstill.

[Therapist's Commentary]: Albert's defense mechanisms are over-control, perfectionism, and rigidity. Albert focused more on his thoughts, not how he felt, a hallmark of an obsessional character. In the transference, Albert tried to be the perfect patient

yet unconsciously undermined the treatment. He dominated and trivialized the therapy, often ignoring his therapist. The therapist remained engaged and increased treatment frequency to better know Albert causing him, unexpected pleasure when he allowed greater feelings. However, the pleasure also produced powerful feelings of guilt and anxiety that caused inhibition. Albert attempted to ruin the pleasure, fearing the rejection he had experienced in childhood.

The therapist was induced to feel numb, bored, and irritated, but analyzed the meaning of these countertransference reactions. First, there was an overwhelming flood of words. Then Albert's growing anxiety as he felt close and accepted. Then silence. The content was not significant; what was significant was the process, and Albert's growing capacity to feel emotions then abrupt silence. Albert reenacted a bind with his therapist because he believed he didn't deserve pleasure or intimacy. The seeming meaninglessness of the therapeutic situation was what was meaningful. Albert was showing the therapist that they didn't deserve to share something good, and that they would both act as punisher and victim unless something new occurred. The sadomasochistic bind was alive in the transference–countertransference dynamic. Rather than suggest a different treatment or decide that the approach was ineffective, the therapist made himself more available to sort out what was happening and why.

The therapist interpreted that Albert was masochistically sabotaging the treatment because he believed he was unworthy of closeness and pleasure. Albert agreed and said he did this everywhere. He expressed that his therapist's encouragement felt like permission to enjoy the closeness, so he did. He idealized the therapist and revealed more. Each night he drank alcohol and scanned his bank accounts. He then admitted, "I am not a partner. I was ambiguous." He talked about ways he intentionally misled and offended people.

He decided to stop drinking alcohol, and a flood of emotions arose. He was lonely and confided that his wife complained about his bad breath, but he refused to go to the dentist. His therapist pressed the topic, and he recalled going to the dentist for the first time at age 12. By then, he had so many cavities that the experience was traumatic. He felt angry and disappointed in his parents, but was able to describe them more fully. Growing up, his mom worked long hours, coming home tired and grumpy. He found her abrasive and unsavory. Dad was "football obsessed" and worked nights. Albert was bitter and admitted to treating his family poorly. The therapist persisted in confronting Albert about undermining relationships and work. He gradually expressed anger with ease, and ultimately improved his marriage and his career.

[Therapist's Commentary]: Albert's defense mechanisms evolved from reaction-formation (covering a feeling with its opposite), sublimation, and isolation of affect into healthy humility, acceptance, and gratitude. In the early transference, Albert repeated a dynamic from his childhood of outward compliance with a perceived authority figure, but acted out his anger unconsciously or unintentionally through defiance. Albert hid his alcohol use and misrepresented himself as a partner at his investment firm. With his therapist's acceptance, he revealed secrets. Eventually, his therapist became an invaluable partner with whom he could be genuine. Early in the countertransference, the therapist was irritated and felt misled but also sympathetic. The therapist understood that Albert felt a need to pretend things, which added to his feelings of inadequacy and anger. The clinical challenge was to balance confrontation with kindness in the face of Albert's provocative behavior. By the end of the treatment, the therapist experienced Albert as direct, engaging, and authentically connected.

Cooper writes about obsessional thinking as a defense against loss.[54] She suggests a family constellation of "an emotionally absent father coupled with inadequate mothering." Ambivalence is high for obsessional individuals, and decisions are difficult. The doing and undoing is an effort to avoid inevitable losses when making a decision.

Levels of Evidence for Effectiveness of Treatment

Currently, there are no widely accepted, empirically based treatments for OCPD. Some studies examine the effectiveness of psychological therapies compared to pharmacological treatments. Few studies investigate OCPD in the absence of other psychiatric disorders, and only one randomized control study compares psychological treatments in OCPD in the absence of other personality disorders.[55] Review Table 24.5, Table 24.6 (see p. 604), and Table 24.7 (see p. 605) for a summary of the evidence for treatment of OCPD. More and better data are needed.

Table 24.5. Evidence for Psychological Treatment of OCPD

Psychological Studies				
Study	Intervention	Sample	Design	Results
Enero et al. (2013) [56]	Group CBT	116 OP with OCPD	Longitudinal (10 sessions) Level C	Distress level found to be predictor of treatment response
Barber and Muenz (1996) [55]	CT vs IPT	139 OP with MDD and elevation of OCPD/AVPD	Comparative study (≥12 sessions) Level C	IPT found superior over CT for depression symptoms for patients with MDD and elevated OCPD levels
Bamelis, Evers, Spinhoven, Arntz (2014) [57]	ST vs COT	313 OP with PD	RCT (Weekly sessions) Level B	ST superior to COT and TAU in recovery rate and reduction of dropout
Barber, Morse, Krakauer, Chittams, and Crits-Christoph (1997) [58]	SEDP	38 OP with AVDP/OCPD and depressive and/or anxiety disorder	Longitudinal (52 weekly sessions) Level B	Following treatment only 15 percent retained their diagnosis, improvements on personality disorder symptoms, depression, general functioning, interpersonal problems, and anxiety

Abbreviation key: CBT = Cognitive behavioral therapy, CT = Cognitive Therapy, IPT = Interpersonal psychotherapy, ST = Schema therapy, COT = Clarification-oriented therapy, SEDP = Supportive-expressive dynamic psychotherapy, OP = Outpatients, OCPD = Obsessive-compulsive personality disorder, MDD = Major depressive disorder, AVPD = Avoidant personality disorder, RCT = Randomized Control Trial, TAU = Treatment as Usual

Key: Levels of Evidence; Strength of recommendation taxonomy (SORT)*

Level of Evidence A: Good quality patient-oriented evidence.

Level of Evidence B: Limited quality patient-oriented evidence

Level of Evidence C: Based on consensus, usual practice, opinion, disease-oriented evidence, or case series for studies of diagnosis

*Ebell MH, Siwek J, Weiss BD, Woolf SH, Susman J, Ewigman B, Bowman M. Simplifying the language of evidence to improve patient care. *J Fam Pract.* 2004 Feb 1;53(2):111–120.

Table 24.6. Evidence for Psychological and Pharmacologic Treatment of OCPD

Psychological & Pharmacological Studies				
Study	Intervention	Sample	Design	Results
Smith, et al. (2016)[59]	MM	52 OCPD IP, 56 IP with other PD, 52 IP with no PD	PSM (average: 59.4 hrs of programming a week, 45.85 days in treatment) Level B	MM resulted in clinically significant improvements for all groups but OCPD IP experience the lowest anxiety remission rate at discharge
Popa, (2013)[60]	CBT and SSRI	31 IP & OP with OCPD and GAD	Pre-post test (40 sessions + escitalopram) Level B	Improvements in extroversion, anxiety levels, agreeableness, and emotional stability

Abbreviation key: MM = Intensive multimodal psychiatric approach, CBT = Cognitive behavioral therapy, SSRI = Selective serotonin reuptake inhibitor, OCPD = Obsessive-compulsive personality disorder, IP = Inpatient, OP = Outpatients, GAD: Generalized anxiety disorder, PSM = Propensity score matching
Key: Levels of Evidence; Strength of recommendation taxonomy (SORT)*

Level of Evidence A: Good quality patient-oriented evidence.

Level of Evidence B: Limited quality patient-oriented evidence

Level of Evidence C: Based on consensus, usual practice, opinion, disease-oriented evidence, or case series for studies of diagnosis

*Ebell MH, Siwek J, Weiss BD, Woolf SH, Susman J, Ewigman B, Bowman M. Simplifying the language of evidence to improve patient care. *J Fam Pract.* 2004 Feb 1;53(2):111–120.

Evidence for Psychological Treatment

While the pertinent data depicted in Table 24.5 (see p. 603) supports cognitive-behavioral and various psychotherapy models as providing significant reductions in symptom severity of personality pathology, depression, and anxiety, the data does not account for co-occurring personality disorders alongside OCPD. While some argue that CBT is the best validated psychological treatment for OCPD,[56] interpersonal psychotherapy has been proven superior in reducing depressive symptoms in a randomized controlled trial in individuals with OCPD.[55] Additionally, Schema Therapy, a behavioral/relationship theory-based treatment, was superior to clarification-oriented therapies (CBT-like) at decreasing depressive disorders and increasing social and occupational functioning.[57] One study provided 52 sessions of "time-limited Supportive-Expressive dynamic psychotherapy," at the end of which only 155 of OCPD patients retained their diagnosis.[58]

Evidence for Psychological and Pharmacological Treatment

One study specifically assessed OCPD inpatients who benefited from an intensive multimodal treatment approach (medication management, educational groups, individual and group psychotherapy, and recreational activities).[59] Another study assessed both an SSRI (citalopram) and CBT in 31 outpatients with OCPD and generalized anxiety disorder (GAD), with significant improvements in anxiety, extroversion, agreeableness, and emotional stability from pre- to post-treatment.[60]

Table 24.7. Evidence for Pharmacologic Treatment of OCPD

Pharmacological Studies

Study	Intervention	Sample	Design	Results
Ansseau (1994)[61]	Fluvoxamine (50-100 mg/day)	4 OP with OCPD with no significant depressive symptoms	Longitudinal (3 month) Level C	Significant decrease in OCPD symptoms
Ansseau M, Troisfontaines B, Papart P, Von Frenckell R. (1991)[62]	Fluvoxamine (100-200 mg/day)	22 OP with MDD, 24 OP with MDD and OCPD	Longitudinal (8 weeks) Level C	Greater decrease in depressive symptoms for those with OCPD than those without
Greve KW, Adams D. (2002)[63]	Carbamazepine (100-200 mg/day)	1 OP with OCPD and OCD features	Case Study (8 month) Level C	Significant decrease in OCPD symptoms
Ekselius L, von Knorring L. (1998)[64]	Sertraline (50-150 mg/day) vs. Citalopram (20-60 mg/day)	308 OP with OCPD, MDD, and OCD	RCT (24 weeks) Level B	Citalopram resulted in significant reduction in OCPD diagnosis, Sertraline also had significant reduction in symptoms but not to a level of remission

Abbreviation key: OP = Outpatients, OCPD = Obsessive-Compulsive Personality Disorder, OCD = Obsessive-Compulsive Disorder, MDD = Major depressive disorder RCT = Randomized Control
Key: Levels of Evidence; Strength of recommendation taxonomy (SORT)*

Level of Evidence A: Good quality patient-oriented evidence.

Level of Evidence B: Limited quality patient-oriented evidence

Level of Evidence C: Based on consensus, usual practice, opinion, disease-oriented evidence, or case series for studies of diagnosis

*Ebell MH, Siwek J, Weiss BD, Woolf SH, Susman J, Ewigman B, Bowman M. Simplifying the language of evidence to improve patient care. *J Fam Pract.* 2004 Feb 1;53(2):111–120.

Evidence for Psychopharmacological Treatment

SSRIs are the most studied medications for OCPD, followed by tricyclic antidepressants, serotonin-norepinephrine reuptake inhibitors, and antipsychotics. There are two studies using fluvoxamine in patients with OCPD without other psychiatric disorders. The first study, by Ansseau, an open-labeled pilot with four participants, showed a statistical decrease in OCPD severity.[61] The second study (the only double-blind, randomized controlled trial) had 24 participants and also showed a reduction in OCPD severity.[62] However, both of these studies used an unvalidated criterion scale. A case report (n = 1) of OCPD showed a decrease in aggression with the use of carbamazepine.[63] One study, in patients with OCPD and major depressive symptoms, found a reduction in symptoms of OCPD with citalopram.[64]

No specific medication is indicated or approved by the U.S. Food and Drug Administration to treat OCPD. However, treatment of concomitant conditions, such as depression or anxiety, provide an OCPD patient with some relief and strengthen the alliance while psychological treatment is underway. SSRIs are commonly used when OCPD is comorbid with OCD. It is useful to clarify medication's limitations and set realistic expectations that a lengthy psychotherapeutic treatment will likely bring the most benefit.[65]

Treatment Modalities for OCPD

Individual Therapy

Psychodynamic psychotherapy (PDP) and CBT are the two most common forms of therapy offered to OCPD patients. Despite a lack of clear evidence, PDP has historically been considered the treatment of choice.[66] It is common practice to use either PDP or CBT augmenting the treatment of OPCD with medication and behavioral interventions.[65] In OCPD, CBT aims to change maladaptive behavior, cognition, and relational patterns while increasing adaptive patterns through a detailed examination of real-life situations.

Experienced clinicians and this author find that interpersonal psychotherapy effectively treats patients with OCPD by focusing on maladaptive preconceptions of the self, others, and the patient's relationship in the world, limited by early experiences. Patterns arise between the therapist and patient that represent old patterns, allowing for change. For example, patients have an irrational expectations of criticism from a therapist related to early experiences with a critical parent, allowing for a positive reconfiguration of how they feel about themselves and how they experience others.

Group Therapy

There are multiple benefits to group therapy for patients with OCPD.[67] They learn vicariously as other patients express emotions they deny. They receive feedback from group members about problematic aspects of their behavior and interpersonal style. Group therapy increases a capacity for vulnerability, spontaneity, and experiencing acceptance. However, OCPD patients might become socially overwhelmed and withdrawn from the group milieu. Alternatively, they may dominate the group dynamics and inhibit other members, or flood the group with details, intellectualizing the process. For these reasons, the group leader is advised to be active and engaged.

Marital and Family Therapy

Often a complaining partner or family member compels a person with OCPD into couple's treatment. Yudofsky describes three phases for partners of patients with OCPD.[68] Early on, there is deep admiration for the patient's intellectual and organizational abilities, followed by a second period of insecurity as the partner experiences chronic criticism. Eventually, the patient with OCPD is experienced as cold and impossible to please. The couple's therapist validates the partner's experience of the OCPD patient's cold and critical behavior, breaking through the denial system.

Conclusion

The diagnostic criteria in the DSM-5 require a pervasive pattern of orderliness, perfectionism, and control, beginning in young adulthood, alongside four or more additional symptoms. OCPD is one of the most common personality disorders. While causing long-standing disability, it is less functionally impairing than other personality disorders. OCPD is highly comorbid with psychiatric disorders, including major depression, anxiety disorders, alcohol abuse/dependence, OCD, hoarding disorder, eating disorders, and other personality disorders. Our current etiological understanding of OCPD is an additive genetic effect and unique environmental factors. Clinically, individuals with OCPD often operate at a higher level of functioning within the continuum of personality disorders, as illustrated in a theoretical model of personality disorders called "Personality Lane." Clinical assessment of OCPD includes an interview, collateral information from others, and psychometric tests when necessary. OCD is clinically confused and co-occurs with OCPD; however, it requires a vastly different treatment approach. People with OCPD often wish to be "the perfect patient" but unconsciously undermine treatment by avoiding emotions. Therapist countertransferences often oscillate between boredom and frustration. A two-part treatment strategy first involves establishing trust and a relational base, then clarifying distorted thought patterns and interpreting sadomasochistic binds. As the patient experiences new intimacy and empathy in the relationship with a therapist and loved ones over time, something they never had, a lengthy grief process ensues followed by a more adaptive and often happier life. While multiple treatment modalities exist, few studies have investigated OCPD in the absence of other psychiatric disorders. More data is needed to determine the most effective treatment. In the meantime, there is historical clinical experience which supports long-term psychodynamic therapy or CBT, adding medication and behavioral interventions as indicated. Review relevant resources for patients, families, and clinicians in Box 24.1.

Conflict of Interest/Disclosure: The author of this chapter has no financial conflicts and nothing to disclose.

Box 24.1 Resources for Patients, and Families and Clinicians

Patients and Families

- Trosclair, G. *The Healthy Compulsive: Healing Obsessive Compulsive Personality Disorder and Taking the Wheel of the Driven Personality.* Lanham, MD: Rowman and Littlefield; 2020 Outlines a four-step program for positive outcomes.
- Brown, B. *The Gifts of Imperfection: Let Go of Who You Think You're Supposed to Be and Embrace Who You Are.* Center City, MN: Hazelden Publishing; 2010, is a guide to embracing a perfectly imperfect life.
- OCPD Online. https://ocpd.org.
- Website: The Healthy Compulsive. http://www.thehealthycompulsive.com.

Clinicians

- *Obsessive-compulsive Personality Disorder.* Washington, DC: American Psychiatric Association Publishing; 2019
- Gabbard GO. *Psychodynamic Psychiatry in Clinical Practice.* 4th ed. Washington, DC: American Psychiatric Publishing; 2014: 571–599.
- Centre for Clinical Interventions. https://www.cci.health.wa.gov.au/Resources/Looking-After-Yourself/Perfectionism.

References

1. Reich W. *Character Analysis*. 3rd ed. New York, NY: Orgone Institute Press; 1949.

2. *Diagnostic and Statistical Manual: Mental Disorders*. Washington, DC: American Psychiatric Association; 1952.

3. *Diagnostic and Statistical Manual: Mental Disorders*. 2nd ed. Washington, DC: American Psychiatric Association; 1968.

4. *Diagnostic and Statistical Manual: Mental Disorders*. 3rd ed. Washington, DC: American Psychiatric Association; 1980.

5. *Diagnostic and Statistical Manual: Mental Disorders: DSM III-R*. 3rd ed., rev. Washington, DC: American Psychiatric Association; 1987.

6. *Diagnostic and Statistical Manual: Mental Disorders: DSM-IV*. 4th ed. Washington, DC: American Psychiatric Association; 1994.

7. *Diagnostic and Statistical Manual: Mental Disorders: DSM-5*. 5th ed. Washington, DC: American Psychiatric Association; 2013.

8. Bach B, Sellbom M, Skjernov M, Simonsen E. ICD-11 and DSM-5 personality trait domains capture categorical personality disorders: finding a common ground. *Aust NZ J Psychiatry*. 2017; 52(5): 425–434. doi:10.1177/0004867417727867

9. Grant JE, Mooney ME, Kushner MG. Prevalence, correlates, and comorbidity of DSM-IV obsessive-compulsive personality disorder: results from the National Epidemiologic Survey on Alcohol and Related Conditions. *J Psychiatric Res*. 2012; 46(4): 469–475. doi:10.1016/j.jpsychires.2012.01.009

10. Oldham JM, Skodol AE, Bender DS. *The American Psychiatric Publishing Textbook of Personality Disorders*. 2nd ed. Washington, DC: American Psychiatric Publishing; 2014.

11. Zimmerman M, Rothschild L, Chelminski I. The prevalence of DSM-IV personality disorders in psychiatric outpatients. *Am J Psychiatry*. 2005; 162(10): 1911–1918. doi:10.1176/appi.ajp.162.10.1911.

12. Ansell EB, Pinto A, Crosby RD, et al. The prevalence and structure of obsessive-compulsive personality disorder in Hispanic psychiatric outpatients. *J Behav Ther Exp Psychiatry*. 2010; 41(3): 275–281. doi:10.1016/j.jbtep.2010.02.005

13. Rossi A, Marinangeli MG, Butti G, et al. Personality disorders in bipolar and depressive disorders. *J Affect Disord*. 2001; 65(1): 3–8. doi:10.1016/S0165-0327(00)00230-

14. Grilo CM, Stout RL, Markowitz JC, et al. Personality disorders predict relapse after remission from an episode of major depressive disorder: a 6-year prospective study. *J Clin Psychiatry*. 2010; 71(12): 1629–1635. doi:10.4088/JCP.08m04200gre

15. Pinto A, Mancebo MC, Eisen JL, Pagano ME, Rasmussen SA. The Brown Longitudinal Obsessive Compulsive Study: clinical features and symptoms of the sample at intake. *J Clin Psychiatry*. 2006; 67(5): 703–711. doi:10.4088/jcp.v67n0503

16. Gadelkarim W, Shahper S, Reid J, et al. Overlap of obsessive-compulsive personality disorder and autism spectrum disorder traits among OCD outpatients: an exploratory study. *Int J Psychiatry Clin Pract*. 2019; 23(4): 297–306. doi:10.1080/13651501.2019.1638939

17. Ansell EB, Pinto A, Edelen MO, et al. The association of personality disorders with the prospective 7-year course of anxiety disorders. *Psychol Med*. 2011; 41(5): 1019–1028. doi:10.1017/S0033291710001777

18. Skodol AE, Gunderson JG, McGlashan TH, et al. Functional impairment in patients with schizotypal, borderline, avoidant, or obsessive-compulsive personality disorder. *Am J Psychiatry*. 2002; 159(2): 276–283. doi:10.1176/appi.ajp.159.2.276

19. Samuels J, Nestadt G, Bienvenu O, et al. Personality disorders and normal personality dimensions in obsessive-compulsive disorder. *Brit J Psychiatry*, 2000; 177(5): 457–462. doi:10.1192/bjp.177.5.457

20. Pinto A, Greene AL, Storch EA, Simpson HB. Prevalence of childhood obsessive-compulsive personality traits in adults with obsessive compulsive disorder versus obsessive compulsive personality disorder. *J Obsessive Compuls Relat Disord*. 2015; 4: 25–29. doi:10.1016/j.jocrd.2014.11.002

21. Frost RO, Steketee G, Tolin DF. Comorbidity in hoarding disorder. *Depress Anxiety*. 2011; 28(10): 876–884. doi:10.1002/da.20861

22. Phillips KA, McElroy SL. Personality disorders and traits in patients with body dysmorphic disorder. *Compr Psychiatry*. 2000; 41(4): 229–236. doi:10.1053/comp.2000.7429

23. Halmi KA, Tozzi F, Thornton LM, et al. The relation among perfectionism, obsessive-compulsive personality disorder and obsessive-compulsive disorder in individuals with eating disorders. *Int J Eat Disord*. 2005; 38(4): 371–374. doi:10.1002/eat.20190

24. Gadelkarim W, Shahper S, Reid J, et al. Overlap of obsessive-compulsive personality disorder and autism spectrum disorder traits among OCD outpatients: an exploratory study. *Int J Psychiatry Clin Pract*. 2019; 23(4): 297–306. doi:10.1080/13651501.2019.1638939

25. McGlashan, Thomas H, et al. The collaborative longitudinal personality disorders study: baseline axis i/ii and ii/ii diagnostic co-occurrence. *Acta Psychiatrica Scandinavica*. 2000; 102(4): 256–264. doi: 10.1034/j.1600-0447.2000.102004256.x

26. Sjåstad HN, Gråwe RW, Egeland J. Affective disorders among patients with borderline personality disorder. *PLoS One*. 2012; 7(12). p.e50930. doi:10.1371/journal.pone.0050930

27. Freud S. *The Standard Edition of Complete Psychological Works of Sigmund Freud: Character and Anal Eroticism*. London: Hogarth Press; 1908:167–176.

28. Reichborn-Kjennerud T, Czajkowski N, Neale MC, et al. Genetic and environmental influences on dimensional representations of DSM-IV cluster C personality disorders: a population-based multivariate twin study. *Psychol Med*. 2007; 37: 645–653. doi:10.1017/S0033291706009548

29. Nestadt G, Samuels J, Riddle M, et al. A family study of obsessive-compulsive disorder. *Arch Gen Psychiatry*. 2000; 57(4): 358–363. doi:10.1001/archpsyc.57.4.358

30. Lilenfeld LR, Kaye WH, Greeno CG, et al. A controlled family study of anorexia nervosa and bulimia nervosa: psychiatric disorders in first-degree relatives and effects of proband comorbidity. *Arch Gen Psychiatry*. 1998; 55: 603–610. doi:10.1001/archpsyc.55.7.603

31. Ansari Z, Fadardi JS. Enhanced visual performance in obsessive compulsive personality disorder. *Scand J Psychol*. 2016; 57(6): 542–546.

32. Atmaca M, Korucu T, Kilic MC, Kazgan A, Hulya Yildirim H. Pineal gland volumes are changed in patients with obsessive-compulsive personality disorder. *J Clin Neuroscience*. 2019; 70: 221–225. doi:10.1016/j.jocn.2019.07.047

33. Nicoletti A, Luca A, Raciti L, Contrafatto D, Bruno E, Dibilio V, et al. Obsessive compulsive personality disorder and Parkinson's disease. *PLoS One*. 2013; 8: e54822. doi:10.1371/journal.pone.0054822

34. Nordahl HM, Stiles TC. Perceptions of parental bonding in patients with various personality disorders, lifetime depressive disorders, and healthy controls. *J Personal Disord*. 1997; 11: 391–402. doi:10.1521/pedi.1997.11.4.391

35. Sullivan HS. *The Interpersonal Theory of Psychiatry*. New York: Norton; 1953.

36. Toman W. *Family Constellation: Theory and Practice of a Psychological Game*. New York: Springer; 1961.

37. Landucci J, Foley GN. Couples therapy: treating selected personality-disordered couples within a dynamic therapy framework. *Innov Clin Neurosci.* 2014; 11(3-4): 29–36.

38. Millon T. *Disorders of Personality: DSM-III-Axis II.* New York: Wiley; 1981.

39. Shabad PC. The unconscious wish and psychoanalytic stoicism. *Contemp. Psychoanal.* 1991; 27(2): 332–350. doi:10.1080/00107530.1991.10747170

40. Blatt S, Shichman S. Two primary configurations of psychopathology. *Psychoanal. Contemp. Thought.* 1983; 6(2): 187–254.

41. Fineberg NA, Sharma P, Sivakumaran T, Sahakian B, Chamberlain SR. Does obsessive-compulsive personality disorder belong within the obsessive-compulsive spectrum? *CNS Spectr.* 2007; 12(6): 467–482. doi:10.1017/s1092852900015340

42. Butcher JN, Dahlstrom WG, Graham JR, Tellegen AM, Kaemmer B. *Minnesota Multiphasic Personality Inventory-2 (MMPI-2): Manual for Administration and Scoring.* 2nd ed. Minneapolis, MN: University of Minnesota Press; 1989.

43. Shedler J, Westen D. The Shedler-Westen Assessment Procedure (SWAP): making personality diagnosis clinically meaningful. *J Pers Assess.* 2007; 89(1): 41–55. doi:10.1080/00223890701357092

44. Millon T, Grossman S, Millon, C. *Millon Clinical Multiaxial Inventory-IV.* Minneapolis: Pearson Assessments; 2015.

45. Rorschach H. *Psychodiagnostik: Methodik und ergebnisse eines warhrnehmungsdiagnostischen Experiments (deutenlassen von zufallsformen).* Bern: E. Bircher; 1921.

46. Morgan CD, Murray HA. A method for investigating fantasies: The Thematic Apperception Test. *AMA Arch. Neurol. Psychiatry.* 1935; 34(2): 289–306.

47. Pinto, A. Introducing the POPS (pathological obsessive-compulsive personality scale): Derivation and exploratory factor analysis. Paper presented at Annual Meeting of the Society for Personality Assessment; 2011; Cambridge, MA.

48. Frost, RO, Marten P, Lahart C, Rosenblate R. The dimensions of perfectionism. *Cog Ther and Res.* 1990; 14(5): 449–468.

49. Tolin DF, Gilliam CM, Davis E, et al. Psychometric properties of the hoarding rating scale-interview. *J Obsess Compuls Relat Disord.* 2018; 16: 76–80. doi:10.1016/j.jocrd.2018.01.003

50. Pinto A, Steinglass JE, Greene AL, Weber EU, Simpson HB. Capacity to delay reward differentiates obsessive-compulsive disorder and obsessive-compulsive personality disorder. *Biol Psychiatry.* 2014; 75(8): 653–659. doi:10.1016/j.biopsych.2013.09.007

51. Gabbard GO. *Psychodynamic Psychiatry in Clinical Practice.* 4th ed. Washington, DC: American Psychiatric Publishing; 2005: 579

52. Josephs L. Self-criticism and the psychic surface. *JAPA.* 2000; 48: 255–280. doi:10.1177/00030651000480011101

53. Josephs L. *Character Structure and the Organization of the Self.* New York: Columbia University Press; 1992.

54. Cooper S. Obsessional thinking: a defense against loss. *Brit J Psychotherapy.* 2000: 16(4); 412–423.doi:10.1111/j.1752-0118.2000.tb00537.x

55. Barber JP, Muenz LR. The role of avoidance and obsessiveness in matching patients to cognitive and interpersonal psychotherapy: empirical findings from the treatment for depression collaborative research program. *J Consult Clin Psychol.* 1996; 64: 951–958. doi:10. 1037/0022-006X.64.5.951

56. Enero C, Soler A, Ramos I, et al., 2783: distress level and treatment outcome in obsessive-compulsive personality disorder (OCPD). *Eur Psychiatry.* 2013; 28: 1. doi:10.1016/S0924-9338(13)77373-5

57. Bamelis LL, Evers SM, Spinhoven P, Arntz A. Results of a multicenter randomized controlled trial of the clinical effectiveness of schema therapy for personality disorders. *Am J Psychiatr.* 2014; 171: 305–22. doi:10.1176/appi.ajp.2013.12040518

58. Barber JP, Morse JQ, Krakauer ID, Chittams J, Crits-Christoph K. Change in obsessive-compulsive and avoidant personality disorders following time-limited supportive-expressive therapy. *Psychol. Psychothe.* 1997; 34(2): 133–143. doi:10.1037/h0087774

59. Smith R, Shepard C, Wiltgen A, et al. Treatment outcomes for inpatients with obsessive-compulsive personality disorder: an open comparison trial. *J Affect Disord.* 2016; 209: 273–278. doi:10.1016/j.jad.2016.12.002

60. Popa CO, Nireştean A, Ardelean M, Buicu G, Ile L. Dimensional personality change after combined therapeutic intervention in the obsessive-compulsive personality disorders. *Acta Med Transilvanica.* 2013; 2: 290–292. doi:10.1017/S1352465815000582

61. Ansseau M. Are SSRIs useful in obsessive-compulsive personality disorder? *Eur Neuropsychopharmacol.* 1994; 4(3): 266–267. doi:10.1016/0924-977X(94)90085-X

62. Ansseau M, Troisfontaines B, Papart P, Von Frenckell R. Compulsive personality as predictor of response to serotonergic antidepressants. *Br Med J.* 1991; 303: 760–761. doi:10.1136/bmj.303.6805.760

63. Greve KW, Adams D. Treatment of features of obsessive-compulsive personality disorder using carbamazepine. *Psychiatry Clin Neurosci.* 2002; 56: 207–208. doi:10.1046/j.1440-1819.2002.00946.x

64. Ekselius L, von Knorring L. Personality disorder comorbidity with major depression and response to treatment with sertraline or citalopram. *Int Clin Psychopharmacol.* 1998; 13(5): 205–211. doi:10.1097/00004850-199809000-00003

65. Silk, KR and Feurino III, L. Psychopharmacology of personality disorder. In: Widiger TA, ed. *The Oxford Handbook of Personality Disorders.* NY: Oxford U Press; 2012:713–726. doi:10.1093/oxfordhb/9780199735013.013.003

66. Sperry L. *Handbook of Diagnosis and Treatment of DSM-IV Personality Disorders.* New York: Routledge; 2013.

67. Wells MC, Glickauf-Hughes C, Buzzell V. Treating obsessive-compulsive personalities in psychodynamic/interpersonal group therapy. *Psychol Psychother.* 1990; 27(3): 366–379. doi:10.1037/0033-3204.27.3.366

68. Yudofsky S. *Fatal Flaws: Navigating Destructive Relationships with People with Disorders of Personality and Character.* Washington, DC: American Psychiatric Publishing; 2005.

25

Masochistic/Self-defeating Personality Styles

Robert Alan Glick and Brenda Berger

Key Points

- An appreciation of the profound and tenacious role suffering has in the inner lives of patients with masochistic/self-defeating personality styles is central to developing clinical understanding and therapeutic approaches.
- Diagnosis: Patients with masochistic/self-defeating personality disorder (DSM III- Revised) reveal a chronic and recurrent history of painful relationships, disappointments, and avoidance of pleasurable or successful situations; they reject help from others.
- Three clinical cases of masochistic/self-defeating personality style are presented and describe the typical treatment challenges.
- Arnold Cooper described the masochistic-narcissistic personality disorder as an early developmental and attachment experience of sustained frustration and powerlessness in the face of parental trauma and neglect.
- Otto Kernberg described a general classification of masochistic psychopathology based on the severity of the psychopathological level of personality organization and variations in this type of personality disorder.
- Eve Caligor uses a three-dimensional approach to the assessment of personality disorders: descriptive, structural, and dynamic perspectives.
- The treatment of masochistic patients requires "infinite" patience, humility, unrelenting curiosity, and unfailing respect for the patient's internal world, their psychic reality.
- Clinical challenges in the treatment of masochistic/self-defeating personality style include management of the transference and countertransference, and an understanding of therapeutic action.
- A collaborative treatment perspective, combining elements of cognitive-behavioral therapy (CBT) and psychodynamic therapy is invaluable for improving opportunities for effective treatment.
- Therapeutic effectiveness depends on the clinician's attention to the patient's needs to suffer, their profound trauma, and the unconscious painful attachments that define these patients' inner lives. Managing the difficult countertransference reactions that inevitably arise is essential in sustaining effective treatments.

Introduction

Pain and suffering are inescapable in life, woven into our common experiences of failure, loss, guilt, shame, and regret. As mental health professionals, we seek to alleviate or at least lessen forms of mental and emotional pain. Clinical experience makes clear that our patients come to us because they suffer and seek relief. However, certain patients who present with histories of persistent patterns of pain, suffering, rejection, subjugation, disappointment, defeat, and loss appear paradoxically attached to these experiences, which is at odds with their seeking treatment. Clinicians face the significant challenge of a patient's seeming desire to feel better but who shows little intention or capacity to change. These are features of the masochistic/self-defeating personality style.

The diagnosis and treatment of masochistic personality presents significant clinical challenges for clinicians at the beginning and throughout their careers. It requires a complex, often disquieting, understanding of mental life and its treatment. Clinicians often feel powerless and ineffective after many years of hard therapeutic work; they frequently struggle with the puzzle of why their patients' suffering continues in the various relentless forms that it does.

Central to the clinical understanding and therapeutic approaches to masochistic personality/self-defeating personality style is an appreciation of the profound and tenacious role suffering has in these patients' inner lives. Clinicians, whose very identity is defined by the effort to relieve suffering and foster health, need tools to guide them in sustaining an effective therapeutic relationship. The clinician therefore faces significant psychological obstacles in the effort to improve patients' lives and promote positive change. We will describe psychoanalytic theories that can be helpful, which suggest overpowering unconscious needs, wishes, and motivations tied to suffering. Characteristically, both cognitive-behavioral and psychodynamic treatment strategies are useful synergistically. The strict setting of cognitive and behavioral goals and the premature use of an insight-oriented approach (i.e., encouraging self-reflection about patients' roles in their problems) are experienced by patients respectively as setting them up for failure and as blaming attacks. Both approaches can be experienced and interpreted as further evidence of injustice and reinforce negative senses of self, but both can also be used effectively in long-term treatments.

The etiology of this complicated personality style, and its seemingly intractable relationship to suffering, has not been definitively researched. However, clinical experience suggests a crucial interweaving of temperament and the enduring impact of traumatic developmental experiences. Maladaptive and painful solutions to intrapsychic and interpersonal conflict are the result.

Masochistic Personality/Self-defeating Personality Style

The diagnosis of masochistic/self-defeating personality disorder has not been included in the *Diagnostic and Statistical Manual* (DSM) after the DSM-III-Revised.[1] Issues of diagnostic reliability and the question of misapplication of self-defeating personality disorder (as a "blame the victim" bias against women) have been addressed by several authors elsewhere.[2] The DSM-III-R recommended research on this diagnosis. Despite this decision to remove this disorder from the current DSM, the issues of masochistic and self-defeating style or behavior are ubiquitous. The DSM III-R criteria give us a starting place to define some of the characteristics of this personality style; see Box 25.1, p. 615.

> **Box 25.1. Summary of Masochistic Personality Disorder (DSM III-Revised)**
>
> ---
>
> Patients with masochistic/self-defeating personality disorder reveal a chronic and recurrent history of painful relationships, disappointments, and avoidance of pleasurable or successful situations and of seeking help from others. Pain, suffering, depression, and guilt characterize their life experience. These patients tend to provoke rejection and anger, often feeling hurt, victimized, and treated unfairly. They fail to meet appropriate expectations in school, work, or social situations, prompting criticism, humiliation, and rejection. These patients have a pattern of injustice collecting, rejecting people who attempt to treat them well, and of self-sacrifice leading to further disappointment and grievance. They sabotage positive opportunities in relationships, work, and academic advancement.

Despite these ongoing diagnostic questions, masochistic/self-defeating patients, male and female, continue to ask for treatment. They describe their life experiences as full of repetitive pain, suffering, disappointment, and defeat. They also present patterns of interpersonal subjugation, rejection, and loss. Their self-experiences typically involve negative self-images and feelings of inferiority. Patients with this disorder often feel aggrieved, unfairly victimized, and alone in their unfortunate state. They tend to view themselves as altruistic and self-sacrificing when addressing the needs of others, and then will see themselves as victims, suffering injustices at the hands of uncaring others. Some are intensely self-critical, believing they deserve their misery for some reason. Their anger can be self-directed or, at times, intensely focused on others who have hurt and rejected them. They also often have difficulty acknowledging and expressing their anger for fear of retaliation. Patients with this character pathology tend to "snatch defeat from the jaws of victory." They search for the negative in a wide array of positive possibilities, focusing on what is missing rather than what is available. They are often also depressed but not helped by antidepressant medications.

Clinical Presentations of Masochistic/Self-defeating Personality Style

The Masochistic/Self-defeating Personality Style with Features of Other Personality Styles

Case 1. Ms. B: Masochistic or Self-Defeating Personality Style with Histrionic Features; Recurrent Victimization in Romantic Relationships

Ms. B, a long-divorced woman in her late 40s, sought help in a state of acute distress, because of an impending disruption of a romantic relationship of several months' duration. She presented as attractive and engaging in appearance but anxious and despairing. She felt that she had finally met her "long-sought soulmate" and feared that recent fights would end the relationship. She saw herself as intensely giving, generous, and attentive to others, including this man. He seemed to have suddenly grown intensely selfish, withholding, and now rejecting. When they fought, she lost control of her temper and shouted hurtful remarks. He became cold and distant. She desperately wanted help to salvage this relationship.

Ms. B's history revealed a recurrent pattern of crisis and rejection in relationships. Her family history suggested that her mother was very self-effacing and self-sacrificing in her relationship with a volatile and demanding husband. The patient saw herself, among her siblings, as the chosen mediator in the family. Ms. B experienced herself in her adult life as the victim of selfish and cruel men who hurt and rejected her when she sought affection and intimacy. While effective and talented in her professional life, her crisis-ridden personal life interfered with her work. She was intensely dramatic in both her history and self-presentation, easily crying, laughing, and soliciting approval. She had little self-awareness of her role in these problems. Prior treatments had been ineffective in improving her relationship patterns. As she began psychotherapy, she described an immediate sense of relief that "someone wise and compassionate is seeking to help me." She described her painful childhood, her relationships with her parents, and how she suffered at the "hands of selfish men" like her father. After a few weeks, the history of her provocative dramatic, self-sacrificing behavior became evident. The therapist attempted to explore her problems controlling her intense responses and the confrontations and disruptions these reactions prompted. She became uncomfortable and slightly irritated with this exploration. After approximately three months of treatment, she announced that her schedule and finances demanded she end the treatment. She said that she hoped to return as soon as possible since the therapist "seemed so understanding and sympathetic." There was no further contact.

Case 2. Mr. S: Masochistic or Self-Defeating Personality Style with Obsessive and Dependent Features; Victimization and Pervasive Disappointment in a Man with Chronic Depressive Traits

Mr. S was a 44-year-old man in twice-weekly psychodynamic therapy for 12 years. Well-educated and talented in his creative field, he entered his regularly attended sessions in the way he seemed to live, like a wound up, overly busy robot. He spoke through gritted teeth, unaware of the substantial contempt that his style revealed. He was joyless, even when he talked about something he liked doing. He gave himself few "happy" opportunities. When asked about the competitive job he successfully landed, he described his daily life at the office as if it he was a prisoner on a chain gang. Unaware of this punitive behavior, he frequently made work assignments more difficult by eating poorly and not sleeping for days at a stretch.

Mr. S. saw himself as nerdy and inadequate despite being a good-looking, smart, and interesting person. He very much wanted to feel "normal," like somebody who could marry and have children. But care and warmth toward the women he met was missing from how he spoke of them. Over time in treatment, he began to approach women and ask them out. However, he repeatedly chose unavailable women who were narcissistic or cruel. Mr. S told his therapist about the "red flags" he saw in women when he began dating them, including how disinterested they were in commitment. He ignored what he knew, and then took up an insistent mission of trying to make his dates into viable wives, ending up rejected, devastated, and clinging to them like a terrified child. As he clung, he also actively fought with them about their role, versus his own, in the breakups, offering magical ideas about how he could fix things. Like a "good," angry little soldier, he tried unsuccessfully to undo whatever they disliked about him.

Mr. S. was an only child, born to a severely depressed mother who was extremely anxious and prone to psychotic ruminations about being poverty stricken. Mr. S. always felt a huge pressure coming from her to cure her, and to succeed in various ways so that she could "worry less." Remaining unmarried and without children was just one of several ways in which he enacted his battle with her. This made his treatment (elaborated further later in this chapter) long and arduous.

Case 3. Mr. R: Obsessional Character with Depressive and Masochistic Features; the Need to Suffer as the Price of Pleasure

Mr. R was a married businessman, father of four, in his mid-40s. He came to treatment because he felt guilty and quietly depressed most of his life. He loved his wife and children, and had a lovely, comfortable life. He had features of an obsessional character with depressive and masochistic qualities. Resisting treatments for a long time, implicitly afraid of "opening up," he entered psychotherapy. He slowly did better, became less obsessed with guilt and punitive fantasies, but remained miserable in his work life and unable to find or risk a change. An antidepressant helped some. After several months into the course of the treatment, with a painful anguish, he revealed a crucial secret: he had become involved in an extramarital affair and was consumed with guilt over this passionate illicit relationship. (His treatment is elaborated later in this chapter.)

All three of these patients experienced significant childhood trauma. Ms. B had an abusive, but seductive, father. She believed she should be able to "bring peace to the family" by calming her dangerous father. Mr. S was invaded by his mother's need for him to cure her desperate depressions. Mr. R had severely damaged older brothers who completely dominated his family and caused him deep shame and guilt, and a wish for reparations.

Other Common Behavioral Patterns in Patients with Masochistic/Self-defeating Style

These case examples reveal several behavioral patterns commonly seen with the masochistic personality style. However, there are other variations that include the following:

1. Long painful relationships, for example marriages in which the patient constantly feels hurt and unappreciated by their partner and forced to submit to their partner's "selfishness." They wish they could leave, but are fearful of being alone.
2. Recurrent failed relationships and work failures, in which patients cannot express their own desires without fear of punishment and rejection. These include repetitive patterns of dysfunctional, unhappy relationships, and academic, vocational, or professional failures in which performance expectations are not met despite opportunity for success.

Psychodynamic Theories of Masochism as a Guide to Treatment

Evaluation and diagnosis of the clinical phenomenology of masochistic/self-defeating personality styles requires a combination of clinical inference and empirical observation. Given that treatments are so challenging, the use of psychodynamic theory to better understand these patients is helpful.

Masochism has remained a theoretical and clinical challenge for the mental health field since the term was originally described. It was introduced for scientific exploration by Krafft-Ebing in his encyclopedic text, *Psychopathia Sexualis*,[3] as a form of sexual desire and expression associated with passion, physical pain, humiliation, and subjugation. Drawing on the 1870 publication of Leopold Von Sacher-Masoch's novel *Venus in Furs*,[4] Kraft-Ebing coined the term "masochism" and added it to the classification of sexuality. The novel portrays a male lover's passionate submission to forms of enslavement, failure, deprivation, humiliation, cruelty, and physical and psychological abuse for the sake of "love" and "sexual" pleasure. Interestingly, Krafft-Ebing viewed masochism as an intensification of normal passivity and dependence. He considered masochism a congenital disorder of sexual instincts—the wish for pain, humiliation, abuse, and sexual subjugation equating passivity and femininity—as Freud problematically did.

The psychological investigation of non-sexual forms of masochism can be traced to Freud's 1905 monograph *Three Essays on Sexuality*.[5] He described the instinctually driven phases in the development of normal human sexuality. This established oral, anal, phallic, and genital (oedipal) as stages in psychological maturation. Freud took up the issue early in the development of his psychosexual instinct theory, and wrestled with it throughout his career in a series of papers. He coined the term "moral masochism"[6] to describe the role of unconscious guilt and the characterological need for punishment.

Historically, the various approaches to understanding masochism have been described as reflecting "the developmental vicissitudes of psychoanalytic theory as it moved from its earliest focus on instinct to considerations of psychic structure and oedipal dynamics, object relations, separation-individuation, self-organization, and self-esteem regulation, and as it progressed into more systematic investigation of child development and attachment."[7] One central psychoanalytic construct is:

> Masochism is a complex configuration, multiply determined from different developmental levels, and serves various functions. The essence of masochism is conceptualized as *pleasure in pain* . . . because the pain is unconsciously considered the necessary, indispensable condition for need satisfaction or "pleasure," and becomes inextricably associated with it.[7]

For an additional and extensive historical review of psychoanalytic understanding of masochism, see Glick and Meyers.[7]

Arnold Copper: On Masochism

Arnold Cooper developed a particular, in-depth understanding of the development of masochistic/self-defeating personality disorder. He believed it was rooted in the early developmental experience of sustained frustration and powerlessness in the face of parental trauma and neglect.[8] The masochistic character is understood as a deeply necessary psychological defense. As revealed in the case studies, masochism, in its many forms and degrees, is often forged in the crucible of severe childhood traumatic development. The deformation of self-development, self-regulation, and self-organization comes from the fearful dependence on overly abusive, inconsistent, unpredictable, cruel, and exploitative caregivers. This creates profound pathological attachments, with a primitive form of omnipotent control, and with self-directed rage as an adaptive survival response.

To live as a child constantly afraid, helpless, and traumatized changes both the mind and brain. Being abused by narcissistic parents (e.g., fragile unstable narcissists or rigid insatiable narcissists) damages a child's healthy, resilient sense of self. A traumatized child creates vigilance as a form of protective, omnipotent control against the terror of the unexpected, and of helplessness in the face of pain. This can lead to the child's loyal attachment to the tortured, torturing, and deeply suffering parent. Trauma creates a life-long, recurrent pattern of seeking out and repeating these attachments in the illusory hope of mastery and change. For individuals with such histories, it is crucial to understand and respect the tenacity of their unconscious attachments to severely narcissistic family members who, due to their own fragility, behaved with them in selfish, cruel, critical, and demanding ways.

Issues of boundaries, identity, and impulse control shape these patients' lives. They cling to an apparently wretched early relationship, which remains essential to maintaining self-cohesion and self-regulation. As a consequence, they develop complex identifications with the suffering of the primary objects: "keeping them alive through suffering."[8] These are among the most persistent and severe forms of masochism, and they are therefore often heartbreaking and challenging treatments. The process of "transplanting"[8] one pathological attachment with a new, healthy analytic attachment can feel interminable.

Dr. Arnold Cooper, a seminal contributor to the psychodynamic theory of masochism, is particularly helpful in understanding treatments in which suffering was central, intractable, and seemingly endless. In his paper "The Narcissistic Masochistic Character,"[9] Copper describes how the wish for omnipotent control in masochism reflects the pathological narcissism inseparable in this character structure. Summarizing the explanatory theories of masochism, Cooper wrote:

1. Attitudes of passivity, harmlessness, and nonaggression are unconsciously adopted as a defense against dangerous competitive impulses and fears of retaliation.
2. Suffering, helplessness, and defeat represent a cry for love and are unconsciously intended to ensure loving care, which is otherwise perceived not to be available.
3. Early, severe, inescapable painful traumas lead to defensive efforts to cope with the trauma by learning to enjoy it, adopting it as one's own.
4. Early injuries to the infantile sense of omnipotent control are adapted to defensive style, by the fantasy of control over disappointing, powerful parents and by defensively claiming the disappointment as directed by oneself.
5. Experiences of pain result in endorphin release in the attempt to ease the pain, and one becomes self-addicted to endorphin release, pursuing painful events for this end.
6. Children reared under abusive conditions nonetheless attach to their abusing caretakers. For these persons with damaged self-esteem and fears of abandonment, maintaining the safety of familiarity takes precedence over potential pleasure that entails the anxiety of the new.[9]

Otto Kernberg: On Masochism

Otto Kernberg[10] offers other perspectives to help guide clinicians' assessments and treatments of masochism. He evaluates levels of personality organization, ego organization, anxiety tolerance, impulse control, and defenses. His focus is also on ego and superego integration. This approach is based on assumptions of unconscious mental structures and functions, which include desires/impulses and fears (e.g., fears of punishment, guilt, shame, humiliation, conflict, and competing impulses and desires). Kernberg sees the core defense of splitting as an essential component of borderline personality organization, not always seen in the masochistic personality style. But an example of splitting can be seen in what Mr. S did in the way he reported his dates' unavailability: He split off his anger about this situation, and transformed it by enacting masochistically against the women he dated, and himself.

Using this approach, psychopathology can be assessed along a spectrum of structural organization: normal, neurotic personality organization, or borderline personality organization. This psychodynamic perspective has particular importance when approaching treatment of this disorder[11] because it highlights the crucial place of different personality organizations in determining the difficulty of treatment, and especially highlights different therapeutic approaches.

Kernberg[11] offers a general classification of masochistic psychopathology based on the severity of the psychopathological levels of personality organization and the kind of personality disorder. His taxonomy of masochistic character pathology includes:

1. Normal masochism. This involves universal minor, self-defeating behaviors, including obsessional acts to "ward off" unconsciously feared punishments for victories. The extension of appropriate self-criticism deepens into negative and depressive moods.

2. The neurotic level of personality organization. It is commonly linked with obsessive-compulsive and histrionic personality traits or disorders. Some of these patients can show intense, harshly self-critical, conscientious, and judgmental attitudes. They can be humorless and given to moral indignation and grievance collecting. Many patients are easily disappointed in others. They may be overly "needy" and dependent on others for support, attention, and acceptance, and are intensely rejection sensitive.

3. Patients who have an intense avoidance of any awareness and acceptance of their own anger. When potentially enraged by hurt and disappointment, they can become self-defeating, self-deprecating, submissive, and compliant.

4. Patients with a sadomasochistic personality disorder, with a borderline personality organization. They are sadistic, alternating with masochistic functioning. They have chaotic personal relationships, act sadistically or feel constantly victimized, and feel rejected by others who offer to help them.

5. Syndrome of pathological infatuation. This involves intense obsessions and idealization of the loved one, and an unrelenting and self-defeating compulsion to gain the affection of the loved one despite the impossibility of these efforts that usually leads to crisis and failure.

Eve Caligor: On Masochism

Eve Caligor[12] offers a three-dimensional approach to the assessment of personality disorders that is useful both in diagnosis and treatment: descriptive, structural, and dynamic perspectives.

Using the descriptive perspective, an individual's normal personality is described as clusters of personality traits which are relatively stable with durable patterns of behavior, thoughts, emotions, and interpersonal relationships. (Review Box 25.1 (see p. 615) for the descriptive approach for masochistic personality disorder.)

From a structural perspective, an individual's personality can be described in terms of the relatively stable and enduring patterns of psychological functions and processes that underlie and organize the individual's behaviors, perceptions, and subjective experience in predictable ways.[12] Patients with masochistic PD can function at the neurotic, borderline, or narcissistic personality organization levels. These different levels of personality organization determine the intensity and relative difficulty of managing the transference and countertransference and the predominant defense used (e.g., splitting versus repression) by the patient.

Within the psychodynamic framework, object-relations theory describes the severity of personality pathology as defined through the lens of the individual's experience of self and significant others, the quality of relationships and the internal representation of these relationships, the nature of defensive operations, and the stability of reality testing.[11] For masochistic/self-defeating personality style, this object-relations perspective emphasizes the depth and tenacity of the pathological object relationship, namely the unconscious, unyielding bond to a hostile, rejecting, or punishing internal object-representation. Unconscious hostility toward the object-representation is turned back on the self-representation, which leads to intensification of self-punishing attack, despair, and humiliation.

From a self-psychological perspective,[13] the use of a narcissistic grandiose self-object determines the persistent pattern of failure to achieve recognition and a stable, mature self-organization.

Central to all these theoretical frames of reference is the fundamental assumption of pathological attachment, based on forms of developmental trauma and failure of healthy emotional nurturance.

Analysis of the Three Case Studies

In order to illustrate the clinical application of these descriptions and theories of masochistic/self-defeating personality styles, consider again the three case studies. In each of them, we can see how the defensive structure serves to maintain the infantile, masochistic object attachment.

In the case of Ms. B, one can infer the primary unconscious defenses of denial and avoidance, particularly of her provocative hostility and demands for attack. Her seductive "wish to please" and histrionic style cover her unconscious grandiosity, and her self-dramatization expressed as her desire to be "center stage" in all situations. Unconsciously, she seeks an attachment to her hostile and rejecting father, while identifying with her "noble," self-sacrificing mother.

In the case of Mr. S, one can infer several of the unconscious functions of the sado-masochistic defense. Using this defense, he internally holds onto and protects his very troubled mother, punishing his dates with the disavowed rage toward his mother. He also tortures himself out of his unremitting guilt for that rage, and enacts the obedient/defiant attachment he has to his mother. Over the years, he demonstrated that he would, and would not, obey her and become a "normal" married man. Here, the bond to his mother dominates his entire emotional life.

In the case of Mr. R, the primary masochistic defense appears as self-punishment and guilt for the rage toward his parents and brothers, and for the passion and sexual satisfaction he experienced in his extramarital relationship. Additionally, his passionate pleasures are an unconscious compensation to which he felt entitled, because of what he endured growing up with his defective brothers and the attention they demanded.

Clinical Challenges in the Treatment of Masochistic/Self-defeating Personality Styles

In dynamic psychotherapies, therapists seek to discover what drives patients in their suffering masochistic attachments and self-defeating behaviors, and to use the therapeutic relationship to help the patients know themselves more deeply. This effort is made in the hope of lessening that suffering and improving their lives. Through the therapeutic alliance, therapists seek to aid patients in their liberation from pain and self-defeating inhibitions, to facilitate healing from the traumas of damaging childhoods, thereby restoring healthy self-regard and self-regulation.

Transference, Countertransference, and Therapeutic Action

Central to working psychodynamically are the concepts of transference, countertransference, and therapeutic action. These concepts help guide the clinician through the challenges of particularly difficult treatments, both in the immediate and the longer phases of the treatment.

Common transferences include the patient's insistent conviction that the therapist is critical and rejecting or, alternatively, that the therapist will somehow repair all injustice and rejection. When the therapist inevitably fails to gratify this wish, the patient experiences the therapist as an uncaring, punitive, cruel, and shaming authority.

Common countertransferences involve therapist feelings of frustration, disappointment, and being misunderstood as angry, rejecting, or indifferent to the patient's suffering. Problematic anger in the therapist, in response to the patient's attacks, is a frequent occurrence in the therapeutic process. Other patient-generated countertransferences include unconscious and disavowed sadistic aggression toward the therapist and the wish to reverse roles and defeat, punish, and humiliate the therapist. These are transmitted to the therapist via projective identification. This reflects the unconscious grandiosity of the patient as supreme victim, and poses severe challenges in the maintenance of the treatment relationship because of the intense countertransference reactions engendered.

Therapeutic action in the treatment of masochistic patients involves maintaining the therapeutic relationship through the phases of profound frustration and absence of positive change, as well as the patient's provocations. The goal is the patient's slow internalization of an attachment to a more benign and caring object that replaces the pathological attachment. This crucially reflects the long-term resilience of the relationship between therapist and patient.

Transference, countertransference, and therapeutic action serve the clinician as inferential tools or "stencils" for making sense of the continuous flow of the clinical process:

the stream of feelings, thoughts, and behaviors of both participants. Dynamically oriented clinicians attend to these feelings in both the micro-process of the moment-to-moment interactions with the patient and in the macro-process of the phases of the patient's treatment over weeks, months, or years. (An excellent and comprehensive discussion and review of these concepts is available elsewhere.)[14] Nothing reveals as much as a patient's masochism does about the power of psychic reality (unconscious motivations, fears, and narratives) over external reality. Given the tenacity of this pattern, and because the clinical process is often so difficult, the clinician must guard against countertransference reactions of unrealistic expectations and frustration with the pace of the therapy. The process can feel especially arduous and painful, and it can prompt interventions that will compound a shared sense of failure and disappointment.

Other Psychodynamic Considerations with Masochistic Patients

Another important element in treating masochism is the clinician's attention to the possible meanings of the patient's behaviors both within and outside the treatment setting. These meanings are offered by the explanatory, dynamic theories of masochism that can serve as guides during the differing phases of the treatment process.

Collaborative Treatments

A collaborative treatment perspective, combining elements of cognitive-behavioral therapy (CBT) and psychodynamic therapy, is an invaluable approach that may improve the possibility of effective treatment over long periods of time. Useful elements of CBT include setting goals for changes in conscious cognitions from negative to positive (e.g., seeing oneself as a participant, collaborator, or a person of value, and not as a victim) and suggesting novel, more-adaptive behaviors that could offer more positive outcomes, such as completing assignments, meeting expectations, and showing initiative. CBT interventions can serve as opportunities to test the patient's motivation and alliance in the treatment, suggesting the current state of therapeutic leverage and possibilities for positive change. Measuring modest patient behavioral goals such as showing up on time for appointments or not missing sessions can reveal the incremental effectiveness of the treatment relationship. For example, CBT interventions can focus on setting schedules for getting work done on time, taking more positive stances in relationships, avoiding provocative passive-aggressiveness, or shifting from a conscious sense of being or acting like a victim in a relationship.

Successful CBT interventions can provide opportunities to demonstrate to patients an empathic understanding of the severity of their difficulties, and demonstrate the effectiveness of the therapeutic alliance. These interventions can also serve as markers of the underlying, dynamic elements in the treatment process itself, especially the state of the transference relationship (e.g., the conflict between patients' wishes to please the therapist, and their powerful insistence on failure). These dynamic inferences may aid the clinician's understanding of the patient's complex motivations and defensive organization. They can facilitate awareness of the patient's largely unconscious experience of the therapist, the therapeutic relationship, and what is "at stake" for them in the treatment process.

Eye Movement Desensitization and Reprocessing (EMDR)

In addition to CBT, EMDR offers another kind of collaborative treatment that can be useful clinically. It was suggested to Mr. S by his therapist because his sexual inhibitions revealed themselves as more severe over time, seeming more like a phobia based on past trauma. Surprisingly, Mr. S agreed; through EMDR targeting his early trauma, he gained some greater kindness toward, and engagement with, the engulfed boy within him.

EMDR posits that when children experience traumatic events which are more than their systems can handle, these experiences are recorded in the limbic system, rather than being stored in the prefrontal cortex where factual nonaffective memory gets housed.[15] When situations in the present trigger old traumatic experiences, they can trigger body sensations like heart pounding, throat tightening, and stomach upset. Traumatic thoughts which are more related to the past than the present may also intrude. For example, Mr. S, with a deeply troubled attachment to his mother, was terrified in dating situations. He rejected interested women despite his conscious desire to find a partner. EMDR targeted feeder memories from his past, like those of being trapped, panicked, and helpless in the hands of a mother who set him up to date inappropriate older women in invasive, asphyxiating ways. The treatment technique involved having the patient vividly describe a current dating situation that was very upsetting, and encouraged him to free-associate to a memory in the past that somehow evoked the same emotions or bodily sensations. The older memory was discussed in such a way as to make it affectively alive in the patient. He was then asked to hold this experience in mind while the therapist used various techniques (eye movements, sounds, tapping patterns) to interrupt his working memory. Research has shown that EMDR decreases the intensity and vividness of the old memories and facilitates access to rational thoughts when triggering events occur in the present.[15] The way EMDR worked with Mr. S was evident in his growing ability to find a space to think more clearly about his provocative rejecting behavior with women rather than becoming trapped by fear, responding defensively, and thereby falling into abandonment terror and loss.

Psychodynamic Treatment Process

Throughout these treatments, clinicians should be recurrently asking themselves, as they examine their experience of the therapeutic relationship, these questions:

1. Why does the patient want to hold on to this pain, impoverishment, or an empty life, rather than have success or pleasure?
2. What makes this a better choice?
3. What does masochism preserve and protect?
4. What ideal self is maintained through masochism?
5. What victory is obtained, what guilt or destruction is avoided?

Secrecy

Masochistic patients' tendency toward secrecy can be ever-present in the therapeutic relationship. Even when the patient relinquishes some masochistic pleasure or triumph, the therapist may be the last to know. Perhaps more than most patients, the masochist has the biggest investment in keeping secrets; once the patient has engaged and established the needed masochistic transference, any shift, any little success, pleasure, assertion, or non-victimized experience must be kept secret. Secrets also embody the patient's (omnipotent) power over the therapist. Therapists may feel cheated of any success, which may be precisely what the patient seeks the therapist to experience. Acknowledging any improvement or gain from the treatment may signal for the patient various dangers: an intolerable sense of failing and the therapist winning; the potential and dreaded, but always anticipated, end of the treatment relationship; and/or the gratification of the needed but failing therapist. Gains from the treatment are fragile; they can feel like they are written in sand or made of smoke. This is the essence of the "negative therapeutic reaction."

Further Treatment Considerations

The treatment of masochistic patients requires "infinite" patience, humility, unrelenting curiosity, and unfailing respect for the patient's internal world, their psychic reality. The therapist may also need to examine feeling demoralized when offering therapy. Demoralization may be manifest in feelings of deadness, hopelessness, and powerlessness. These are the inevitable countertransference reactions that arise in the course of these often-protracted treatments. The therapist may struggle with feelings of anger at, and frustration with, the patient; she or he may have a troubling wish to punish "the impossible patient" or find a way to reject or abandon the patient. When recognized, the therapist can consequently have painful feelings of inadequacy, shame, guilt, isolation, and despair. When this happens, it can be quite helpful to consider how these countertransference reactions reflect the patient's ways of unconsciously communicating their inner experiences of their impossible childhoods, and the intolerable emotions they were too young to adequately manage. Recognizing this form of projective communication can lighten the therapist's tortured, hostile feelings. Clinicians at all levels of experience often seek helpful consultations with colleagues to assist them in untangling dauntingly painful therapeutic stalemates or impasses.

Therapeutic Effectiveness

In the most general sense, the treatment works, to the extent that it can work, with modest expectations, through the very slow acceptance of the patient's need to preserve their self-image and position in relationships. Clinicians understandably hope to facilitate positive change; but the patient may be deeply (and unconsciously) motivated to "simply" hold onto the masochistic attachment to the therapist. In a significant sense, these treatments are effective inasmuch as the treatment relationship survives the deeply agonizing mutual frustration, disappointment, pain, and latent hostility.

The internal world of patients with masochistic/self-defeating personality styles is dominated by internal unconscious representations of harsh, punitive, rejecting others (objects), and of their sense of self as hurt, powerless, and victimized. Clinicians must demonstrate through tolerance, persistence, lack of traumatizing imposition of per-ceived demands (like getting better), the long, slow disconfirmation of the patient's te-nacious perceptions and modes of relating. Patients with this personality style are not particularly self-reflective and have powerful resistances to recognizing and acknow-ledging their role in their suffering and disappointments.

As suggested by Cooper,[9] significant masochistic character pathology always involves narcissistic pathology (and often the reverse is true as well). Masochism becomes an early developmental "fortress" and serves to protect and defend the internal, injured, and ever-fragile child. Much to the vexation of the therapist, the apparent "weakness and vulnerability" of the masochist is secretly a resilient and well-protected strength. This makes them especially resistant to awareness of their own sadistic aggression, particu-larly in the treatment relationship. Appreciating this dilemma allows therapists to work at accepting the steadfastly maintained rewards in the pain and suffering.

In a crucial sense, the fate of the treatment rests on the capacity and awareness of the clinician to preserve the therapeutic relationship through the ruptures and repairs that come with patients living out their masochistic/self-defeating patterns in the treatment process. The therapeutic relationship must survive in order for there to be any incre-mental internalization of the healthy relationship with a therapist who ultimately does not punish or reject the patient. The resilience of the clinician and an empathic and pos-itive therapeutic relationship "over the long haul" can contribute to the gradual modifi-cation of the patient's insistent pain and suffering. In a deep sense, the treatment survives the masochism. Clearly, many factors determine and influence the degree and nature of any successful outcome of the treatment.

Theoretically, treatment works because of a long, slow disconfirmation of the transfer-ence; the incremental internalization of robust, benign, independent superego represen-tation; and a new object-relationship. Over the long haul, the impact of the relationship with the therapist or self-object allows some modified sense of self to evolve in the pa-tient, a shift that no longer relies on a self-definition ruled by suffering, unhappiness, and the virtue of pain.[16]

A central and invaluable feature of all psychodynamic treatments is the therapist's on-going attention to, and consideration of, the unconscious meanings of the interaction in the therapeutic process. While not necessarily sharing these reflections with the patient, awareness of these unconscious meanings allow the therapist to manage the intensity of the treatment situation. For example, psychotherapies may often have a honeymoon pe-riod where the patient feels better and starts to accomplish long-avoided or difficult life tasks or makes positive changes in relationships. Then, for reasons that are not clear to patient or therapist, improvements and gains evaporate and "victories go up in smoke." The patient insists that they are either incapable of being helped, or that the therapist is attacking them and harboring unjustified expectations. For the therapist, recognizing the possible unconscious motives in a sudden treatment stalemate or negative thera-peutic reaction calls for patience and a "recalibration" of the current therapeutic efforts. Patients' unconscious motives function as tightly held defenses that are experienced as crucially important for them. The defenses protect patients against early guilt, shame, and vulnerability. They also provide, among other needs, ways of remaining attached to depriving parents or difficult siblings. The defense is a kind of autonomy–the claiming of the victory of the victim—suggesting the forms of narcissistic grandiosity deeply woven into masochistic pathology.

Treatments of the Case Studies

The treatments of Ms. B, Mr. S, and Mr. R show how theory can be applied in practice. They also reveal how arduous these therapeutic processes can be.

Case 2: Mr. S

After six years of treatment (and to his therapist's relief), Mr. S finally agreed that he might benefit from an antidepressant, because his self-esteem suffered repeatedly after multiple dating rejections. He tried medication gingerly, reporting unheard-of side effects at tiny doses, and he conveyed the experience as if he were being poisoned. This was similar to the way he approached sex with women: gingerly, with terrible anxiety, a feeling of being on high alert. Once an effective medication dose was reached, his mood and feelings of self-loathing actually improved. However, he then went on a trip with his mother, and without discussion in his therapy, he stopped the antidepressant. Mr. S. became quite depressed again a few weeks later, and said he discontinued the medication because his mother would disapprove of it.

In the countertransference, the therapist felt punished, disappointed, helpless, and pain and anger. He also felt set up to fail. These were emotions he felt throughout a long treatment. They were all affects which he needed to manage quietly internally. This induced countertransference emotion captured Mr. S's life-long relationship with his mother and the various women he dated. It took 10 treatment years before Mr. S. could begin to see how he repeated a torturous experience: playing both the villain and the victim. He was only conscious of being the rejected child he once was, not of the adult torturer he had become.

Mr. S's whole being exemplified the capturing of a person by the enduring effects of early traumatic experience. For many years, he was suffused with rage, unconscious about what lay inside him. His furies, fears, and guilt had a massive impact on his psyche, deeply compromising his ability to enjoy life, women, and work. Locked in an internal no-win battle with his mother, Mr. S. externalized it through numerous "who is crazy and reject-able battles" with the women he dated. He sadly needed to prove, and disprove at once, that he was "It."

Case 3: Mr. R

Mr. R's case also shed a light on what makes the therapeutic process so difficult. He seemed immovably stuck in his passivity and victimhood, feeling both lucky and short-changed in life. Then, maybe as a result of the treatment and maybe not, he fell passionately in love with a woman with whom he worked. This was a relationship he had never expected to find. He knew that he could not hurt his wife and children by leaving them. But he could not give up his lover who understood him deeply, with whom he felt unique passion and a deep intimacy.

Tellingly, both he and his lover grew up in deeply compromised families dominated by physically and emotionally handicapped family members. He felt he had found a soulmate.

For him, they had both been oppressed by a tragic fate, in a way that he felt he could not share with his happy wife.

Three years into this parallel life, Mr. R lived in unremitting guilty fear of getting caught. He was both happier and more miserable than before. In a way, these feelings mirrored his pathology: He seemed to believe that his pleasure needed to be contingent on suffering. He felt like a "bad person" because of this affair, but had no desire to give it up. After exploring their therapeutic stalemate, both the patient and therapist agreed to end the treatment, with the understanding that the patient could return when he wished. At the termination, the therapist was left with a manageable but nonetheless significant sense of sad disappointment and frustration.

Conclusion

Patients with masochistic/self-defeating personality styles show recurrent and persistent patterns of pain, suffering, failure, loss, and disappointment in many facets of their lives. Psychodynamic explanatory theories of masochism can guide the clinician through the slow, difficult, and often discouraging treatment process. Combining aspects of cognitive-behavioral and psychodynamic treatment approaches may offer significant tools in the therapeutic process over long periods of time. Clinicians must pay close attention to the profound unconscious, painful attachments that define the inner lives of these patients, and consequently to the significant, difficult countertransference reactions that inevitably arise. This recognition is essential in sustaining effective treatments.

See Box 25.2 for relevant resources for patients, families, and clinicians.

Conflict of Interest/Disclosure: The authors of this chapter have no financial conflicts and nothing to disclose.

Box 25.2 Additional Resources for Patients, Families, and Clinicians

Patients and Families

- Are You A Masochist? https://theawarenesscentre.com/are-you-a-masochist/.
- Self-Destructive Personality Disorder Symptoms: Self-Destructive Personality Disorder Symptoms. https://www.google.com/search?sxsrf = ALeKk0398wsmn-GtuqFCs1SenjZ3aaug2Q:1589767685747&q = self-destructive + personality+disorder + symptoms&sa = X&ved = 2ahUKEwjturyRqrz-pAhVST6wKHU0MDRAQ1QIoAXoECAwQAg&biw = 1276&bih = 727.
- Goulston M, Goldberg P. *Get Out of Your Own Way: Overcoming Self-Defeating Behavior*. London, UK: Penguin; 1996.

Clinicians

- Glick RA, Meyers DI. *Masochism: Current Clinical Perspectives*. Hillsdale, NJ: The Analytic Press; 1988.
- Holtzman D, Kulish N., eds. *The Clinical Problem of Masochism*. Lanham, MD: The Analytic Press; 2018.

References

1. *Psychodynamic Diagnostic Manual (PDM)*. Silver Spring, MD: American Psychoanalytic Association and Alliance of Psychoanalytic Organizations; 2006.

2. Fiester SJ. Self-defeating personality disorder: a review of data and recommendations for DSM-IV. *J Pers. Disord.* 1991;5:194–209.

3. Krafft-von Ebing R. *Psychopathia Sexualis*. New York, NY: Physicians & Surgeons; 1931.

4. Von Sacher-Masoch L, Neugroschel, J. *Venus in Furs*. London, UK: Penguin Books; 2000.

5. Freud S. *Three Essays in Sexuality*. Std. ed., vol. 7. London: Hogarth Press; [1905] 1956: 135–243.

6. Freud S. The Economic Problem of Masochism. Std. ed., volume 19. London, UK: Hogarth Press; [1924] 1961:159–170.

7. Glick RA, Meyers DI. *Masochism: Current Clinical Perspectives*. Hillsdale, NJ: The Analytic Press; 1988.

8. Cooper AM. Psychotherapeutic approaches to masochism. *J Psychother Pract Res.* 1992;2: 51–63.

9. Cooper AM. Feature: The narcissistic-masochistic character. *Psychiatr Ann.* 2009;39:904–912.

10. Kernberg OF. Clinical dimensions of masochism. *JAPA*. 1988;36:1005–1029.

11. Kernberg OF. *Severe Personality Disorders: Psychotherapeutic Strategies*. New Haven, CT: Yale University Press; 1984.

12. Caligor E, Kernberg O, Clarkin J, Yeomans F. *Psychodynamic Therapy for Personality Pathology: Treating Self and Interpersonal Functioning*. Washington DC: American Psychiatric Association Publishing; 2018: 22–24.

13. Kohut H. *The Analysis of the Self: A Systematic Approach to the Treatment of Narcissistic Personality Disorders*. New York, NY: International Universities Press; 1971.

14. Gabbard G0, Litowitz BE, Williams P, eds. *The Textbook of Psychoanalysis*. 2nd ed. Washington, DC: American Psychiatric Publishing; 2012.

15. Gibbs R. Eye movement desensitization and reprocessing. In: Cabaniss D, Holoshitz Y, eds. *Different Patients, Different Therapies*. New York, NY: WW Norton; 2019:266–273.

16. Holtzman D, Kulish N, eds. *The Clinical Problem of Masochism*. Lanham, MD: Jason Aronson; 2018.

Index

Printed in the USA
CPSIA information can be obtained
at www.ICGtesting.com
CBHW080121210324
5457CB00010B/9